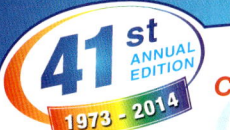

41st ANNUAL EDITION
1973 – 2014

A Calori

Alcoholic Drinks (with Alcohol Counts)	3
Baking Ingredients	4
Bars (Breakfast, Muesli, Meal)	5
Beverages: Cocoa, Hot Chocolate	7
Coffee & Coffee Drinks	,+9
Energy, Protein, Sports Drinks	39
Fruit & Vegetable Juices	40
Milk (Plain, Flavored, Mixes)	44
Non-Dairy (Soy, Rice/Cereal/Nut)	47
Soda/Soft Drinks	48
Tea & Iced Tea	50
Biscuits/Cookies/Crackers	52
Bread & Bread Products, Bagels	56
Breakfast Cereals (Hot & Cold)	60
Cakes, Donuts, Muffins, Pastries	64
Cheese & Cheese Products	72
Chicken, Duck, Goose, Turkey	75
Chocolate, Confectionery, Lollies, Gum	79
Cream, Custard	89
Desserts (Puddings, Gelatin), Toppings	90
Dips	92
Eggs, Egg Substitutes, Egg Dishes	93
Fats, Butter, Spreads, Oils	94
Fish, Shellfish	95
Flour, Grains	101
Fruit (Fresh/Packaged/Dried/Snacks)	103
Ice Cream & Frozen Yoghurt	109
Meals: Canned & Packaged, Frozen	115
CalorieKing Recipe Dishes	129
Meats: Beef, Lamb, Pork, Game	130
Sausages/Franks/Hot Dogs	137
Deli/Lunch Meats	139
Milk ~ *See Beverages*	
Noodles	140
Nuts, Seeds	141
Pasta & Spaghetti	142
Snacks (Popcorn, Chips, Pretzels)	159
Soups	161
Soy, Tofu	165
Spreads, Honey, Jam, Peanut Butter, Tahini	167
Sugar, Sugar Substitutes, Syrup	166
Vegetables (Fresh, Frozen, Canned)	168
Yoghurt, Drinking Yoghurt	173

Eating Out & Fast-Food Chains:

Index	177
Cafe-Style Meals & Take-Away	179
International Foods	180
Fast-Foods Restaurant Chains	185
A-Z Foods Index	222

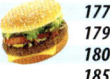

BONUS DIET GUIDES & COUNTERS

Alcohol Guide & Counter	23-30
Caffeine Guide & Counter	210
Calcium Guide & Counter	211
Diabetes Diet Guide	16-21
Fats & Cholesterol Guide	214-218
Fibre Guide & Counter	219-222
Protein Guide & Counter	223-226
Salt & High Blood Pressure with Sodium Counter	227-233
Weight Control Guide	2-15

Weight Control Tips

✅ **Eat & Drink Sensibly**
- Avoid fad diets. Eat 3 sensible portion-controlled meals daily.
- Limit fats, high-fat foods/snacks and sugar. Eat adequate fresh fruit and vegetables.
- Limit soft drinks, energy drinks, fruit juice and alcohol. Quench your thirst on water. *(See Sample Meal Plan ~ Page 10)*

✅ **Exercise Daily**
- Aim for at least 30 minutes daily – even in 5-10 minute lots. For motivation, find an exercise buddy, personal trainer or join a gym. *(Extra Notes ~ Page 12)*

✅ **Reshape Eating Behaviours**
- Be aware of eating and shopping behaviours that lead to overeating.
- Also focus on social and emotional situations that may trigger compulsive eating. *(Extra notes - Page 14)*

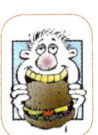

✅ **Keep a Food & Exercise Diary**
- A diary helps you see exactly what you eat and drink, and how much you really exercise.
- An excellent motivator that keeps you honest! *(See Page 15)*

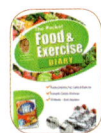

✅ **Arrange Moral Support**
- Gain the support of family and friends. Get extra professional help if required from your doctor, dietitian, psychologist, exercise trainer, or slimming group.
- Beware of saboteurs (family/friends) who may discourage you from adopting a healthier lifestyle!

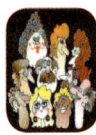

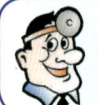

DOCTOR CHECK-UP
Ask your doctor to check you for high blood pressure, diabetes, high blood cholesterol and thyroid function.

HEALTHY WEIGHTS ~ MEN & WOMEN ~ (Over 18 Years)

Based on weights with least risk of disease or death from heart disease, diabetes, stroke and cancer.

Based on Body Mass Index of 20-25

BMI calculated as: $\frac{\text{Weight (kg)}}{\text{Height (m)}^2}$

Height (No Shoes)		Healthy Weight Range (kg)
Cm	Ft Ins	
140	4'7"	39-49
142	4'8"	40-50
145	4'9"	42-52
148	4'10"	44-55
150	4'11"	45-56
152	5'0"	46-58
155	5'1"	48-60
158	5'2"	50-62
160	5'3"	51-64
162	5'4"	52-66
165	5'5"	54-68
168	5'6"	56-71
170	5'7"	58-72
173	5'8"	59-74
175	5'9"	61-76
178	5'10"	63-79
180	5'11"	65-81
183	6'0"	66-83
185	6'1"	68-85
188	6'2"	71-88
190	6'3"	72-90
193	6'4"	74-92
196	6'5"	77-96
198	6'6"	78-98
200	6'7"	80-100

Body Fat Distribution ♦ BMI

Body Fat Distribution & Health

Fat above the hips carries a far greater health risk than fat on or below the hips – better to be a **'pear-shape'** than an **'apple-shape'**.

Abdominal obesity greatly increases the risk of developing diabetes, heart disease, high blood fats, hypertension, stroke and some cancers. So-called 'cellulite' carries no extra health risk.

Waist Measurement ~ High Health Risk:
Men: Over 102cm (40 inches)
Women: Over 88cm (35 inches)

Women who become obsessed with dieting away their thighs and buttocks on an otherwise lean body, are fighting mother nature and may well be inviting health problems.

If you are within a healthy weight range, it is better to exercise regularly to maintain body shape, rather than to be constantly dieting and lacking in energy. Accept your body shape and focus on other pursuits and enjoying life!

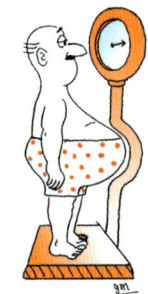

Abdominal obesity greatly increases the risk of ill-health and earlier death.

Body Mass Index (BMI)

BMI is a general indicator of body fatness. The higher the BMI, the greater the health risk of developing diabetes, high blood pressure and heart disease.

Formula for BMI = $\dfrac{\text{Weight (kg)}}{\text{Height (m)}^2}$

Example BMI Calculation:
75kg person, 1.7m tall
BMI = $75 \div (1.7 \times 1.7) = 26$

BMI Classification (Adults):

- **Less than 18** – Underweight
- **20-25** – Healthy Weight (Low Health Risk)
- **25-30** – Overweight (Moderate Health Risk)
- **30-40** – Obese (High Health Risk)
- **Over 40** – Morbid Obesity (Very High Risk)

Note: BMI does not apply to heavily muscled persons. For children, BMI is interpreted differently.

Calorie Levels for Weight Loss

Commence with a well-balanced eating plan that allows for gradual weight loss of ½-1 kg per week. Weight loss is usually much larger in the first few weeks due to extra fluid losses.

The more active you are, the more calories you can eat - as shown in the chart below.

Note: It is better to increase exercise rather than lessen food calories too drastically.

SUGGESTED FOOD CALORIES FOR WEIGHT LOSS

Women:	Non-active	1000-1200
	Active	1200-1500
	Very Active	1400-1800
Men:	Non-active	1200-1500
	Active	1500-1800
	Very Active	1800-2100
Teenagers:	Non-active	1200-1500
	Active	1400-1800
	Very Active	1600-2000

(1 Calorie = 4.2 Kilojoules)

Calories & Weight Loss

- Different people require different amounts of calories - even between two people of the same age, weight and physical activity.

- Allow up to 400 calories (1700 kilojoules) above or below the figures below, for normal variations between individuals.

- The charts below are for persons who are largely inactive or office workers. Any extra calories required for moderate or strenuous activity, and for pregnancy and lactation, must be added to these figures. (See Calorie Adjustments Chart below.)

1 CALORIE = 4.2 KILOJOULES (kJ)

WOMEN	**18-35 Yrs**	**36-55 Yrs**	**Over 55**
45kg	1760 Cals (7400 kJ)	1570 Cals (6600kJ)	1430 Cals (6000 kJ)
50kg	1860 Cals (7800kJ)	1660 Cals (7000kJ)	1500 Cals (6300kJ)
55kg	1950 Cals (8100kJ)	1760 Cals (7400kJ)	1550 Cals (6500kJ)
60kg	2050 Cals (8600kJ)	1860 Cals (7800kJ)	1600 Cals (6800kJ)
65kg	2150 Cals (9000kJ)	1960 Cals (8200kJ)	1630 Cals (6800kJ)
70kg	2250 Cals (9400kJ)	2050 Cals (8600kJ)	1660 Cals (7000kJ)
75kg	2400 Cals (10,000kJ)	2150 Cals (9000kJ)	1720 Cals (7200kJ)

MEN	**18-35 Yrs**	**36-55 Yrs**	**Over 55**
60kg	2480 Cals (10,400kJ)	2300 Cals (9600kJ)	1900 Cals (7900kJ)
65kg	2620 Cals (11,000kJ)	2400 Cals (10,000kJ)	2000 Cals (8400kJ)
70kg	2760 Cals (11,500kJ)	2480 Cals (10,400kJ)	2100 Cals (8800kJ)
75kg	2900 Cals (12,100kJ)	2560 Cals (10,700kJ)	2200 Cals (9200kJ)
80kg	3050 Cals (12,800kJ)	2670 Cals (11,200kJ)	2300 Cals (9600kJ)
85kg	3200 Cals (13,400kJ)	2760 Cals (11,500kJ)	2400 Cals (10,000kJ)
90kg	3500 Cals (14,600kJ)	3000 Cals (12,500kJ)	2600 Cals (10,900kJ)

CALORIE ADJUSTMENTS FOR ACTIVITY (Per Day)

Body Weight (Kg)	Inactive Bedridden Subtract from Charts Above ▼	Moderate Activity Skilled Trades, Heavy Gardening Add to Charts Above ▼	Strenuous or Heavy Activity Heavy Labouring Strenuous Sports Add to Charts Above ▼
41-50kg	-480 Cals (2000kJ)	+240 Cals (1000kJ)	+480 Cals (2000kJ)
51-60kg	-570 Cals (2400kJ)	+290 Cals (1210kJ)	+570 Cals (2400kJ)
61-70kg	-670 Cals (2800kJ)	+340 Cals (1420kJ)	+670 Cals (2800kJ)
71-80kg	-760 Cals (3200kJ)	+380 Cals (1600kJ)	+760 Cals (3200kJ)
81-90kg	-960 Cals (4000kJ)	+430 Cals (1800kJ)	+860 Cals (3600kJ)

PREGNANCY: Add 300 calories (from 4th month). **LACTATION:** Add up to 500 calories.
Note: Strict dieting during pregnancy is not recommended unless medically directed.
Adequate weight gain lessens the risk of a low birth weight baby.

Portion Size Counts!

Portion Size Counts!

Food portion size is critical to controlling calorie intake for weight control.

Super-sized food servings have become more common when eating out and in the home. This can mean a day's worth of calories being consumed in one meal; or a snack being equivalent to a full meal.

It is easy to underestimate portion size of foods and drinks, and unwittingly consume excess calories – even if the fat content is low or even zero!

To more accurately estimate portion size of different foods, weigh and measure your food with food scales, measuring spoons and cups. Better control of calories will result.

For a visual idea of portion sizes, visit www.CalorieKing.com.au See examples (fries and cola) on this page.

Allow for Extra Calories in Packaged Food!

The actual weight of packaged foods is usually 5-10% more than the label net weight (the minimum legal weight) – and in some cases up to 30% more (particularly in some baked cakes and snacks). However, manufacturers calculate the calories based on the net weight so, calories can be underestimated.

For actual calories, weigh the product and calculate the extra calories.

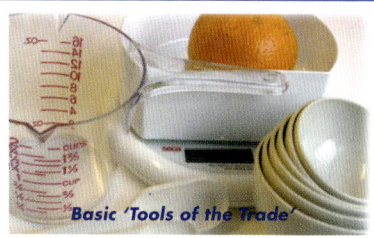

Basic 'Tools of the Trade'

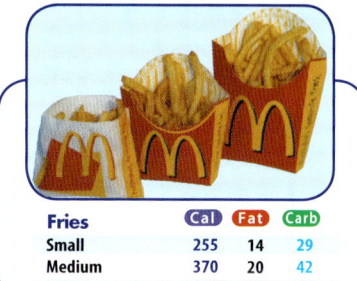

Fries	Cal	Fat	Carb
Small	255	14	29
Medium	370	20	42
Large	455	25	51

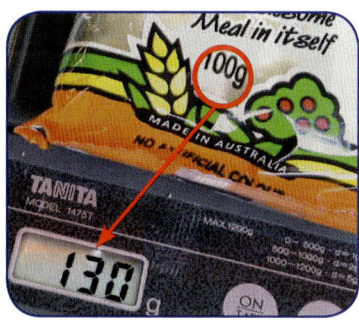

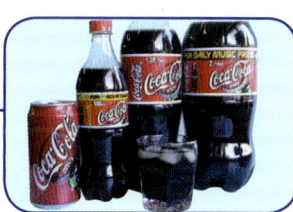

Cola	Cal	Fat	Carb
250ml Glass	100	0	27
375ml Can	155	0	40
600ml Bottle	250	0	65
1.25 Litre Bottle	515	0	135
2 Litre Bottle	820	0	215

Recommended Fat Intake

Fat in the Diet

- Some fat in the diet is essential for good health. However, too much fat can contribute to obesity, and a higher risk of heart disease, high blood pressure, diabetes, gall stones and certain cancers.
- Dietary fats/oils have over double the energy of carbohydrate and protein.

ENERGY VALUES PER GRAM

Carbohydrate:	4 Calories ●	17 kilojoules
Protein:	4 Calories ●	16 kilojoules
Fat/Oil:	9 Calories ●	37 kilojoules
Alcohol:	7 Calories ●	29 kilojoules

- Dietary fat is more readily converted to and stored as body fat compared to carbohydrates and protein.

MAXIMUM DESIRABLE DAILY FAT INTAKE FOR ADULTS

Calories ~ kJoules	Fat
1200 cals ~ 4800kJ ▶	30g fat
1500 cals ~ 6300kJ ▶	40g fat
1800 cals ~ 7500kJ ▶	50g fat
2000 cals ~ 8400kJ ▶	60g fat
2200 cals ~ 9200kJ ▶	70g fat
2500 cals ~ 10,500kJ ▶	80g fat
3000 cals ~ 12,500kJ ▶	110g fat

Note: Fat intake should be quite low at lower calorie levels used for weight loss (in adults). This allows extra calories for protein which has nutritional priority over fat.

Infants Fat Intake

Infants and toddlers under 3 years should not be restricted in their fat intake because much larger volumes of food would be required to guarantee adequate energy intake and growth. Whole milk should be used rather than low-fat milk.

Similarly, a high-fibre diet is also not suitable for infants.

Beware Low-Fat Food Claims

Beware of low-fat and fat-free promotional claims. The food may not be any healthier and may be high in sugar and calories. '98% Fat-Free' can simply mean '98% Sugar' (or other refined carbohydrate).

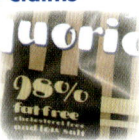

Don't mistakenly think you can consume extra quantities of low-fat or fat-free foods. It is easy to consume excess calories and gain weight.

Remember, food products which are fat-free but high in calories include soft drinks, fruit juices, sugar confectionery, beer, spirits and sugar itself. Bread, rice and pasta also have negligible fat and need to be eaten in controlled amounts.

Ultimately, it is food portion size as well as total calories that count whether from fat, carbohydrate or protein. Remember, cows get fat on grass!

LOW-FAT LABEL CLAIMS

Food Products claiming a reduction in fat content must meet the following guidelines:

'Reduced Fat': At least a 25% reduction from the original product

'Low Fat': Less than 3% fat for solid foods, and 1.5% for liquid foods

'Fat Free': Less than 0.15% fat

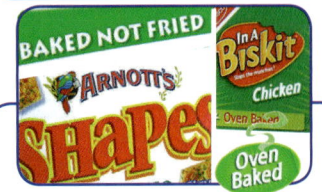

Don't be fooled by 'Baked Not Fried' or 'Oven Baked' on the packs of savoury snack biscuits.
They still have up to 25% fat – similar to fried potato crisps!

Hints to Reduce Fat

Fats, Oils, Dressings
- **Use minimal amounts.** Choose reduced-fat or 'light' margarine spreads.
- **Limit** mayonnaise, and oil dressings. Choose low-fat or fat-free dressings (e.g. *Kraft Free*).

Milk, Dairy, Cheese, Soy Drinks
- **Choose** low-fat (1%) and nonfat milks, low-fat soy milk drinks (e.g *So Good Lite*); and yoghurts (e.g. *Nestle Diet*).
- **Choose** fat-reduced cheeses; (e.g. *Kraft Light*), cottage, ricotta. Limit cream cheese.
- **Ice Cream:** Choose low-fat ice creams (e.g. *Nestle Light 'N Creamy,* water ices and water-based gelati.

Meats, Poultry, Fish
- **Choose lean cuts** of meat with little marbling, chicken breast. Trim off skin and fat. Limit serving size to 100-120g (cooked weight). Add extra beans, baked beans, lentils, vegetables, potatoes or rice.
- **Avoid fatty sausages,** ham, bacon, salami. Choose low-fat varieties.
- **Avoid fried fish in batter.** Choose grilled or baked fish, and canned fish in water pack.

Frozen Meals & Pies
Choose low-fat varieties (e.g. *Lean Cuisine, Lite n' Easy*) and meals with the Heart Foundation Red Tick. Avoid high-fat pies, quiches etc.

Breads, Breakfast Cereals
Most are low-fat but still exercise portion control. Avoid croissants and high-fat toasted muesli.

Fruits, Vegetables, Vegetarian
- **Choose** all types. Normal serves of avocado and olives are fine. Choose baked beans, soybeans, dried beans, lentils. Limit nuts. Avoid potato chips, veggies in cream sauces.
- **Choose** vegetarian burgers (e.g. *Sanitarium Vegie Delights*).

Desserts
- **Avoid high-fat desserts,** e.g. fruit pies, pastries, cheesecake, cheese board. Choose fresh fruit, light canned fruit, low-fat ice cream, yoghurt, gelati (water), diet jelly (e.g *Aeroplane Jelly•Lite*).

> ### FRYING ADDS FAT!
> The greater the surface area of potato exposed to fat or oil, the higher the fat content and calories.
>
>
> **Whole Potato (100g)**
> **0g Fat** 70 Cals/290 kJ
>
>
> **Roasted Potato (100g)**
> **5g Fat** 140 Cals/585 kJ
>
>
> **Fries (Large cut, 100g)**
> **12g Fat** 220 Cals/020 kJ
>
>
> **Fries (Small, 100g)**
> **15g Fat** 290 Cals/1210 kJ
>
>
> **Potato Chips (100g)**
> **30g Fat** 500 Cals/2090 kJ

Snacks, Cookies
- **Limit high-fat snacks** such as potato crisps, Cheezel-types and chocolate. Choose pretzels (e.g. *Parker's*), low-fat cookies (e.g. *Paradise Lites);* and plain popcorn. Ideally substitute with fruit.

Fast-Foods & Take-Away
- **Avoid high-fat foods** such as deep-fried chips/fish/chicken, fried onion rings, pies, sausage rolls, quiche, high-fat pizzas. (Check the Fast-Foods Section of this book.)

> ### COOKING METHODS
> - **Choose cooking methods** that use minimal fat or oil such as microwaving, grilling or *ActiFry* Cooker *(Tefal)* for chips.
> - **Modify recipes** to contain less fat/oil Substitute high-fat ingredients with low-fat alternatives (e.g. yoghurt for sour cream, whipped ricotta cheese for fresh cream).
> - **When baking cakes,** use prune or apple puree as a part-substitute for fat or oil.
>
> *ActiFry Cooker*

Carbohydrates ~ Friend or Foe?

Naturally-Friendly Carbs

- **Carbohydrate foods in their more natural forms (not overly processed) are essential to good health.** They are the main source of fuel for the body, and also provide important vitamins, minerals, antioxidants and fibre – all of which help protect against heart disease, diabetes, hypertension, constipation-related ailments and many other diseases.

- Carbohydrates even help the body produce serotonin, the 'feel good' brain chemical that helps control appetite and overeating. Too little serotonin can lead to mood swings and depression.

Carbohydrates are found in different forms in food as:

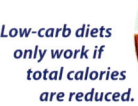

- Sugars in fruit, sugar cane, milk
- Starches in whole grains, legumes, nuts, seeds and vegetables
- Dietary fiber (See Fibre Guide ~ Page 219)

Low-carb diets only work if total calories are reduced.

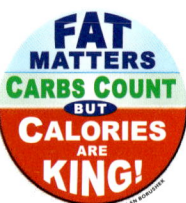

RECOMMENDED DAILY CARBOHYDRATE INTAKE

Calories (Daily)	Carbohydrate (Grams)	Percent Carbohydrate Calories
1200 cals	100-120g	35-40%
1500 cals	140-170g	40-45%
1800 cals	180-200g	40-45%
2000 cals	200-250g	40-50%
2500 cals	310-350g	50-55%
3000 cals	410-450g	55-65%

How Much Do We Need?

- As shown in the chart, well-balanced diets above 2000 calories contain 50-60% of total calories from carbohydrates.
- At lower calorie levels used for weight control (1200-1500 calories), carbohydrates account for as little as 40% of total calories. This is because protein calories have nutritional priority.
- Carbohydrates & Diabetes ~ See Page 19-21

Low-Carbohydrate Diets

- Popular low-carbohydrate diets can be extreme in their recommendations.

  This may lead to overly restricting carb-containing foods such as fruit, vegetables and even milk (which contains lactose sugar).

  Eliminating these foods greatly increases the risk of nutritional deficiencies and compromises health, particularly if fat intake is excessive through fatty meats, high-fat dairy products, and fried foods.

- While overweight Australians may need to reduce carbohydrate intake, it should be done sensibly as part of reducing portion sizes and total calories.
- Simply eating 'low-carb' food products without regard to portion size, calories or fats, will do little to promote weight loss or good health.
- Low-carb diets (and indeed any diet) only work if total calories are reduced.
- Refined sugars should be one of the first targets in moderating carbohydrate intake.

Extra Info ~ www.CalorieKing.com.au

Carbohydrate foods (minimally processed) are essential to good health.

Be sure to eat adequate fruit (2 serves) and vegetables (5 serves) every day.

Hints to Reduce Sugar

- **Australians consume, on average, around 40 kg of refined sugar** per person per year – more than is considered healthy.

  This is equivalent to a daily intake of 22 teaspoons sugar; and provides some 440 calories or 1840 kilojoules each day – a significant amount in weight control terms. Cutting this intake by at least half would be reasonable and worthwhile.

- **Most sugar in our diet is 'hidden'** in processed foods such as soft drinks, cordials, fruit drinks, canned fruits in syrup, confectionery, biscuits, cakes, jam, sauces, ice cream, jelly and breakfast cereals.

  Certainly enjoy moderate quantities of these foods but for serious weight control, look for 'low joule', 'diet', sugar-free alternatives. Be careful not to substitute high-sugar foods with high-fat foods which might boost calories even more.

- **Sweeteners** such as *Equal, Sugarine* and *Splenda* make it easy to cut down on sugar we add to drinks and dessert recipes.

- The body can obtain sufficient sugar for its needs from carbohydrate-rich foods such as bread, rice, pasta, potatoes, corn, fruit, vegetables, beans, nuts, seeds, and lactose in milk.

- **These foods are also rich in other nutrients.** Refined sugar is called 'empty calorie' because it supplies calories but negligible nutrients and no fibre.

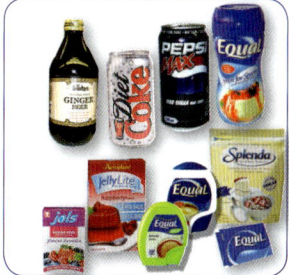

Sugar substitutes and sugar-free products can save hundreds of calories. Still limit these products to prevent developing an oversweet tooth.

Teaspoons Of Sugar In Some Common Foods

Soft drinks: 375ml can	~ 10 tsp
600 ml bottle	~ 15 tsp
Ribena, 1 glass, 250ml	~ 8 tsp
Flavoured Milk, 600ml ctn	~ 12 tsp
Chocolate, 50g bar	~ 7 tsp
Mars Bar, 53g	~ 9 tsp
Jelly Beans, 50g	~ 10 tsp
Cornetto, Trumpet, Drumstick	~ 6 tsp
Jelly, regular, ½ cup	~ 4 tsp
Canned Fruit in Syrup	~ 3 tsp
Tomato Sauce, 1 Tbsp	~ 1 tsp
Nutella, 1 Tbsp, 20g	~ 2 tsp
Coco Pops, 1 cup, 30g	~ 2 tsp
Nutri-Grain, 1 cup, 40g	~ 2 tsp
Cream Biscuit, *Tim Tam*	~ 2 tsp

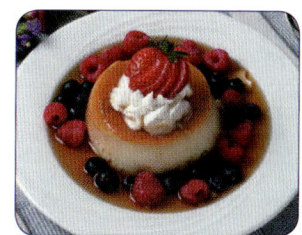

Most recipes can be adapted to contain less sugar with little effect on taste or quality.

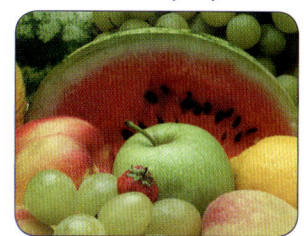

Reach for fresh fruit when you want to snack instead of confectionery or snack products rich in sugar and fat.

Sample Meal Plan ~ 1400 Calories

~ 1400 Calories (5800 kJ) Meal Plan ~
For Overweight Persons Without Any Medical Condition. Check With Your Doctor & Dietitian

Breakfast (Approx. 300 Cal/1200kJ)

1 medium Fruit or 30g Dried Fruits
Plus   Cereal: 50g Dry (high fibre)
     or 1 cup cooked (e.g. Oats Porridge)
Plus   Milk (from daily allowance) or Yogurt (low-fat)

Daily Milk Allowance (160 Calories/670kJ)
2 cups Skim Milk or 1½ cups Low-Fat Milk
or equivalent Soy Drink, Yoghurt, Cheese, Tofu

Daily Fat Allowance (140 Calories/590kJ)
4 tsp Fat or 6 tsp reduced-fat Marg. or 3 tsp Oil
or 1½ Tbsp Mayonnaise or ½ medium Avocado
or 1½ Tbsp Peanut Butter or 30g Nuts/Seeds

Breakfast ~ Choice 2

1 small Fruit
Plus   2 Eggs (minimal fat added)
     or 40g Cheese or 50g 'Light' Cheese
     or 120g Cottage Cheese
     or 150g (½ cup) Baked Beans
Plus   1 Tomato
Plus   1 slice Toast (wholegrain)
     or ½ English Muffin

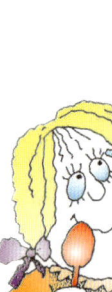

Lunch (Approx. 440 calories/1840kJ)

2 slices Bread (60g) or 4 Crispbreads/Crackers
Plus   60g lean Meat, Chicken or Turkey
     or 100g Tuna (in water) or 70g Salmon
     or 30g Cheese or 100g Cottage Cheese
     or 75g Ricotta Cheese
     or ½ cup, 120g Fruit Yoghurt (low-fat)
     or ½ cup, Baked Beans or Bean Salad
Plus   Large Salad (Oil-free dressing)
Plus   1 small Fruit or 20g Dried Fruit

Dinner (Approx. 360 calories/1500kJ)

Soup (fat-free)
Plus   100g lean Meat (cooked weight)
     or 125g Chicken Breast (no skin)
     or 90g Chicken Thigh/Leg (no skin)
     or 150g Fish (grilled, no fat)
     or 200g Beans (Soy, Baked, Haricot etc)/Lentils
     or Low-Fat Recipe Dish (e.g. Lean Cuisine, Lite n' Easy)
Plus   1 small Potato or ½ cup Rice/Pasta or 1 slice Wholegrain Bread
Plus   2-3 servings Vegetables/Salad
Plus   1 small Fruit + Diet (Low Joule) Jelly

Between Meals
Water, Coffee, Tea, Diet (Low joule) drinks,
Fruit from main meals; Raw vegetable pieces, Milk from Daily Allowance
Note: Take a multivitamin/mineral supplement daily while dieting.

For extra flexibility in meal planning, or to meet special dietary requirements,
seek referral to a registered dietitian through your doctor.

Exercise & Weight Control

- **Persons who exercise regularly lose more weight** and keep it off longer than non-exercisers.
- **Exercise also improves general health and well-being.** Mood, confidence and self-esteem are enhanced by a sense of control and accomplishment.
- **Exercise is a good way to 'wake up' a sluggish metabolism** and burn extra fat tissue.
- **Aerobic (huff and puff) exercise most days** is great for burning calories and for cardiovascular fitness. But, it is strength training that mainly builds the muscles that burn calories even while we sleep.
- **Strength training is the key to retaining or rebuilding muscles.** As we age, we lose some 2-3 kg of muscle per decade. This results in a lower metabolism and fewer calories being burnt.
- **Muscles are the furnaces that burn calories.** The more muscle you have, the more calories you will burn.
- **Regular strength training (2-3 times weekly)** can increase metabolic rate for several days following exercise. This can mean an extra 100 calories (400 kilojoules) per day being burnt. While 1-2 kg of muscle may be gained in the first 8-10 weeks, weight from exercised muscles is okay. It is excess fat (particularly abdominal fat) that is a potential health hazard. Gaining muscle and losing fat also helps body reshaping – even if the scales don't show it.
- **Avoid injury** by beginning with walking, low impact aerobics, or weight-supported exercise (e.g. swimming, cycling). Avoid competitive sports. Allow 2-3 days of recovery between strength training sessions. Get professional advice – particularly if you have a medical condition.
- **How Much?** Start with 10-20 minutes of walking and progress to 30-60 minutes per day. Also walk up stairs instead of using elevators. Take a brisk walk at lunch. Stand instead of sitting. Use an exercise bike, treadmill or stair machine while watching TV. Walk the dog.
- **How Often?** While aerobic fitness requires only 3-4 sessions weekly, weight control is a daily event which requires daily exercise to burn calories. Add in strength training 2-3 times weekly.
- **For motivation,** find an exercise buddy, personal trainer or join a gym.

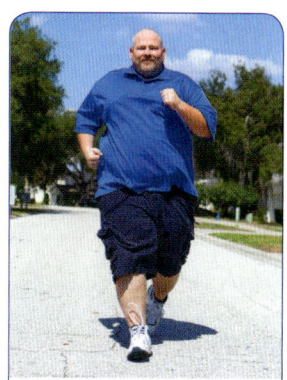

Brisk walking each day is a safe and effective way to burn calories and keep fit.
Try it – you'll like it!

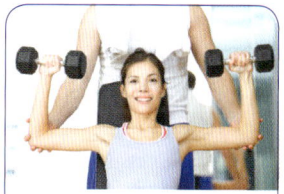

Strength training is the key to retain or rebuild muscles.

Muscles burn extra calories even while you sleep.

For extra guidance, seek a qualified trainer or join a gym.

Exercise Calories ~ Walking

Calories Used in Exercise

LIGHT
60kg ~ 3 Cals/Min.	
80kg ~ 4 Cals/Min.	
100kg ~ 5 Cals/Min.	

▼

Walking, slow
Cycling, light
Gardening light
Golf, social
Tennis, doubles
Housework, cleaning
Callisthenics, Yoga
Ten Pin Bowling
Table Tennis, Social
Tai Chi
Aquarobics, light
Line/Square Dancing
Skate Boarding

MODERATE
60kg ~ 5 Cals/Min.	
80kg ~ 6 Cals/Min.	
100kg ~ 7 Cals/Min.	

▼

Walking, brisk
Cycling, moderate
Swimming, crawl
Weight-training, light
Tennis, singles
Squash, Badminton
Rebounding, moderate
Football
Basketball
Volleyball, advanced
Snow Skiing (downhill)
Canoeing
Dancing, vigorous

HEAVY
60kg ~ 8 Cals/Min.	
80kg ~ 10 Cals/Min.	
100kg ~ 12 Cals/Min.	

▼

Walking (power),
Jogging
Cycling, vigorous
Swimming, strenuous advanced
Football training
Skipping
Kick Boxing, Tae Bo
Basketball (Pro)
Climbing Stairs
Skiing (cross country)
Aquarobics, advanced
Dancing, strenuous

Note: Only those sports or activities that are sustained over a period of time (e.g jogging) qualify for heavy exercise. Stop-start sports such as tennis are considered 'moderate'.

Interactive Calculations ~ www.CalorieKing.com.au/tools

WALKING PROGRAM

USE DISTANCE OR STEPS OR TIME

Weeks	Distance	Steps (Pedometer)	Time
1-2	1.5 km	2000	20 mins
3-5	2 km	3000	28 mins
6-8	3 km	3500	35 mins
9-10	4 km	4500	45 mins
11+	5.5 km	6000	60 mins

10,000 STEPS PER DAY

A pedometer can motivate you to be more active. It clips to your belt or waist band and registers each step.

Aim for 8,000 - 10,000 steps per day, instead of an average of only 3,000 - 4,000 steps.

Extra Info: www.CalorieKing.com.au

Reshaping Eating Behaviour

- **Eating is a behaviour** that is largely controlled by people with whom we live or socialise, places in which we carry out our lives, and our emotions. Become aware of those situations that commonly lead to extra food being eaten.

- We may also be unaware of 'bad' eating habits that can lead to excess calorie intake; e.g. eating quickly, large mouthfuls, eating when tense or bored, finishing a large serving of food when not hungry.

Tips to help uncover and correct those 'bad' eating habits include:

- **Don't eat while engaged in other activities;** e.g. watching TV, reading. Eat only at the table, not at the fridge or while standing.

- **Don't eat quickly.** Chewing slowly allows time to register a feeling of fullness. Don't use fingers, only utensils. Cut food into smaller pieces. Don't load your fork until the previous mouthful is finished.

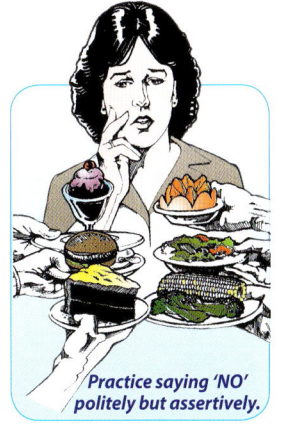
Practice saying 'NO' politely but assertively.

- **Don't purchase problem high calorie foods.** Shop from a set list to prevent impulse buying. Avoid shopping with children. Plan meals in advance. Stick to a set menu.

- **Buy snack foods in the smallest package size.** The larger the package, the more you are likely to consume.

- **Plan meals in advance.** Stick to a set menu.

- **Plan a strategy to avoid uncontrolled eating** and drinking at social events, or when your emotions urge you to binge.

  Rehearse repeatedly in your mind exactly what you will do in such situations. Remind yourself several times each day that you are in charge of your actions and that you can be strong-willed. Seek counselling or coaching on various strategies.

- **Distract yourself** that when you feel the urge to snack impulsively. Engage in some activity that will distract you from thinking about food. Examples: go for a walk, brush your teeth, phone a friend.

- **If you eat out of boredom,** find some new hobby or interest that regularly gets you out of the house.

Note: Persons with deep-seated emotional problems and eating disorders require counselling. Seek a doctor's referral to a specialist.

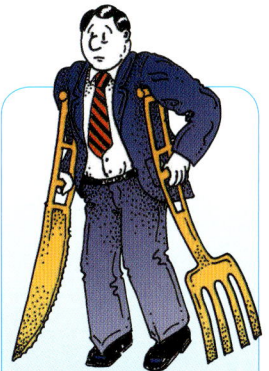
Do you use food as an emotional crutch? If so, professional counselling may be helpful.

The Value of a Food Diary

The food diary is the most powerful proven aid for dieters. Persons who keep a food and exercise diary not only lose more weight they also keep it off. Here are some of the reasons:

- **Recording your eating** and exercise habits jolts you into realizing just what you do eat and drink each day; and also whether you exercise sufficiently.
- **Helps you identify problem foods** and drinks with excessive calories and fat. Also helps plan meals.
- **Helps identify moods,** situations and events that lead to excessive eating of unwanted calories. You can then plan to overcome or avoid them.
- **Prevents 'calorie amnesia',** the forgetfulness that leads to rebound weight gain after successful weight loss. Recording puts you back on the right track.
- **Helps you develop greater self-discipline.** You will think twice about over indulging if you have to record it – especially if someone checks your diary regularly. It certainly keeps you honest!
- **Motivates you** to carefully plan your meals and to exercise each day.
- **Serves as a check system** for your doctor, dietitian or counsellor to assess your progress and make recommendations.

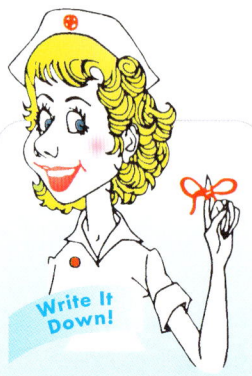

"Keeping a diary gives me feedback on exactly what I eat and drink each day.

It helps prevent 'calorie amnesia' and reminds me to exercise each day.

It's a must for successful weight control!"

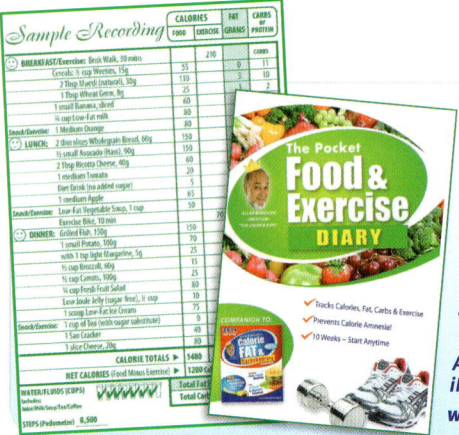

Sample Page from
The Pocket
Food & Exercise Diary

- 10-week diary to record food and exercise.
- At day's end, exercise calories are deducted from food calories.
- Includes Weekly Summary Page & Progress Checklist.

Also check the CalorieKing iPhone app. (ControlMyWeight)
www.CalorieKing.com.au

Tips for Overweight Kids & Parents

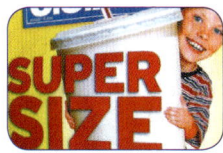

The XL Generation

Some 25% of Australian kids and adolescents are over-weight; and childhood obesity has doubled over the last 20 years. Diabetes, high blood pressure and high cholesterol are major problem areas for overweight children and adolescents, as are depression, low self-esteem, sleep apnoea and bone joint problems.

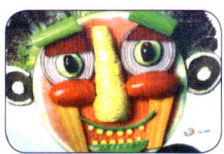

To address this problem, cooperation is required between kids, parents, schools and regulators. Weight control (i.e. what we eat, drink and do) is a family and community affair.

Some Simple Tips To Get Started:

❶ Watch Soft Drink Intake

Limit soft drinks and sugary drinks to a few cups on weekends. Soft drinks should not be an everyday beverage – water should be. When eating out, choose small serves with extra ice or choose diet/sugar-free brands instead. Schools should provide water and restrict access to soft drinks – as should parents when eating out or at home. Fruit juices, cordials and sports drinks should also be limited in overweight kids.

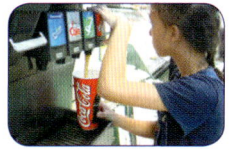

❷ Cut back on Fast-Foods and Eating Out

Many more calories are usually consumed when eating out. Healthy meals prepared at home are best for the whole family. Choose sensible portion sizes (the smallest) for kids. Resist the temptation to upsize soft drinks and french fries.

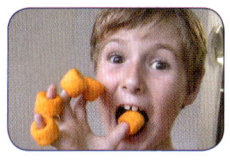

❸ Limit Between-Meal Snacking ~ Eat Fruit!

Watch out for high-fat and high-calorie snacks. Choose fresh fruit and vegetables instead. Keep your eye on portion sizes and limit foods like potato crisps, salty fried snacks and lollies to parties and special occasions. Don't keep them at home.

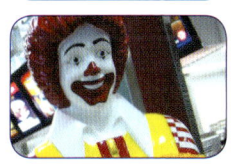

❹ Get Moving ~ Watch Less TV

Kids need at least 60 minutes of physical activity every day. It's critical for their fitness and greatly lessens the risk of obesity, diabetes, high blood pressure and high blood cholesterol.

Encourage kids to be active out of school hours. Limit TV and non-active computer games to just one hour per day. Dance video games such as *Dance Dance Revolution and The Wiggles Dance Party* provide fun and motivation for kids to move – as can *Wii Fit (Nintendo)*. Wearing a pedometer to record daily steps is also a useful motivator.

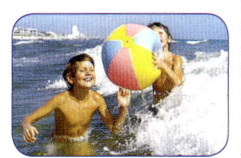

Include exercise in family activities and take water with you.

Extra Information and Tips ~ www.CalorieKing.com.au/library

Diabetes Guide

What is Diabetes?

Diabetes occurs when the body has difficulty processing glucose sugar in the blood.

- **After digestion,** sugar and starches are changed into **glucose** – the simplest form of sugar vital for body energy and growth.
- **Insulin** is the hormone which acts like a key that opens the door to body cells and allows glucose to enter.
- **Without enough insulin,** glucose builds up in the blood and passes into the urine. High blood glucose levels lead to frequent urination, extreme thirst, and tiredness.
- **Untreated diabetes increases the risk of damage to nerves and blood vessels.** This, in turn, increases the risk of heart disease, stroke, blindness, kidney damage, foot ulcers and gangrene (with amputation), impotence and other complications.

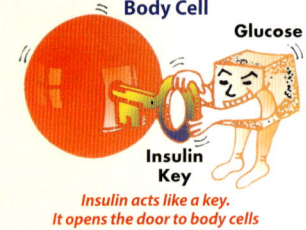

Insulin acts like a key. It opens the door to body cells and allows glucose to enter.

People with type 1 diabetes and some with type 2 have too few or no insulin keys and require insulin injections.

Others (primarily type 2) make enough insulin but the body doesn't use it as well as it should – particularly if overweight and physically inactive.

SYMPTOMS OF DIABETES

- Frequent urination
- Extreme thirst
- Unusual hunger
- Rapid weight loss
- Extreme fatigue
- Blurred vision
- Skin infections that are slow to heal
- Tingling/numbness in feet

Note: Diabetes can be present even with no symptoms.

DON'T IGNORE DIABETES – IT'S A SERIOUS DISEASE

TYPE 2 DIABETES

- Occurs in 90% of diabetes cases
- Occurs mainly in adults - particularly in overweight and inactive persons
- Insulin is produced but body cells resist its action and glucose cannot enter cells
- Usually treated with meal planning and physical activity. Sometimes requires medication (pills or insulin)

TYPE 1 DIABETES

- Occurs in 10% of diabetes cases
- Usually in children and young adults
- Pancreas produces little or no insulin. Daily insulin injections (or use of an insulin pump) are necessary, as well as:
  - matching pre-meal insulin to the amount of carbohydrate eaten
  - weight control and regular physical activity

GESTATIONAL DIABETES

- Occurs in some women during pregnancy. It usually disappears after the baby's birth.
- Women who have had gestational diabetes still have a high risk of developing type 2 diabetes within 5 to 10 years.
- Requires weight control, a healthy lifestyle and regular medical checks.

Diabetes Guide (Cont)

Are You At Risk for Diabetes?

Pre-Diabetes ~ an Early Warning!
Pre-diabetes means that your blood glucose levels are higher than normal, but not high enough to be called diabetes.

If you have pre-diabetes, you have a higher risk for getting diabetes later on.

The good news is that you can start taking steps to prevent diabetes by making healthy lifestyle changes – such as losing weight if overweight, and being more physically active.

BLOOD GLUCOSE CLASSIFICATION OF DIABETES

- **Normal:** Below 5.9 mmol/L*
- **Pre-Diabetes:** 6 – 7 mmol/L*
- **Diabetes:** Over 7 mmol/L*

(*Fasting Blood Glucose)

KNOW YOUR BGL
(Blood Glucose Level)
Everyone over the age of 45 should have a blood glucose test every three years

WHAT'S YOUR RISK?
Find out if you're at risk for diabetes by answering the following questions:

- ☐ I have been told I have pre-diabetes
- ☐ I have a family history of diabetes
- ☐ I am over 35 y.o. and I am from an Aboriginal, Torres Strait Island, Pacific Island, Indian sub-continent, or Chinese cultural background
- ☐ I had diabetes when pregnant
- ☐ I am over age 65
- ☐ I am overweight
- ☐ My waist is larger than: 80cm for a woman or 94 cm for a man
- ☐ I get little or no physical activity
- ☐ My blood pressure is higher than 130 over 85
- ☐ My HDL (good cholesterol) is too low
- ☐ My triglycerides (blood fats) are too high

 CHECK YOUR RESULT

- If you've put a check mark in two or more of the boxes, you may be more likely to develop type 2 diabetes.
- Talk with your doctor to see if you should have a blood test for diabetes.

Importance of Weight Control

- **Type 2 diabetes** is more common in people who are overweight.
- **Being overweight** means that your insulin doesn't work as well to control blood glucose levels.
- **Losing just 5 to 10 kilograms** can help you better manage your diabetes and lower your risk for heart disease.
- **Keys to weight control include:**
  - Following a healthy eating plan
  - Controlling food portions
  - Being physically active most days of the week
  - Keeping food records
  - Setting realistic goals
- **Work with your doctor and dietitian** who can help you reach a weight that's ideal for you.

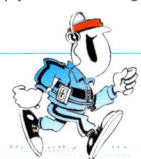

KEEP MOVING!
Every day, do at least 30 minutes of moderate intensity exercise.
(even in 5-minute lots)

It's the key to improving insulin action.
Add muscle strength training 2-3 times a week for extra benefits.

Diabetes Guide (Cont)

Managing Diabetes

Don't battle diabetes alone. Establish a partnership with your doctor, dietitian, diabetes educator, and pharmacist. For extra information and support, contact *Diabetes Australia* in your state.

- **To find an Accredited Practising Dietitian (APD),** check www.daa.asn.au or call toll free on 1-800-812-942
- **To find an Accredited Diabetes Educator (CDE),** contact the *Australian Diabetes Educators Association:* www.adea.com.au or phone (02) 6287 4822

Tips to keep blood glucose within safe limits:

- **Control your food intake.** Know what and when you will eat. Seek referral to a dietitian for expert advice.
- **Exercise regularly.** It assists weight control and can improve sensitivity of body cells to insulin. Plan physical activity into your daily routine.
- **Monitor your blood glucose** at home and work with a blood glucose meter. It will help you become familiar with your blood glucose patterns, and the effects of food, activity and medication.
- **Take insulin or oral medication as prescribed.** If on insulin, know what action to take if hypoglycemia (low blood glucose) occurs. Also educate your family and friends.

Blood glucose meters and insulin pumps can greatly improve control of diabetes

BLOOD GLUCOSE METERS (EXAMPLES)

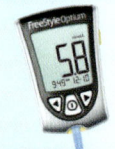
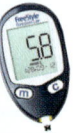

INSULIN PUMPS (EXAMPLES)

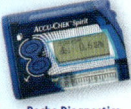
Roche Diagnostics Accu-Chek

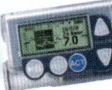
Medtronic MiniMed

Be Heart Smart ~ Know Your ABC's

If you have diabetes, you are at high risk for heart attack and stroke. Heart disease is more likely to strike you – and at an early age – than someone without diabetes.

But you can fight back. Be smart about your heart.
Take control of the ABC's of diabetes and live a long and healthy life. Talk to your doctor about your ABC targets.

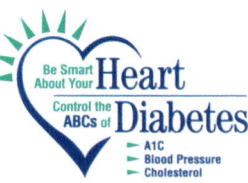

Be Smart About Your **Heart**
Control the ABCs of **Diabetes**
- A1C
- Blood Pressure
- Cholesterol

Ⓐ is for A1c
The A1c (A-one-c) test – short for haemoglobin A1c. It reflects your average blood glucose (sugar) level over the last 3 months.
Suggested Target: Below 7%

Ⓑ is for Blood Pressure
High blood pressure makes your heart work too hard. **Suggested Target: Below 130/80**

Ⓒ is for Cholesterol
Bad cholesterol, or LDL, can build up and clog your arteries.
Suggested Target: Below 2 mmol/L

A1C VALUES ▼	AVERAGE DAILY BLOOD GLUCOSE ▼
6% ►	**6.5 mmol/L** Excellent Control
8% ►	**10 mmol/L** Needs Treatment Change
10% ►	**13 mmol/L** Poor Control
13% ►	**18 mmol/L** Seriously Out of Control

Diabetes Guide ~ Meal Planning Tips

Guidelines for choosing a healthy diet apply equally to people with or without diabetes. Eating a wide variety of foods that are mainly low in fat and refined sugars, and high in fibre, is recommended.

However, actual food quantities, as well as when you eat, will also influence control of blood glucose. Your dietitian will individualize a meal plan to suit your food preferences, lifestyle and medical status.

Here are a few tips:

- **Maintain a healthy weight.** If overweight, even a modest weight loss plus daily physical activity can help manage blood glucose in type 2 diabetes.

- **Don't skip meals.** If you take insulin or an oral hypoglycemic agent, regular meals are important.

- **Know how much carbohydrate you should eat** at your meals and snacks.

- **Know which foods contain carbohydrate;** and learn how to check the Nutrition Information Panel on food labels. Check the serving size and total carbohydrate – not just the sugar content. All carbohydrate breaks down to sugars after digestion.

- **If you are on fixed doses of insulin,** you should try to eat your meals at the same time each day, with the same amount of carbohydrate at each meal and snack.

- **If you are on a flexible insulin regimen** (or an insulin pump), counting your carbohydrate intake will allow you to adjust your insulin to varying meal times and meal size.

- **Choose wholegrain breads, cereals and pasta.** Eat fresh fruits, vegetables and legumes. These foods contain more fibre and slow the release of glucose into your blood after a meal.

- **Limit foods high in saturated fat, trans fat and cholesterol.** Enjoy fish, soy foods, and other foods rich in omega-3 fats. *(Extra Notes: Page 203)*

- **Limit sugars and foods high in added sugar** particularly if overweight. Small amounts of sugar as part of a meal may occasionally be okay. Check with your dietitian. *(Extra Notes: Page 9)*

Eat a well-balanced diet with foods high in fibre and low in saturated fat.

The Plate Method is an easy way to eat healthfully. (See next page)

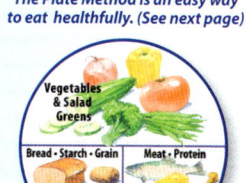

ALCOHOL TIPS

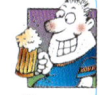

- **If you drink alcohol, have only moderate amounts:**
  Men ~ 1-2 drinks/day
  Women ~ 1 drink/day
  For some people, safe drinking will mean no alcoholic drinks at all.
  (Also see Alcohol Guide ~ Page 27)

- **Drink together with food** – especially if you use insulin or diabetes pills.

- **Do not omit any carb food** in exchange for an alcoholic drink.

- **Alcohol increases the risk of hypoglycemia** (low blood sugar) and drug interactions if you take insulin and certain types of diabetes pills.

- **Check with your doctor and dietitian.**

Diabetes Guide ~ The Plate Method

The Plate Method — An Easy Way to Eat Healthfully

The plate method is a helpful tool to guide your food choices until you see a dietitian for your own meal plan.

For a healthy meal:
- **Fill half of your plate** with **non-starchy** vegetables (broccoli, green beans, carrots).
- **Fill a quarter of your plate** with carbohydrate (wholegrain bread, pasta, potato, brown rice).
- **Fill the other quarter of your plate** with 90-120g of lean meat, poultry, or fish.
- **Use 1-2 teaspoons of margarine** (mainly Canola or olive oil) or a heart-healthy vegetable oil.
- **Add a small piece of fruit** or 1 cup of skim/low-fat milk or yogurt.

How Much Carbohydrate Should You Eat?

A dietitian can best determine how much carbohydrate you need at each of your meals, based on your lifestyle, food preferences, and overall diabetes control. Until you see a dietitian, aim to keep the amount of carbohydrate you eat the same at each of your meals.

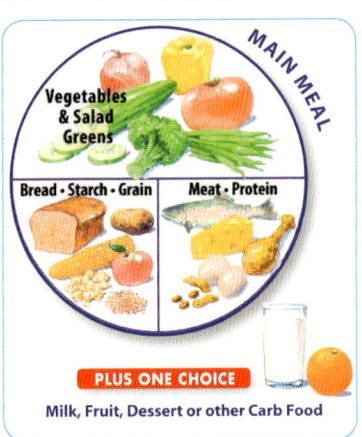

CARB CHOICES MEAL PLAN
One Carb Choice = 15 Grams of Carb

15 grams carbohydrate is the amount in: *1 thin slice Bread or ¾ cup Cereal (unsweetened) or 1 small Potato or 1 small Fruit*

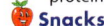 **Breakfast**
- Eat 2-4 carb choices (30-60 grams)
- Include a low-fat protein source such as egg whites or skim milk.

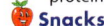 **Lunch and Dinner**
- Eat 2-4 carb choices (30-60 grams carb)
- Include fruit and non-starchy vegetables. Choose small portions of low-fat protein foods.

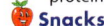 **Snacks**
- If needed, eat 1-2 carb choices (15-30 grams carb).

Note: Above plan is for adults. Carbohydrate amounts will vary with your physical activity level.

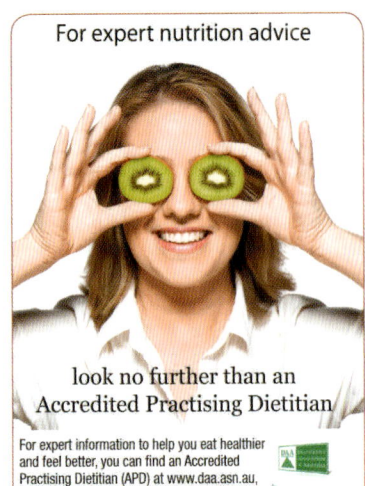

Diabetes ~ Carbs & Glycemic Index

Carb Type Affects Blood Glucose

The various forms of carbohydrate affect blood glucose levels in different ways. It is difficult to predict the effect of particular foods, sugars, or meals, simply by their carbohydrate content.

Thus, the same amount of carbohydrate from different foods may affect blood sugar levels very differently. **Many factors affect the rate of digestion and absorption such as:**

- the type of sugar, starch, and fibre
- the degree of processing and cooking (which increases digestion rate)
- the amount of protein and fat. Indeed, one can lower the GI of a high-GI food by adding fat/oil (which slows down stomach emptying and digestion).

Glycemic Index (GI)

The GI is a method of ranking carbohydrate foods on a scale (0-100) according to how they affect blood glucose levels. *(See next column)*.

The higher the GI value, the greater the food's ability to rapidly raise blood glucose levels, and the more insulin needed by the body (not desirable).

Eating low-GI foods may lead to better control of blood glucose and insulin levels (which in turn lowers the risk of damage to blood vessels and nerves). The slower digestion of low-GI foods may also help to delay hunger pangs and benefit weight control.

Cautionary Notes

Choosing low-GI foods is not a licence to eat unlimited amounts. Calorie restriction and portion control for weight control is of prime importance.

Also remember, Low-GI foods are carbohydrate foods and must still be counted as part of any dietetic carbohydrate plan.

While GI may be a helpful tool for people with diabetes, what is most important is to control the total amount of carbohydrate that you eat.

Extra Info: www.glycemicindex.com
*(The New Glucose Revolution) Diabetes &
Pre-Diabetes Handbook (Publisher: Hatchette Aust.)*

LOWER-GLYCEMIC FOODS
Slower-Acting Carbohydrates

These foods are more slowly digested and absorbed. They help maintain more even blood glucose levels, as long as excessive amounts are not eaten. Eat these foods regularly but limit portion size for weight control.

Examples:
- Dense wholegrain breads
- Bran cereals, oats, muesli
- Fresh fruit: apples, avocados, bananas (firm), cherries, grapefruit, grapes, olives, oranges, peaches, pears, plums. Fresh juices
- Pasta, basmati rice
- Potato *(Carisma in Coles)*, sweet potatoes, yams
- Sweet corn, barley, buckwheat
- Butternut Pumpkin
- Dried beans, peas, lentils, nuts and seeds
- Milk, yogurt, soy drinks
- Dark chocolate

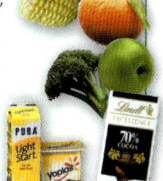

HIGHER-GLYCEMIC FOODS
Quicker-Acting Carbohydrates

These foods more rapidly raise blood glucose levels. Eat only in moderation.

- White bread, rice cakes, bagels, plain crackers
- Low-fibre cereals: Cornflakes, Rice Bubbles, Froot Loops
- Watermelon, ripe bananas, cantaloupe, pineapple
- White potatoes (except *Carisma*), white rice (most types), parsnips
- Soft drinks, cordials, sugar-sweetened sports and energy drinks
- Sugar, confectionery, popcorn (plain)
- Ice cream (low-fat), frozen yogurt

High-GI fruits and potatoes are still healthy choices when eaten in moderate amounts.

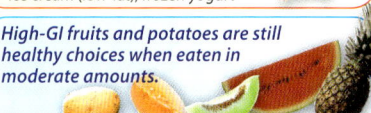

Abbreviations, Measures & Disclaimer

- **Calorie and fat values have been rounded off.**
  Calories – to the nearest 5 or 10 calories.
  Kilojoules – to the nearest 5 or 10.
  Fat – to the nearest half gram.

  Note: Trace amounts of fat or carbohydrate (less than 0.3 grams per serving) have been treated as zero.

- Figures in this publication are generally rounded off and therefore may differ slightly from the label. Serving sizes may also vary from that shown on the package.

Disclaimer ~ Seek Professional Advice

This book is intended for educational purposes only. It is not a substitute for professional advice. Users should consult their medical professional before making any health, medical or other decisions based on the material contained herein. Therapeutic diets are best planned by a dietitian (APD) through a doctor's referral.

- Persons using the information herein for any medical purposes, such as matching insulin dosage to carbohydrate intake, should not rely solely on the accuracy of figures herein and should independently check food labels or contact the food manufacturer for the latest data.

- Because nutritional data for food products is subject to change, users should consult the most recent edition of this book, and the author's website www.calorieking.com.au for the most up-to-date information.

C ~ Calories
kJ ~ Kilojoules
F ~ Fat (grams)

Abbreviations

tsp	=	teaspoon
Tbsp	=	Tablespoon
c	=	cup
ml	=	millilitre(s)
g	=	gram(s)
kJ	=	kilojoule(s)
<1	=	less than 1

Volume Measures

1 tsp	=	5ml
1 Tbsp	=	20ml
½ cup	=	125ml
1 cup	=	250ml
4 cups	=	1 litre

(All measures are level)

Note: 250g weight is not the same as 250ml volume (space occupied). Dense foods weigh more per set volume.

Examples of Cup Weights:
1 cup popcorn weighs 10g
1 cup milk weighs 260g
1 cup honey weighs 580g

Metric Conversion

1 oz	=	28.4 grams
1 fl.oz	=	30 mls
1 calorie	=	4.2 kilojoules

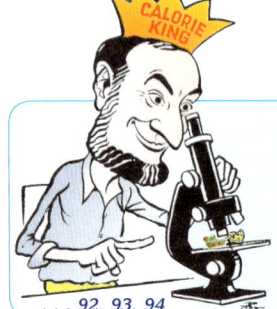

. . . 92, 93, 94

𝒥eedback 𝒲elcome!

Please contact the author directly with your queries, and suggestions for foods to be included in future editions.

Write to: Allan Borushek,
PO Box 3100, Nedlands WA 6009
Email: feedback@CalorieKing.com.au

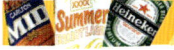

Alcohol Guide

- **Health Hazards:** Excess alcohol contributes to obesity, high blood pressure, stroke, heart and liver disease, some cancers, and even impotence.
- **Concentration, short-term memory,** and sporting performance are also reduced.
- **Other alcohol hazards include** menstrual problems, anxiety, headaches, insomnia, work absenteeism and engaging in risky behaviour. Drinking during pregnancy increases the risk of Foetal Alcohol Spectrum Disorder.
- **Alcohol contributes to obesity,** through its high calories/kilojoules; and by lessening the body's ability to burn fat. Fat storage is promoted, particularly in the belly – a health danger zone.
- **Alcohol is potentially more harmful while dieting.** Blood sugar levels may drop with resultant tiredness and further impairment of concentration, reflexes and driving skills – and maybe the dieter's resolve!

LOWER RISK ALCOHOL LIMITS

 WOMEN: No more than **1-2 drinks** per day.

 MEN: No more than **2 drinks** per day.

(At least 2 days a week should be alcohol-free.)

1 STANDARD DRINK CONTAINS 10 GRAMS ALCOHOL
- 1 Middy Beer (¾ of 375ml can) (4.8% Alc.)
- OR 1 Can (375ml) Mid Strength (3.5%)
- OR 100ml Wine (12% Alc.)
- OR 30ml Spirits (40% Alc.)

Note: You cannot save daily drinks for one occasion.
Binge drinking is particularly harmful ~
4-6 drinks for males, or 3-4 drinks for females (within 2 hours).

Note: For some people, safe drinking means no alcohol at all. Even one drink may impair driving skills, particularly if tired. For women who drink frequently, breast cancer risk is increased by 9% for each drink after the first drink. In men, just 2 drinks a day doubles the risk of cancers of the mouth and throat.

It is advisable not to drink at all if you are:
- pregnant, trying to conceive or breast-feeding
- taking medication or have liver or heart disease (unless approved by your doctor or pharmacist)
- planning to drive, use machinery or play sport
- studying or needing to concentrate
- a child or teenager under 18 year old.

 Note: Women and adolescents are more prone to alcohol's ill-effects due to their lower body weight, smaller livers and lesser capacity to metabolise alcohol.

STANDARD DRINKS

 1 **One Standard Drink (Australia) contains 10 Grams of Alcohol**

The 'Standard Drink' is a simple way to keep track of your alcohol intake. In Australia, the labels of all packaged alcoholic drinks must state the number of standard drinks.

EXAMPLES OF STANDARD DRINKS

Beer:
Full Strength - **1 middy (285ml)**
Mid Strength (3.5%) - **1 can (375ml)**
Light (2.7%) - **1¼ cans (470ml)**

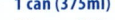

Table Wine (12%): **100ml**
or ⅔ small 150ml glass
or ½ large 200ml glass

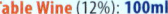

Sherry (18%): **60ml**
Spirits (40%): **1 shot (30ml)**
Cocktails: **1 cocktail glass**
Alcoholic Soda (5%): **250ml**
or ⅔ of 375 ml can

HOW TO CALCULATE ALCOHOL CONTENT

Alcohol percentage on label refers to alcohol volume (ml alcohol/100ml).

To convert to grams (weight) of alcohol:
1. Calculate total alcohol volume (ml) in drink.
2. Multiply by 0.8 - since 1 ml of alcohol weighs only 0.8g (actually 0.789g).

Example:
375ml Can Beer (4.6% alcohol)
4.6% alc.volume = 4.6% of 375ml
= 17ml alcohol
Weight (17 x 0.8) = **13.6g alcohol**

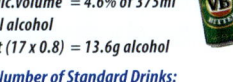

 1.4 *Number of Standard Drinks:*
Divide total grams of alcohol weight by 10
(1.36 standard drinks in 375ml can).

A. Alcohol ~ Beers (with Alcohol Counts)

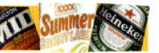

Beer Quick Guide ~ Average all Brands

- **Alc** ~ Alcohol (grams)
- **C** ~ Calories
- **kJ** ~ Kilojoules
- **Cb** ~ Carbohydrate (g)

	FULL STRENGTH 4.8% Alc.				MID STRENGTH 3.5% Alc.				LIGHT ALCOHOL 2.7% Alc.			
	C	kJ	Alc	Cb	C	kJ	Alc	Cb	C	kJ	Alc	Cb
Pony, 140 ml (5 oz)	55	230	5.5	4.5	45	195	4	4.5	35	155	3	3
Glass/Seven, 200 ml (7oz)	75	315	7.5	6.5	65	280	6	6.5	55	225	4	5
Middy/Pot, 285 ml (10 oz)	110	460	11	9	95	400	9	9	75	315	6	7
Stubbie/Can, 375 ml	145	605	14	12	125	520	11	12	100	420	8	9
Schooner/Pint, 425 ml (15 oz)	165	690	16	14	140	385	12	13	115	480	9	10
Bottle, 800 ml	310	1300	30	26	265	1110	23	25	215	900	18	20
Jug, 1140 ml (40 oz)	440	1840	43	36	380	1580	35	36	305	1285	25	27

Beer ~ Brands

Beer Contains No Fat
% = Percent Alcohol (By Volume)

Per 375ml Can/Stubbie Unless Indicated

	C	kJ	Alc	Cb
Amstel, Lager, 4.7%, 330ml	105	435	13	5.5
Arvo, Brew 34/51, 4.9%, 330ml	120	500	13	9
Asahi, 5%, 330ml	140	580	13	10
Ballarat Bitter, 4.6%, 375ml	140	590	14	11
Barecove Radler, 4.2%, 330ml	115	490	11	10
Beck's, 5%, 330ml	135	570	13	11
Beez Neez, 4.7%, 345ml	130	540	13	10
Bighead (Burleigh Brewing)				
No Carb, 4.2%, 330ml	90	370	11	0.5
Bintang, 4.7%, 330ml	130	545	13	10
Blue Bitter, 2.3%, 375ml	100	430	6	16
Bluetongue: Lager, 4.9%, 330ml	155	640	13	9
Light, 2.7%, 330ml	110	450	7	11
Boag's:				
Classic Blonde, 4.5%, 375 ml	115	475	14	4
Draught, 4.6%, 375ml	140	580	14	10
Light Draught, 2.7%, 375ml	100	400	8	9
Premium, 5%, 375ml	150	625	15	10
Prem. Light, 2.9%, 375ml	100	410	9	8
Pure, 4.5%, 330ml	120	510	12	9
St George, 4.8%, 375ml	130	550	14	7
XXX Ale, 4.8%, 375ml	145	610	14	11
Boddington's, Pub Ale, 4.7%, 440ml	180	750	17	16
Budweiser, 4.9%, 355ml	145	605	15	11
Byron Bay, Prem. Ale, 5%, 330ml	100	430	13	4
Caffrey's, Irish Beer, 4.8%, 440ml	175	730	16	10
Canterbury Draught, 4%, 375ml	120	505	12	11

Per 375ml Can/Stubbie Unless Indicated

	C	kJ	Alc	Cb
Carlsberg: Regular, 4.8%, 330ml	130	545	13	10
Elephant, 7.2%, 330ml	200	825	21	13
Carlton: Black Ale, 4.4%, 375ml	145	605	13	13
Cold Filtered, 4%, 375ml	120	500	12	10
Draught, 4.6%, 375ml	140	585	14	10
Dry (Lower Carb), 4.5% 355ml	120	500	13	7
Dry Fusion: 4.2%, 355ml				
Black; Lemon, 355ml	125	520	12	10
With Lime, 355ml	115	490	12	8
Light, 2.7%, 375ml	100	425	9	10
Mid, 3.5%, 375ml	135	570	11	15
Natural, 4.5%, 355ml	110	455	13	4.5
Sterling, 5%, 375ml	100	430	13	12
Cascade: Bitter Ale, 4.4%, 375ml	130	550	13	9
Blonde, 4.8%, 375ml	155	650	14	13
Draught, 4.7%, 375ml	145	595	14	10
First Harvest, 5.5%, 330ml	155	655	14	13
Lager, 4.8%, 375ml	145	605	14	10
Pale Ale, 5%, 375ml	150	640	15	12
Premium, 5%, 375ml	150	635	15	12
Premium Light, 2.6%, 375ml	105	445	8	12
Cintra Pilsner (Portugal), 4.8% 330ml	130	545	13	10
Classic Blonde, 4.5%, 375ml	115	475	13	4
Cold Filtered, 4%, 375ml	120	500	12	9
Coopers: Birrell, 0.5%, 375ml	80	325	1.5	16
Clear, Low Carb, 4.5%, 355ml	110	460	13	3.5
Dark Ale, 4.5%, 375ml	130	535	14	6
Premium Light, 2.9%, 375ml	100	405	9	5
Mild Ale, 3.5%, 375ml	115	470	11	6
Original Pale Ale, 4.5%, 375ml	130	545	15	6
Sparkling Ale, 5.8%, 375ml	165	695	19	8

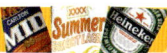

Alcohol ~ Beers (with Alcohol Counts)

Beer ~ Brands (Cont)

Ale ~ *Alcohol (grams)*

Beer Contains No Fat

Per 375ml Can/Stubbie Unless Indicated

	C	kJ	Ale	Cb
Coors, Draft, 5%, 355ml	140	595	13	11
Corona, Extra, 4.6%, 330ml	140	585	12	13
Crown: Gold, 3.5%, 375ml	125	520	11	12
Lager, 4.9%, 375ml	150	630	15	12
Cruiser: Humm. Blonde, 4%, 275ml	105	430	9	3.5
With Passionfruit, 4%, 375ml	95	410	9	3.5
DB (NZ): Bitter, 3.5% 330ml	105	430	9	9
Draught, 4%, 330ml	110	465	11	9.5
Emu: Bitter, 4%, 375ml	150	625	12	11
Draught, Midstrength, 3%, 375ml	115	470	9	11
Export, 4.4%, 375ml	135	565	13	10
Eumundi, Lager, 4.8%, 375ml	145	620	15	11
Fiji: Bitter, 4.6%, 375ml	145	600	14	10
Gold, 4.6%, 375ml	125	510	14	6
Fosters:				
Lager, 4.9%: 375ml can	150	630	15	12
355ml Long Neck bottle	140	585	14	11
Light Ice, 2.3%, 375ml	105	435	9	13
Gage Roads, Pils, 3.5%, 330ml bottle	110	465	9	10
Gold Bitter, 3%, 375ml	105	440	9	10
Grolsch Premium, 5%, 330ml	130	545	13	10
Guinness: Draught, 4.2%:				
375ml can/bottle	135	570	13	12
440ml can	160	670	15	14
Stout, 6%, 375ml	200	845	19	19
Hahn:				
Harvest, 4.2%, 375ml	120	510	11	9
Premium, 5%, 375ml	155	645	15	12
Premium Light, 2.6%, 375ml	100	430	8	11
Super Dry, 3.5%, 330ml	85	345	10	3.5
Heineken, 5%:				
330ml stubbie	140	580	13	11
375ml can	160	655	15	13
5 litre keg	2100	8750	200	165
Hopman, Premium Pale, 0.5%, 375ml	60	230	0.5	12
James Squire:				
Amber Ale, 5%, 345ml	155	630	14	14
Golden Ale, 4.5%, 345ml	140	575	12	12
Pilsener, 5%, 345ml	160	660	14	15
Porter, 5%, 345ml	165	675	14	16
Sundown Lager, 4.4%, 345ml	130	545	13	12
KB Lager, 4.4%, 375ml	145	590	13	12
Kent Old Brown, 4.4%, 375ml	145	595	13	12
Kirin, (Japan), 5%, 330ml	135	560	13	10
Kronenbourg 1664, 5%, 330ml	145	590	14	12

Per 375ml Can/Stubbie Unless Indicated

	C	kJ	Ale	Cb
Lion (New Zealand): Red, 4%, 355ml	110	455	11	10
Ice, 4.5%, 355ml	130	550	13	9
Matilda Bay: Beez Neez, 4.7%, 375ml	140	590	14	10
Bohemian Pilsner, 4.7%, 345ml	145	600	13	10
Dogbolter, 5.2%, 375ml	190	775	16	19
Fat Yak, 4.7%, 345ml	140	585	13	12
Maxx (Coles Brand), Low Carb:				
Blonde, 4.6%, 330ml	100	425	12	4.5
Dry, 5%, 330ml	130	545	13	10
Melbourne Bitter (Fosters), 4.6%, 375ml	145	595	14	11
Michelob, 5%, 355ml	155	650	15	14
Miller: Draft, 4.7%, 355ml	145	600	13	13
Chill, 4.2%, 355ml	105	445	12	7
Monteith's, Original Ale, 4%, 330ml	150	630	11	10
Pilsner, 5%, 330ml	130	545	13	10
Newcastle Brown Ale, 4.7%, 330ml	130	545	14	10
NT Draught (Carlton),				
Darwin Stubby, 4.9%, 2 litres	820	3420	80	64
Pepperjack Ale, 4.7%, 375ml	150	630	13	15
Peroni: Leggera, 3.5%, 330ml	95	390	9	7
Nastro Azzurro, 5.1%, 330ml	150	620	15	12
Platinum Blonde (Woolworths), 4.6%, 330ml	110	455	11	4.5
Power's: Bitter, 4.4%, 375ml	135	565	13	10
Gold, 3%, 375ml	100	430	9	9
Ice, 4.5%, 375ml	130	555	14	9
Pure Blonde:				
Premium (Low Carb), 4.6%:				
355ml bottle	105	445	13	3
375ml can	115	470	13	3.5
Premium Mid, 3.5%:				
355ml bottle	90	385	10	5
375ml can	100	410	12	4
Redback (Matilda Bay):				
Original, 4.7%, 375ml	155	645	14	14
Cristal, 4.5%, 354 ml	140	575	12	12
Mild, 3.4%, 375ml	115	470	10	10
Red Bitter, 4%, 375ml	135	565	12	11
Reschs: Draught, 4.5%, 375ml	140	580	13	12
Pilsener, 4.4%, 375ml	140	580	13	11
Real Bitter, 4%, 375ml	125	520	12	11
Richmond Lager, 4.5%, 375ml	135	570	13	12
Rogers (Little Creatures), 3.8%, 330ml	120	500	11	11
Sail & Anchor, Dry Dock, 5%, 330ml	130	545	13	10
Sapporo (Japan): 5.2%, 350ml	135	570	15	10
650ml can	255	1065	26	19

Updated Nutrition Data ~ www.CalorieKing.com.au
Persons with Diabetes ~ See Disclaimer (Page 22)

Alcohol ~ Beer ◇ Cider ◇ Stout

Beer ~ Brands (Cont) — Alc ~ Alcohol (grams)

Per 375ml Unless Indicated	C	kJ	Alc	Cb
Schlossgold, Ultra Light, 0.4%, 330ml	65	260	1	12
Singha, Lager, 5%, 330 ml	155	645	13	16
Sol, 4.6%, 330ml	145	595	13	12
Southwark, Bitter, 4.5%, 375ml	145	585	15	11
Speight's: Distinction, 5%, 330ml	140	580	13	13
Old Dark, 4%, 330ml	125	520	11	14
Pale Ale, 4.5%, 330ml	125	520	12	10
Steinlager (New Zealand):				
Classic, 5%, 330ml	135	570	13	11
Pure 5%, 330ml	140	575	13	11
Stella Artois, 5%, 330ml	145	600	14	12
Swan Draught, 4.5%, 375ml	140	575	14	10
Tiger, 5%, 375ml	155	645	13	16
Tooheys: Extra Dry, 4.6%: 375ml	145	605	14	10
345ml bottle	130	555	13	9
Extra Dry Platinum, 5.2%, 345ml	175	720	15	11
New, 4.6%, 375ml	145	605	14	12
Old, 4.4%, 375ml	150	585	13	12
Pils, 4.5%, 345ml	120	505	13	8
White Stag (Low Carb), 4.4%, 345ml	105	435	13	9
Tsingtao, 4.8%, 330ml	145	605	13	14
VB/Victoria Bitter (Carlton):				
Mid Strength, 3.5%, 375ml	120	500	11	11
Original, Full Strength, 4.9%, 375ml	145	610	15	11
Raw, 4.5%, 355ml	120	495	13	7
WA Gold, 3%, 375ml	145	605	9	20
Waikato, Draught, 4%, 330ml	105	445	11	9
West End, Draught, 4.5%, 375ml	140	575	13	10
XXXX: Bitter, 4.6%, 375ml	140	570	14	10
Light Bitter, 2.3%, 375ml	90	370	7	10
Gold, 3.5%, 375ml	110	460	11	7
Summer Bright, 4.2%, 330ml	100	415	11	4

Shandy

Beer diluted 1:1 with Lemonade:

	C	kJ	Alc	Cb
Full Strength Beer, 200ml	85	350	4	13
with Low Joule Lemon/Soda	40	165	4	2
Mid Strength, 3.3%, 200ml	70	290	3	12
with Low Joule Lemon/Soda	30	125	3	1
Tesco, Shandy, 330ml bottle	70	290	1.5	15

Non-Alcoholic Brew

	C	kJ	Alc	Cb
Coopers, Birell, 0.5%, 375ml	80	325	1.5	16

Stout

	C	kJ	Alc	Cb
Abbotsford, Invalid, 5.2%, 375ml	170	700	17	14
Brass Monkey, 6%, 375ml	195	810	18	17
Cascade, 5.8%, 375ml	190	795	17	17
Coopers Best, 6.3%, 375ml	175	735	19	12
Guinness Stout, 6%, 375ml	200	845	18	18
Sheaf, 5.7%, 375ml	200	835	17	20
Southwark Old, 7.4%, 375ml	225	945	21	18
Swan, 7.4%, 375ml	220	895	22	14

Cider ~ Alcoholic

	C	kJ	Alc	Cb
5 Seeds *(Tooheys)*:				
Extra Dry, 5%, 345ml	170	710	14	17
Batlow Premium, 5.5%, 330ml	190	800	16	19
Bulmers: Orig. Apple, 4.7%, 330ml	135	570	12	15
Pear, 4.7%, 330ml	150	630	14	12
Castaway *(Sail & Anchor)*, 5%, 330ml	170	710	13	20
Cruiser, Apparella, 4%, 275ml	130	545	9	13
James Squire,				
Orchard Crush Apple, 4.8%, 500ml	210	875	19	19
Kingstone Press: 5.3%:				
Dry Cider, 660ml	285	1190	28	22
Pear Cider, 660ml	345	1440	28	37
Magners:				
Original, 4.7%: 330 ml	135	565	13	12
568ml bottle	230	960	21	21
Pear, 4.7%, 568ml bottle	300	1255	21	32
Mercury: Draught, 5.2%, 375ml	190	795	16	23
Dry, 5.2%, 375ml	160	660	14	14
Sweet, 5.2%, 375ml	180	760	16	20
Monarch Apple Cider:				
Draught, 7%, 330ml	205	855	19	18
Dry, 7%, 330ml	180	750	19	11
Sweet, 7%, 330ml	225	940	19	23
Monteith's, Apple, 4.5%, 330ml	135	560	12	13
Old Mont Scrumpy, 8%, 330ml	185	775	21	10
Pipsqueak: Best Cider,				
5.2%, 330ml	145	605	14	12
Rekorderlig: Apple, 4.5%, 500ml	240	1005	18	28
Pear, 4.5%, 500ml	250	1045	18	30
Strawberry-Lime, 4%, 500ml	210	880	16	25
Scrumpy, Dry, 6%, average, 345ml	155	645	17	10
Strongbow: Clear, 5%, 355ml	145	600	14	13
Dry, 5%, 355ml	150	625	14	15
Original, 5%, 355ml	180	735	14	22
Pear, 5%, 355ml	170	695	14	20
Sweet, 5%, 355ml	205	850	14	29
Three Kings, 4.6%, 330ml	135	565	12	12
Westons: Old Rosie Cloudy Scrumpy,				
7.3%, 500ml bottle	275	1150	29	18
Stowford Press, Med. Dry, 4.5%, 500ml	250	1045	18	30

Alcohol ~ Cocktails

Cocktails

	C	kJ	Alc	Cb

Most cocktails listed are made to standard recipes followed by The Australian Bartenders' Guild.

	C	kJ	Alc	Cb
Absolut Madam (with Vodka/Midori)	210	880	15	26
Australian Crawl	190	795	20	13
B and B	135	565	15	4
B52 (2.5g fat)	140	585	11	10
Baileys On Ice (5g fat)	95	400	4	6
Bananas in Pyjamas (6g fat)	240	1005	14	22
Between The Sheets	240	1005	30	7.5
Bloody Mary	120	495	14	5
Brandy Alexander (16g fat)	300	1255	16	11
Brown Cow	240	1005	7	48
Caipirinha (w. 60ml Cachaca)	230	960	19	24
Champagne Cocktail	125	520	13	9
Chastity Belt	275	1150	20	34
Chupa Nuranjas (with 45ml Tequila)	150	630	16	8
Collins	180	770	20	11
Cosmopolitan	150	630	15	11
Creme de Menthe Frappe	120	500	7	18
Daiquiri	110	460	14	3
Dry Martini (On-The-Rocks)	125	520	18	0
Flaming Lamborghini, (7g fat)	250	1045	16	19
Frappe (w. Cointreau/Midori)	180	755	15	19
Gin Sling	145	605	15	10
Godfather; Godmother	180	750	16	17
Grasshopper (22g fat)	420	1755	13	33
Hard On (Cocktail)	290	1210	13	50
Island Lei (22g fat)	380	1590	11	26
Japanese Slipper (with Midori)	190	800	15	21
Jo Jo Ivory (14g fat)	340	1420	12	33
Kahlua & Milk (4g fat)	170	710	7	21
Kamikaze	160	670	20	5
Mai Tai	260	1075	27	17
Manhattan	260	1075	27	17
Mardi Gras	200	835	15	24
Margarita	110	460	15	1
Memphis Meltdown (17g fat)	350	1465	13	27
Menage à Trois; Mint Julep	160	670	19	5
Midori & Lemonade	130	545	5	24
Midori Margarita	220	920	20	20
Mojito (with 60ml Rum)	170	710	19	9
Monk's Madness	410	1715	15	76
Moscow Rule (with Vodka)	160	670	15	14
Pimm's	140	585	10	18
Planters Punch	90	375	10	5
Pina Colada: (6g fat)	210	880	15	12
With Cream (17g fat)	290	1210	10	16

Cocktails (Cont)

	C	kJ	Alc	Cb
Prairie Oyster (Pick-Me-Up)	85	360	3	3
Raffles Bar Sling	330	1380	30	30
Red Bull & Vodka	210	880	14	28
with sugar free Red Bull	105	440	14	3
Screwdriver	140	585	20	0
Seabreeze (with Vodka)	125	525	15	5
Serengeti Sunset	160	670	10	23
Silk Stockings	370	1545	16	65
Singapore Sling	150	630	18	6
Slippery Nipple	200	835	14	26
Sloe Comfortable Screw	170	710	19	9
Spritzer (Wine & Soda)	20	85	3	0
Strawberry Daiquiri (Aust)	160	670	16	12
Tequila Sunrise, Long Drink	160	670	10	23
Vodkatini (with fruit)	120	500	13	7
Whiskey Highball	140	585	10	13
Whiskey Sour	145	605	15	10
Whisky Mac	120	500	13	14
White Russian (22g fat)	370	1545	16	15
Zombie	300	1255	35	64
Zulu Warrior	190	795	11	28

Shooters

	C	kJ	Alc	Cb

30ml shot of 2-3 liqueurs/spirits

	C	kJ	Alc	Cb
5 Best Friends	75	315	11	2
Angry Fijian; B 52 Shooter	100	420	5	12
Flaming Lamborghini; Oil Slick	100	420	10	11
Fruit Tingles	255	1070	20	36
Jelly Shot:				
Small, 30ml (with15 ml Vodka)	55	230	5	5
Large, 60ml (with 30ml Vodka)	110	460	10	10
Liquid Cocaine	80	345	10	7
Slippery Nipple	100	420	7	9
Windex Shooter	85	350	9	5

Mocktails~Non Alcoholic

	C	kJ	Alc	Cb
Bora Bora	120	500	0	30
Cool Cow (32g fat)	550	2300	0	40
Egg Nog (16g fat)	290	1200	0	29
Lemon, Lime & Bitters	90	375	0	21
Mickey Mouse	20	70	0	5
Roy Rogers	80	330	0	20
Schmooze	315	1320	0	77
Shirley Temple	145	605	0	5
Southern Belle	130	545	0	8
Strawberry Kiss	95	395	0	17
Tomato Juice Cocktail	20	85	0	5

Updated Nutrition Data ~ www.CalorieKing.com.au
Persons with Diabetes ~ See Disclaimer (Page 22)

Alcohol ~ Liqueurs ◆ Spirits

Liqueurs

	C	kJ	Alc	Cb
Per 30 ml				
Advocaat, 18% alc., (2g fat/30ml)	85	355	4	9
Alizé Gold Passion, 16% alcohol	90	375	4	11
Amaretto, Anisette, 28% alcohol	110	460	6	19
Apricot Brandy, 35% alcohol	85	355	8	9
B & B, 43% alcohol	95	400	10	4
Baileys Irish Cream, 17%, (4g fat):				
Original/Flavours, avg	100	410	4	8
Mini's 70ml bottle	220	920	9.5	17
Baitz Island Cream, 17%, (0.6g fat)	60	250	4	7
Benedictine, 40% alcohol	90	375	11	5
Bundaberg Royal, 32% alcohol	100	420	8	11
Cassis, 20% alcohol	70	295	5	12
Chartreuse: Green/Aniseed, 55%	105	435	16	11
Yellow/Liquorice, 40% alcohol	100	420	10	11
Cherry Brandy, 24% alcohol	80	335	6	9
Cointreau, 40% alcohol	100	420	10	8
Creme de Banane/Cacao, 26%	100	420	6	11
Creme de Menthe, 30% alcohol	120	500	7	14
Curacao, 35% alcohol	95	395	8	6
Drambuie, 40% alcohol	105	440	10	9
Frangelico (Hazelnut), 24% alcohol	80	335	6	11
Galliano, 40%	100	420	10	11
Grand Marnier, 40% alcohol	100	420	10	11
Godiva, Chocolate, 17% alcohol	105	435	5	11
Hpnotiq, 17.5% alcohol	105	435	5	11
Kahlua, 20% alcohol	80	335	5	12
Kilkenny Cream, 16.5% alc., (2g fat)	75	310	4	7
Kirsh, 34% alcohol	80	335	8	6
Malibu, 21% alcohol	60	240	5	6
Mandarin, 28% alcohol	90	375	6.5	11
Maraschino, 30% alcohol	80	335	7	8
Midori Melon, 20% alcohol	70	280	5	9
Opal Nera Sambuca, 40% alcohol	100	420	10	11
Ouzo, 40% alcohol	105	435	11	11
Peach, 35% alcohol	65	270	10	3
Pernod, 40% alcohol	75	315	10	11
Port Liqueur (Morris Old), 17.6% alc.	45	190	4	4
Sabra, 30% alcohol	80	335	7	6
Sambuca, 40% alcohol	100	420	10	11
Sloe Gin, 28% alcohol	80	335	6.5	8
Southern Comfort, 30% alcohol	80	335	7	9
Strawberry Liqueur, 23% alcohol	80	335	5.5	10
Tia Maria, 32% alcohol	90	375	7.5	0
Triple Sec, 30% alcohol	105	435	8.5	11

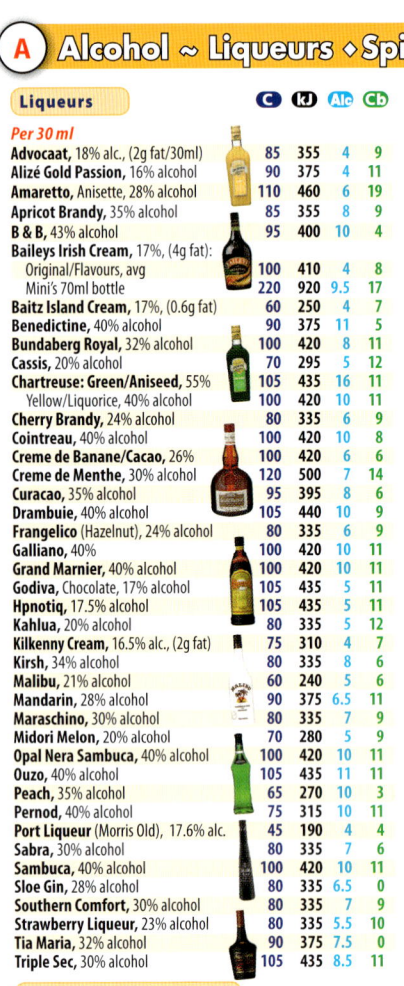

Cordials/Fruit Syrups

Grenadine, Cassis, Strawb., Raspb., Almond	75	315	0	19
Margarita Mix, 100ml	90	380	0	20

Alc ~ Alcohol (grams)
Spirits Contain No Fat

Quick Guide ~ Spirits

Spirits, Brandy, Vodka, Whisky
Includes: Brandy, Rum, Whisky, Gin, Vodka, Bourbon, Cachaca, Cognac, Scotch, Tequila

Average (40% alcohol):	C	kJ	Alc	Cb
1 Shot/Nip, 30ml	65	275	10	0
1 Double Shot/Jigger, 60ml	130	550	19	0
½ Bottle, 350ml	760	3180	112	1
1 Bottle, 700ml	1520	6360	224	2

Aperitifs

Campari, (25%), 300ml	65	270	6	5
Pimm's No. 1, (25%), 30ml	50	210	6	2
Pernod, (40%), 30ml	70	295	10	1
Shochu, (Japanese, 25% alc.), 60ml	85	355	12	0

Spirits ~ Bar Drinks

	C	kJ	Alc	Cb
Includes 30ml (1 Shot/Nip) of Spirits				
Coke Mixers include ½ cup (125ml) Coke				
Bacardi/Bourbon & Coke	120	500	10	7.5
with Diet Coke	70	290	10	0
Brandy, Lime & Soda	110	460	10	11
Bundy on Ice	70	290	10	0
Bundy & Coke	120	500	10	13
Gin & Tonic	110	460	10	11
Rum/Scotch & Coke	120	500	10	13
with Diet Coke	70	290	10	0
Whisky & Dry Ginger Ale	120	500	10	13
Cocktails ~ *See Page 27*				

Angostura, Claytons

Angostura Bitters, ¼ tsp	3	10	0	0
Claytons (Non-alcoholic), 30ml	40	175	0	11
Lemon Lime & Bitters, 200ml	85	360	0	21

Liqueur Coffees

Benedictine (10g fat)	200	835	10	10
Cointreau, Galliano (10g fat)	200	835	10	10
Egg Nog (16g fat)	290	1200	10	29
Hot Toddy	100	420	10	11
Irish Coffee, +1 tsp sugar (10g fat)	190	795	10	6
Kahlua/Tia Maria (10g fat)	190	795	7	13

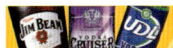

Alcoholic Sodas (Pre-Mixed)

Alcoholic Soda ~ Ready To Drink

Pre-Mixed Cans or Bottles	C	kJ	Alc	Cb
Bacardi & Cola (4.5%), 375ml	230	960	14	34
Bacardi Breezer (4.4%), 275ml:				
Blueberry Guava; Raspberry	155	645	10	20
Lemon; Lime; Orange; P'Apple	165	680	10	23
Pink Grapefruit	170	710	10	25
Watermelon	140	585	10	17
Bearded Lady, Bourb. w. cola (6.5%), 375ml	255	1065	19	30
Black Douglas: & Cola (4.7%), 375ml	235	975	14	34
& Dry (4.7%), 375ml	210	865	14	28
Zero Scotch & Cola (4.7%), 375ml	100	410	14	0
Bluetongue,				
Ginger Beer (4%), 330ml bottle	135	565	13	8
Bulleit Bourbon & Cola:				
Original (4.6%), 375ml	220	910	13	30
Black (6.5%), 375ml	255	1065	19	30
Bundaberg Rum: *Per 375ml*				
& Cola (4.6%)	250	1040	15	37
Bare, No Sugar Cola (4.6%)	100	420	14	0.5
Dark & Stormy (4.6%)	250	1035	13	40
Mid 3.5 & Cola (3.5%)	225	940	11	37
Soda, Red (4.6%)	225	940	14	32
Canadian Club Whisky:				
Dry (4.8%), 330ml	190	790	13	25
Cola, (4.8%), 330ml	195	815	13	26
Cougar: *Per 375ml*				
Bourbon & Cola (4.7%)	235	970	14	34
With Cola Zero (4.7%)	100	410	14	0.5
XS Bourbon & Cola (6%)	265	1110	18	36
CS Cowboy, Butterscotch & Cream, (4%), 270ml	245	1025	9	29
Elevate, (8%), 300ml	260	1090	19	32
Gordon's: Gin & Tonic (6%), 275ml	250	1040	13	39
Haig & Cola, (5%), 275ml	260	1085	15	39
Haig & Dry, (5%), 375ml	230	960	15	31
Hi NRG, Vodka Energy (6.5%), 250ml	200	835	13	26
Jack Daniels & Cola, (6%), 375ml	255	1070	18	32
Jagermeister, Raw (6.5%), 330ml	230	950	18	27
Jim Beam & Cola: *Per 375ml*				
Black Label (6%)	220	920	18	23
Devil's Cut & Cola (6.66%)	230	960	20	23
Mid Strength & Cola (3.5%)	150	625	10	19
White Label (4.8%)	190	800	15	23
Zero Sugar Cola (4.8%)	100	425	15	0
Jim Beam, & Dry, (4.8%), 375ml	175	735	15	20
Johnnie Walker: & Cola (4.6%), 375ml	235	970	14	34
& Dry (4.8%), 375ml	185	780	14	22
Premium Strength (6.5%), 375ml	260	1090	19	31
Kilt, Whiskey & Cola (8%), 375ml	290	1210	24	30

Pre-Mixed Cans or Bottles (Cont)	C	kJ	Alc	Cb
Midori: Illusion (4.5%), 275ml	195	805	10	30
Lemonade (4%), 275ml	200	840	8.5	36
Splice (4.5%), 275ml	215	900	10	37
Pulse: Vodka with,				
Ginseng & Berry (4.8%), 250ml	95	390	10	6
Guarana (6.5%), 300ml	270	1130	16	39
Pure Platinum, (4.5%), 355ml	210	875	13	30
Rebellion Bay, Rum w. Cola (4.8%), 375ml	235	975	14	34
Rum & Cola, (6%), 375ml	260	1085	18	34
Rush, (Infused Vodka), 4%, 275ml	165	690	9	25
Ruski, Lemon (4.5%), 300ml	180	750	11	25
Skyy Blue, (4.8%), avg. all, 275m	140	590	16	17
Smirnoff Ice: Red (4.5%), 335ml	200	835	13	25
Double Black: (6.5%): 335ml bottle	230	950	18	27
375ml can	255	1070	19	30
& Guarana (6.5%), 250ml	180	740	13	22
Super Dry (3.5%), 375 ml	145	605	11	18
Smirnoff Cocktails: *Per 120ml of 700ml Bottle*				
Grand Cosmopolitan (14%), 120ml	145	605	14	11
Pomegranate Martini (15%), 120ml	185	775	15	23
Vodka Mojito (15%), 120ml	160	675	15	19
Casks (6.4%), avg., 200ml	150	625	10	19
Southern Comfort & Cola, (4.5%), 375ml	240	1005	14	36
Stone's, Ginger Beer, (4.8%), 330ml	210	880	13	30
Three Kings, Vodka Ginger (4.6%), 330ml	190	795	12	26
UDL Cans, (4.2%), 375ml can:				
Gin & Tonic	180	755	13	23
Ouzo Cola, average	220	910	13	31
Vodka Green Apple	215	895	13	30
Vodka Lemon Lime & Soda	190	805	13	25
Vodka Raspberry	235	970	13	36
Vickers, London Gin/Grapefruit (4.8%), 250ml	160	670	10	23
Vodka, Russian Standard, Citrus:				
Single Can (in bars), (5%), 300ml	190	800	12	27
4-Pack can/bottle (6.5%), 300ml	215	900	16	27
Vodka Cruiser (4.6%): Avg., 275ml	175	725	10	25
Sugar Free (4.6%), avg., 275ml	75	310	10	0
Ice (4.8%), 275ml	180	750	11	25
West Coast Cooler, (3.5%), 250ml	135	565	7	22
Wild Turkey & Cola:				
(5%), 375ml	235	980	15	32
American Honey (4.8%), 340ml	220	920	13	32
Premium 101 (6.5%), 375ml	270	1130	20	32
WKD: Vodka Blue (4.5%), 275ml	215	900	10	36
Vodka Iron Brew (4.5%), 275ml	160	670	10	26
Woodstock Bourbon & Cola:				
(4.8%): 375ml can	255	1060	15	37
440ml can	300	1250	17	43

Updated Nutrition Data ~ www.CalorieKing.com.au
Persons with Diabetes ~ See Disclaimer (Page 22)

Alcohol ~ Wine

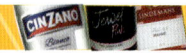

Table Wine ~ Quick Guide   Alc ~ Alcohol (grams)

Average All Varieties, 12% Alcohol

	C	kJ	Alc	Cb
100ml, (½ of 200ml Glass)	75	315	10	2
120ml serve, (⅔ of 180ml Glass)	90	375	12	2.5
160ml serve, (⅔ of 240ml Glass)	120	500	15	3
½ Bottle, 375ml	280	1170	35	7.5
1 Bottle, 750ml	560	2340	70	15

Note: Wines contain no fat.

Table Wines

Per 120ml Serve
Average All Brands (12% Alcohol)

	C	kJ	Alc	Cb
Red: Claret/Burgundy/Chianti	80	335	12	0
Sparkling Reds	90	375	12	2.5
Rose, Medium, 120ml	80	335	12	2
White: Dry (Chablis/Hock/Riesling)	75	315	12	0
Sweet (Moselle/Sauternes)	85	355	12	3
Sparkling (Rhinegold/Mardi Gras)	95	395	12	1
Passion Pop, (9.5%), 120ml	120	500	9	10
Green Ginger Wine (Stone's), Original, 13.9%, 120ml	180	765	13	24

Champagne

	C	kJ	Alc	Cb
Average: (11.5%), 1 glass, 120ml	85	355	11	2
With Orange Juice (3:1 orange)	70	290	8	4
With Orange Juice (1:1 orange)	55	230	6	6
Sparkling Moscato, Red/White, 120ml	95	395	8.5	1

Fortified Wines

	C	kJ	Alc	Cb
Cinzano, 14.4%: Bianco, 60ml	80	335	7	8
Extra Dry, 60ml	55	230	7	1
Rosso, 60ml	75	315	7	6
Madeira, 18% alcohol, 60ml	85	355	9	7
Marsala, 18% alc., av., 60ml	110	460	9	10
Muscatel; Port, 18% alc., 60ml	95	395	9	8
Sherry, 18% alcohol: Dry, 1 sherry glass, 60ml	60	260	9	0.5
Sweet/Cream average, 60ml	85	355	9	7
Vermouth: Dry, 18% alc., 60ml	70	290	9	1.5
Sweet, 15% alc., 60ml	85	355	7	8

Mead, Mulled Wine

Flavoured/Spiced Wines, warmed to serve.
Heat is insufficient to evaporate alcohol

	C	kJ	Alc	Cb
Mulled Wine (Gluhwein), 150ml	230	960	18	26
Maxwell Mead: Spiced/Honey, 12.5%, 120ml	120	500	12	9
Liqueur Mead, 22.5%, 30ml	60	250	5	6

Reduced Alcohol Wines

Per 120ml Serve

	C	kJ	Alc	Cb
Brown Bros., Moscato, 5.5%	95	400	5.5	15
Lindemans: Early Harvest: Dry White, 8.5%	60	255	8	1
Rose, 8.5%	65	270	8	2
Semillon Sauv Blanc, 8.5%	60	245	8	0.5
Sparkling, 7.5%	60	240	7	2
Sparkling Rose 7.5%	60	240	7	2
Shiraz, 9%	65	270	8.5	1
Sweet Seasons: Blancello, 8.5%, 150ml	110	455	10	20
Dulciana, 9.5%, 150ml	125	530	12	12
Zibibbo, 7.5%, 150ml	105	440	9	11
McWilliam's: Balance: Brut Cuvee, 8%, 120ml	55	230	8	0.5
Shiraz, 9%, 120ml	80	325	8	5
Sauvignon Blanc, 8%, 120ml	65	270	8	1
Trentham, Semillon Sauv. Blanc, 8.5%	60	260	8	3
Verdi, Spumante, 4.8%	50	210	4.5	19
Yellowglen: Bella, 7.5%	85	350	6.5	9
Jewel: 'Light on Calories', 6% Pink/Yellow, average	50	215	6	3

Non-Alcoholic Wines/Juice

Per 120ml Serve

	C	kJ	Alc	Cb
Ariel: Blanc	90	380	0	22
Rouge	60	260	0	15
Edenvale: Chardonnay; Sparkling Cuvee	30	130	0	7.5
Shiraz	25	105	0	6
Fronti, Lambrusco	65	265	0	16
Maison *(Orlando),* Grape Juice	65	265	0	16
Norfolk Punch, Herbal Wine	30	135	0	10
Rose River: Pearl	70	280	0	16
Ruby	80	335	0	19

Japanese Sake ~ Rice Wine

	C	kJ	Alc	Cb
Hana Kohaku (12.6%), 300ml	300	1250	30	21
Snow Beauty (15%), 300ml	310	1300	36	15

Cooking with Wine

Table Wines (Unsweetened): Negligible cal/kJ if sufficient heat and cooking time (at least 30 minutes simmering) for alcohol to evaporate.

Sweetened Wines (e.g. Sherry): Residual cal/kJ after adequate cooking – **10 cal/42 kJ per 30ml** of wine used.

Flambé Desserts: Only surface alcohol is burnt off.

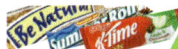

Bars ~ Breakfast, Diet, Sports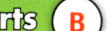

Bars ~ Brands

Note: Some bars weigh up to 30% more than stated net weight. For accuracy, weigh bar and recalculate.

Per Bar/Cookie	Cal	kJ	Fat	Cb
All Natural Bakery: *Per 100g*				
Organic Oat Slice: Almond & Apple	430	1800	20	53
Banana	425	1770	19	54
Yogurt, Almond & Apricot	435	1820	21	53
Amway ~ *See Nutriway*				
Aribar, average all flavours, 22g	90	370	2	17
Artisse: *Per 40g Bar*				
All About Nuts	205	850	13	18
Almond Nougat	185	770	6	29
Berry, Cherry & Almonds	160	670	6	22
Coconut & Almond	165	695	7	21
Cranberry Crunch	185	765	11	19
Seed Delight	190	800	11	19
Walnut & Acai	175	725	7	22
Atkins:				
Note: Carbohydrate figures do not include sugar alcohols.				
Advantage: *Per 60g Bar*				
Chocolate Brownie	220	925	10	3
Chocolate Decadence	250	1055	13	4
Chocolate Hazelnut Crunch	240	1000	10	3
Day Break: *Per 37g Bar*				
Almond Cranberry	185	765	10	4
Cappuccino Nut	175	730	8.5	4
Chocolate Chip Crisp	145	600	7	2
Strawberry Crisp	155	645	8	3
Endulge: Choc Coconut, 40g	180	750	12	3
Peanut Caramel, 34g	150	615	9	4
Aussie Bodies:				
HPLC, avg. all flavours, 100g	375	1560	10	7
Protein FX:				
All Flavours, avg., 65g	260	1080	7	12
Lo Carb, Choc-coated, 60g	200	835	6	4
Note: Contains 8.5g Polydextrose & 7.3g Maltitol				
Mini Bar, 30g	100	420	3	2
Super, Choc Caramel, 85g	365	1530	14	16
Balance: Fuel 2Go, av. all flavours, 60g	210	880	4	19
Muscle 2Go, 90g	295	1220	6.5	11
Be Good To Yourself: *(Amcal/Guardian)*				
Lunch Bars, avg., 45g	165	690	5	3
Snack Bars, avg., 30g	110	460	3	2
Be Light *(Aldi):*				
Grains Delight, 30g bar	110	455	1	21
Orange, 30g bar	110	465	1	23

Per Bar/Cookie	Cal	kJ	Fat	Cb
Be Natural:				
Nut: Almond Apricot, 40g	185	775	10	20
Nut Delight, 40g	215	890	14	12
Nut, Macadamia Honey, 40g	255	1060	22	11
Four: Apple, Flame Raisin, Alm. & Pepita	145	600	7	15
Currant, Berry, Oats & Pepita, 32g	140	575	6	17
Coconut, Apricot, Oats & Chia, 50g	150	615	8	15
Lunchbox: Amazing Apple, 22g	80	330	1	16
Bouncing Berry, 22g	80	325	1	15
Trail Bars: Berry, 32g	110	465	1.5	20
Dark Chocolate, 32g	120	500	3	19
Honey Nut, 32g	120	485	2	18
Nut & Fruit, 32g	115	480	2	19
Bellis, School Bars, 20g	85	325	1	16
Betty Baxter:				
Meal Replacement Bars: *Per 58g*				
Cherry Choc	220	920	6.5	28
Choc Mint; Strawb., avg	210	875	5	29
Biggest Loser:				
Meal Replacement Bars: *Per Bar*				
Double Choc, 55g	210	880	6.5	19
Strawb. & White Choc., 60g	225	930	6.5	20
Toffee & Chocolate, 60g	225	940	6.5	20
Snack Bars: *Per 30g Bar*				
Lo Carb Choc Honey	120	500	4	2.5
Protein Bites: *Per Bite*				
Choc Honeycomb (1), 12g	45	190	1.5	0.5
B.Sc *(Body Science):*				
Fuel 01, 40g	155	640	4	22
High Protien, Choc, 65g	230	965	5	7
Cadbury Brunch Bars:				
Peanut, 35g	180	755	11	18
Avg. other varieties, 35g	160	665	6.5	20
Carman's:				
Muesli Bites, avg., 20g	85	350	3	12
Muesli Bar: Apricot & Almond, 45g	200	840	10	25
Classic Fruit, 45g	195	820	8	26
Dark Choc: Blueberry, 35g	145	600	4	23
Cranberry & Almond 35g	155	650	7	21
Yoghurt, Apricot & Almond, 35g	160	670	8	19

Updated Nutrition Data ~ www.CalorieKing.com.au
Persons with Diabetes ~ See Disclaimer (Page 22)

B Bars ~ Breakfast, Diet, Sports

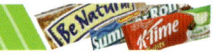

Per Bar/Cookie	Cal	kJ	Fat	Cb
Coles:				
Chewy Bars: *Per 31g Bar*				
Apricot & Coconut	120	505	2.5	22
Chocolate	135	560	4	21
Mixed Berry	125	515	3	22
Cocoa Puffs, Choc Chip Rainbow, 22g	90	375	2.5	16
Fruit Filled, Apple; Apricot, 38g	125	530	1	24
Yoghurt Topped Bars,				
Apricot; Strawberry, 31g	135	560	4	22
Emma & Tom's, Life Bars, avg, 40 g	170	690	8	18
Europe: Nougat Honey Log	195	820	9	26
Summer Roll, 40g	190	795	8	26
Extendbar,				
Choc. Delight, 40g	150	630	3	20
FindingForm:				
Meal Replacement Bars,				
avg, 55g	215	900	9	11
Snack Bars, average, 30g	110	460	2.5	7
Flapjack (Reflex), 80g	250	1050	11	25
Fontelle:				
Fibre Fix, 35g, average	140	575	4.5	19
Collagen Fix, 30g, avg	120	490	3	14
Mini Meal, 100g, average	450	1880	20	55
Food For Health:				
Gluten Free Bar: W/ Fruit, 35g	120	510	4.5	21
Fruit Free, 25g	90	370	3	15
Freedom Foods:				
Nut Free: Ancient Grains, 32g	125	515	3.5	21
Berry Good Delight, 35g	130	535	2	25
Muesli, 35g	140	585	5	22
Free Oats Chewy, average all flav., 35g	130	545	3	23
Go Natural:				
Fruit Nut, Soft Eating,				
Choc Macadamia, 40g	145	615	6.5	21
High Protein: Almond & Apricot, 80g	320	1330	11	43
Nut Crunch, Original, 50g	230	960	13	16
Popcorn Bar, Apple, Apricot. Ban., 35g	120	490	1	27
Premium Natural: Macadamia Divine	270	1130	19	23
Macadamia Dream, 50g	275	1145	20	23
Nut Fantastic, 60g	315	1320	22	24
Savoury Snack: Almond & Cashew, 45g	225	945	16	15
Macadamia & Hazelnut, 45g	240	995	18	13
Chia Sesame Crisp, 40g	180	760	8	25

Per Bar/Cookie	Cal	kJ	Fat	Cb
Go Natural (Cont):				
Snack Bars: Almond & Apricot, 40g	180	760	12	16
Fruit & Nut Delight: 50g	220	915	13	22
With Dark Choc Ripple, 50g	225	930	13	23
Macadamia & Apricot, 40g	195	810	14	17
Nut Delight, 40g	210	870	16	11
97% Fat-Free:				
Apricot & Coconut, 35g	115	480	1	26
Superfood Breakfast: Mixed Berries, 40g	160	665	6.5	22
Walnut Date & Maple, 40g	170	705	7	23
Superfood Meal Bars: Apricot, 80g	285	1190	6	53
Apple & Sultana Ripple, 80g	305	1260	8	54
Apple Strawb. Cranberry, 80g	305	1275	8	55
Chocolate Banana, 80g	305	1280	8	54
Choc Berry, 80g	300	1250	8	53
Peach & Apricot, 80g	300	1250	7.5	53
Superfood Snack Bars: Alm. Cranb., 50g	245	1015	16	20
Walnut Date with Chia, 50g	240	1010	16	21
Superfood Trail Mix:				
Almond Brazil Berries w. 9 Grains, 35g	155	640	7.5	19
Mixed Berry w. 8 Grains, 40g	160	665	5	26
Golden Days:				
Peanut Snaps (1), 15g	80	320	3.5	9
Sesame Snaps: Original (1), 40g	215	895	12	22
Mini, Original (3), 30g	160	670	9	17
Dark Chocolate (1), 13.3g	75	300	4	7.5
Healtheries:				
Simple Cherry Bliss, 40g	200	835	11	22
Simple Nougat Roll, 40g	185	770	7.5	28
Hillcrest (Aldi):				
Bubble Bars:				
Choc Rainbow/Vanilla, 20g	80	340	2	14
Choc Squiggle, 20g	85	350	3	14
Chewy Muesli:				
Choc Squiggle, 31g	125	525	4	20
Honeycomb & Nut, 31g	135	560	5	20
Chewy: Apricot & Yoghurt, 31g	135	565	5	20
Strawb./Tropical & Yog., 31g	140	570	5.5	19
Fruit Filled Bars:				
Apricot, 38.5g	125	520	1	25
Mixed Berry, 37.5g	120	505	1	23
Muffin Bars: Choc Fudge, 40g	140	595	4	20
Apple & Cinnamon/Fruit Explosion, 35g	140	590	6	20
Williams, Muesli Bars, avg., 45g	200	845	8	26

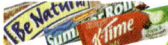

Bars ~ Breakfast, Diet, Sports

Per Bar/Cookie	Cal	kJ	Fat	Cb
Horley's				
Carb Less, 55g	165	680	3.5	6
Carb Less Crunch, 50g	175	730	7	7
Carb Less Deluxe, 35g	130	545	4.5	4
Protein 33, 60g	220	915	3	28
Sculpt Protein Bars, 45g	155	650	3.5	15
IGA:				
Active Start: Fruit & Nut, 36.7g	145	615	2.5	27
Oven Baked: Apple; Apricot, 37.5g	110	460	1	24
Way of Life:				
Apple; Apricot, 37.5g	105	440	3.5	18
Fruit & Nut, 50g	245	1015	15	21
Macadamia & Apricot, 50g	245	1020	17	21
Nut Delight, 50g	260	1085	18	18
IsoWhey Complete:				
Functional:				
Choc Berry, Pom. & Green Tea	210	865	5.5	12
Strawberry Yoghurt, 55g	200	840	4.5	11
Snack:				
Choc Mint Crunch, 55g	160	665	6	6.5
Double Choc Crunch, 55g	165	685	6	8
Vanilla Yoghurt & Apricot, 55g	170	705	6	15
Kellogg's:				
Crunchy Nut,				
All varieties, 30g	150	620	8.5	14
K-Time Twists: *Per 37g Bar*				
All varieties	130	530	2.5	24
LCMs: 4D Choc, 29g	120	500	3	22
Choc Chip, 22g	90	380	2.5	17
Corn Flakes, 23g	95	390	2	19
Kaleidos, 22g	90	385	2	18
Rice Bubbles, 22g	90	380	2	18
Strawbubbles, 22g	90	380	2	18
Split Stix: Chocolatey, 23g	100	410	3	17
Mash-ups, 23g	105	425	3.5	17
Yoghurty, 23g	100	420	3	17
Nutri-Grain Bars:				
Original: Multi-Pack, 30g	125	525	3	22
Single-Wrapped, 35g	145	615	3.5	25

Note: Bars are not vitamin-fortified like the breakfast cereal

	Cal	kJ	Fat	Cb
Special K:				
Chocolatey: Caramel, 22g	90	370	1.5	16
Raspberry, 22g	90	370	1.5	16
Dessert Inspired: Berry Cheesecake, 21.5g	85	355	1.5	16
Lemon Meringue Pie, 21.5g	90	365	1.5	15
Fruit & Nut, all varieties, 28g	115	485	4	17

Updated Nutrition Data ~ www.CalorieKing.com.au
Persons with Diabetes ~ See Disclaimer (Page 22)

Per Bar/Cookie	Cal	kJ	Fat	Cb
Kuranda:				
Almond & Cherry, 40g	190	800	14	12
Almond Nut Snax, 40g	200	820	15	13
Brazil Nut & Date, 40g	200	845	15	11
Cashew & Almond, 45g	235	980	17	13
Chia & Berry, 40g	190	800	13	11
Chinoa, 40g	195	815	14	8
Nut & Berry, 45g	205	855	14	13
Macadamia & Apricot, 40g	200	840	15	10
Macadamia & Hazelnut, 40g	240	1005	18	13
Pecan & Pistachio, 45g	240	1000	18	13
Walnut & Fig, 40g	200	845	15	11
Yummy Choc Bites, average, 30g	150	625	11	10
Leda: *Per Bar*				
Apple & Cinnamon, 85g	265	1100	1	56
Apricot, 85g	300	1240	4	56
Banana, 85g	300	1250	3.5	55
Fruit Filled, all flavours, 38g	120	495	0.5	27
Twist, Apple & Blueberry, 38g	130	545	2.5	21
Lite n' Easy:				
Cinnamon Oat, 30g	120	490	3.5	19
Classic Choc & Oats, 32g	130	530	4	20
Little Kids: *(Heinz),*				
Yoghurt Muesli Fingers	60	240	1.5	10
Milo:				
Energy Bars: Original, 21g	80	335	1	15
Snack with Milk, 27g	110	450	2.5	18
Oatie, 35g	140	570	3	23
Mother Earth: Baked Fruit Sticks, 19g	60	255	0.5	13
Baked Oaty Slices, Average, 40g	170	710	8.5	20
Musashi:				
Bulk Bars: Mass Gain, 80g	295	1235	7	10
Mass Gain Deluxe, av all flav., 90g	330	1385	13	23
Energy Bar, Growling Dog, 65g	245	1030	4	35
Protein Bars:				
P, Choc Hazelnut, 90g	365	1530	10	28
P10, Low Carb, avg., all flav., 40g	160	660	7	8
P20, Low Carb, avg., all flav., 65g	220	925	5	7
Nana Diver's: *Per 120g Bar*				
Mini Meal: Apple & Blueberry	500	2075	18	71
Apricot & Yoghurt	485	2015	21	63
Chocolate Chip	565	2355	31	59
Roasted Almond	540	2255	24	66
Nature Valley:				
Crunchy, average, 42g	195	820	8.5	13
Sweet & Nutty, average, 30g	150	620	8	16
Nature's Goodness,				
Goji Rite, 40g	135	565	9	15

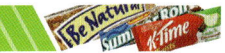

Bars ~ Breakfast, Diet, Sports

Per Bar/Cookie	Cal	kJ	Fat	Cb
Nature's Way:				
SlimRight, Fruit & Nut, 40g	155	645	6	19
Protein Bars, average all flavours, 30g	85	355	2	3
Nice & Natural:				
Nut Chocolate: Almond; Original, 30g	160	650	10	12
Apricot, 30g	150	625	9	12
Nut Natural: Almond, 32g	165	690	11	12
Apricot, 32g	160	660	10	12
Chocolate; Trailmix, 32g	165	685	10	13
Original; Yoghurt, 32g	160	670	10	12
Not a Trace:				
Wholegrain: Apple, 25g	85	345	1	17
Chocolate Custard, 25g	90	385	2	15
Vanilla Custard, 25g	85	360	1	16
Nutriway/Amway:				
Protein Bars: Fuel Factor, all var., 40g bar	150	650	4.5	5.5
Positrim, all varieties, 60g bar	250	1045	9	4
XS, Energy, all varieties, avg., 46g bar	175	735	4	14
OptiSlim VLCD, average, 60g bar	240	1015	8	25
PowerBar: Performance, 60g bar	220	925	2	40
Protein Plus, 55g	175	740	4.5	17
Ride, av. all flavours, 55g	215	890	9	23
Protein 33 (Horleys), 60g	220	915	3	28
Sanitarium: Per Bar, ½ Meal				
One Square Meal:				
Apricot w. Manuka Honey	350	1460	12	45
Cranberry w. Manuka Honey	350	1455	12	45
Simply Less (Coles): Per 40g Bar Unless Otherwise Stated				
Apricot & Peach, 21.5g	85	355	1	16
Date, Sesame & Chia Seed	160	680	7	17
Fruit, Oat & Quinoa	145	605	3.5	24
Trio Nut	190	780	9	21
Slim Secrets:				
Fit Balls, Choc Mint Chip, 50g	180	740	6	2
Milk Active:				
Bombs, Choc Mint, 60g	210	890	7	2
White Choc & Caramel, 60g	210	865	6	2
Protein Bars, average all varieties, 40g	140	580	4	8
Wanted! less than 100 Calories,				
Av. all varieties, 28g	85	355	2.5	7
Supa Wired Chewy, avg., 30g	115	480	3.5	19

Per Bar/Cookie	Cal	kJ	Fat	Cb
Slimmm:				
Meal Replacement, 55g Bar	205	850	7	10
Snack Bars: Choc Mint, 30g	110	460	2.5	5.5
Forest Fruits, 30g	100	415	2	6
SLM:				
Petite, average all flavours, 35g	110	455	3.5	1.5
Toning, average all flavours, 55g	195	815	5	5.5
Wholegrain Energy, avg., 40g	145	610	3.5	25
Sun Health Foods: Per 40g Bar				
HiFi Plus: Almond & Apricot	160	675	7.5	18
Macadamia & Apricot, 40g	165	690	9	17
Premium Nut	190	785	13	14
Yoghurt, Almond & Apricot	165	690	8	18
Indulgence: Almond & Honey	200	830	12	18
Macadamia & Honey	230	960	18	17
Oxi+: Goji Berry & Cranberry	150	620	5.5	23
Olive Leaf & Cashew	195	810	11	20
Prota+, Apricot & Almond	120	500	3.5	18
Rice Syrup: Almond & Honey	200	825	12	16
Apricot	130	545	3.5	25
Cashew & Honey	200	820	12	20
Macadamia & Honey	240	1010	20	15
Sesame	190	780	9	23
Sunibrite:				
Cookies, Big One, Chocolate Chip, 100g	480	2000	22	65
Slices: Muesli, 90g	405	1685	19	52
Apricot & Muesli, 90g	405	1685	19	52
Slim 'N' Trim: Average, 90g	280	1170	1.5	58
Based on actual weight, 110g	345	1430	2	70
Yoghurt Coated:				
Apricot & Muesli, 90g	435	1810	22	55
Strawberry & Muesli, 90g	380	1575	13	58
Swisse:				
Active Recover: Choc Coconut, 30g	120	510	4	3
Choc Goji, 30g	120	500	3	3
Tasti Bars:				
Mega Nuts: Double Choc, 40g	210	890	13	17
Peanut Buter, 40g	215	905	14	15
Milkies, Choc Vanilla, 20g	70	280	2	11
Muffin Bakes, Choc Fudge	145	605	4.5	21
Nut Bar, Choc. Peanut, 35g	180	750	11	15
Tony Ferguson:				
Munch High Protein Bars:				
Apricot Munch, 60g	205	850	4	26
Berry Munch, 60g	205	860	4	28
Honey Soy, 60g	210	865	5	22
Pizza, 60g	210	880	5	21

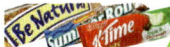

Bars ~ Breakfast, Diet, Sports

Per Bar/Cookie	Cal	kJ	Fat	Cb
Tony Ferguson (Cont):				
Munch Meal, Chilli & Sour Cream, 60g	210	880	5	21
Snack Bars: Berry Delite, 25g	100	410	4	12
Chocolate, 30g	135	555	7	13
Mixed Nut, 30g	140	585	8	13
The Ministry of Muffins: *Per Twin Pack, 2 Muffins*				
Little Bites: Choc Chip, 32g	145	595	7	18
Choc Fudge Brownies, 40g	195	810	9.5	24
Cookies & Cream, 38g	180	755	10	21
Ultra Slim, Dark Cherry, 40g	140	580	5	24
Uncle Tobys: *Per Bar*				
BodyWise Bars:				
Apple Delight, 35g	110	465	2	18
Heart Wellbeing, Cranberry & Rasp., 30g	110	445	2	22
Omega 3 Boost, Alm. Cinn. & Honey, 30g	125	515	4.5	17
Chewy Bars: Choc Chip, 31g	135	565	5	20
Forest Fruits, 31g	130	545	4	21
White Choc Chip, 31g	130	540	4	21
Crunchy Bars: Choc Chip, 20g	90	365	3	13
Nut Crumble, 20g	90	370	3.5	12
Oat Slice: Alm. & Honey, 35g	150	630	6.5	19
Apple & Cinnamon, 35g	150	625	6.5	20
Puffs, Caramel, average all flavours	90	375	2.5	15
Yoghurt Topps: Apricot, 31g	130	545	5	20
Honeycomb, 31g	140	575	5.5	20
Mango & Passionfruit, 31g	135	560	5	20
Raspberry; Strawberry, 31g	135	560	5	20
Wallaby Natural:				
Superbars:				
Macadamia & Cashew, 40g	205	845	14	16
Macadamia & Fruit, 40g	185	775	10	23
Macadamia & Ginger, 50g	225	930	10	31
Macadamia, Sesame & Honey, 40g	215	895	14	19
Mango Passionfruit & Guava, 40g	130	535	3	22
Yoghurty: Cranberry, Fruit & Nut, 50g	210	870	6.5	33
Fruit & Nut, 40g	190	795	10	21
Macadamia & Ginger, 40g	195	810	10	20
Orange Almond & Poppy, 50g	225	940	8.5	31

Updated Nutrition Data ~ www.CalorieKing.com.au
Persons with Diabetes ~ See Disclaimer (Page 22)

Per Bar/Cookie	Cal	kJ	Fat	Cb
Weight Watchers: *Per 40g Bar*				
Cereal Bars:				
Apple Crumble	125	515	0.5	23
Custard & Apple, 37.5	115	480	0.5	22
Raspberry Pie	125	515	0.5	23
Strawberry & Blueberry, 37.5g	120	490	0.5	22
Baked Bar:				
Caramel Shortcake, 22g	90	365	3	14
Chewy Chocolate, 22g	90	380	2.5	15
Muffin Bar, Ginger Kiss, 35g	110	470	2.5	17
Nut Bars: Almond & Apricot, 34g	150	630	6.5	19
Hazelnut & Orange, 34g	155	650	7.5	19
Macadamia & Cranberry, 34g	155	640	7	19
Nut Deluxe, 34g	150	635	6	19
Well, Naturally:				
AntiOx Bar, Acai/Goji, 40g	160	675	7.5	19
High Protein Mini Bars: *Per Bar, 25g*				
Banana Fudge	90	380	2.5	3.5
Caramel Fudge	100	410	2.5	3
Cherry Delight	100	410	3	3.5
Double Choc	100	420	3	3
French Vanilla	100	410	2.5	3
Peppermint Surprise	85	355	3	3.5
Winners:				
Energy: Apple Berry Crumble, 55g	185	760	2	37
Choc Berry, 50g	185	770	4.5	28
Choc Nut Honey, 50g	200	830	7	26
Gym Protein, Choc Peanut, 75g	270	1125	8	20
Woolworths:				
Select Fruit Bars: Custard & Banana, 37.5g	135	560	3	23
Custard & Blueberry, 37.5	130	545	2	24
Select Muesli Bars: Chewy Choc Chip, 31g	125	525	4	19
Yoghurt Apricot, 31g	125	520	4	20
Yoghurt Strawberry, 31g	130	545	4.5	20
Select Nut Bars: *Per 40g Bar*				
Choc & Nut	210	870	13	15
Macadamia & Cranberry	200	845	12	19
Nut & Fruit	180	760	9	20
Select Premium Muesli:				
Berry Burst, 35g	130	550	2	24
Oats & Seeds, 35g	150	640	7	16
Select Rice Bars, average all flavours, 22g	90	380	2	17
Woolworths Homebrand:				
Muesli: Choc Chip, 25g	100	420	3	15
Chocolate Honeycomb, 31g	130	540	5	18
Strawberry & Yoghurt, 25g	105	435	3.5	16
Oven Baked, average all flavours, 37g	120	505	1	26

35

B Beverages ~ Coffee Shops

Coffee ~ Instant

	Cal	kJ	Fat	Cb
Instant Coffee: *Granulated/Ground:*				
1 teaspoon	0	0	0	0
Brewed/Percolated, 1 cup	0	0	0	0
Black: + 1 rounded tsp sugar	20	85	0	5
+ 2 rounded tsp sugar	40	170	0	10
White: With whole milk, 1 T, 20ml	15	65	1	1.5
With reduced-fat, 2 Tbsp, 40ml	20	85	0.5	2
With skim milk, 2 Tbsp, 40ml	20	80	0	2

Coffee ~ Dry Mixes, Brands

Jarrah: *Prepared as Directed*

	Cal	kJ	Fat	Cb
Coffee Sensations; *Per 12.5g*				
Bavarian Bliss; French Liaison	60	250	2	9
Brazil Delight; Swiss Moments	55	240	2	10
Cappuccino, Cheeky Cino, 15g powder	65	265	2	10
Latte: *Per 15g powder*				
Mocha Indulgence	65	265	2	10
Vanilla Thriller	65	270	2.5	10
White Choc-a-mocha	60	255	2	9

Moccona:

	Cal	kJ	Fat	Cb
Cafe Classics:				
Cappuccino: Regular, 14.4g sachet	70	295	3.5	7.5
Lite, 14.2g sachet	55	225	2	6
Latte, 15g sachet	80	325	4.5	7.5

Nescafe:

	Cal	kJ	Fat	Cb
Cafe Menu:				
Cappuccino:, 12.5g sachet	60	250	3	6.5
Skim, 12.5g sachet	45	180	0.5	8.5
Latte: Regular, 18g sachet	90	375	5.5	8
Skim, 12.5g sachet	45	175	1	6.5
Flavoured, average, 18g sachet	75	315	2.5	13

Robert Timms:

	Cal	kJ	Fat	Cb
Cafe Moments:				
Cappuccino, 12.5g sachet	55	230	1.5	9
Latte, 17g sachet	75	305	1.5	13
Mocha, 17g sachet	75	305	1.5	14

Coffee Flavoured Milk ~ *See Page 45*

Coffee Alternatives

Roasted Cereals & Caffeine-Free:

	Cal	kJ	Fat	Cb
Caro; Ecco, 1 heaped tsp, 3g	10	40	0	2
Dandelion, 1 heaped tsp, 3g	10	40	0	2
Teeccino, 1 heaped tsp, 3g	10	40	0	2

Caffeine Guide & Counter ~ *See Page 210*

Coffee Shops ~ Generic

	Cal	kJ	Fat	Cb
Coffee: *Per 250ml Cup Unless Indicated*				
Afogatto, (Espresso + Ice Cream)	80	340	3	13
Cappuccino: With whole milk	100	420	5.5	7.5
With skim milk	55	230	0.5	8
With Soy milk	95	395	4.5	8
350ml Mug/Take-Away Cup:				
With whole milk	140	585	7.5	11
With skim milk	75	315	0.5	11
With Soy milk	135	555	6.5	11
Caffe Latte: *Same as Cappuccino*				
Flat White: With whole milk	130	545	7.5	10
With skim milk	70	295	0.5	10
With Soy milk	125	525	6.5	10
350ml Mug/Take-Away Cup:				
With whole milk	180	750	11	14
With skim milk	100	420	11	14
With Soy milk	175	730	9	14
Espresso, black	5	15	0	0
Iced Coffee:				
With whole milk, 350ml	180	760	9	17
+ ice cream + cream, 350ml	410	1720	27	34
Iced Frappe, 350ml	225	940	0	65
Long Black	0	0	0	0
Macchiato, (2 shots + milk), 100ml	10	40	0.5	1
Mocha: With whole milk	195	815	7	24
With skim milk	125	525	1	21
With Soy milk	170	710	5.5	22
Turkish Coffee, 120ml	18	75	0	4.5
Vienna, (black + 1 oz wh. cream), 250ml	105	435	12	1

Gloria Jean's/ Starbucks ~ *See Next Page*
Liqueur Coffees ~ *See Page 28*

Coffee Shops ~ Chocolate Drinks

Per 250ml Cup

	Cal	kJ	Fat	Cb
Hot: All milk (whole milk)	230	950	8.5	29
With reduced-fat milk	225	945	3	31
Iced Chocolate: All milk	265	1100	13	33
With ice cream + cream	500	2095	30	51
Mocha, (with whole milk)	160	670	6	21
Vienna Chocolate	230	960	12	29
Marshmallows, 2 small, 10 g	35	140	0	8.5

Coffee Shops ~ Milkshakes

	Cal	kJ	Fat	Cb
Milk + flavouring	300	1255	11	33
With whipped cream	350	1465	15	34
With ice cream	400	1670	17	35

Beverages ~ Coffee Shops

Coffee Shops ~ Brands | Cal | kJ | Fat | Cb

Gloria Jean's:
Chocolate: Per Regular, Without Cream
- **Regular:** With Whole Milk — 245 | 1030 | 10 | 29
- With Skim Milk — 170 | 715 | 1 | 29
- With Soy Milk — 180 | 745 | 4.5 | 24
- **White Chocolate:** With Whole Milk — 365 | 1530 | 16 | 45
- With Skim Milk — 285 | 1200 | 6.5 | 45
- With Soy Milk — 295 | 1230 | 10 | 40

Coffee: Per Regular
- **Cafe Latte/Flate White:**
- With Whole Milk — 175 | 740 | 9 | 14
- With Skim Milk — 100 | 425 | 0.5 | 14
- With Soy Milk — 110 | 455 | 4 | 9
- **Cafe Mocha:** With Whole Milk — 235 | 975 | 9 | 28
- With Skim Milk — 165 | 685 | 0.5 | 28
- With Soy Milk — 170 | 710 | 4.5 | 23
- **Cappuccino:** With Whole Milk — 150 | 625 | 7.5 | 12
- With Skim Milk — 85 | 360 | 0.5 | 12
- With Soy Milk — 90 | 385 | 3.5 | 8
- **Espresso:** Long Black, 242ml — 5 | 10 | 0 | 0.5
- Short Black — 5 | 25 | 0 | 1
- **Flat White** ~ *See Cafe Latte*
- **Macchiato,** with Whole Milk, 80ml — 20 | 75 | 1 | 2
- **Minicino:** Caramel, w. Whole Milk, 241ml — 180 | 755 | 7.5 | 21
- Vanilla, with Whole Milk, 242ml — 190 | 805 | 7.5 | 21
- **Piccola Latte,** with Whole Milk, 85ml — 45 | 190 | 2.5 | 4
- **Very Vanilla Latte:** With Whole Milk — 290 | 1210 | 11 | 41
- With Skim Milk — 230 | 960 | 3.5 | 41
- With Soy Milk — 235 | 985 | 6.5 | 36

Add Whipped Cream:
- Small, 22g cream — 60 | 250 | 6.5 | 1
- Regular/Large drinks, 28g cream — 80 | 325 | 8 | 1
- **Tea:** Chai Tea, with Whole Milk — 130 | 540 | 7 | 10
- Black Tea, without sugar — 5 | 20 | 0.5 | 0

Cold Drinks: *Per Regular Size, With Whole Milk, Without Cream*
- **Espresso Chillers:** Creme Brulee — 360 | 1505 | 9 | 65
- Very Vanilla — 375 | 1560 | 14 | 57
- Voltage — 410 | 1715 | 16 | 60
- **Fruzies:** Banana — 295 | 1230 | 1.5 | 70
- Mango — 325 | 1350 | 1.5 | 78
- Strawberry — 280 | 1165 | 1.5 | 65
- **Fruzie Smoothie:** Banana — 455 | 1905 | 5.5 | 99
- **Iced Chocolate:** Arnott's Tim Tam — 475 | 1985 | 19 | 70
- Original — 410 | 1710 | 13 | 64
- **Iced Coffee:** Signature — 310 | 1290 | 12 | 41
- **Iced Mocha** — 315 | 1310 | 12 | 39
- **Mocha Chiller:** Cookies 'N Cream — 510 | 2115 | 21 | 71
- Mudslide Mocha — 375 | 1555 | 13 | 56
- **Italian Soda:** Small — 155 | 655 | 0 | 38
- Regular — 210 | 870 | 0 | 50
- Large — 310 | 1310 | 0 | 75

Coffee Shops ~ Brands (Cont) | Cal | kJ | Fat | Cb

Hudsons Coffee: *Drinks Based on Low Fat Milk, Without Cream or Ice Cream Unless Indicated*

Hot Drinks: *Per Small Take-Away Cup*
- **Chocolate:** Choc Mocha — 190 | 800 | 3.5 | 34
- Marble Mocha — 200 | 835 | 5.5 | 32
- Traditional — 195 | 815 | 4 | 34
- White — 215 | 895 | 5 | 35

Coffee:
- Cappuccino — 65 | 265 | 2 | 7
- Espresso — 0 | 0 | 0 | 0
- Flat White — 90 | 375 | 3 | 10
- Latte — 105 | 435 | 3 | 11
- Long Black — 0 | 0 | 0 | 0
- Long Machiato — 5 | 25 | 0 | 0.5
- Short Machiato — 5 | 20 | 0 | 0.5
- Vienna Cream — 270 | 1120 | 26 | 8

Tea:
- Traditional — 130 | 550 | 3 | 19
- Chai — 130 | 545 | 4 | 19

Cold Drinks:
IceStorm:
- Caramel Crunch with Cream — 655 | 2735 | 36 | 47
- Chocolate Crunch with Cream — 655 | 2735 | 36 | 47
- Coffee — 330 | 1370 | 10 | 22
- Mocha — 345 | 1430 | 11 | 23

Iced Chocolate: *Per 340ml*
- Traditional, with Cream & Ice Cream — 645 | 2695 | 41 | 62
- White, with Mocha Cream & Ice Cream — 745 | 3110 | 43 | 82

Iced Coffee:
- Traditional, w. Mocha Cream
  & Ice Cream, 340ml — 445 | 1855 | 35 | 25
- Iced Latte, 240ml — 80 | 345 | 2.5 | 9
- Iced Mocha with Cream & Ice Cream, 340ml — 585 | 2445 | 37 | 56

Smoothie with Skim Milk: *Per 473ml*
- Banana Mango — 170 | 710 | 0.5 | 35
- Berry — 220 | 925 | 0.5 | 48
- Mango — 195 | 810 | 0.5 | 42

For Full Nutritional Data and Product Updates
~ See Author's Website
www.CalorieKing.com.au

Updated Nutrition Data ~ www.CalorieKing.com.au
Persons with Diabetes ~ See Disclaimer (Page 22)

37

Beverages ~ Coffee Shops

Coffee Shops ~ Brands (Cont) | Cal | kJ | Fat | Cb

Starbucks:
Coffee: *Per Grande, 470ml*

	Cal	kJ	Fat	Cb
Cappuccino: With Whole Milk	135	570	7	11
With Non-Fat Milk	80	345	0.5	12
With Soy Milk	90	385	3.5	8
Caffe Latte/Flat White: *Per Grande, 470ml*				
With Whole Milk	225	935	12	18
With Non-Fat Milk	130	550	0.5	19
With Soy Milk	150	620	5.5	13
Caffe Mocha: *Per Grande, 470ml, With Whipped Cream*				
With Whole Milk	365	1525	19	42
With Non-Fat Milk	290	1205	10	44
With Soy Milk	300	1265	14	38
Frappuccino: *Blended Coffee, With Whipped Cream*				
Caramel, Grande, 470ml	380	1600	15	57
Mocha, Grande, 470ml	380	1580	15	57
Iced Coffee: *Per Grande, 470ml, with Whole Milk Unless Indicated*				
Americano, without milk	15	70	0	3
Caffe Mocha w. Whipped Cream	335	1390	19	38
Latte	150	625	7.5	12
Hot Chocolate: *Per Tall, 355ml, with Whipped Cream*				
With Whole Milk	435	1800	26	45
With Non-Fat Milk	395	1645	21	46
With Soy Milk	400	1680	24	43

Extra Items ~ See CalorieKing.com.au

CALORIE KING TIP!
Reduce the Calories in Your Coffee Drinks:
- Request low-fat milk in place of whole.
- Downsize to a 250ml cup.
- Avoid Iced Coffees/Chocolate/Mocha and Frappuccinos made with whole milk milk and cream.
- Avoid the cream on Mochas.
- Replace sugar with *Equal, Splenda Stevia* or *Sweet 'N Low*.
- Avoid syrup add-ons.

Coffee Shops ~ Brands (Cont) | Cal | kJ | Fat | Cb

The Coffee Club: *Drinks Based on Whole Milk, No Whipped Cream*
Hot Drinks: *Per Large Take-Away Cup*

	Cal	kJ	Fat	Cb
Coffee: Caffe Latte	230	955	13	17
Cappuccino	230	965	13	18
Chai Latte	335	1395	13	40
Flat White	255	1065	15	19
Per Small Take-Away Cup				
Coffee: Affogato	75	315	4	8
Black, Short/Long	0	0	0	0
Cappuccino	140	585	7.5	12
Flat White	140	580	8	10
Hot Mocha	235	980	7.5	34
Latte	140	580	8	10
Liqueur	345	1435	30	10
Melloccino	185	770	7.5	23
Macchiato: Long	15	55	1	1
Short	10	30	0.5	0.5
Muggaccino	170	715	10	13
Piccolo Latte	35	140	2	2.5
Ristretto	0	0	0	0
Vienna with Cream	290	1200	30	3.5
Others:				
Chai Latte: Long	220	925	9	25
Short	195	805	7.5	23
Chai Tea	175	730	10	13
Hot Chocolate	265	1105	8.5	37
White Hot Chocolate	290	1220	11	36
Cold Drinks:				
Iced Chocolate	840	3520	58	65
Iced Coffee	835	3490	58	69
Ice Frappes:				
Latte, small	190	790	6	29
Mango, small	210	875	0	50
Mocha, small	275	1150	6	47
Pine Lime, small	200	840	0	49
Tropicana, large	470	1950	5.5	99
Milkshakes: Caramel	330	1365	11	49
Chocolate	370	1545	12	54
Strawberry	330	1365	11	49
Spider, with Coke	160	670	4	31
Thickshake: Caramel	415	1740	16	59
Chocolate	465	1925	17	64
Strawberry	415	1740	17	59

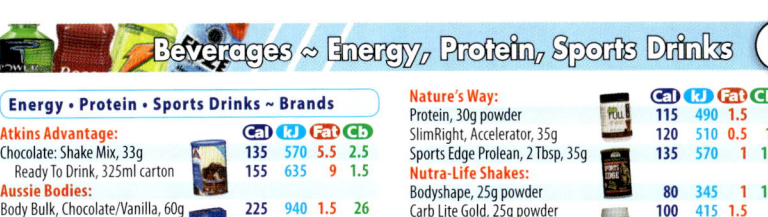

Beverages ~ Energy, Protein, Sports Drinks

Energy • Protein • Sports Drinks ~ Brands

Item	Cal	kJ	Fat	Cb
Atkins Advantage:				
Chocolate: Shake Mix, 33g	135	570	5.5	2.5
Ready To Drink, 325ml carton	155	635	9	1.5
Aussie Bodies:				
Body Bulk, Chocolate/Vanilla, 60g	225	940	1.5	26
Perfect Protein Natural, 40g	155	635	2	3.5
Protein FX, Lo Carb Shake, avg., 30g	110	465	1.5	3
HPLC Protein, Vanilla, 45g	170	710	2.5	4.5
Protein FX, Lo Carb, Choc., 250ml	150	620	3.5	6
Protein Revival: 375ml ctn	275	1150	2	31
Lo Carb, Chocolate	290	1200	7	10
Balance, 100% Whey Protein, 30g	120	500	1.5	0
Be Good To Yourself (Amcal/Guardian):				
Shakes, So Slim, avg. all flavours, 275ml	120	510	1.5	11
Shakes, average, 45g sachet	155	645	2	16
Berocca Performance,				
Twist n Go, 250ml	5	20	0	0
Dextro Energy: Liquid Gel, 60ml	115	485	0	28
Powder, 56g sachet (makes 750ml)	210	880	0	49
Ensure: Liquid, 250ml can	270	1120	6.5	43
Ensure Plus, 237ml can	355	1485	12	50
Powder, 1 scoop, 9g	40	165	1.5	5
G-Force, 650ml bottle	295	1215	0	73
Gatorade:				
G Series: 01 Prime, 118ml	100	420	0	25
02 Perform: Powder, 250ml prep'd	65	260	0	15
Ready to Drink, 600ml bottle	150	620	0	36
Endurance, Blackberry, 600ml	155	650	0	37
03 Recovery, all flavours, 500ml	130	545	0	14
Horleys: Awesome Mass, Van., 75g	295	1230	5.5	35
Body Build, all flav., 2 scoops, 27g	105	425	1	15
Hydralyte Sports, 1 sachet (makes 600ml)	45	190	0	11
Insane Energy, Original, 500ml	230	950	0	56
Lucozade, Lemon/Orange, 300ml	215	895	0	52
Mizone, Sportswater, avg., 750ml	120	490	0	8
Monster Energy:				
Original, 500ml	230	970	0	57
Anti Gravity, Extra Strength, 340ml	150	625	0	37
Mother:				
Original, 500ml can	235	980	0	52
Sugar Free, 500ml can	25	095	0	0.5
Big Shot, 150ml	90	365	0	19
Musashi:				
Bulk, Mass Gain, 500ml	375	1570	4	43
EShot, Raspberry Cola, 300ml	105	435	0	25
P25, Lean Muscle, avg. all flav. 500ml	115	480	0.5	5
P30, Protein Drink, 375ml	250	1040	1.5	28
Protein H2O, avg. all flav., 500ml	140	595	2.5	22
SLM, Protein Milk, avg. all flav., 250ml	165	695	1	19
Nature's Way:				
Protein, 30g powder	115	490	1.5	4
SlimRight, Accelerator, 35g	120	510	0.5	19
Sports Edge Prolean, 2 Tbsp, 35g	135	570	1	1.5
Nutra-Life Shakes:				
Bodyshape, 25g powder	80	345	1	1.5
Carb Lite Gold, 25g powder	100	415	1.5	4
Load Up, average, 20g	75	305	0	17
Nutriway/Amway:				
Positrim, 51g sachet w/ 250ml skim milk	260	1085	2	30
Protein Powder, Berry, 10g	40	170	1	4.5
Powerade Drinks:				
Isotonic: Avg. all flav., 375ml	120	490	0	29
600ml bottle	190	800	0	46
Fuel+, avg. all flavours, 300ml can	105	540	0	25
Sports Drink, Zero, avg all flavours, 600ml	6	35	0	0.5
Red Bull, all flavours:				
250ml bottle	115	480	0	28
330ml bottle	150	635	0	37
473ml can	220	910	0	52
Sugar Free, 250ml	10	35	0	0
Zero	0	0	0	0
Red Eye, 330ml bottle	150	640	0	37
Sanitarium Up & Go:				
Energize, avg. all flav., 350ml	295	1230	5.5	38
Liquid Breakfast, 250ml	200	825	4	31
Vive, avg. all flavours, 250ml	175	735	4	24
Smart Water, 500ml	120	500	0	28
Staminade, 600ml bottle	185	770	0	45
Sustagen:				
Powder, 3 tsp, 15g	60	245	0	11
Tetra Pack, average, 250ml	250	1050	3.5	42
Sport, powder, 60g	225	940	0.5	40
Hospital Formula, powder, 60g	230	955	1.5	39
Swisse:				
Active Recover, Choc., 2 heaped scoops, 45g	160	675	1.5	10
Tony Ferguson:				
Meal Shakes: 53g sachet	205	855	2	29
RTD Shakes, 375ml	215	890	2.5	31
TwoCal HN, 237ml can	475	1985	21	51
'V' Energy Drink:				
Blue, 250ml can	150	620	0	35
Green: 250ml can	120	490	0	27
350ml bottle	165	685	0	37
Sugarfree, 250ml can	10	30	0	9
Berry/Black, 250ml can	115	480	0	26
Isokinetic, 600ml bottle	175	740	0	42
Wicked Energy Drink, 500ml can	475	1975	0	116
XS/Amway, Energy, avg. all flavous, 250ml	10	40	0	0

Weight Loss Meal Replacement Shakes ~ *See Page 50*

Updated Nutrition Data ~ www.CalorieKing.com.au
Persons with Diabetes ~ See Disclaimer (Page 22)

B. Beverages ~ Fruit & Vegetable Juices

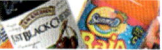

Quick Guide

	Cal	kJ	Fat	Cb
Fruit & Vegetable Juices & Drinks				
Average All Brands:				
Apple Juice, 200ml	80	340	0	20
Appletiser, sparkling, 200ml	90	365	0	21
Blackcurrant Drinks ~ See Page 50				
Carrot Juice, 200ml	80	330	0	11
Coconut Water, (100%), 200ml	35	150	0	9
Cranberry Juice, (100%), 200ml	75	315	0	18
Goji Juice, 30ml	20	85	0	5
Grape Juice, average, 200ml	105	440	0	27
Grapefruit Juice: Sweetened, 200ml	90	385	0	22
Unsweetened, 200ml	55	240	0	12
Lemon Juice: Sweetened/carton, 200ml	85	360	0	20
Unsweetened, fresh, 30ml	10	35	0	1
Lime Juice, unsweetened, 30ml	5	30	0	0.5
Noni Juice, unsweetened, 30ml	5	20	0	1
Orange Juice: Average				
150ml glass (small)	55	225	0	12
250ml cup	90	375	0.5	19
300ml carton/bottle	110	450	0.5	24
500ml carton	180	750	1	40
1 Litre (4 cups)	360	1500	2	80
2 Litres (8 cups)	720	3000	4	160
Pomegranate Juice, 200ml	130	540	1	32
Tomato Juice, average, 150ml	30	120	0	6.5
V8 Vegetable Juice, Reg., 250ml	45	190	0	8.5
Wheat Grass Juice: 1 Shot, 30ml	5	20	0	1
2 Shots, 60ml	10	40	0	2

Juices & Fruit Drinks ~ Brands

	Cal	kJ	Fat	Cb
5+2: *Per 250ml*				
Vegetable Juice:				
Tropical Fusion	90	375	0	22
Vegie Kick	75	300	0.5	18
Ayam:				
Coconut Water, 320ml can	75	310	0	17
Berri: *Per 200ml Unless Indicated*				
Apricot Nectar	145	590	0	34
No Added Sugar: Apple	85	360	0	21
Apple & Pear	90	375	0	21
Orange; Pineapple	85	360	0	19
Tropical	85	360	0	20
Truly: Oranges & Guava Puree	90	370	0	21
Oranges with Pulp	100	430	0	23
Lime/Lemon Squeeze, 2 tsp, 10ml	5	10	0	1
Tomato	50	200	0	11

Brands (Cont)

	Cal	kJ	Fat	Cb
Berri (Cont):				
Australian Grown Juices: *No Added Sugar, Per 200ml*				
Apple	85	360	0	21
Apple & Mango	100	430	0	25
Apple & Passionfruit/Strawberry	110	460	0	26
Apple & Pineapple	85	360	0	21
Breakfast Time	90	370	0	22
Orange; Orange, pulp free	75	320	0	17
UHT/Longlife, DeLuxe, avg. all flavours	90	380	0	21
Super Juice: Clarity	100	425	0	24
Immune	95	395	0	22
Fruit Smoothie: Eyesight, 200ml	80	315	0	16
Guard, 200ml	120	500	0	27
Bickford's: *Per 250ml*				
Applemaid (sparkling)	120	500	0.5	30
Blackcurrant, 250ml diluted	110	460	0	27
Coconut Juice	50	200	0	12
Pomegranate Juice	160	675	0.5	40
Prune Juice	165	695	0	38
Boost Juice: *Per 610 ml*				
Crushes: Berry	280	1185	0.5	70
Lemon	190	790	0.5	43
Tropical	320	1325	0.5	72
Juices: Energiser	255	1080	0.5	58
Two & Five	170	705	0.5	37
Wild Berry	225	955	0.5	56
Low-Fat Smoothies: All Berry Bang	345	1420	7	64
Banana Buzz	460	1925	7	77
Blueberry Blast	440	1835	4	96
King William Chocolate	465	1935	7.5	75
Passion Mango	380	1595	4.5	78
Strawberry Squeeze	400	1650	7	74
Tropical Storm	400	1650	7.5	69
Shooters, fresh Wheatgrass, 1 shot, 30ml	15	60	0	1.5
Skinny Smoothies: Berry Berry Light	220	920	2	48
Mini Me Mango	215	890	2	46
Skinny Minnie Melon	180	745	2	37
Sports Smoothies: Banana Sports	410	1695	3	58
Berry Sports	275	1150	3	40
Chocolate Sports	365	1525	4	48
Mango Sports	345	1440	3	54
Super Smoothies:				
Brekkie To Go Go, Original	630	2625	14	99
Brekkie to Go: Mango; Strawberry, av.	635	2655	14	101
Energy Lift	400	1665	7	71
Green Tea Mango Mantra	415	1740	4	91
Gym Junkie	440	1830	7.5	69

For Complete Nutritional Data ~ See CalorieKing.com.au

Beverages ~ Fruit & Vegetable Juices

Brands (Cont)

	Cal	kJ	Fat	Cb
Biotta, Beetroot Juice, 250ml	110	480	0	25
Brownes (WA),				
Orange C 25%, 200ml	85	355	0	20
Cascade: Ultra-C, 375ml	160	655	1	38
Apple Isle Sparkling, 375ml	155	650	1	41
Cawston Press, average all flavours, 250ml	115	485	1	24
Cocobella, Coconut Water, 250ml	50	215	0	13
CocosNoni, Noni Juice, 30ml	5	20	0	1
Coles: *Per 200ml*				
No Added Sugar: Apple Juice	85	360	0	22
Orange Juice	75	320	0	17
Tomato Juice	50	200	0	9
Tropical	85	360	0	20
Viten	95	400	0	23
Daily Juice: *Per 200ml*				
Breakfast with A, C & E	100	430	0	25
Classic Orange	90	370	0	19
Orange & Mango	95	390	0	22
Orange Passionfruit	80	350	0	18
No Added Sugar:				
Apple	85	360	0	21
Five Fruits	90	370	0	21
Orange, Pulp Free	75	320	0	17
Emma & Tom's: *Per 350ml*				
Carrot Top	145	595	0.5	35
Cloudy Apple	175	725	2	37
Extreme C	155	640	1	33
Go-Fusion	160	670	0.5	40
Green Power	200	840	1	42
Karmarama	190	795	1	42
Radical Action	140	580	0.5	31
Straight OJ	150	615	1.5	27
Eskal: *Per 250ml*				
Pomdelicous:				
100% Pomegranate	140	575	0	35
100% Pomegrante & Blueb. Juice	145	605	0	35
Go Coco, Coconut Water Drink,				
all flavours, 500ml	85	365	0	22
Goji Juice:				
30ml quantity	20	85	0	5
60ml quantity	40	170	0	10
Golden Circle:				
100% Juices: *Per 250ml Cup*				
Apple	125	515	0	29
Orange	110	450	0	23
Tomato	50	210	0	7.5
Fruit Drinks, (35% Juice), avg.	120	510	0	28

Brands (Cont)

	Cal	kJ	Fat	Cb
Golden Circle (Cont):				
Healthy Life: *Per 300ml Bottle*				
Probiotic: Apple Mango	155	645	0.5	36
Breakfast	140	585	0.5	32
Raw: *Per 400ml*				
Berry Burst	175	720	0	40
Citrus Crush	195	800	0	42
Goulburn Valley: *Per 250ml*				
Premium:				
Apple; Apple & Blackcurrant	120	495	0	28
Five Fruits	115	475	0	27
Orange, 200ml	85	355	0	20
Orange & Mango	110	460	0	26
Pineapple	110	465	0	28
Quencher: Lemon, 420ml Bottle	135	565	0	32
Mixed Berry, 420ml Bottle	145	600	0	34
Blood Orange & Passionfruit, 420ml Bottle	140	575	0	33
Grapetiser: *Per 250ml*				
Sparkling Red Grape	130	545	0	32
Appletiser, Sparkling White Grape	120	495	0	28
Grove Juice: *Per 250ml*				
25% Juice Drinks: Orange; Passion	100	415	0	24
Orange Mango; Tropical	105	440	0	25
White Bottle: Mandarin	110	455	0.5	21
Orange	105	435	0.5	24
Premium Juice:				
Apple & Blackcurrant	120	500	0	28
Lemon; Tomato	55	225	0	11
Orange; Orange & Mango	100	420	0	23
H2COCO,				
Coconut Water, average all flav., 330ml pak	80	335	0.5	19
Harvey Fresh (WA): *Per 250ml*				
Fruit Drinks:				
35% Juice, average	100	415	0	25
Lemon Brew	95	400	0	25
Tempt, all flavours	115	475	0	28
Fruit Juices:				
100%: Apple Blackcurrant/Guava	115	475	0	25
Carrot	80	340	0	20
Southwest Orange	95	390	0	21
Tomato	60	250	1	12
Longlife: Apple & Blackcurrant	120	500	0	30
Orange	125	525	0	30
Just Juice:				
Fruit Juices, No Added Sugar: *Per 250ml Carton*				
Apple & Mango	110	450	0	28
Breakfast Juice	105	440	1	25
Orange; Orange & Mango	95	400	1	22
Tomato Juice, 200ml	50	200	0	9

Updated Nutrition Data ~ www.CalorieKing.com.au
Persons with Diabetes ~ See Disclaimer (Page 22)

Beverages ~ Fruit & Vegetable Juices
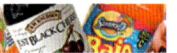

Brands (Cont)

	Cal	kJ	Fat	Cb
Lakewood:				
Cranberry Jce (100%), ½ cup, 125ml	40	170	0	10
Pomegranate w. Blueberry, 200ml	110	460	0	26
LOL, average all flav., 250ml can	120	505	0	29
Macquarie Valley: *Per 375ml Bottle*				
100% Orange Juice	120	505	0	24
Fruit Drinks (35%): Lemon; Orange	140	575	0	33
Orange Mango; Orange Passio	155	640	0	36
No Added Sugar: Apple	175	735	0	43
Orange	130	550	0	29
Pineapple	185	760	0	44
Mildura: *Per 200ml*				
Concentrate, 25%	75	320	0	19
25% Juice:				
Apple & Guava	85	345	0	20
Orange/Orange Mango	85	360	0	21
Orange Passionfruit	80	340	0	20
Pineapple & Coconut	90	375	0	23
Tropical	80	335	0	20
Mountain Fresh:				
Premium Juice: *Per 400ml Bottle*				
Apple; Apple & Cherry	220	920	1	53
Apple & Blackcurrant	235	985	1	54
Apple & Guava; Tropical Cocktail	200	840	1	47
Apple & Mango; Orange & Mango	195	825	1	45
Apple & Pear	215	895	1	50
Apple & Pineapple Crush	210	880	0.5	48
Nekta,				
Liquid Kiwi Fruit, 250ml cup	115	480	0	28
Nippy's:				
Fruit Juices: *Per 500ml*				
Apple/Blackcurrant	265	1100	1	61
Orange/Orange & Mango	240	1000	1	56
Orange & Passionfruit	225	950	1	53
No Added Sugar:				
Apple	265	1100	1	63
Orange	195	825	1	43
Pineapple	250	1050	1	60
Tropical	215	900	1	50
Fruitylicious: *Per 300ml*				
Apple	125	515	1	29
Apple Blackcurrant	150	635	0	34
Orange	110	460	1	25
Tomato	90	365	1	14

Brands (Cont)

	Cal	kJ	Fat	Cb
Nippy's (Cont):				
UHT / Longlife Fruit Juice: *Per 250ml Carton*				
Apple & Blackcurrant	125	525	0	30
Pineapple	105	445	0	22
Unsweetened: Apple; Orange & Mango	120	495	0	29
Orange	100	415	0	22
Nudie:				
Coconut Water: *Per 350ml Bottle*				
Lychee & Lime	90	385	2	21
Pineapple, Orange & Passionfruit	110	455	2	25
Straight Up	75	315	2	18
Crushies: *Per 250ml Bottle*				
Chia Juice	220	920	3	42
Blueberry, Blackberry & More	150	625	1.5	35
Cranberry, Raspberry & More	125	510	0.5	28
Green	180	750	1.5	43
Mango, Passionfruit & More	135	565	0.5	31
Orange, Mango & Pineapple	110	460	0.5	25
Strawberry, Banana & More	140	575	1.5	33
Juicies, Orange, Carrot & Ginger	80	330	2.5	17
Nothing But: *Per 250ml*				
Apple, Cucumber & Kiwifruit	145	605	0.5	34
Beetroot, Pineapple, Mint & More	130	540	0.5	27
Carrot, Apple, Orange & Ginger	110	450	0.5	25
Nothing But 20 Apples,				
Cloudy Apple	115	480	1.5	29
Nothing But 21 Oranges,				
with or without pulp	105	425	1.5	23
Smoothies: *Per 250ml*				
Mango, Banana, Passion Fruit, Yoghurt	160	675	2	34
Ocean Spray: *Per 250ml*				
Cranberry Blackcurrant	135	560	0	34
Cranberry Classic	125	520	0	31
Cranberry Light	20	85	0	5
Raspberry Cranberry	120	505	0	30
Ruby Red Grapefruit	125	525	0	31
Pom Wonderful: *Per 250ml*				
100% Pomegranate	160	670	0	40
Lite, all flavours	85	355	0	21
Preshafruit: *Per 250ml*				
Fruit Juices: Apple & Lemon	110	465	0.5	27
Apple & Pear	125	520	0.5	31
Avg., other flavours	105	440	0.5	27
Prima: *Per 200 ml*				
Apple; Apple Razzberry	85	355	0	21
Average other flavours	90	370	0	22
Raw ~ *See Golden Circle*				

Beverages ~ Fruit & Vegetable Juices

Brands (Cont)	Cal	kJ	Fat	Cb
Ribena Blackcurrant:				
Syrups:				
Regular, 40ml (240ml, diluted)	120	505	0	30
Light, 40ml (240ml, diluted)	20	85	0	4.5
Fruit Drinks (Ready To Drink):				
250ml multipack	105	445	0	26
500ml bottle	210	885	0	51
Squeezepak, 330ml	140	585	0	34
Rosie: *Per 250ml*				
Apple & Cranberry	160	660	0	38
Apple, Raspberry & Cranberry	105	440	0	25
Cranberry Lite	25	95	0	6.5
So Juicy:				
Fruit Juice: Apple, 300ml	150	620	0	36
Orange, 300ml	125	515	0	27
Fruit Drinks (35%): Orange	135	550	0	31
Orange Mango	140	580	0	33
Orange Passionfruit, 300ml	135	550	0.5	31
Spring Valley: *Per 375ml Bottle*				
Crushes:				
Apples & Berries	140	585	0	34
Citrus & Peaches	160	660	0	38
Pineapple & Guavas	155	640	0	36
Tropical & Goji Berries	130	550	0	31
Nectar, Mango & Banana	220	925	0	52
Fruit Juices:				
Apple, 375ml	190	790	0	47
Apple & Blackcurrant, 375ml	185	775	0	45
Orange, 375ml	160	670	0	39
Tomato, 250ml	45	190	0	7
Sunraysia: *Per 250ml*				
Fruit Drinks:				
Blueberry (20% Juice)	140	585	0	33
Cranberry (30% Juice)	195	820	0	48
Fruit Juices (100%):				
Australian Mango	140	575	0	33
Beetroot & Apple	85	360	0.5	19
Prune	150	630	0	37

Brands (Cont)	Cal	kJ	Fat	Cb
Tahitian Gold, Pure Org. Noni Juice, 5ml	5	20	0	1
The Cidery,				
Apple Kiss, 330ml bottle	170	705	0	42
The Switch: *Per 250ml Can*				
Fruit Juices:				
Citrus Weld	150	630	1.5	37
Lemon Rush	200	835	1.5	49
Orange Fusion	130	535	1.5	32
Solar Splash	160	660	1.5	39
Strawberry Melon Crush	155	635	1.5	38
V8: *Per 250ml*				
V8, Original, Vegetable Juice	50	215	0	9.5
V8 Fruit & Veg Juices:				
Apple & Blackcurrant	110	445	0.5	25
Apple, Carrot & Ginger; Tropical	120	495	0	27
Orange Mango Passion	105	440	0	24
Vegetable, Low Sodium	50	215	0.5	9
Low Sodium Vegetable Juice	50	215	0	9
V8, Hot 'n' Spicy; Original	55	230	0	10
V8 Fruit & Veg: Apple Berry Fusion	115	470	0.5	27
Berry Refresh	105	430	0	24
Breakfast	120	490	0	28
Citrus Splash	125	510	0	29
Tropical	120	495	0.5	27
V8 Smoothies: Mango, Peach & Pear	125	520	6.5	29
Pineapple, Passionfruit & Banana	135	550	0.5	31
Strawberry, Raspberry & Banana	130	540	0.5	30
Well Naturally, Antiox Shots,				
Mangosteen & Pomegranate, 900ml bottle	55	225	0.5	12

FRUIT JUICE & DRINKS COMPARISON
Choose fruit drinks wisely. Some are high in added sugar and very low in fruit.

250ml Cartons	Ribena	Orange Fruit Drink	Just Juice
Calories:	105	120	95
Added Sugar:	6 tsp	4 tsp	0
Vitamin C:	20mg	50mg	100mg
Percent Fruit:	6%	35%	100%

Note: 'Fruit juice' must contain 100% fruit, whereas 'fruit drinks' need only contain 5% fruit.

Updated Nutrition Data ~ www.CalorieKing.com.au
Persons with Diabetes ~ See Disclaimer (Page 22)

B. Beverages ~ Milk

MILK ~ Quick Guide

- Cal ~ Calories
- kJ ~ Kilojoules
- Fat ~ Fat
- Cb ~ Carbohydrates

	FULL CREAM 3.6% FAT				**REDUCED FAT** 1.4% FAT				**NON-FAT/SKIM** 0.1% FAT			
	Cal	kJ	Fat	Cb	Cal	kJ	Fat	Cb	Cal	kJ	Fat	Cb
1 Tbsp, 20ml	13	55	0.5	1	10	40	0.5	1	10	40	0	1
100ml Measure	65	270	3.5	5	50	210	1.5	5.5	40	180	0.1	5.5
½ Cup, 125ml	80	340	4.5	7	65	265	2	7	50	220	0.1	7
1 Cup, 250ml	165	680	9	12	125	525	3.5	14	105	440	0.3	14
600ml Carton	390	1630	22	28	300	1260	8.5	33	250	1050	0.7	33
1 Litre (1000ml)	650	2720	36	47	500	2100	14	55	420	1760	1	55

Fresh Milk

Per 250ml Cup

	Cal	kJ	Fat	Cb
Full Cream: Regular (3.6%)	165	680	9	12
Pura (3.6%)	165	680	9	13
Froth Top *(Paul's)*, (3.8%)	185	770	9.5	15
Permeate Free, Original	160	665	8.5	12
Pure Organic (4%)	175	720	10	12
Higher Fat *(Pauls)*,				
Farmhouse (4.9%), 250 ml	190	790	12	12
Reduced-Fat: *Per 250ml Cup*				
A2, Light, (1.3%)	115	475	3.5	13
Anlene *(Fonterra)*, (1.4%)	140	575	3.5	17
Boost *(Pura)*, (1.4%)	130	540	3.5	14
Farmdale, Light *(Aldi)*, (1.5%)	120	500	3.8	13
Farmers Best *(Dairy Farmers)*, (1.4%)	140	575	3.5	16
Farmers Best *(Dairy Farmers)*, (With Omega 3)	155	635	3.5	13
Heart Plus *(Brownes WA)*	135	550	4	15
HI-Lo, (1.4%)	115	475	3.5	13
Lite White, (1.4%)	120	495	3.5	13
Lite *(Riverina Fresh)*, (1.3%)	130	535	4	15
PhysiCAL *(Paul's)*, (1.4%)	130	530	3.5	14
Rev *(Paul's)*, (1.3%)	115	480	3.5	13
Skimmer, (1.5%)	125	525	4	14
Smarter White *(Pauls)*, (2%)	145	595	5	14
Low-Fat: *Per 250ml Cup*				
All Lite *(Bannister Downs)*, (0.8%)	100	415	2	13
Calcium Plus *(Brownes WA)*, (0.8%)	135	565	2	18
Farmdale Light *(Aldi)*	120	500	4	13
Heart Active *(Pura)*, (1%)	105	435	2.5	12
Light Start *(Pura)*, (1%)	110	460	2.5	13
Pure Organic, (1%)	110	455	2.5	13

Fresh Milk (Cont)

Skim/Nonfat: *Per 250ml Cup*

	Cal	kJ	Fat	Cb
Anlene, No-Fat *(Fonterra)*	135	555	0	20
Permeate Free	90	370	0.5	12
PhysiCAL, No-Fat *(Paul's)*	105	440	0	15
Tone, No-Fat *(Pura)*	100	410	0	14
Shape *(Dairy Farmers)*	100	410	0	14
Skinny *(Paul's)*	100	405	0	14

UHT/Longlife Milk

Per 250ml Cup

	Cal	kJ	Fat	Cb
Fullcream *(Devondale)*	160	660	8.5	13
Reduced Fat: Average	135	560	3.5	16
Reduce One *(Devondale)*	130	540	3	16
Skim	90	380	0	14
Smart One *(Devondale)*	125	530	3	16
Smart Plus One *(Devondale)*	135	550	3	17
Low-Fat, Light Start	110	460	2.5	13
Lactose Free: *Per 250ml Cup*				
Liddells: Full Cream	160	665	9	12
Low-Fat	100	440	2.5	12
Zymil: Easy To Digest:				
Full Cream	165	680	9	12
Low Fat	115	475	3.5	13
Skim	90	365	0.5	13

OTHER MILKS & MILK DRINKS
- Condensed/Evaporated ~ Page 46
- Milo/Powdered Milk Drinks ~ Page 46
- Flavoured Milks ~ Page 45
- Soy & Rice Drinks ~ Page 47

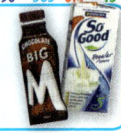

44

Beverages ~ Milk, Flavoured

Milk ~ Brands

	Cal	kJ	Fat	Cb
Big M, Regular, average, 300ml	200	840	5.5	29
Brownes (W.A.):				
Chill: *Per 300ml*				
Banana; Caramel	200	830	5	28
Choc	200	845	4.5	29
Choc Mint	210	880	4.5	31
Coffee/Iced Coffee, average	180	750	4.5	24
Coffee, Extra Strength, 600ml	375	1555	9	50
Light Iced Coffee	130	550	1	18
Fuel, Banana/Berry/Vanilla, 250ml	155	650	3	25
Kick: Cappuccino, 500ml	435	1810	19	49
Double Espresso, 500ml	475	1985	19	49
Mocha, 500ml	460	1920	21	49
Dare: *Per 500ml*				
Iced Coffee: Cappuccino	340	1415	8.5	47
Espresso	425	1780	19	48
Double Espresso	440	1845	19	51
Devondale:				
Moo, Chocolate, 200ml	160	665	7	19
Our Real Chocolate Milk, 250ml	160	665	2.5	25
Our Real Coffee/Strawberry Milk, 250ml	150	615	2.5	23
Farmers Union: *Per 375ml*				
Feel Good Choc; Coffee, average	160	655	2	21
Iced Coffee	255	1075	6.5	37
Light Iced Coffee	180	750	3.5	25
Goulburn Valley: *Per 600ml*				
Iced Coffee	420	1795	11	65
Milk Chocolate	440	1830	11	68
Smooth Banana	445	1855	11	70
Wild Strawberry	455	1915	11	74
Harvey Fresh (WA):				
Chocolate/Cappuccino, 500ml	310	1300	10	24
Extra, average, 600ml	400	1680	11	51
Moolish, 200ml	120	500	4.5	16
Just Natural: Iced Coffee, 500ml	330	1370	8	45
Banana & Honey, 500ml	395	1645	8	58
Malt, Honey & Chocolate, 500ml	390	1640	8	58
Masters (WA):				
Edge, average, 500ml	310	1305	8	38
Iced Coffee, 600ml	360	1510	11	46
Light: Chocolate, 600ml	335	1390	5.5	49
Iced Coffee, 600ml	325	1345	5.5	46
Mocha, 600ml	360	1495	5.5	55
Moove: *Per 600ml*				
Chocolate	420	1760	11	60
Iced Coffee	390	1630	11	53
Strawberry; Vanilla, average	410	1715	11	58
Muscle Milk, 2 scoops, 70g	300	1255	12	16

Brands (Cont)

	Cal	kJ	Fat	Cb
Nippy's: *Per 375ml Carton*				
Banana; Honeycomb	235	985	7.5	31
Ice Coffee	250	1030	8	33
Iced Chocolate	250	1045	7	34
Strawberry	235	970	7.5	30
Vanilla Malt	245	1015	7.5	33
Oak:				
Banana, 600ml	510	2140	22	59
Chocolate, 300ml	270	1130	10	33
Egg Nog, 250 ml	275	1150	14	27
Iced Coffee, 600ml	495	2060	22	55
Strawberry, 600ml	535	2220	21	68
The Max, 600ml	395	1655	11	55
Vanilla Malt, 600ml	540	2265	22	67
Light, Chocolate, 300ml	200	830	4.5	30
Pauls:				
Breaka:				
Chocolate: 300ml bottle	240	990	6	33
500ml carton	395	1645	10	55
600ml carton	475	1975	12	66
Strawberry: 300ml bottle	220	915	6	29
500ml carton	365	1520	10	58
Iced Coffee, 500ml	380	1590	10	53
Chocolate Milk, (UHT, 8-Pack), 160ml	140	575	6	16
Choc Shake, 500ml	475	1990	18	56
Egg Nog, 250ml	190	790	4.5	27
Rush: *Per 500ml Bottle*				
Low Fat: Iced Chocolate	240	1000	4	29
Iced Latte	230	955	3.5	27
Iced Strong Iced Coffee	245	1020	3.5	30
Iced Vanilla Malt	240	995	3.5	30
Sipahh: *Flavouring Straws*				
All flavours: 1 straw	15	60	0	3
With 250ml low-fat milk (1%)	135	560	2.5	16
With 250ml non-fat milk	125	520	0	13
SupaShake: *Per 500ml*				
Choc Honeycomb	405	1690	5	70
Chocolate	400	1680	6	67
Jaffa	405	1685	5.5	69
Vanilla Malt	405	1685	6	68

Shakes, Smoothies

	Cal	kJ	Fat	Cb
Shake (McDonald's), medium, average	380	1590	9	65
Smoothie (McCafe), medium, average	290	1210	1	65
Boost Juice ~ See Page 40				

Updated Nutrition Data ~ www.CalorieKing.com.au
Persons with Diabetes ~ See Disclaimer (Page 22)

Beverages ~ Milk, Powdered, Cocoa

Powdered Milk

	Cal	kJ	Fat	Cb
Full Cream, 4 Tbsp, 30g	150	625	8	12
Skim/Non-Fat, 2 heaped Tbsp, 25g	90	380	0.3	13
Goats Milk (Healtheries), 2 level tablespoons, 15g	75	315	4.5	5

Coffee-Mate (Non-Dairy)

	Cal	kJ	Fat	Cb
Powder: 1 level teaspoon, 4g	20	90	1.5	2.5
1 heaped teaspoon, 6g	35	140	2	3.5
Liquid, all flavours, 1 sachet, 15 ml	40	160	2	5

Condensed & Evaporated Milk

	Cal	kJ	Fat	Cb
Condensed Milk:				
Whole, Full Fat:				
1 Tbsp, 20g	65	275	1.5	11
¼ cup, 63g	210	870	5	35
Skim, Non-Fat:				
1 Tbsp, 20g	55	240	0	12
¼ cup, 63g	180	755	0	38
Evaporated Milk:				
Full Cream:				
1 Tbsp, 20ml	30	130	1.5	2.5
½ cup, 125ml	195	820	11	16
100ml quantity	155	655	8.5	13
Light & Creamy/Reduced-Fat:				
1 Tbsp, 20ml	20	80	0.5	2.5
½ cup, 125ml	120	510	2	16
100ml quantity	95	405	1.5	13

Other Milks

	Cal	kJ	Fat	Cb
Buttermilk:				
Paul's (0.9%), 250ml	120	495	2.5	14
Casa (1.9%), 250ml	110	465	5	10
Coconut Milk ~ See Page 47				
Goat Milk:				
Paul's, 250ml	155	645	10	10
Powder (Healtheries), 20g in 200ml water	100	425	6	7
Human Milk, (4.1% fat), 250ml	180	740	10	17
Lactose Free (Liddells), 250ml	160	665	9	12
Low Fat, 250ml	100	440	2.5	12
Oat Milk (Pureharvest), 250ml	145	605	5	20
Sheep Milk (7% fat), 250ml	270	1130	18	14
Whey Powder, 1 Tbsp, 11g	40	165	0	2
Yakult ~ See Page 176				

Powdered Drinks ~ Brands

	Cal	kJ	Fat	Cb
Cocoa: Unsweetened, 5g	15	60	0.5	1
1 level Tbsp, 8g	25	100	1	2
Malted Milk; Malt Extract,				
Nestlé; Horlicks, 1 heaped tsp, 5g	20	90	0.5	4
Protein/Slimming Shakes ~ See Page 39 & 50				
Akta-Vite,				
3 heaped tsp, 15g	55	225	0.5	12
Alpen Blend (Nestlé),				
3 heaped tsp, 15g	60	245	0.5	13
Cadbury: Drinking Chocolate, 15g	60	250	0.5	14
Bournville Cocoa, 2 tsp. 10g	30	130	1.5	2.5
Dick Smith, OzeChoc, 2 tsp, 15g	60	240	0.5	13
Horlicks, 1 Tbsp, 25g	95	390	1	19
Jarrah: *200ml, Prep'd as Directed*				
Choc o' Lait	45	190	1	7
Chocolatte:				
Choc L'Orange	60	240	1.5	8.5
Frothy Classic	45	190	1	7
Extreme Choc	55	225	1.5	8.5
Mint Madness	70	290	1.5	9
White Delight	60	255	2	8.5
Milo:				
1 heaped tsp, 5g	20	90	0.5	3.5
3 heaped tsp, 15g	65	265	1.5	10
With whole milk, 250ml	270	1130	12	24
With reduced-fat milk, 200ml	185	770	5	24
With skim milk, 200ml	155	650	2	23
Nesquik:				
Chocolate, 3 tsp, 12g	50	200	0.5	11
Other flavours, 3 tsp, 12g	50	200	0	12
Nestle: Cocoa, 20g	70	285	2	5
Dolce Gusto,				
Hot Chocolate, capsule & 210ml water	150	630	5.5	20
Ovaltine: 3 heaped tsp, 15g	60	250	0.5	13
Light Break, 200ml prepared	80	335	1.5	14
Vittoria:				
Chocochino: *Per 3 Heaped Teaspoons*				
Dark	80	320	1	14
Original	80	320	0.5	17
White	90	390	2	19
Weight Watchers,				
Drinking Chocolate, 200ml prepared	35	130	0.5	4.5

Beverages ~ Non-Dairy ◊ Rice ◊ Cereal ◊ Soy

Soy Drinks ~ Brands

	Cal	kJ	Fat	Cb
Per 250ml Cup				
Australia's Own:				
Premium	130	535	7.5	7.5
Malt Free Soy	130	535	7.5	5
Organic Unsweetened	110	450	7.5	5
Bonsoy, 250ml	150	630	6	14
Coles: Original	145	610	5	12
Lite	100	420	2.5	12
Freedom Foods,				
Wholebean Soy, Original	140	585	7.5	12
Macro *(Woolworths):* Organic	185	780	12	13
Light	130	540	4.5	15
Nature's Soy *(Pureharvest):*				
Original	185	765	8	17
Lite	140	580	4	18
Enriched with Calcium	140	585	6	14
Malt Free	110	455	7	3
So Good *(Sanitarium):*				
Regular	155	650	8.5	13
Lite	95	400	2.5	12
Fat Free	85	350	0.5	13
Essential	135	550	4	16
Flavours: So Good Bliss: Vanilla	150	625	4	20
Chocolate	150	625	4	21
So Nice: Regular	155	650	7.5	14
Lite	120	500	3.5	14
Vitasoy: Original, 250ml	165	680	7.5	16
Calci-Plus	160	675	7.5	15
High-Fibre	130	540	3.5	14
Light	50	205	1.5	7.5
Soy Milky: Regular	135	550	7.5	8
Lite	95	400	4	7.5
Chocolate	140	585	4	19
Vanilla	135	560	4	17
Vita Cafe, 240ml	90	385	3.5	7.5
Vitality	110	465	4.5	9
Woolworths, Homebrand, 250ml	180	750	12	13

Condensed/Creamy Soy ~ Brands

	Cal	kJ	Fat	Cb
Carnation, Soy, ½ cup, 125ml	115	470	4	13

Rice Milk Drinks ~ Brands

Dairy-free/Lactose-free: Per 250ml Cup

	Cal	kJ	Fat	Cb
Australia's Own, Original, Organic	165	680	2.5	34
Pureharvest, Aussie Dream	140	585	3.5	26
So Good, Rice Milk	130	535	2	26
Vitasoy: Original	125	525	3	24
Protein Enriched	140	580	3	24

Soy Powder ~ Brands

	Cal	kJ	Fat	Cb
Bonvit, 30g, (makes 200ml)	130	545	6	5
F.G. Roberts, 2 scoops, 29g	115	480	3.5	9.5

Almond & Oat Milk Drinks ~ Brands

	Cal	kJ	Fat	Cb
Australia's Own: Honey Oat Milk, 250ml	145	600	2.5	25
Longlife Milk, Almond, 250ml	90	375	7	7.5
Blue Diamond:				
Almond Breeze: Chocolate, 250ml	120	505	3	22
Original, 250ml	65	265	3	8
Original Unsweetened, 250ml	40	170	3	2
Dairy Farmers,				
Oats Express, all flavours, 250ml	175	735	1.5	30
Devondale,				
Fast Start, all flavours	195	815	2.5	30
So Good, Almond Milk, 250ml	80	325	3	12
Vitasoy, Oat Milk	155	645	5	25

Breakfast Drinks ~ Brands

	Cal	kJ	Fat	Cb
Up & Go *(Sanitarium):*				
Average all flavours, 250ml	200	825	4	30
Energize, all flavours, 350ml	295	1230	5.5	35
Vita Go *(Vitasoy),* avg. 250ml	200	835	5	29
Vive, all flavours, 250ml	180	740	4	26

Coconut Milk ~ Brands

Per ½ Cup, 125ml

	Cal	kJ	Fat	Cb
Ayam: (24.3% Fat)	305	1280	31	5
Light (13.4% Fat)	175	725	17	4
Pandaroo: (12% Fat)	140	590	15	1.5
Lite (5% Fat)	65	265	6.5	0.5
Carnation, Light & Creamy	120	510	2	16
Trident Lite, (5.8% Fat)	110	450	9	6
Woolworths, (25.7% Fat)	305	1275	32	4

Coconut Cream ~ Brands

Top thick layer of liquid expressed from grated coconut

	Cal	kJ	Fat	Cb
Raw/Natural, (35% Fat), ½ cup, 130g	430	1795	45	8.5
Canned: Per ½ Cup, 125ml				
Admiral: Regular, 21% Fat	255	1065	26	3
Lite, 12% fat	150	625	15	2.5
Ayam: Regular, 29.3% Fat	365	1520	37	4
Lite, 16.7% Fat	215	890	21	4
Coles *(Smart Buy)* 15% Fat	190	790	19	3.5
Trident: Regular, 125ml	325	1350	35	2
Lite, 125ml	110	455	11	2
Coconut Water, 1 cup, 250ml	50	200	0.5	12
Coconut Fibre Drinks, 330ml can	130	540	0.5	30

Updated Nutrition Data ~ www.CalorieKing.com.au
Persons with Diabetes ~ See Disclaimer (Page 22)

B. Beverages ~ Soft Drinks ◊ Soda ◊ Mineral Water

Cola Drinks ~ Quick Guide

Cans/Bottles	Cal	kJ	Cb	Sugar Teaspoons
250ml Cup/Can	105	440	27	6
375ml Can	160	670	40	10
600ml Bottle	260	1085	64	15
1 litre Bottle	425	1770	106	25
1.25 litre Bottle	540	2255	133	32
1.5 litre Bottle	635	2655	160	38
2 litre Bottle	860	3540	212	52

Note: 1 level teaspoon sugar weighs 4 grams
Soft Drinks contain no fat.

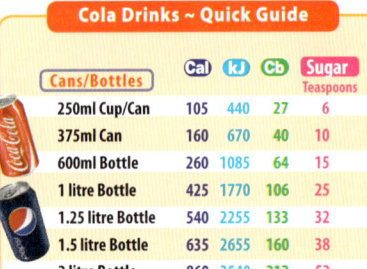

THEATRE CUPS

	Cal	kJ	Cb	Sugar Teaspoons*
Without Ice:				
Small, 420ml	175	730	44	11
Medium Cup, 685ml	285	1190	72	18
Large Cup, 800ml	335	1400	82	20
Extra Large, 1 Litre	425	1770	106	26
With Ice (⅓ Cup):				
Small, 420ml	130	545	30	8
Medium, 685ml	215	900	53	13
Large Cup, 800ml	250	1045	63	15
Extra Large, 1 Litre	310	1300	77	19

*1 level teaspoon sugar = 4 grams

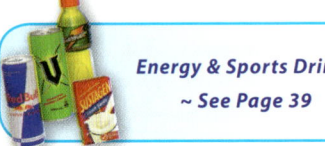

Energy & Sports Drinks ~ See Page 39

Per 375ml Unless Indicated

	Cal	kJ	Fat	Cb
A&W Root Beer, 330ml	160	670	0	40
Angostura, Lem. Lime & Bitters, 330ml	135	570	0	34
Appletiser, 275ml	130	545	0	31
Aqua Pura, Fruit Splash, av, all flav., 600ml	115	480	0	28
Bitter Lemon *(Schweppes)*	200	830	0	49
Bitters/Lemon Soda	200	830	0	49
Bundaberg: Apple Ale, 340ml	170	695	0	41
Blood Orange, 340ml	170	695	0	41
Burgundee, 340ml	155	645	0	37
Ginger Beer: Regular, 340ml	150	630	0	37
Diet, 340ml	30	120	0	6
Guava, 340ml	160	665	0	39
Lemon; Lime Bitters, 340ml	165	685	0	40
Peachee, 340ml	160	665	0	39
Pink Grapefruit, 340ml	155	655	0	39
Sarsparilla: Regular	190	790	0	46
Diet, 340ml	30	115	0	7
Cascade Ultra C, (Sparkling)	160	655	0	39
Chinotto *(Bisleri),* 200ml glass	90	370	0	22
Classic Berry, Clear Cola	150	630	0	40
Club Lemon Squash *(Kirks)*	175	27	0	43
Coca-Cola: 375ml	160	675	0	40
330ml bottle	140	585	0	35
Diet Coke	2	10	0	0
Coca-Cola Zero	1	5	0	0
Cola, avg. all brands, 375ml	150	630	0	40
Coles Mineral/Spring Water: Natural	0	0	0	0
With Juice, 375ml	160	675	0	40
Creaming Soda, avg., 375ml	145	590	0	37
Deep Spring: Lemon, 375ml	145	595	0	34
Lemon/Lime & Orange, 375ml	125	515	0	30
Natural, 375ml	0	0	0	0
Or. Mango/Passionfruit, 375ml	115	490	0	28
Diet Cola (Aust. Choice/K-Mart)	1	5	0	1
Diet Coke, 375ml	2	10	0	0
Dry Ginger Ale *(Schweppes):* Regular	120	505	0	29
Diet/Low Joule	5	20	0	0
Emma & Tom, Well Being Water, all flav., 600ml	60	255	0	15
Esprit: Raspberry, 300ml	130	555	0	33
Other flavours, average, 300ml	140	585	0	35
Mineral/Spring Water, 300ml	0	0	0	0
Fanta, 375ml	175	730	0	43
Ginger Ale, 375ml	145	590	0	37
Ginger Beer: Regular, 375ml	190	805	0	47
Diet Ginger Beer, 375ml	5	15	0	0
Natural, 375ml	0	0	0	0

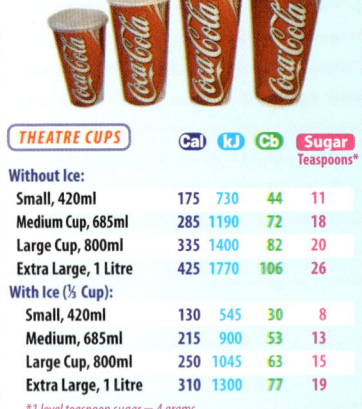

Beverages ~ Soft Drinks ◆ Soda ◆ Mineral Water

Per 375ml Unless Indicated

Item	Cal	kJ	Fat	Cb
Grenada (Schweppes)	160	675	0	40
H2GO, all flavours, 375ml	40	160	0	9.5
Kyneton, 5% Juice, 375ml	140	590	0	35
Kole Beer (Kirks), 375ml	165	680	0	41
La Ice Cola, 300ml	140	590	0	35
Lemonade: Average	150	630	0	39
Light/Diet/Low Joule	5	20	0	0
Lemon Lime Bitters & Soda	165	700	0	39
Lemon Soda Squash	175	735	0	42
Lift: Sparkling Lemon, 375ml	175	735	0	42
Diet	10	30	0	1
Lime & Soda, 375ml	75	310	0	18
LOL ~ See Page 42				
Margaret River (WA):				
Berry Fusion, 330ml	140	590	0	34
Chilli Cola, 330ml	140	590	0	34
Citron Presse, 330ml	140	585	0	35
Triple G (Ginger Beer), 330ml	155	650	0	38
Mineral/Spring Water	0	0	0	0
Mountain Dew, Original, 375ml	180	750	0	47
Energized	175	740	0	46
Nutrient Water, all flavours	75	320	0	19
Orange: Average all brands	190	790	0	49
Low Joule	9	35	0	0
Orange Soda Squash, 375ml	75	310	0	18
Pasito (Kirks), 375ml	175	725	0	42
Passiona (Schweppes), 375ml	170	720	0	41
Pepsi: Regular, 375ml	160	655	0	42
Caffeine Free, 375ml	1	5	0	0
Light, 375ml	1	5	0	0
Pepsi Max, 375ml	5	10	0	0
Pepsi Next, 375ml	105	445	0	28
Perrier: Plain	0	0	0	0
Twist of Lemon/Lime	0	0	0	0
Portello; Pub Squash	150	630	0	42
Red Creaming Soda	160	660	0	39
7-Up (Schweppes), Regular, 375ml	165	685	0	43
Sarsparilla (Schweppes)	175	735	0	43
Schweppes: Agrum, avg., all flav., 300ml	140	575	0	33
Dry Ginger Ale, 250ml	80	340	0	19
Lemonade: Regular, 375ml	175	735	0	42
Sugar Free, 250ml	5	20	0	0
Lemon, Lime & Bitters, 375ml	160	660	0	39
Orangeade, 250ml	80	340	0	20
Mineral Water: Natural	0	0	0	0
Flavoured, average, 375ml	115	470	0	28
Tonic Water, 250ml	95	390	0	22

Per 375ml Unless Indicated

Item	Cal	kJ	Fat	Cb
Saxbys: Orig. Ginger Beer, 375ml	200	835	0	49
Diet Ginger Beer, 375ml	2	10	0	0.5
Soda Stream, reconstituted:				
Classics: Avg., all flav., 250ml	35	140	0	9
Sugar Free, 250ml	1	5	0	0
Sparkling Goodness, avg., all flav	100	405	0	24
Soda Water	0	0	0	0
Solo (Schweppes): 375ml	190	785	0	46
600ml bottle	300	1255	0	74
Low Carb, 375ml	10	40	0	1.5
Lemon Lime, 375ml	175	730	0	43
Sparkling Lemon, 375ml	170	715	0	44
Spring Valley, Smart Water	90	375	0	21
Sprite: Regular, 375ml	160	665	0	38
Zero	5	15	0	0.5
Summit, 375ml	0	0	0	0
Sunkist: 375ml can	200	835	0	49
600ml bottle	320	1335	0	78
Sugar Free, 375ml	5	20	0	0
Spritz, avg. all flavours, 330ml	130	540	0	32
Tarax, Soda, 375ml	15	55	0	32
Tonic Water:				
Average, 375ml	135	565	0	30
Low Joule	5	30	0	0
Torquay, 330ml	120	510	0	30
Tru-Blu:				
Brewer's Choice, Ginger Beer, 300ml	105	440	0	26
Club, Lemon Lime Bitters, 300ml	125	520	0	31
Crush, Orange, 300ml	130	530	0	32
Dry Ginger ale, 300ml	85	360	0	21
Pub Squash: The Original, 300ml	105	445	0	26
Diet, 300ml	20	93	0	5.5
Waterfords: Diet	10	40	0	2.5
Sparkling, average, 375ml	0	0	0	0

Granita, Slurpees

Item	Cal	kJ	Fat	Cb
Granita, 250ml	90	375	0	21
Slurpees (7-Eleven): Small, 250ml	90	375	0	21
Medium, 500ml	180	750	0	42
Slush Puppie, 225ml	85	350	0	21

Energy & Sports Drinks ~ Page 39

Updated Nutrition Data ~ www.CalorieKing.com.au
Persons with Diabetes ~ See Disclaimer (Page 22)

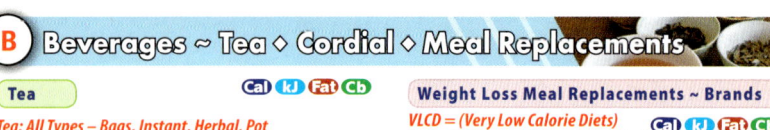

B — Beverages ~ Tea ◊ Cordial ◊ Meal Replacements

Tea

	Cal	kJ	Fat	Cb
Tea: All Types – Bags, Instant, Herbal, Pot				
Black, No sugar, 1 cup	2	10	0	1
White: *Per Cup, Add extra for sugar*				
With Whole Milk, 1½ Tbsp, 30ml	20	90	1.5	2.5
Reduced-Fat Milk, 1½ Tbsp, 30ml	15	70	0.5	2.5
Skim/Nonfat, 1½ Tbsp, 30ml	15	55	0	2.5

Iced Tea • Bubble Tea ~ Brands

	Cal	kJ	Fat	Cb
Tea Bag/Brewed:				
Unsweetened, 1 glass	2	10	0	0
Sweetened, average, 200ml	65	270	0	12
Bubble Tea, average, 375ml	210	865	3.5	45
Bickfords:				
Iced Tea: Lemon; Peach, 250ml	70	300	0	17
Mango, 250ml	80	320	0	19
Lipton: Ice Tea, all flavours, average:				
325ml bottle	90	380	0	22
500ml bottle	140	585	0	34
Light, Green/Peach (Sugar Free):				
500ml	5	20	0	0.5
325ml	0	0	0	0
Virgin Cocktails, all flav., av., 325ml bottle	95	400	0	23
Nestea, average, 250ml	65	270	0	15
Spring Valley, Juicy Tea, 500ml	125	530	0	29
Twinings, all flavours, 200ml	5	10	0	0

Cordials, Ribena, Tang ~ Brands

	Cal	kJ	Fat	Cb
Average All Brands				
Cordials *(Sugar or Fruit-base):*				
Undiluted: 1 Tbsp, 20ml	35	145	0	10
50ml (⅛ cup)	80	335	0	23
Diluted (1:4), 1 cup, 250ml	80	335	0	24
Low Joule Cordials *(diluted 1:4):*				
Bickford's, Diet Lime, 250ml	10	30	0	1.5
Cottees:				
Double Concentrate: (1L Bottle),				
(diluted 1:9, 250ml)	65	265	0	16
No Added Sugar (dil 1:9), 250ml	10	30	0	1.5
Golden Circle Sports, 22ml, (220ml diluted)	60	245	0	15
Flavoured Syrups: *diluted 1:4*				
Bickford's: Mixed Berry, 200ml	75	320	0	19
Blackcurrant, 200ml	90	370	0	22
Ribena: Blackcurrant Syrup				
Original, 33ml (200ml, diluted)	100	420	0	25
Light, 33ml (200ml, diluted)	20	70	0	4
Fruit Drinks (Ready To Drink) ~ *Page 40*				
Tang: Orange Flav'd (made up), 250ml	95	390	0	23
Reduced Sugar (made up), 250ml	35	150	0	9
Ultra-C *(Cascade):* 40ml (200ml dil.)	75	320	0	19
Sparkling, 375ml diluted	160	655	0	38

Weight Loss Meal Replacements ~ Brands

VLCD = (Very Low Calorie Diets)

	Cal	kJ	Fat	Cb
Be Good To Yourself (Amcal/Guardian),				
Shakes, average, 45g sachet	155	645	2	16
Betty Baxter:				
Shakes, 50g sachet	205	850	3	31
Soups, 50g sachet	205	855	5.5	26
Biggest Loser,				
Shakes, 55g sachet	210	870	2.5	25
Blackmores:				
Super Fruit Smoothies,				
avg. all flavours, 45g sachet	165	685	1	18
Body Talk Meal Shakes,				
2 rounded scoops, 50g	210	880	2	35
FindingForm: Shakes, average	210	880	2.5	29
Soups, average, 1 sachet	210	870	3	28
KicStart VLCD:				
Shakes, Average, 55g sachet	205	850	4	17
Soup, Pumpkin & Herb, 55g	205	850	4.5	19
Nutriway/Amway:				
Positrim, Chocolate Drink Mix,				
51g sachet & 250ml skim milk	260	1085	2	30
Optifast:				
VLCD: 54g sachet	210	875	4.5	23
Shakes, 40g sachet	150	635	2.5	16
Soup, Chicken, 48g sachet	175	725	3	17

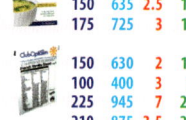

	Cal	kJ	Fat	Cb
OptiSlim VLCD: *Per Sachet*				
Shakes: Chocolate/Vanilla	150	630	2	17
Platinum, Vanilla/Chocolate	100	400	3	8
Soups: Chicken, 55g	225	945	7	20
Pumpkin; Tomato, 55g	210	875	3.5	23
VLCD Bars ~ *See Page 34*				
VLCD Meals ~ *See Page 123*				
Reducta, Meal, 2 heaped T., 40g	135	570	0.5	22
Simply Less *(Coles),*				
Meal Shake, 1 sachet, 56g	50	200	0.5	5
Slimmm, Meal, 55g	215	890	2.5	27
SLM *(Musashi),*				
Meal, 3 scoops, 40g	130	530	1	7
So Slim *(Amcal/Guardian),*				
All Flavours, 275ml	120	510	1.5	11
Tony Ferguson:				
Shakes, 53g sachet	205	855	2	29
Shake Away: 250ml pack				
Chocolate; Espresso	205	850	3	28

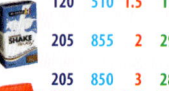

	Cal	kJ	Fat	Cb
Soups, 55g sachet	205	850	3.5	27
Ultra Slim, Powder, 33g	130	530	2.5	21
XS/Amway, Protein Blast,				
all flavours, average, 375ml	205	860	3	17

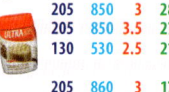

Biscuits ◆ Cookies ◆ Crackers

Biscuits, Cookies, Crackers ~ Brands

Per Biscuit/Cookie Unless Indicated

Always Fresh:

	Cal	kJ	Fat	Cb
Grissini Breadsticks, average, 14g	60	250	2	10
Crackers, wafer, all flavours	40	170	1	7.5

Arnott's, Crackers ~ *See Next Page*

Arnott's ~ Sweet Biscuits:

	Cal	kJ	Fat	Cb
Arno Shortbread	60	255	3	8
Butternut Snaps, Reg.	55	235	2.5	8
Choc Ripple	40	165	1.5	6.5
Chocolate: Big Tedz, Chocolate	90	370	3.5	13
Butternut Snaps	80	335	4	11
Caramel Crowns	75	320	3.5	11
Chip, Premier	75	305	3.5	10
Mint Slice	80	335	5	9
Monte	60	260	3	9
Royals Dark/Milk, average	70	295	2.5	11
Teddy Bear	80	335	3.5	11
Wagon Wheels,				
Snack Pack, Orig., 24g pk	105	435	4	16
Wheaten, average	60	255	3	7.5
Chocolate Tee Vee Snacks: Orig.	25	105	1	3.5
Malt Sticks, average	15	55	0.5	2
Wafer Bites	40	160	2	4.5
Creamy Chocolate	75	310	3	11
Custard Cream	75	305	3	10
Delta Cream	75	305	3	10
Farmbake: Butter Shortbread	65	265	3	9
Chocolate Chip/Fudge	60	245	2.5	9
Crunchy Oat & Fruit	60	245	2.5	8
Peanut Brownie	65	260	3	8
Full 'O' Fruit	40	160	0.5	7.5
Fun Sticks, all flavours, 18g	85	355	3.5	13
Ginger Nut	50	210	1	9
Granita	55	220	2.5	7
Honey Jumbles	40	170	0.5	8
Hundreds & Thousands	35	145	0.5	6.5
Iced Vo Vo	55	225	1.5	9.5
Kingston	65	280	3.5	8
Lattice	50	215	2.5	5.5
Lemon Crisp	70	285	3.5	8.5
Malt 'O' Milk	30	135	1	5.5
Marie	35	150	1	6
Milk Arrowroot: Regular	35	145	1	6
Mini Packet, 1 pkt, 25g	105	440	2.5	18
Milk Coffee	35	155	1	6.5

Per Biscuit/Cookie Unless Indicated

Arnott's (Cont):

	Cal	kJ	Fat	Cb
Mint Slice, Choc	80	335	5	9
Monte Carlo	105	430	5	14
Nice	55	225	1.5	9.5
Orange Slice	70	300	3	11
Raspberry Shortcake	70	290	3	11
Raspberry Tartlet	55	230	2	8.5
Rice Cookies	35	155	2	4
Scalliwag	45	185	1.5	7.5
Tiny Teddy: Choc/Chip	10	35	0.3	1.5
25g packet	115	485	3.5	18
Choc Coated	15	55	0.5	2
25g packet	115	490	4.5	17
Honey, 25g	115	475	3.5	18
Scotch Finger: Original	90	365	4	12
Chocolate-Coated	115	475	5.5	15
Shortbread Cream	85	355	4	11
Shredded Wheatmeal	30	135	1	5
Snack Right: Fruit Pillows	65	260	1	12
Fruit Slices, Sultana, 10g	35	150	0.5	7.5
Sultana Choc: 1 piece, 13g	50	210	1	9
1 strip, 5 pieces, 65g	250	1050	6	45
Spicy Fruit Roll	60	260	1	12
Sport (Coles), Snack Pack, 23g	105	430	3.5	17
Teddy Bear: Plain	45	195	1.5	8
Chocolate	80	335	3.5	11
Tic Toc	40	165	1.5	6.5
Tim Tam:				
Original (1), 18.3g	95	395	5	12
1 packet, 11 Tim Tams	1050	4390	55	130
Snack Pack, 17g	95	395	5	12
Black Forest: (1),	95	400	4.5	13
1 packet, 175g	875	3640	41	117
Chewy Caramel (1)	100	405	5	13
Dark Chocolate, Mint (1)	95	395	5	12
Double Coat (1)	115	485	6	14
Fingers (2), 40g	210	870	11	25
Rum & Raisin (1)	100	405	5	13
Other varieties, average	95	400	5	13
Tina Wafer	45	180	2	5.5
Tiny Teddy, Big Tedz	90	370	3	13
Triple Wafer, all flavours	40	155	2	8
Venetian	65	270	3.5	8
Wagon Wheels:				
Regular, average	210	865	8	32
Mini, average	110	455	4	17
Double Choc, Large, 48g	220	905	9	32
Yo Yo	40	170	1.5	6.5

Updated Nutrition Data ~ www.CalorieKing.com.au
Persons with Diabetes ~ See Disclaimer (Page 22)

Biscuits ◆ Cookies ◆ Crackers

Per Biscuit/Cookie Unless Indicated	Cal	kJ	Fat	Cb
Arnott's ~ Crackers:				
Breton	20	90	1	2.5
Cheds	40	165	2	4
Counter Cracker	10	45	0.5	2
Country Cheese	20	90	1	3
Jatz: Original; Cracked Pepper	20	80	1	2.5
Clix	15	65	0.5	2
Salada: *Per Biscuit, 4 squares*				
Original	60	250	1.5	10
Light	55	230	0.5	11
Multigrain	55	230	0.5	11
Wholemeal	55	230	1	9
Sao	40	165	1.5	5.5
Savoy: Original	20	90	1	4
97% Fat-Free	20	75	0	3.5
Sesame Wheat	30	125	1.5	4
Shapes: Biscuits, average all varieties,				
1 biscuit	10	45	0.5	1
10 biscuits, 20g	110	455	5	12
Roadies: 15 Crackers	110	465	3.5	17
200g Box	980	4095	32	150
Thin Captain	25	100	0.5	4
Vita-Weat:				
9 Grains/Sesame (1), avg.	50	205	1.5	8
Lunch Slices (1), avg. 19g	80	325	2	11
Original/Cracked Pepper (1)	15	60	0.5	2.5
Rice (1)	10	50	0.5	2
Soy & Linseed (1)	45	190	1	6.5
Water Crackers, (1), avg. all varieties	15	55	0.2	2.5
Artisse:				
Crackers:				
Grissini: Classic, 9.2g	40	160	1	6
Sesame, 13.3g	70	290	3	9
Aunty Kath's:				
Choc, Chip, 25g portion	105	440	4.5	16
M&M's, 25g portion	105	440	4.5	16
Australia's Choice (Kmart):				
Decadent Choc Chip Cookie, 16g	80	340	4	11
Belmont (Aldi):				
Mini Cookies, Triple Choc Chip,				
1 snack pack, 30g	145	605	6	20
Blue Cow,				
Crispbreads (5), 7g	30	120	0.5	6
Cadbury:				
Fingers: Chocolate/Honeycomb, 5.3g	25	105	1	3
Mini, Milk Choc./Honeycomb, 2.8g	15	55	0.5	1.5
Freddo, Choc/Vanilla, 11g	55	225	3	7
Carr's:				
Table Water Crackers, all flavours	15	60	0.5	3

Per Biscuit/Cookie Unless Indicated	Cal	kJ	Fat	Cb
Coles:				
Biscuits: Anzac	80	330	4	9
Butternut Creams	75	315	3	9.5
Caramel Deluxe	80	335	4	11
Gingernut, 12g	50	210	1.5	9
Honeycomb/Candy Whirlz, average	85	360	4.5	11
Milk Arrowroot	40	160	1	6.5
Milk Coffee, 9g	40	170	1	6
Raspberry Tartletts	55	220	1	10
Chocolate Biscuits: Chocolate Chip	80	340	3.5	11
Choc Chip	80	325	4	10
Choc. Butternut Snaps	120	500	6.5	14
Chocolate Koalas	75	315	3	10
Chocolate Digestives	115	480	5.5	15
Chocolate Nobles	90	370	3.5	14
Chocolate Fingers	95	390	4	13
Chocolate Sensation	90	400	5	10
Chocolate Surrenders	100	4202	5	13
Mini Toffee Jaffas, 4 pieces, 22g	105	440	5	14
Crackers: Seed 'N' Wheat (2)	65	270	3	8.5
Skipton (2)	80	330	2.5	12
Vitabites (5), average	150	630	3.5	25
Watercrackers (4)	55	235	1	10
Rice Crackers, 10 pieces, average, 25g	100	420	0	21
Coles Smart Buy:				
Milk Arrowroot	35	150	1	6.5
Scotch Finger	85	360	3.5	13
Crackers: Family Cracker (2)	80	335	2.5	13
Water Crackers (4)	65	270	2.5	9
Dick Smith,				
Water Crackers (1)	10	50	0.2	2
Freedom Foods:				
Blissful Berry	70	295	3	10
Chocolate Blitz	100	405	3.5	13
Cranberry Crave	90	375	3	14
Crunchy Coconut	70	280	3	9
Sultana Splitz	95	400	3	16
Triple Treat Brownie	75	305	4	9
Griffin's:				
Chocolate Macaroon	85	350	4	11
Choc Thins	40	160	1.5	5
Gingernuts	55	230	1	11
Mallow Puffs	90	370	3.5	14
Guides Australia:				
Original Cookie	40	170	1.5	7
Chocolate Cookie	60	255	2.5	9

Biscuits ◆ Cookies ◆ Crackers B

Per Biscuit/Cookie Unless Indicated	Cal	kJ	Fat	Cb
Gullon (Aldi),				
Maria, Sugar Free (1), 6g	30	110	1	3.5
Harvest Kitchen,				
Soft Centres, avg all flavours	80	325	3.5	10
Holland House:				
Almond Fingers	185	770	6.5	29
Almond Rounds; Delight	195	815	7.5	29
Peanut Round Biscuits	65	270	3.5	7.5
Speculaas; Spiced Cookies	60	250	2.5	9
ITAL:				
Almond Toscani	40	160	1	5.5
Biscotti Di Frutta	15	70	0.5	3
Lingue Di Gatto	45	180	2.5	5
Kez's				
Free: Almond Bread, 5g	20	80	0.5	3.5
Almond Toffee, 22g	120	490	7	10
Chocolate Chip, 1 pkt, 20g	95	395	4	14
Melting Moments, 32g	150	630	6	24
Indulgence: Almond Bread, 5g	20	90	0.5	3.5
Florentine, 31g	130	545	4.5	19
Melting Moments, 32g	165	690	8.5	22
Viennese Eclairs, 32g	155	640	7.5	19
Jumbo: Chocolate Chip, 80g	390	1625	19	49
Indulgence, Chocolate Bites, 5g	25	105	1	3
Monster Choc, 80g	405	1685	19	52
Moorish Muesli Munch, 60g	295	1235	16	36
Kurrajong Kitchen ~ Lavosh:				
Lavosh Bites, Original, 8 bites 21g	90	385	2.5	15
Lavosh Thins, Caramelized On. & Sea Salt	45	180	1	7

	Cal	kJ	Fat	Cb
Leda:				
Choc Chip, 10g	50	205	3	6
Choculence, 20g	100	410	5.5	12
Gingernut, 10g	40	175	1.5	7
Minton, 17.5g	90	385	5.5	10
McVites:				
Digestive: Dark/Milk Choc.	80	335	4	10
Original	70	300	3.5	9.5
Light	65	275	2.5	11
Wholemeal	70	280	3	8.5
Hob Nobs: Milk Chocolate	90	385	4.5	12
Original	70	285	3	10
Nabisco:				
Chips Ahoy: Origin, 10.5g	55	220	2.5	6.5
Chunky, 17g	90	380	6	8.5
Captains Table, average,	15	55	0.3	2
In A Biskit, average all varieties:				
1 biscuit	10	50	0.5	1.5
10 Biscuits, 25g	115	490	5	15
½ Box, 90g	425	1770	18	56
1 Box, 175g	825	3450	35	110
Crackers: Original (4), 29g	135	555	4.5	20
98% Fat-Free (4), 26g	100	420	0.5	21
High Fibre (4), 27g	100	410	0.5	18
Wholemeal (4), 29g	125	530	4	18
Oreo:				
Average all flavours,				
2 cookies, 21g	100	420	4.5	14
150g pack	730	3045	32	101
Mini Oreo, 115g Cup	540	2260	23	75
Wafer Sticks (1), 18g	95	385	5	12
Orgran:				
Biscotti, Amaretti/Choc Classic	35	155	2	5
Itsy Bitsy Bears, 17g	70	295	2.5	12
Outback Animals: Choc, 17g	70	290	2	12
Vanilla, 17g	70	300	2.5	12
Mini, 22g	90	370	2.5	15
Shortbread Hearts	45	190	2.5	6
Wild Raspberry	70	290	3	10
Paradise:				
Addictions	80	330	3.5	10
Cream Assorted	90	365	4.5	11
Family Assorted	50	200	2	7
Highland Oatmeal	40	170	1.5	6.5

Don't be fooled by *'Baked Not Fried'* or *'Oven Baked'* on the packs of savoury snack biscuits.

They still have up to 25% fat – similar to fried potato crisps!

Biscuits ◆ Cookies ◆ Crackers

Per Biscuit/Cookie/Cracker Unless Indicated

Paradise (Cont):	Cal	kJ	Fat	Cb
Cottage: Choc. Chip Indulgence (2)	100	425	4.5	14
Heavenly Chocolate Hazelnut (2)	100	420	4.5	13
More-ish Macadamia (2)	110	455	6	13
Triple Chocolate Temptation (2)	105	430	4.5	14
Minis: Choc Chip, 30g	145	610	6.5	20
Triple Chocolate, 30g	145	605	6	20
Fancies, Strawberry Mallows	65	260	2	11
Kidz: Choc Pinkie Fingers (6)	125	520	5.5	17
Uglies (8)	120	505	5	17
Plain Sweet: Malt (2)	75	310	2	12
B'Scotch/Rich Shortbread (2)	90	380	4	12
Rich Tea (2)	75	320	2.5	12
Veri Deli: *Per 10 Biscuits*				
Crackers: Cheddar & Chives	90	370	3	13
Fig & Mixed Grain	140	585	3.5	23
Italian Roast Tomato	95	385	3.5	12
Original, with Sea Salt	185	780	7.5	25
Sesame & Poppyseed	185	770	8.5	22
Soy & Linseed	180	755	7.5	23
Wholewheat	160	675	6.5	20
Vive Lites: All varieties	45	185	1	8
Vive Minis, Lites, avg., 30g	125	520	2.5	24
Ritz:				
Regular: 2 crackers, 7g	35	150	2	4.5
6 crackers, 20g	100	425	5	13
Reduced Fat, (50% less fat) (6), 18g	80	335	2.5	13
Sticks, 15 sticks, 25g	115	485	4.5	18
Stern's,				
Pfeffernusse Gingerbread, (1)	45	185	1	9
SuniBrite:				
Chocolate Chip, 70g	345	1450	17	44
Big One, Choc. Chip/Chunka, 100g	480	2000	22	65
Tucker's Natural:				
MultiFibre, all flavours,				
¼ of 100g packet, 25g	100	405	3	12
Vita-Weat ~ *See Arnott's, Page 55*				
Walker's:				
Shortbread: Rounds	90	380	5	10
Finger	85	350	5	9
Oatcakes, average	60	240	3	7
Triangles	80	330	4.5	9

Per Biscuit/Cookie/Cracker Unless Indicated

Weight Watchers:	Cal	kJ	Fat	Cb
Choc Chip	35	140	1	5.5
Raspberry Tartlets	40	155	1	7
Fruit Slice: 2 pieces	80	335	0.5	17
1 row (9 pieces), 90g	315	1310	2	65
White Wings:				
Chunkies: Choc Chunk (1)	70	285	3	9.5
Creamies, average all flavours	135	560	7.5	16
Splits, avg., all flavours, 21g	105	440	5	13
Triple Choc Chunk (1)	70	285	3	9
White Choc & Macadamia (1)	70	295	3.5	9
Minis, average, 25g	120	500	5	17
Drizzles (1), average	85	360	4	11
Woolworths:				
Homebrand: Choc Chip	90	385	4	13
Choc Mint Slice	95	390	5	10
Choc Monty	65	265	3.5	7
Choc Scotch Finger	105	435	4.5	14
Gingernut (1)	55	215	1.5	9
Milk Arrowroot	40	160	1	6.5
Scotch Finger	90	365	4	12
Tiny Bears: Chocolate (5)	50	200	2	7.5
Honey (5)	45	195	1.5	7
Triple Choc, 20g	100	420	5	14
Wafers: Chocolate Creme	30	125	1.5	4
Strawberry/Vanilla Creme	30	130	1.5	4
Macro: Choc Coated	85	345	4	12
Choc Chip Double	60	240	2.5	7.5
Choc Coated Orange	80	325	3	12
Double Choc	105	440	6	12
Golden Choc Filled	90	380	5.5	10
Gluten Free: Mini Choc, snack pack, 25g	115	480	4	17
Orange & Poppyseed, Choc Coated, 17g	80	330	3	12
Select:				
Choc Chunk; Chocolate Macadamia	65	265	3	9
Chocolate Finger	35	145	1.5	5
Chocolate Sandwich	90	375	4	13
Double Chocolate; Stem Ginger, average	65	260	3	8.5
Fruit & Nut	105	440	5	14
Honeycomb Crunch	85	360	4	12
Mint Creme	90	375	5	12
Orange Creams	70	300	2.5	11
Toffee Caramel	80	335	4	12

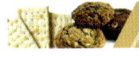

Crispbreads ◆ Ricecakes ◆ Crumpets B

Crispbreads ~ Brands | Cal | kJ | Fat | Cb

Per Crispbread

Item	Cal	kJ	Fat	Cb
Coles, Simply Less (1)	30	130	0	6
Cruskits *(Arnott's):* Original	25	115	1	4
Light	20	90	0	4
Rye	20	85	0	4
Damora *(Aldi):*				
Crispetts (1), 7g	30	115	0.5	5.5
Prista: Hi Fibre (1), 6.8g	25	105	0.5	4.5
Lite (1), 6.3g	25	100	0	5
Wholemeal Crispbread (1), 6.8g	30	125	1	4
VitaGrain Crackers (1), avg., 7g	30	120	1	4
Falwasser, all varieties (1)	20	85	0.5	4
Finn Crisp: Original (2)	40	170	0.2	8.5
Multigrain; Garlic (2)	45	180	0.5	8
Kurrajong Kitchen, Lavosh (2)	60	255	1.5	10
Kavli: Crispy Thin	15	65	0.5	3
Golden Rye	30	135	0.5	6
Hearty Thick	35	140	0.5	6.5
Melba Toast	20	80	0	4
Orgran: Crispbread, average	25	95	0	4.5
Essential Fibre, 12.5g	35	150	0.5	7
Toasted Corn	20	90	0.5	4.5
Ryvita:				
Multi-Grain, (2)	80	330	1	13
Fruit & Seed with Honey (2)	120	495	2	21
Pumpkin Seeds & Oats (2)	95	395	2	14
Rye Original (2)	70	290	0.5	13
Sesame Rye (2)	80	320	2	11
Sunflower Seeds & Oats (2)	90	385	2.5	13
Crackerbread, Original (1)	20	90	0.2	6
Simply Less *(Coles),* Crispbread (1) 14g	65	265	0.5	11
Vita-Weat *(Arnott's):* Original (1)	25	95	0.5	4
9 Grains (1)	20	90	0.5	3.5
Grain Snacks (17), 20g	85	355	2.5	13
Sandwich Size, each	50	205	1	8
WASA: Light	20	85	0.5	4
Original	35	145	0.5	7.5
Weight Watchers,				
Original (1)	25	105	0	5
Wheatsworth, 2 biscuits	65	270	2	9

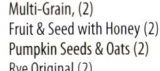
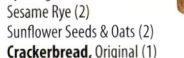
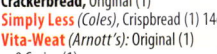
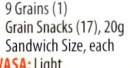
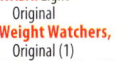
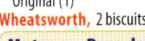
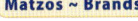

Matzos ~ Brands

Item	Cal	kJ	Fat	Cb
Solomon's: White/Wholemeal, Regular Size (17.5cm), average 1 Matzo, 34g	135	570	0.5	28
Afternoon Tea Matzos, 1 Matzo, (10cm), 13g	50	220	0	11
Matzo Meal: Coarse, 1 cup, 90g	330	1380	1	69
Flour, superfine, 1 cup, 150g	560	2340	2	120

Updated Nutrition Data ~ www.CalorieKing.com.au
Persons with Diabetes ~ See Disclaimer (Page 22)

Rice/Corncakes ~ Brands | Cal | kJ | Fat | Cb

Per Serving

Item	Cal	kJ	Fat	Cb
Damora *(Aldi),* Thin Rice/Corn (1)	20	90	0	4
Pure Harvest, average, 1 cake, 11g	45	180	0.5	9
Real Foods: Corn Thins (1), 6g	20	95	0.2	4
Rice Thins (1), 6g	25	100	0	5
SunRice: Rice & Corn (1), 6g	25	95	0.2	4.5
Rice Cakes: Thin, average (1), 6g	25	100	0.2	4.5
Thick	40	160	0.3	8
Flavoured: Savoury, avg., (1)	30	125	0.5	5.5
Sweet, avg., (1)	35	150	0.5	7.5

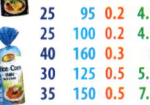

Rice Crackers ~ Brands

Average All Brands: Round, 45mm diameter

Item	Cal	kJ	Fat	Cb
2 crackers, 4g	15	65	0	3
5 crackers, 10g	40	170	0.5	8
12-14 crackers, 25g	100	420	1	20
1 packet, 100g	400	1670	4	80
Coles, avg., 14 pieces, 25g	100	420	0	21
Fantastic: Avg., 13 pcs, 25g	90	380	0	20
Bursts, avg., all flavours, 12 crackers, 23g	100	405	2.5	18
Crisp'ns, avg., all flavours, 1 pkt, 25g	110	455	2	21
Delites, ¼ pkt, 25g	105	430	3	18
Sakata, avg., 13 pcs, 25g	100	425	1.5	20
Trident, avg., 14 pcs, 25g	105	435	1	22
Vita-Weat, avg., 10 pcs, 25g	115	490	3	19

Crumpets, Muffins (English) ~ Brands

Item	Cal	kJ	Fat	Cb
Crumpets: Average All Brands (1), 50g	85	345	0.5	16
with 3 tsp butter/margarine	190	795	13	16
Bakers Life *(Aldi):*				
Crumpets (1), 50g	90	375	0.5	17
Muffins: 97% fat free (1), 67g	160	665	2	27
Fruit (1), 67g	170	705	1.5	31
Golden: Round; Wholemeal (1), 50g	95	390	0.5	19
Breaks (1), 71g	120	490	0.5	23
Finger (1), 34g	55	235	0.5	11
Mighty Soft: Rounds (1)	100	410	0.5	19
Splits (1), 69g	150	615	1	29
Muffins: *English Style*				
IGA, English (1)	150	625	1.5	27
Mighty Soft: English (1)	165	695	2	30
Fruit 'n' Spice (1)	175	735	2.5	32
Tip Top: Multigrain (1)	150	625	2.5	23
English (1)	170	710	2	28
Spicy Fruit (1)	180	745	2	30
Wonder White, Hi Fibre (1)	140	590	1.5	24
Cake Muffins ~ *See Page 66-69*				

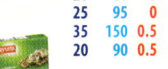
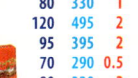
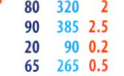
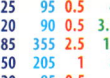
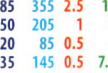
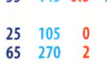

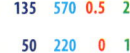
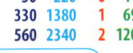
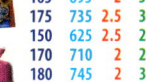

55

Bread & Bread Products

Breads ~ Quick Guide

	Cal	kJ	Fat	Cb
Average All Brands				
White Bread: *Per Slice*				
Plain: Thin slice, 30g	75	305	1	14
Toasting slice, 35g	85	355	1	17
Thick slice: 40g	95	405	1	19
Double thick (home-made), 60g	140	580	2	29
Toast: Same cal/kJ/fat as bread used.				
Thin slice + 1 tsp fat	100	420	5	14
Thick slice, 35g: With 2 tsp fat (10g)	160	670	9	17
With 1 Tbsp fat (20g)	230	960	17	17
Wholemeal: Brown/Mixed Grain/Soy				
Average all types, thin slice, 30g	70	300	1	13
Toasting slice, 40g	90	375	1	17
Thick slice, 45g	105	445	1.5	20
Double thick, 70g	165	695	2	30
Rye: Light, 1 slice, 30g	75	315	1	14
Dark, 1 thin slice, 30g	70	295	1	13
1 medium slice, 45g	105	440	1	19
Soy & Linseed, thick slice, 40g	90	375	1.5	14

Notes: All breads have similar cal/kJ/fat on a weight for weight basis. However, volume may vary. For example, 30g of bread may equal 1 slice of normal bread or 2 slices of a lighter bread. It is best to weigh bread used and calculate on 30g = 65 cal, 270 kJ, 1g fat.

Brands ~ See Pages 58-59

Breads

	Cal	kJ	Fat	Cb
Baguette:				
2 slices, 30g	80	330	0.5	16
1 whole (25cm), 300g	790	3300	3	159
Challah, 55g slice	180	760	5	29
Chapati, average, 45g	110	460	2	19
Puris (deep-fried Chapati), 50g	190	800	13	19
Ciabatta, 1 slice, 20g	50	210	0.5	9
Corn Bread, 1 slice, 65g	180	750	7	28
Damper, 30g piece	80	335	2	13
Dumpling, 100g	165	680	6.5	25
Focaccia: Plain, 50g piece	120	510	2	22
With Olives, 50g piece	120	490	2.5	19
French Stick, 2 slices, 30g	80	345	1	16
Fruit Loaf: Light, 1 slice, 30g	80	330	1	17
Heavy, 1 slice, 45g	120	500	1.5	23
Garlic Bread, avg., 1 slice with 8g fat	100	420	8.5	11
Supermarket brands, average:				
1 stick (8 slices), with butter, 185g	580	2420	23	79
Slice: Middle slices (1)	85	355	7	13
End Slice (has less butter)	65	270	5.5	9

Breads (Cont)

	Cal	kJ	Fat	Cb
Gluten-Free, white, 35g slice	80	340	1.5	14
Lavash, 50g	145	610	2	27
Lebanese Flatbread:				
Med. (24cm diam.), 75g	205	860	2	39
Large, 100g	275	1145	3	51
Lupin Loaf, 20g	45	180	1	5
Melba Toast, 5 pieces	20	80	0	4
Mountain Bread, 25g slice	70	300	0.5	14
Naan Bread: 50g piece	135	565	3	24
Mission, (1), 70g	225	930	5	36
Patak, 115g	320	1335	6.5	55
Panini, small, 100g	250	1050	2	40
Pappadums, (Patak), 6" average, 10g	25	115	0	4.5
Pita: White, 50g	140	585	1	29
Wholemeal, 75g	190	790	1	35
Poppadum *(Chang's),* fried, 3g	15	65	0.5	2
Puppodums *(Sharwoods),* 15g	45	185	0	7
Pumpernickel, small, 25g slice	45	195	0.5	9.5
Raisin Bread, 1 slice, 30g	80	330	1	17
Rice Bread ~ same as regular bread				
Roti *(New Deli),* 1 slice, 45g	160	665	4	22
Sorj Bread, 1 sheet, 70g	195	810	1	38
Sourdough/Soy Bread, 30g	65	270	1	15
Sweet & Sour/Latvian, 30g	65	270	1	15
Tortilla: Small, 25g	80	335	2	13
Large, 45g	150	620	3.5	24
Jumbo, 75g	250	1040	5.5	40
Turkish/Mediterranean: 50g piece	135	565	2	25
½ Large Loaf, 390g	860	3600	6.5	195
1 Large Piece, (11x19cm),150g	330	1380	2.5	75
Pide, 1 roll, 180g	445	1860	2	85

Breadcrumbs, Sticks, Croutons

Per Serving

	Cal	kJ	Fat	Cb
Breadcrumbs, ¼ cup, 30g	110	450	1	20
Breadsticks:				
Plain, 1 stick, average, 7g	30	125	1	4
Grissini *(Always Fresh),* 1 stick, 7g	30	125	1	4
Sesame, 1 large stick	55	230	2	4.5
Cornflake Crumbs, ½ cup, 30g	115	475	0	18
Croutons:				
Plain: ¼ cup, 10g	40	165	0.5	7
1 cup, 40g	150	625	1	28
Seasoned, Caesar *(Cardini's),* 25g	95	390	2	15
Pretzels, (10), thin, 10g	40	170	0.5	8

Bread & Bread Products

Bread Rolls & Buns | Cal | kJ | Fat | Cb

Baker's Delight /Brumby's ~ *See Next Page*

	Cal	kJ	Fat	Cb
Bread Rolls, White:				
Medium (6"/15cm), 75g	190	800	2	38
Large (8½"/22cm), 110g	280	1170	3	56
Brioche, 1 only	180	760	10	27
Ciabatta Roll, medium, 150g	340	1430	3.5	66
Cheese & Bacon Roll, 90g	265	1100	10	32
Damper Roll, 75g	190	800	2	36
Dinner Rolls: Small, 30g	70	290	1	17
Large, 45g	105	430	1.5	25
Easter Buns, average, 56g	150	625	2.5	30
Focaccia Roll, 120g	330	1380	3	52
Frankfurter Roll, 75g	210	875	3	37
French Rolls:				
Small, 40g	110	460	1	21
Large, 85g	240	1005	2	45
Fruit Bun, 60g	145	605	2	28
Hamburger Buns:				
Medium, 65g	180	760	3	32
Large (Tip Top), 87g	235	985	3	43
Hot Cross Buns ~ *See Page 65*				
Hotdog Rolls:				
Medium (6"/15cm), 50g	140	585	2.5	25
Large (Tip Top), (9"/23cm), 75g	195	820	2	36
Kamut, 83g	195	820	3.5	31
Knot Rolls:				
Small, 60g	155	655	1	31
Large, 90g	235	985	1.5	46
Lupin, 65g	140	575	2.5	17
Pide ~ *See Turkish*				
Rye, 1 roll, 113g	250	1040	3	38
Sourdough Bun, 55g	150	625	1.5	29
Spelt: White, 1 roll, 98g	285	1195	5	43
Wholemeal: 1 roll, 90g	185	780	1.5	35
Large, 170g	430	1800	6	67
Submarine Roll, (6"/15cm), 135g	320	1340	3	73
Turkish: White, 85g roll	210	880	2	210
150g roll	370	1550	4	68
Whole-Grain Buns:				
Small/Dinner, 30g	75	320	1	12
Medium, 65g	165	690	2.5	26
Large, 100g	255	1060	3.5	40

Updated Nutrition Data ~ www.CalorieKing.com.au
Persons with Diabetes ~ See Disclaimer (Page 22)

Bagels | Cal | kJ | Fat | Cb

	Cal	kJ	Fat	Cb
Bagels: *Average All Brands*				
Small/Bagelette, 30g	80	325	0.5	15
Medium, 55g	145	600	1	28
Large, 85g	220	925	1.5	43
Bagel Chips/Crisps, 30g	120	500	3.5	19

Croissants ~ Brands

	Cal	kJ	Fat	Cb
Croissants (Plain): *Average all Brands*				
Medium, 50g	200	820	12	25
Large, 70g	280	1150	17	35
Golden: 53g	200	840	9.5	24
Mini, 17g	65	270	3	8
Coles: Fresh, 75g	305	1265	13	37
Frozen, 50g	185	775	8.5	23
Sara Lee, 50g	185	760	8.5	22
Woolworths, 50g	220	920	14	19

Bread Mixes ~ Brands

	Cal	kJ	Fat	Cb
Basco: *Per 35g Slice*				
Gluten-Free	95	385	1.5	19
Defiance:				
Easy Bake: *Per Slicep*				
White, 50g	120	505	1	24
Crusty White, 50g	120	495	1	23
Hi-Fibre Grain, 50g	120	500	1	22
Laucke: *Per Slice*				
Barossa Sourdough Rye, 85g	195	815	1.5	36
Multigrain, 75g	185	770	2.5	33
White, Crusty, 80g	195	805	1	38
Orgran: *Per 27g Dry*				
Bread Mix: Easy Bake	95	385	0.5	21
Wholemeal Alternative Grain	90	380	0.5	21
Simply Wize,				
Crusty, Gluten Free, 50g slice	80	335	2	19
Tip Top Kitchen Collection: *Per 50g Slice*				
Grain Bread	130	545	2.5	20
White Bread	120	495	2	22
Wholemeal	115	480	1.5	19

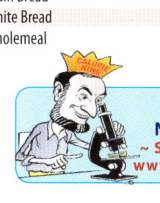

For Full Nutritional Data
~ See Author's Website
www.CalorieKing.com.au

Bread

Bread ~ Brands

	Cal	kJ	Fat	Cb
Abbott's Village Bakery: *Per Slice*				
Country Grains	120	500	1.5	20
Farmhouse Wholemeal	100	425	1	18
Light Rye	95	390	0.5	17
Rustic White	100	430	1	20
Bakers Delight: *Per Slice, Unless Indicated*				
Baguette, 100g	265	1110	1.5	52
Breadstick: Pane di Casa, slice, 29g	75	315	0.5	14
White, slice, 14g	40	170	0.5	7.5
Cape Seed: Thin slice, 33g	100	410	4.5	14
Thick slice, 45g	135	565	6.5	13
Chia:				
Block: White 40g	100	420	1.5	18
Wholemeal, 39g	95	385	1.5	14
Roll: White 70g	185	780	3	31
Wholemeal, 65g	165	695	3	25
Continental: Baguette, 62g	160	670	0.5	31
Dark Rye, 28g	75	315	0.5	13
French Cob, 28g	75	310	0.5	15
Italian, 36g	95	390	0.5	19
Light Rye Vienna 22.5g	60	240	0.5	10
Country Grain, Vienna, 38g	105	430	1.5	19
Damper, Traditional, piece, 63g	190	780	4.5	32
Hi-Fibre Lo-GI, White Block, 2 sl., 79g	170	720	1	30
Linseed & Soy, 48g	130	545	5	13
Pullapart:				
Cheese, Spinach & Feta, 65g	185	775	5.5	26
Cheese & Sundried Tomato, 78g	225	945	6.5	32
Rye, 41g	105	430	1	18
Sourdough, White Vienna, 33g	80	320	0.5	15
Traditional Fruit, 30g	95	400	1.5	18
Turkish, average, 88g	285	1190	10	40
White, Block, 2 slices, 62g	160	670	1.5	30
Wholemeal: Block/Cob, 31g	75	305	1	12
Croissants/Cakes/Pastries/Sweetbuns ~ *See Page 66*				
Savoury Items ~ *See Page 185*				
Bakers Life (Aldi): *Per Slice*				
Bakehouse: Light Rye, 38g	100	415	1	18
Mixed Grain, 47.5g	120	485	2	19
Soy & Linseed, 47.5g	125	510	3	16
Wholemeal, 42g	100	405	1	16
Grainwise, Orig. with 9 grains/seeds, 37g	90	370	1	14
Multigrain, Sandwich, 1 slice, 34g	90	370	1	16
Raisin Toast, 1 slice, 35g	90	380	1	16
Turkish, average, 50g piece	120	500	1	22
Viva Active: White, 37g	80	335	1	14
Wholemeal, 37g	95	390	1	16
White: Sandwich, 1 slice, 34g	90	370	0.5	17
Toast, 1 slice, 39g	100	425	1	20
Wholemeal, sandwich, 1 slice, 34g	85	360	1	14
Be Light (Aldi):				
German Dark Bread: *Per Slice*				
Four Grains/Rye, avg., 63g	120	505	1	22
With Sunflower Seeds, 63g	125	525	2.5	20
Bodhi's Bakehouse (WA):				
Bread: *Per Slice*				
Barley, Honey & Oats	100	420	2.5	11
Chia + More	110	450	2	12
Chia Linseed, 39g	95	400	2.5	14
Dinkelbrot, 32g	80	335	1.5	13
Gluten & Yeast Free, 39g	85	360	1	18
Low Carbo Flatbrot, 1 pita, 88g	195	820	2.5	30
Organic Rye, 49g	105	445	1	16
Vollkornbrot with Green Tea, 38g	90	380	1.5	11
White Spelt, 28g	80	340	1.5	12
Wupper, Soft with Lupin	95	395	2	10
Wupper: Flatbrot Pitta, 100g	220	920	2.5	34
Fruit, 40g	95	395	1	16
Rye Light, 40g	90	370	0.5	14
Bovell's (WA): *Per Slice*				
Soft Wholemeal, Toast, 40g	90	385	1	16
Soy 'n' Linseed with Folate, 35g	95	385	2.5	13
Soft White Sandwich, 33g	80	330	0.5	15
Brumby's:				
White Breads: *Includes All White Loaves*				
1 thin slice, 30g	70	290	0.5	14
1 thick slice, 40g	90	375	1	17
Other Breads: *Per 31g Slice*				
12-Cereal	70	295	1	11
Aegean Apricot Loaf	75	315	0	16
Banana Bread	65	270	1	13
Bavarian Rye	65	270	1	11
Fruit & Walnut Rye	80	345	2.5	12
Wholemeal Vienna	65	270	1	11
Swiss Fig & Date	75	315	1	13
Wholemeal Grain, Mini, 21g	55	230	1	8
Rolls: *Per Roll*				
12-Cereal, Round, 70g	160	660	2.5	25
Omega Wholemeal, 75g	165	695	2.5	27
Cakes/Pastries ~ *Page 69*				
Savouries ~ *Page 187*				
Burgen: *Per Slice*				
Antioxidant, Fruit & Muesli, 42g	110	460	2.5	17
Digestive, Rye, 42g	100	425	2	16
Energy, Pumpkin Seeds, 42g	110	460	3	14
Gluten Free, White, 43	105	445	2	19
Heart, Wholegrain & Oats, 42g	95	400	2	14
Weight, Wholemeal & Seeds, 42g	100	425	1.5	13
Women's, Soy-Lin, 42g	100	420	2	13

Bread

Country Life: Per Slice	Cal	kJ	Fat	Cb
Country Grain Organic Rye, 33g	80	335	1	11
Gluten Free: Multigrain, 39g	95	400	2	17
Low GI White, 39g	95	405	3	15
Fruit, 39g	105	425	3	16
White, 35g	80	340	1.5	16
Gluten & Yeast Free, White, 44g	100	425	2	19
Heartwise Mixed Grain & Oat, 36g	80	345	1	14
Organic Rye, 45g	105	430	1	15

Healthybake: Per Slice	Cal	kJ	Fat	Cb
Organic: Barley, 43g	115	480	2.5	16
Gluten Free, 40g	95	395	1.5	18
Honey & Oat Sourdough, 43g	110	455	2.5	15
Rye, Fruit, Nut & Seed, 46g	160	670	8	16
Rye & Carraway, 43g	115	475	2.5	16
Spelt, 32g	90	385	1.5	14
Spelt Fruit, 42g	115	485	2	18
Vintage Sourdough Cob, 43g	115	485	2	19

Helga's: Per Slice	Cal	kJ	Fat	Cb
Golden Linseed & Barley, 38g slice	105	440	2	18
Light Rye, 34g slice	85	350	1	15
Mixed Grain, 43g slice	105	440	2	19
Pumpkin Five Seed, 40g slice	110	460	2	17
Soy & Linseed, 43g	115	475	2	16
Spelt & Sunflower Seed, 34g slice	95	390	1.5	16
Wholemeal Grain, 42g	105	435	1.5	19
Wholegrain Quinoa and Flaxseed, 39g	100	420	2	15
Sandwich Thins: Mixed Grain/Soy & Lins.	120	495	1.5	22
Traditional Wholemeal, 43g	115	475	1	20
Traditional: White, 42g	105	435	1	19
Wholemeal, 42g	95	400	1	17
Wraps, Mixed Grain, White, (1), 70g	205	860	4	35

Mighty Soft: Per Slice	Cal	kJ	Fat	Cb
Multigrain, 30g	75	310	0.5	13
White, 30g	75	320	0.5	14
White Thick, 36g	90	380	0.5	18
Wholemeal, 30g	70	295	0.5	12
Cafe Style: Extra Thick Fruit, 75g	190	790	1.5	35
Raisin Toast, 35g	95	390	1	17

Molenberg Swiss Bake: Per 2 Slices	Cal	kJ	Fat	Cb
Chia	180	760	2	32
Original	190	795	2	33
Original Toast	210	880	2	37
Soy & Linseed	200	840	4	31

New Norcia (WA): Per 45g Slice, Unless Indicated	Cal	kJ	Fat	Cb
Casalinga Sourdough	115	480	0.5	24
Dark/Light Rye/Wholemeal	110	455	0.5	21
Fig and Fennel/Olive	110	450	0.5	21
Raisin and Walnut	130	545	4	20
Multigrain Fruit, 68g	205	850	4	35
Seven Grain Sourdough	135	560	1.5	25
Sourdough Fruit, 68g	175	740	0.5	37

Tip Top/Sunblest: Per Slice	Cal	kJ	Fat	Cb
Raisin Toast, 33g	100	410	1	19
Spicy Fruit Loaf, 36g	100	420	1	19
9 Grain: 9 Seeds, 37g	100	405	2	14
Original, 37g	95	385	2	13
Pumpkin Seeds, 37g	95	405	2.5	13
Wholemeal, 40g	100	410	2.5	12
Cafe: Raisin, 65g	235	980	3	43
Scone Toast, Classic Buttermilk, 70g	170	700	2	28
Gold Split: White, 24g	65	280	1	11
Sunblest: Multigrain: Sandwich, 30g	80	330	1	14
Thick, 34g	90	375	1	16
White, Sandwich, 30g	75	305	1	14
Thick, 35g	85	350	1	16
Wholemeal: Sandwich, 30g	75	310	1	12
Thick, 34g	85	355	1	14
The One: Sandwich, 37g	90	360	1	14
Toast, 39g	95	380	1	16
UP: Omega 3: White, 37g	100	415	1	18
Smooth Oats, 37g	95	400	2	14
White & 25% Wholegrain, 39g	95	400	1	17
White Lower GI, 37g	95	385	1	17
Wholemeal, 37g	100	405	1.5	16
UP Wraps: Per 45g Wrap				
High Fibre + Calcium	130	545	3	20
High Fibre + Oats with Iron	135	555	3	21
High Fibre + Omega 3	135	565	3.5	22

Wonder: Per Slice	Cal	kJ	Fat	Cb
+ Vitamins & Minerals: Sandwich, 35g	80	335	0.5	15
Slice, 52g	145	610	3	25
Toast, 39g	90	375	1	17
Hi Fibre Plus: White Sandwich, 35g	95	390	1	17
Toast, 39g	90	370	1	16
Wholemeal, 35g	80	340	1	14
Smooth Wholemeal + Iron, Sandwich, 35g	85	340	1	13
Wraps, High Fibre Plus, (1), 52g	145	595	2.5	24

Updated Nutrition Data ~ www.CalorieKing.com.au
Persons with Diabetes ~ See Disclaimer (Page 22)

B. Breakfast Cereals

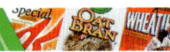

Note: Figures listed here may vary from package data since cup or weight measures on cereal packs are only approximate. People with specific dietary needs should weigh their own serving.

Breakfast Cereals ~ Brands

Brand / Product	Cal	kJ	Fat	Cb
Abundant Earth:				
Organic: Muesli, Bircher, 50g	165	700	3.5	27
Puffed Corn, 1 cup, 30g	115	480	1	24
Puffed Kamut, 1 cup, 30g	95	395	0	21
Puffed Rice, 1 cup, 30g	115	485	1	25
Alpen:				
Muesli: Original, ½ cup, 45g	170	720	2.5	30
No Added Sugar, ½ cup, 45g	170	710	3	29
Back To Nature:				
Bite'z, Cookie, 30g	110	470	0	25
Farmers Choice:				
Apple, Cranb. & Cinn Clusters, 34g	115	480	1.5	20
French Vanilla & Almond Clusters, 34g	90	385	3.5	12
Basco, Gluten Free, avg, 40g	140	585	0.5	30
Be Light *(Aldi)*				
Special Flakes:				
Forest Berries, 30g	110	465	0.5	23
Natural, 30g	115	470	0.5	24
Be Natural: *Per ¾ Cup*				
5 Whole Grain Flakes, 45g	165	690	0.5	34
Apple & Flame Raisin, 45g	170	710	2	32
Cashew, Alm., Hazelnut & Coconut, 45g	195	815	7	26
3 Grain Porridge:				
Honey, ⅓ cup, 35g	140	570	3	23
Original, ⅓ cup, 35g	140	570	3	21
Pink Lady Apple, Raisin & Coconut, 35g	140	570	2.5	23
Brookfarm:				
Muesli:				
Natural Macadamia with Cranberries, 50g	210	870	3.5	37
Gluten Free Macadamia:				
With Apricots & Apples, 35g	160	650	7	17
With Cranberries, 35g	155	640	7	17
Toasted Macadamia:				
With Apricots, 50g	225	935	8.5	31
With Cranberries, 50g	220	925	8	32
Carman's:				
Berries & Flakes, Light, 35g	120	505	1	23
Clusters: Cranberry & Apple, 45g	195	815	6	29
Honey Roasted Nut, 45g	205	850	7.5	27
Muesli: *Per ½ Cup*				
Classic Fruit, 45g	205	850	9	23
Deluxe Fruit, 35g	155	640	6.5	20
Natural Bircher, 45g	190	800	8	24
Original Fruit-Free, 45g	220	910	11	23
Oats,				
Traditional Australian, 45g	170	710	4	26
Carman's (Cont):				
Porridge: Honey Roasted Nut, 50g	200	845	6	30
Fruit & Seed, 50g	215	900	5	31
Coles:				
Bran Flakes with Sultanas, 45g	155	645	0.5	30
Cocoa Puffs, 1 cup, 30g	120	495	0.5	26
Corn Flakes, 1 cup, 30g	110	460	0	23
Honey Crunch, w/ Almonds, 30g	125	510	2	24
Mighty Grain, 30g	115	485	0.5	22
Oat Bran, 1 Tbsp, 10g	40	160	1	6.5
Organic Oats: Instant, 30g	120	500	3	19
Apricot & Grains, 40g	155	650	3	28
Rice Puffs, 30g	115	475	0.5	26
Right Start, ¾ cup, 45g	160	660	1	32
Simply Less, M'grain Flakes, 1 cup, 40g	155	640	2	30
Special Flakes, 30g	110	470	0.5	24
Whole Wheat Biscuits, 2 biscuits, 30g	115	480	0.5	20
Muesli:				
Apricot, Date & Almond, 50g	190	780	5	26
Natural: Summer Fruits, 50g	190	785	4.5	28
Low-Fat, 50g	170	710	1.5	31
Original, Toasted, 50g	210	885	7.5	28
Dick Smith:				
Bush Foods, Breakfast, 30g	110	460	1	22
Food for Health:				
Muesli: Fibre Cleanse, 50g	210	860	10	22
Fruit Free Clusters w. Chia, 50g	220	900	9	27
Gluten Free, 45g	135	565	3	23
Liver Cleansing, 50g	220	910	12	22
Freedom Foods:				
Ancient Grain Flakes, 1 cup, 50g	190	785	1	40
Berry Good Morning, 1 cup, 45g	165	690	1.5	34
FreeOats, all varieties, av., 66g	275	1150	7.5	44
Muesli, Gluten Free, 40g	165	680	7	20
Pro-Teen Crunch, 1 cup 45g	170	700	1	32
Rice Flakes w. Psyllium, 50g	190	795	1	42
Rice Puffs, 1 cup, 35g	130	540	0.5	29
Tropico's, 1 cup, 35g	130	545	1	29
Freelicious:				
Gluten Free: Corn Flakes, 30g	120	485	0	26
Grainfull Flakes, 30g	120	490	1	25
Gaby's:				
Muesli: Original, 50g	240	985	11	25
No Added Sugar, 50g	230	960	10	28

Breakfast Cereals

	Cal	kJ	Fat	Cb
Goldenvale (Aldi):				
Balanced Right, 45g	170	695	1	34
Bran & Sultanas, 30g	110	465	0.5	24
Breakfast Bubbles, 30g	110	465	0.5	24
Choco Balls/Chips, avg., 30g	120	490	1	23
Choco Rice, 30g	115	480	0.5	26
Cornflakes, 30g	115	480	0.5	25
Cornflakes, Honey Nut, 30g	120	495	1	25
Fruity Flakes: Fruit & Fibre, 40g	145	605	1	28
Tropical Fruits, 40g	145	605	1	29
Wild Berry, 40g	150	610	1	30
Healthy Start: Fruit 'n Nut, 45g	185	775	7	24
Summer Burst, 45g	180	755	4	31
Honey Wheats, 30g	120	490	0.5	25
Just Bran, 45g	140	585	2	16
Oats Sensations, avg., 40g Sachet	150	640	2	27
Power Grain, 30g	120	485	0.5	22
Wheat Biscuits (2), 31g	115	470	0.5	21
Wholegrain Hoops, 30g	110	465	1	22
Minute Oats, dry, 40g	155	650	4	24
Muesli: Apricot & Almond, 40g	160	670	5	22
Continental Natural, 50g	220	910	10	25
Mountain, 50g	235	975	11	25
Swiss Toasted, 50g	200	830	5	31
Muesli Clusters: Fruity, 40g	170	710	5.5	25
Maple & Pecan, 40g	180	750	7	24
Goodness Superfoods:				
Barley & Oats 1st:				
Original, sachet, 35g	125	523	3	16
Traditional, ½ cup, 40g	140	590	3	18
Digestive 1st, 45g	160	675	3	21
Fibre Boost 1st Sprinkles, 15g	50	210	1	6.5
Heart 1st, 45g	180	735	5	20
Protein 1st, 45g	170	700	4	17
Healtheries:				
Bircher Muesli:				
Apple & Berry, ½ Cup, 78g	280	1165	6	41
Deluxe, Apple Cinnamon & Almond, 65g	270	1115	12	26
Just Organic (Aldi):				
Toasted Muesli, 50g	195	820	4.5	32
Toasted Muesli Clusters, 50g	215	890	7	32

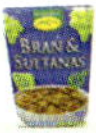

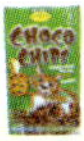

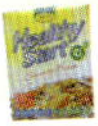

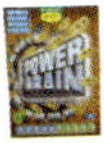

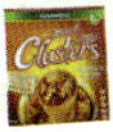

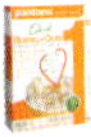

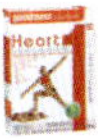

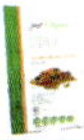

	Cal	kJ	Fat	Cb
Kellogg's:				
All-Bran: Original, ¾ cup, 52g	170	710	1.5	24
Apple Flav. Crunch, ¾ c., 45g	165	680	1.5	29
Dual ¾ cup, 40g	140	585	0.5	26
Fibre Toppers, ½ cup, 25g	75	310	0.5	10
Tropical, ½ cup, 45g	155	640	2	25
Wheat Flakes. Orig., ¾ c., 45g	155	645	1	26
Coco Pops: ¾ cup, 34g	130	545	0	30
1 cup, 45g	175	725	0	40
Chex, 1 cup, 30g	115	470	0	25
Corn Flakes: 1 cup, 30g	115	475	0	25
Crunchy Nut, 1 cup, 45g	180	750	1.5	37
Crispix, Honey, 1 cup, 30g	115	490	0	27
Crunchy Nut Clusters,				
1 cup, 45g	165	690	3	31
Froot Loops, ¾ cup, 30g	120	490	0.5	26
Frosties, 1 cup, 40g	155	645	0	36
Guardian, 1 cup, 60g	205	865	0.5	38
Just Right:				
Barley & Berry, ¾ cup, 45g	160	670	1	32
Clusters & 5 Grains, ¾ c., 45g	170	710	1	35
Original, ¾ cup, 45g	160	670	1	32
Komplete, Oven-Baked Muesli:				
½ cup, 45g	175	730	3	32
1 cup, 90g	350	1460	6	64
Mini-Wheats:				
5 Grains, 1 cup, 60g	215	905	1	41
Blackcurrant, 1 cup, 60g	215	895	1	43
Mixed Berry, 1 cup, 60g	210	870	1	40
Nutri-Grain: ¾ cup, 30g	115	480	0	21
1 cup, 40g	155	640	0	28
1½ cups, 60g	230	960	0.5	42
Rice Bubbles, 1 cup, 30g	115	480	0	26
Special K: Advantage, 1 c., 40g	140	590	0	26
Fruit & Nut Medley, ¾ cup, 40g	155	650	2.5	26
Original: ¾ cup, 30g	115	470	0	21
1 cup, 40g	150	625	0	28
Forest Berries: ¾ cup, 30g	115	470	0.5	21
1 cup, 40g	150	630	0.5	28
Honey Almond: ⅔ cup, 30g	120	500	1	24
1 cup, 45g	180	750	1.5	32
Sultana Bran: 1 cup, 48g	165	680	1	30
Extra, ⅔ cup, 45g	155	655	0.5	33
Buds, 1 cup, 45g	155	645	0	30
Sustain: ¾ cup, 45g	170	705	1.5	34
1 cup, 60g	225	940	2	45

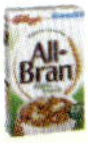

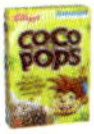

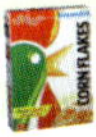

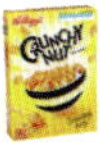

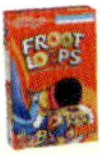

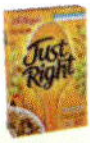

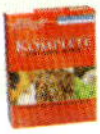

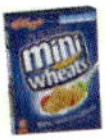

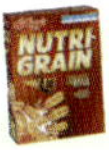

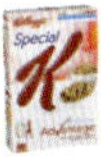

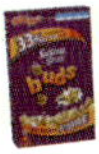

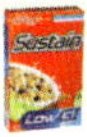

Updated Nutrition Data ~ www.CalorieKing.com.au
Persons with Diabetes ~ See Disclaimer (Page 22)

B. Breakfast Cereals

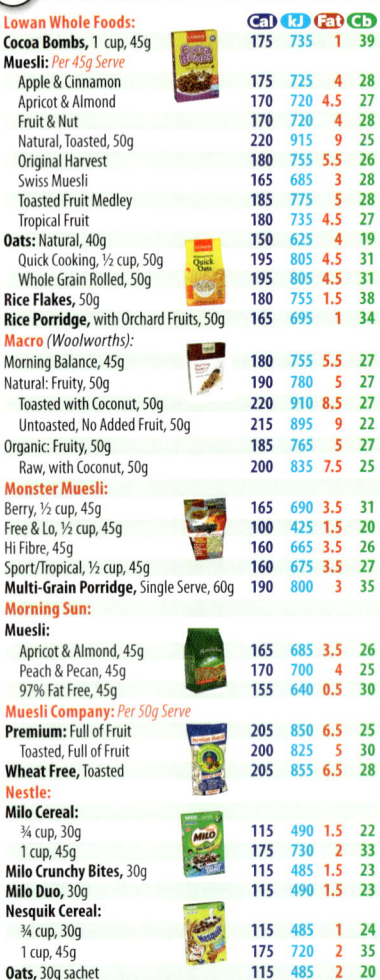

	Cal	kJ	Fat	Cb
Lowan Whole Foods:				
Cocoa Bombs, 1 cup, 45g	175	735	1	39
Muesli: *Per 45g Serve*				
Apple & Cinnamon	175	725	4	28
Apricot & Almond	170	720	4.5	27
Fruit & Nut	170	720	4	28
Natural, Toasted, 50g	220	915	9	25
Original Harvest	180	755	5.5	26
Swiss Muesli	165	685	3	28
Toasted Fruit Medley	185	775	5	28
Tropical Fruit	180	735	4.5	27
Oats: Natural, 40g	150	625	4	19
Quick Cooking, ½ cup, 50g	195	805	4.5	31
Whole Grain Rolled, 50g	195	805	4.5	31
Rice Flakes, 50g	180	755	1.5	38
Rice Porridge, with Orchard Fruits, 50g	165	695	1	34
Macro *(Woolworths):*				
Morning Balance, 45g	180	755	5.5	27
Natural: Fruity, 50g	190	780	5	27
Toasted with Coconut, 50g	220	910	8.5	27
Untoasted, No Added Fruit, 50g	215	895	9	22
Organic: Fruity, 50g	185	765	5	27
Raw, with Coconut, 50g	200	835	7.5	25
Monster Muesli:				
Berry, ½ cup, 45g	165	690	3.5	31
Free & Lo, ½ cup, 45g	100	425	1.5	20
Hi Fibre, 45g	160	665	3.5	26
Sport/Tropical, ½ cup, 45g	160	675	3.5	27
Multi-Grain Porridge, Single Serve, 60g	190	800	3	35
Morning Sun:				
Muesli:				
Apricot & Almond, 45g	165	685	3.5	26
Peach & Pecan, 45g	170	700	4	25
97% Fat Free, 45g	155	640	0.5	30
Muesli Company: *Per 50g Serve*				
Premium: Full of Fruit	205	850	6.5	25
Toasted, Full of Fruit	200	825	5	30
Wheat Free, Toasted	205	855	6.5	28
Nestle:				
Milo Cereal:				
¾ cup, 30g	115	490	1.5	22
1 cup, 45g	175	730	2	33
Milo Crunchy Bites, 30g	115	485	1.5	23
Milo Duo, 30g	115	490	1.5	23
Nesquik Cereal:				
¾ cup, 30g	115	485	1	24
1 cup, 45g	175	720	2	35
Oats, 30g sachet	115	485	2	20
Norganic:				
Ancient Grains, 45g	145	615	1	34
Corn Flakes, 1 cup, 30g	115	470	0.5	24
Nu-Vit:				
Muesli: Natural, 40g	150	635	4.5	23
Fruity, Low-Fat & Gluten Free, 40g	140	595	1	30
Orgran:				
Cocoa O's, ¾ cup, 30g	100	410	0.5	21
Rice O's, ¾ cup, 30g	95	395	1	19
Super Grains:				
100% Amaranth, puffed, 30g	120	500	1.5	22
Multigrain O's (w. Quinoa), 1 cup, 30g	110	455	1	25
Purina:				
Toasted Muesli, ⅔ cup, 60g	260	1100	10	35
Natural Bran, 1 Tbsp, 12g	30	135	0.5	6
Quaker: *Uncooked*				
Oat So Simple: Golden Syrup, 36g Sachet	140	583	2.5	24
Original; Traditional, 27g Sachet	105	430	2.5	16
Sanitarium:				
Granola Oat Clusters:				
Vanilla & Almond, ½ cup, 50g	200	820	5	32
Honey Weets, 1 cup, 30g	110	465	0.5	24
Light 'n Tasty:				
Apricot & Coconut, ¾ cup, 40g	150	630	3	28
Berry, ¾ cup, 40g	150	620	1	29
Macadamia & Honey, ¾ cup, 40g	155	650	3	28
Puffed Wheat, 1 cup, 30g	110	465	0.5	22
Skippy Corn Flakes, 30g	110	460	0	24
Weet-Bix: *Per 1 Biscuit*				
Hi-Bran, 20g	70	300	1	11
Kids, 15g	55	220	0	10
Multi-Grain, 24g	90	380	1	17
Organic, 15g	55	225	0	10
Original, 16g	60	245	0	11
Bites: *14 Pieces, 45g*				
Apricot	155	645	0.5	31
Crispy Grains & Seeds	180	750	3	31
Crunchy Honey	170	710	0.5	34
Rough Crumble	180	750	3.5	30
Schar:				
Corn Flakes, 50g	185	770	0.5	40
Milly Magic Pops, 50g	190	800	1.5	39
Select *(Woolworths):*				
Clusters, avg all flavours, 45g	170	700	1.5	34
Light Choice, 30g	115	480	1	20
Simply Less *(Coles):*				
Multigrain Flakes: With Psyllium, 42g	170	705	1	35
With Psyllium, Corn & Cranberry, 40g	155	640	2	30

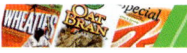

Breakfast Cereals B

Sunsol:	Cal	kJ	Fat	Cb
Breakfast Plus, 30g	120	500	5.5	18
Muesli: Antioxidant w. Strawb. Oats, 45g	190	785	6.5	24
Fibre with Vanilla Oats, 45g	180	745	5	27
Fruity, 40g	150	620	3.5	27
Original, 40g	160	665	6	24
Protein with Cinn. Oats, 45g	180	760	5.5	24
Low-Fat, Apple & Berry, 40g	135	565	1	30
Tropical Breakfast Plus, 30g	95	385	1	20
Table of Plenty:				
Muesli: Heavenly Honey, 45g	155	655	3.5	26
Nicely Nutty, 45g	185	780	6	26
Velvety Vanilla, 45g	170	720	5	27
Tony Ferguson's,				
Muesli, average all flavours, 56g	215	900	3.5	28
Uncle Toby's:				
Bran Plus, ⅔ cup, 45g	140	585	2	16
Cheerios: 1 cup, 30g	115	485	1	23
1½ cups, 45g	175	730	2	35
Fruity Bites, 30g	115	470	1	23
Healthwise, For Heart Wellbeing, 1 c., 35g	135	560	2.5	23
Muesli Natural, Swiss, 60g	220	920	4	36
Oat Brits, 2 biscuits, 42g	160	660	2.5	26
Oat Crisp: Almond, 40g	165	688	6	26
Honey, 30g	120	495	2	21
Oats: Quick; Traditional, 30g	115	480	2.5	17
Multigrain, 40g	150	625	3	23
Quick Sachets, average, 35g	140	570	2.5	24
Smooth & Tasty, average, 30g	120	485	2	20
Weightwise, Original, 40g	150	615	3	19
Cup of Oats: Creamy Honey, 50g tub	60	250	1	11
Berry, 50g	60	245	1	10
Plus: Antioxidant, 45g	165	680	1	34
Calcium, 40g	160	665	3.5	26
Essential For Women, 40g	145	605	1	30
Fibre, 45g	155	645	1	30
Muesli Flakes, 45g	160	680	1	32
Omega 3, 40g	155	645	2.5	28
Protein, 45g	170	700	1	33
Sports, 45g	160	665	1	32
Shredded Wheat, 1 bisc., 24g	85	350	0.5	17
VitaBrits: 1 biscuit	60	250	0	11
2 biscuits	115	490	0.5	23
Weeties: ¾ cup, 28g	100	420	0.5	19
1 cup, 35g	130	535	1	24

	Cal	kJ	Fat	Cb
VitaBrits ~ See Uncle Toby's				
Vogels:				
Cluster Crunch, Classic, 45g	200	820	6.5	29
Muesli: Cluster Spice, 45g	180	755	5	27
Fruit & Nut	190	790	7	24
Ultra Bran Soy & Linseed, 45g	150	635	1.5	22
Weet-Bix ~ See Sanitarium				
Weight Watchers,				
Fruit & Fibre Tropical, 45g	160	680	1	30
Whisk & Pin:				
Winter Porridge, 30g	110	465	3	18
Muesli: Berry Crunch, 50g	260	1100	11	16
Bircher, 50g	190	780	4	29
Gluten Free, 50g	215	890	9	26
Leura Natural, 50g	210	870	7	27
Mountain, 50g	230	945	11	24
Organic, 50g	195	820	6	25
Summer, 50g	200	830	6	28
Woolworths:				
Corn Flakes, 1 cup, 30g	110	460	0	24
Great Start, average, 45g	170	710	1	34
Rice Pops, 1 cup, 30g	120	495	0.5	26
Wheat Biscuits, (1), 16g	60	245	0	11

Brans & Oats

	Cal	kJ	Fat	Cb
Brans: Oat Bran, 1 Tbsp, 12g	45	180	1	6
¼ cup, 36g	130	545	2.5	18
Wheat Bran, natural, 1 Tbsp, 6g	15	65	0.5	1
Oats/Rolled Oats, Dry: 1 T., 10g	40	160	1	6
¼ cup, 30g	115	470	2.5	18
Oatmeal/Porridge:				
Made with water, ¾ cup, 170g	110	465	2.5	18
Quick (Uncle Toby's), 30g	115	480	2.5	24
Instant Oats, Dry, 30g	115	480	2.5	19

Cereal Add-Ons

	Cal	kJ	Fat	Cb
L.S.A., 1 Tbsp, 12g	65	280	5	3.5
Lecithin Granules, 1 Tbsp, 12g	80	325	8	0.5
Lecithin Meal, 25g	115	485	6	11
Pollen Granules, 1 Tbsp, 10g	35	145	1.5	6
Psyllium Husks, 1 Tbsp, 6g	10	50	0	0
Soy Grits (Lowan), 30g	120	500	6	8.5
Wheat Germ, 1 Tbsp, 10g	30	130	1	3

Updated Nutrition Data ~ www.CalorieKing.com.au
Persons with Diabetes ~ See Disclaimer (Page 22)

63

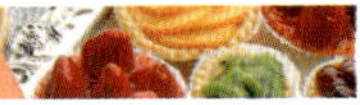

Cakes ~ Baking Ingredients

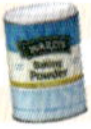

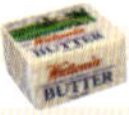

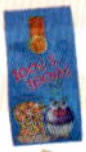

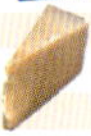

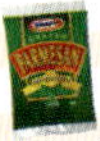

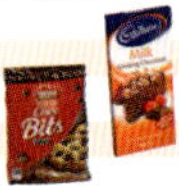

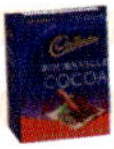

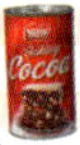

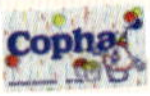

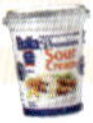

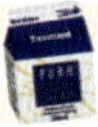

Baking Ingredients

	Cal	kJ	Fat	Cb
Baking Powder, 1 tsp, 5g	10	45	0	2.5
Bi-Carbonate Soda, 1 tsp, 5g	0	0	0	0
Butter:				
1 Tbsp, 20g	150	620	17	1
100g quantity	740	3100	83	1
½ cup, 125g	910	3800	100	1
Cake Decorations:				
100's & 1000's, 1 Tbsp	40	165	0	16
Choc. Hail/Sprinkles, 1 T., 16g	70	285	1.5	14
Cheese:				
Grated/Shredded:				
Cheddar, 1 cup, 120g	490	2040	40	0.5
Goats Cheese (Feta), 100g	250	1040	20	2.5
Mascarpone *(Casa)*, 100g	475	1980	51	2.5
Mozarella, 1 cup, 150g	460	1925	34	1
Parmesan, 4 Tbsp, 30g	140	575	10	0
Philadelphia Cream: 1T., 25g	90	370	8.5	0.5
250g block	880	3675	84	6.5
Chocolate, Cooking: *Average all varieties*				
100g quantity	535	2240	31	57
250g Block	1340	5600	77	142
Chips/Bits/Buttons,				
½ cup, 100g	545	2270	31	57
Cocoa Powder:				
Cadbury Bournville:				
1 Tbsp, 8g	35	135	1.5	2
½ cup, 45g	180	745	7.5	12
100g quantity	395	1650	16	25
Nestle, Baking Cocoa:				
½ cup, 45g	150	630	5	9
100g quantity	335	1400	11	20
Coconut, desiccated, ¼ cup, 25g	165	690	16	6
Copha: 100g quantity	885	3700	100	0
½ cup, 125g	1105	4625	125	0
200g block	1770	7400	200	0
Cornflour, 1 Tbsp, 12g	45	190	0	11
Cream:				
Light/Sour (18% fat),				
200ml carton	390	1638	36	8
Thickened/Sour (35% fat):				
300ml bottle/carton	1005	4200	105	9
Whipping (40% fat):				
½ cup, 60g	205	865	24	2
300ml bottle/carton	1045	4360	110	9
Other Creams ~ *See Page 89*				
Cream of Tartar, 1 tsp, 5g	5	20	0	1

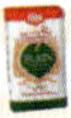

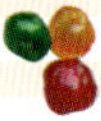

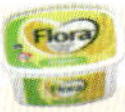

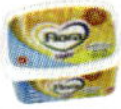

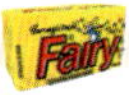

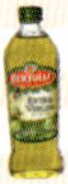

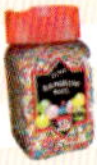

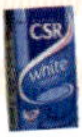

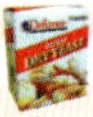

Baking Ingredients (Cont)

	Cal	kJ	Fat	Cb
Flour, All Purpose, 1 cup, 155g	545	2280	2	110
Other Flours ~ *See Page 101*				
Frosting, *(Cake Mate)*, 1 Tbsp, 20g	90	365	4	13
Fruit, dried, mixed, 1 cup, 125g	350	1470	0	82
Fruit Mince *(Robertsons)*, ⅓ cup, 100g	280	1180	3	62
Fruit Pectin, unsweetened, 1 Tbsp	25	110	0	5
Gelatine: Dry, 7g sachet	25	105	0	0
Davis, 10g sachet	35	150	0	0
Detker, leaves, each	5	20	0	0
Glace Cherries/Fruit, 100g	310	1290	0	76
Icing Sugar, avg.,1 Tbsp, 20g	100	420	8	14
Lemon Peel, ¼ cup, 30g	15	60	0	5
Margarine:				
Regular, average:				
1 Tbsp, 20g	115	480	13	0
100g quantity	580	2420	65	0
250g (½ of 500g tub)	1450	6060	163	0
Light (25% less fat):				
1 Tbsp, 20g	85	355	9.5	0
100g quantity	425	1770	47	0.5
Fairy Cooking Margarine:				
100g	715	3000	81	0
250g block	1800	7500	203	0
Marzipan, 30g	125	515	5.5	17
Milk ~ *See Page 44*				
Mixed Peel, 100g	265	1100	1.5	66
Nuts, average, ¼ cup, 35g	210	885	20	2
Oil, average all types:				
1 Tbsp, 20ml	175	730	21	0
¼ cup, 63ml	550	2300	65	0
½ cup, 125ml	1100	4600	125	0
Orange Skin/Zest, 1 Tbsp	0	0	0	0
Pastry ~ *See Page 143*				
Peanut Butter, ½ cup, 125g	800	3340	67	20
Poppy Seeds, ¼ cup, 40g	215	890	14	12
Rainbow Hail, 1 Tbsp, 10g	45	180	1	8.5
Raisins, ½ cup (loose), 75g	230	960	0	56
Rice Paper, 1 sheet (10 x 10cm) 12g	40	175	0	10
Sesame Seeds, 1 Tbsp, 11g	65	270	6	2.5
Sugar: White, granulated,				
1 cup, 230g	920	3845	0	230
500g quantity	1910	8000	0	500
Brown, packed, 1 cup, 240g	960	4010	0	235
Sultanas, ½ cup (loose), 75g	230	960	0	56
Vanilla Essence, 2 tsp, 10ml	5	20	0	1
Whey, sweet, dry, 30g	100	420	0.5	22
Yeast *(Defiance)*, 1 sachet, 8g	30	125	0	3.5

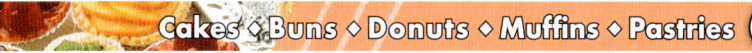

Cakes ◇ Buns ◇ Donuts ◇ Muffins ◇ Pastries

Buns – Sweet

Food	Cal	kJ	Fat	Cb
Cinnamon Bun:				
Medium, 100g	370	1550	16	51
Large, 170g	630	2635	27	86
Cream/Paris, (Cream Bun), 100g	300	1250	25	38
Finger Bun, with Icing, 85g	280	1165	5	53
Fruit Bun: Plain, 75g	195	815	3	36
Iced, 85g	245	1025	7	39
Hot Cross Buns:				
Plain: Medium, 60g	180	750	2	34
Large, 85g	255	1065	3	49

Baker's Delight ~ *See Next Page*
Brumby's ~ *See Page 67*

Cakes & Pastries

Food	Cal	kJ	Fat	Cb
Apple Crumble, 1 piece, 100g	165	700	5.5	27
Apple Danish, 1 piece, 100g	465	1940	27	47
Apple Pie:				
Slices: ⅛ Pie, 120g	335	1405	12	40
Large serve, ⅙ pie, 160g	450	1870	16	53
Individual, 150g	420	1755	15	50
Apple Slice, 100g	300	1045	9	50
Apple Strudel, medium, 150g	350	1460	15	60
Apple Teacake, 1 piece, 43g	120	495	3.5	17
Apple Turnover, medium, 120g	310	1290	12	47
Baklava, average, 50g	200	835	10	26
Banana, 1 piece, 62g	200	830	7.5	36
Bee Sting, medium, 100g	275	1150	9	45
Black Forest: Thin slice, 1/12 cake, 125g	435	1825	25	51
Thick Slice, ⅛ cake, 175g	610	2555	34	71
Buttercake, 1 medium slice, 50g	230	960	10	28
Butterfly Cupcake, 50g				
Caramel Slice, 80g	400	1690	24	44
Carrot Cake: Plain, 1 slice, 88g	295	1225	16	34
With Icing, 100g	375	1565	18	45
Chocolate Brownie, 40g	185	770	10	22
Chocolate Cake, 100g	375	1565	18	45
Chocolate Crackle, each	160	665	13	12
Chocolate Fudge Slice, 70g	370	1550	27	26
Chocolate Eclair: Small, 60g	225	940	14	20
Large, 120g	450	1880	28	40
Extra Large, 240g	900	3760	56	80
Chocolate Mud Cake, 75g	310	1295	17	45
Christmas Cake, medium slice, 75g	270	1130	11	44
Coconut Macaroon, 25g	120	500	5	14
Coconut Slice, 80g	350	1465	12	52
Coffee Scroll, 105g	340	1410	4.5	66
Cream Puff, 33g	110	435	7	12

Cakes & Pastries (Cont)

Food	Cal	kJ	Fat	Cb
Croissant, Choc-filled, 125g	535	2225	24	67
Cronut/Cronot, 100g	415	1740	24	44
Crostoli, 1 stick, 25g	100	415	4.5	13
Cupcakes:				
Plain, average: Small, 40g	60	250	1.5	12
Large, 65g	100	405	2	19
Iced: Small, 50g	185	780	7.5	28
Medium, 80g	300	1245	12	45
Large, 110g	410	1710	17	62
Custard Tart, (9cm diam), 140g	400	1670	23	45
Danish Pastry, avg. all types:				
Medium, 120g	370	1540	18	42
Large, 160g	490	2055	24	56
Donuts, Medium:				
Plain, 50g	185	765	10	20
Iced/Sprinkles: Plain, 70g	295	1240	17	32
Creme filled, 85g	350	1455	20	43
Custard filled, 85g	300	1250	16	45
Jam Donut, average, 100g	360	1505	18	43
Large long donut: Iced, 150g	580	230	20	55
Custard filled, 180g	630	2640	27	81
Eccles, average, 120g	440	1840	20	63
Florentine, medium, 35g	180	750	9	25
Friands, average, 60g	170	710	8	17
Fruit Cake, Dark/Light: Small, 50g	195	815	6.5	31
Medium slice, 75g	295	1225	10	46
Large slice, 100g	390	1630	13	61
Fruit Flan: 100g piece	195	815	7	30
Large, 10cm, 230g	450	1875	17	68
Fruit Mince Pies/Tarts:				
Small, 40g	190	800	8.5	27
Large, 70g	335	1405	15	47
Hedgehog Slice, 135g	700	2925	42	71
Lamingtons: Small, 50g	160	665	6	24
Medium, 80g	255	1060	10	38
Large, 120g	380	1590	14	58
Lamington Roll, 50g slice	180	750	5	27
Lemon Meringue Pie:				
Individual Pie, 140g	570	2380	21	87
Large Pie, 1/12 of pie, 125g	400	1650	14	59
Lemon Meringue Tart, Small, 40g	190	790	7	29
Macaron, French: Avg., all flavours				
Small, 12g	65	270	3	9
Medium, 20g	110	425	5	14
Madeira/Marble: Plain, 45g	165	690	7	24
Iced, 65g	240	990	10	36
Muesli Slice, 70g	355	1490	21	39
Muffins ~ *See Next Page*				

Updated Nutrition Data ~ www.CalorieKing.com.au
Persons with Diabetes ~ See Disclaimer (Page 22)

65

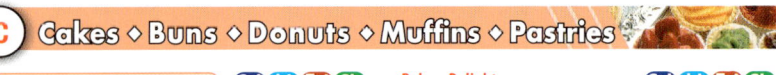

Cakes ◇ Buns ◇ Donuts ◇ Muffins ◇ Pastries

Cakes & Pastries (Cont)

	Cal	kJ	Fat	Cb
Pannettone, medium slice, 100g	365	1520	13	55
Pecan Pie, ⅛ pie, 85g	330	1380	13	42
Profiterole, medium, 35g	120	500	9	11
Rock Cake, large, 90g	335	1400	12	52
Rollettes ~ See Coles ~ Page 68; Top Taste ~ Page 70				
Rum Balls, average, 25g	85	355	3.5	15
Scones:				
Plain: Medium (1), 65g	210	870	5	36
Large (1), 100g	260	1075	6	44
With Date/Sultanas:				
Medium (1), 70g	210	870	3.5	40
Large (1), 100g	290	1210	5	55
Scrolls ~ See Baker's Delight/Brumby's				
Slices: Fruit, average, 100g	300	1045	9	50
Fruit & Nut, average, 100g	360	1085	16	55
Sponge, Plain, ⅛ round layer, 25g	70	300	0.5	14
Sponge Roll, Jam & Cream, 50g piece	145	610	3	23
Stollen Fruit Cake, 1 slice, 50g	215	900	12	26
Strawberry Sponge Gateau, 100g	310	1295	19	40
Sultana Cake, 1 small slice, 50g	175	730	6	24
Swiss Roll/Choc Roll, 1 slice, 40g	120	500	3	25
Tarts: Fruit Mince, 80g	320	1340	11	51
Lemon, 80g	320	1340	14	43
Tiramisu, 100g serve	330	1380	20	32
Torte, average all varieties, 120g	380	1590	29	28
Vanilla Slices: Small, 85g	240	1000	12	28
Large, 170g	480	2000	24	48
Extra Large, 270g	760	3170	38	89

Muffins ~ Quick Guide

Average All Brands

Apple & Cinnamon/Blueberry:

	Cal	kJ	Fat	Cb
Mini/Small, 30g	110	450	5	15
Medium, 60g	215	895	10	29
Large, 100g	355	1490	16	49
Extra Large, 170g	600	2500	27	83
Jumbo, 200g	710	2980	32	97
Chocolate Chip:				
Mini/Small, 30g	125	525	7	16
Medium, 60g	250	1050	14	32
Large, 100g	415	1735	23	54
Extra Large, 170g	705	2945	39	92
Jumbo, 200g	830	3470	46	108
Low-Fat Muffins: *No Added Fat*				
Medium, 60g	155	640	2	31
Extra Large, 150g	385	1610	4.5	78

Bakers Delight:

Note: Weights can vary between stores.

	Cal	kJ	Fat	Cb
Croissant: Chocolate, 75g	290	1220	17	29
Traditional, 70g	255	1070	16	22
Danish Lattice:				
Apple & Sultana, 116g	405	1700	20	36
Apricot, 116g	365	1520	20	41
Custard, 116g	355	1480	20	37
Finger Buns:				
Pink, 100g	340	1420	5.5	64
Coconut, 100g	380	1580	13	42
100's & 1000's, 100g	350	1450	5.5	66
Fruit Bun: 65g	220	920	3.5	40
Iced, 85g	325	1355	9	47
Hot Cross Buns:				
Traditional, 70g	230	965	3.5	43
Choc Chip, 70g	255	1070	8	41
Fruitless, 70g	220	910	5	37
Log, Apple & Walnut, ⅛ slice, 2cm, 80g	300	1250	11	44
Roll, Apricot Delight, 100g	305	1280	1.5	63
Scones: Date, 100g	325	1360	5.5	63
Berry & White Choc, 95g	300	1255	9	48
Fruit, 85g	275	1155	4.5	52
Plain/Traditional, 65g	210	870	5	36
Scrolls: Almond & Custard, 175g	640	2660	26	65
Apple & Cinnamon, 125g	365	1525	6	68
Apple & Walnut, 165g	600	2510	22	88
Apricot Delight, 105g	270	1135	1.5	56
Custard, 165g	585	2445	24	62
Sticky Cinnamon, 93g	385	1600	16	55
Snail/Escargot, 125g	410	1715	9	71
Swirls: Choc Berry, ½ swirl, 57g	180	735	4	31
Sticky Date, ½ swirl, 61g	180	750	3.5	31
Tarts, Fruit Mince, 69g	275	1145	10	45

Breads & Bread Rolls ~ *See Page 57-58*
Savoury Items ~ *See Page 185*

CALORIE KING TIP!

Beware of large muffins. They can have more calories and fat than a burger!

600 Cals / 27g Fat

500 Cals / 27g Fat

Cakes ◊ Buns ◊ Donuts ◊ Muffins ◊ Pastries C

	Cal	kJ	Fat	Cb
Balfours:				
Donut, Choc/Pink, 100g	500	2080	32	47
Better Bite Muffins:				
Blueberry, 75g	215	895	3.5	40
Chocolate, 75g	205	855	5.5	36
Betty Crocker:				
Cake Mix: *Per Slice, Prepared as Directed*				
Decadent Chocolate Mud, 78g	310	1295	14	42
Super Moist: Choc Swirl, 89g	305	1285	14	43
Chocolate Fudge	310	1300	13	46
Devil's Food, 81g	295	1220	12	42
Strawberries & Cream	280	1155	12	37
Vanilla, 89g	305	1280	15	40
Cupcake Mix: Chocolate, 62g	215	895	8	33
Strawberries & Cream, 59g	215	895	7	35
Vanilla, 63g	225	935	8.5	34
Cookie Mix: *Prepared as Directed*				
Milk Chocolate Chunk (1), 37g	175	730	7	26
Rainbow (1), 24g	105	450	4	17
Muffin Mix: *Prepared as Directed*				
Cinnamon Crumble (1), 69g	280	1180	14	35
Triple Chocolate (1), 69g	280	1170	13	39
97% Fat-Free: Apple Cinn., 54g	155	640	1.5	32
Mixed Berry (1), 55g	140	585	1	30
Brownie Mix: *Per Slice, Prepared as Directed*				
Chocolate Fudge, Red. Fat, 58g	205	855	3	42
Frosted Chocolate, 51g	210	875	3	43
Triple Chocolate Fudge, 51g	215	890	7.5	34
Whoopie Pie Mix: *Prepared as Directed*				
Choc Vanilla, 49g	175	725	11	20
Strawberries & Cream, 49g	190	780	8	29
Triple Choc, 49g	200	825	8.5	28
Vanilla Sprinkle, 51g	200	835	9	29
Brumby's:				
Buns: Beesting, 90g	250	1040	9	35
Finger Bun, Iced, 100g	315	1315	10	55
Cakes & Slices: *Per Slice*				
Caramel Slice, 100g	465	1945	22	60
Carrot Cake: Iced, 125g	320	1340	16	40
Loaf, 1 thin slice, 70g				
Cinnamon Log, Iced, 31g	95	380	2	16
Coconut Delight, 80g	250	1040	33	29
Hedgehog, 145g	420	1755	17	65

	Cal	kJ	Fat	Cb
Brumby's (Cont):				
Cakes & Slices (Cont): *Per Slice*				
Lamington: Medium, 120g	240	1005	9	53
Large, 160g	320	1340	12	70
Vanilla Slice: Large, 165g	465	1950	23	54
Medium, 120g	340	1400	18	40
Croissant: Plain, 70g	295	1230	16	29
Chocolate, 85g	340	1420	18	35
Cupcakes: Average all types,				
Iced, large, 110g	410	1710	17	62
Custard Tart, 130g	290	1210	12	39
Danish Lattices:				
Apple & Custard, 110g	335	1400	18	37
Apricot & Custard, 110g	340	1420	16	44
Blueberry & Custard, 110g	345	1440	16	44
Donuts: Plain, with Jam Centre, 100g	300	1260	9	48
Glazed Ring: Regular, 65g	205	850	7.5	32
With Cinnamon Sugar, 50g	165	695	7.5	23
Long John, with Jam, 100g	330	1380	20	35
Muffins:				
Apple & Cinnamon, 125g	390	1640	19	51
Double Choc, Premium, 140g	490	2050	25	63
Jaffa, 125g	455	1910	22	61
Scones: Date, 100g	215	1000	5	47
With Sultanas, 100g	250	1045	5	45
Scrolls: Apple Scroll, 110g	255	1060	3.5	50
American Caramel, 120g	350	1470	9	60
French Custard, 120g	330	1390	9	55
Hazelnut Custard, 120g	310	1300	4.5	59
Low Fat Apricot, 120g	250	1040	1	52
Breads ~ *See Page 58*				
Savoury Items ~ *See Page 186*				
Cheesecake Shop:				
Banana Cake, $\frac{1}{12}$, 165g	510	2130	20	76
Boston Mudcake, $\frac{1}{12}$, 154g	620	2890	37	67
Carrot, $\frac{1}{12}$, 175g	505	2120	31	54
Continental Caramello, $\frac{1}{16}$, 83g	180	755	8	27
Lemon Meringue Pie, $\frac{1}{12}$, 125g	395	1650	14	59
Baked Cheesecake:				
American, $\frac{1}{12}$, 108g	390	1630	26	29
Jamaican, $\frac{1}{12}$, 115g	405	1695	26	34

Updated Nutrition Data ~ www.CalorieKing.com.au
Persons with Diabetes ~ See Disclaimer (Page 22)

Cakes ◆ Buns ◆ Donuts ◆ Muffins ◆ Pastries

Coles:

	Cal	kJ	Fat	Cb
Brandy Snaps, no filling (1)	75	305	2	13
Cup Cakes: Iced Mud, 80g 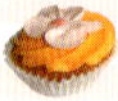	350	1460	17	45
Iced Rainbow, 80g	320	1340	16	41
Fresh Cakes: Apple, ⅛ cake, 46g	120	490	1	25
Carrot, ⅛ cake, 62g	240	995	10	35
Chocolate Mud, ⅛ cake, 75g 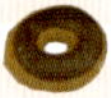	305	1270	16	37
Donut, Mini Iced, 23g	80	340	2	12
Fruit Cake: Average all, 1/16 cake, 50g	205	860	6.5	28
Light, 50g	190	800	7	28
Hedgehog Slice, 42g	200	825	10	24
Loaf, Lemon Drizzle, ⅛ slice, 57g	230	960	10	33
Rich Chocolate, ⅛ slice, 63g	225	940	11	30
Lamingtons: Original, 50g 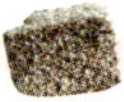	155	655	5.5	25
Fingers, average (1), 19.5g	65	270	3	9
Jam, 75g	255	1070	11	36
Madeira, un-iced, 1/10 cake, 45g	155	640	6.5	22
Muffins: 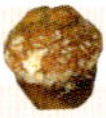				
Large, 173g: Blueberry	610	2545	30	77
Apple & Cinnamon Crumble	585	2440	25	72
Mixed Berry Crumble	620	2595	26	75
Medium, 110g, (4-Pack), Blueberry	390	1620	19	49
Pavlova:				
⅛ of 300g Pavlova, 38g 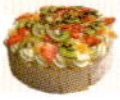	115	480	0	26
1/12 of 500g Pavlova, 42g	125	530	0	29
Profiteroles, Custard (1), 30g	75	305	4	5
Rollettes: Chocolate (1), 42g	150	630	6.5	21
Jam (1), 42g	120	500	1	26
Sponge: Double, Unfilled Double (480g), ⅛ cake, 60g	160	670	3.5	29
Swiss Roll: 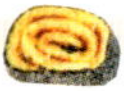				
Chocolate, 1/10 slice, 30g	105	440	4	15
Jam, ⅛ slice, 50g	140	590	1.5	31
Tarts: Lemon, 45g 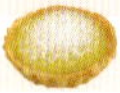	190	790	7	29
Neenish, 55g	275	1150	15	32
Raspberry, 50g	205	855	7.5	24
Frozen Desserts: *Per Serving* 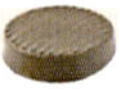				
Black Forrest, ⅙ cake, 100g	235	970	9	35
Cheesecake, French, ⅙ cake, 68g	210	875	11	25
Chocolate Bavarian, ⅙ cake, 68g	220	920	14	22
Strawberry & Cream, 1/10 cake, 95g	210	865	8	31
Triple Chocolate, ⅙ cake, 92g	260	1090	13	30
Melting Middle Cookies:				
Chocolate & Vanilla Creme (2), 114g	500	2090	23	69
Chocolate Chip (2), 114g 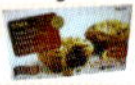	500	2090	23	71
Pies: Apple, 1 slice, ⅛ pie, 75g	180	745	7.5	24
Lite Apple, 1 slice, ⅛ pie, 75g 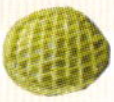	175	725	4.5	31
Snack Pie: Apple, 125g	415	1740	18	59
Apricot, 113g	355	1480	16	49

Donna Hay:

	Cal	kJ	Fat	Cb
Cakes: *Prepared as Directed*				
Molten Chocolate Chunk, slice, 60g	260	1090	12	35

Donut King:

Donuts: Cinnamon Ring, 46g	150	625	6.5	21
Classic Mini, Jam, 36g 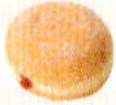	130	550	5.5	18
Iced Cake Ring, 59g	200	820	6.5	32
Iced Donut Ring, 62g	230	960	8.5	34
Iced Jam Ball, 97g	340	1430	10	58

Green's:

Cookie Mix: *Per Cookie, Prepared as Directed*				
Classic Choc Chip, 29g 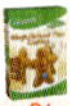	130	545	6	18
Gingerbread Man, 33g	75	310	3.5	10
Essentials: *Per ½ Cake, Prepared as Directed*				
Chocolate; Golden Butter; Vanilla, 49g	160	660	6	23
Indulgent: Caramel Mud, 88g	330	1370	12	52
Choc Mint, 93g 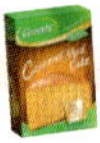	335	1395	15	47
Chocolate, 90g	295	1240	14	40
Chocolate Swirl, 98g	340	1410	14	48
Orange Poppyseed, 94g	325	1360	14	46
Traditional:				
Chocolate, 65g	225	945	9	32
Cinnamon Tea, 60g 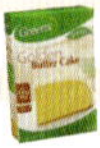	190	780	12	17
Date Loaf, 50g	140	590	2.5	27
Golden Butter, 65g	230	955	9	34
Lemon, 65g	230	950	8.5	34
Orange, 65g 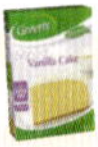	230	950	8.5	34
Smooth Coffee, 58g	210	870	9	29
Sultana, 46g	145	605	5	23
Vanilla, 65g	230	955	9	34
Cupcake Mix: *Per Cupcake, Prepared as Directed*				
Chocolate, 63g	215	900	9	30
Pink, 68g 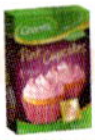	250	1040	11	35
Red Velvet, 60g	205	865	9	29
Vanilla, 54g	190	785	8	27
Muffin Mix: *Per Muffin, Prepared as Directed*				
Low-Fat: Banana Honey, 65g	155	650	1	33
Blueberry, 60g 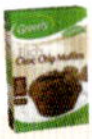	160	660	1	33
Choc Chip, 65g	160	670	1.5	33
Multi-Purpose Base, 64g	210	865	7	33

Kellogg's:

Pop-Tarts: *Per 2 Pastries* 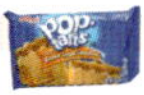				
Brown Sugar Cinnamon	420	1770	14	69

Cakes ◊ Buns ◊ Donuts ◊ Muffins ◊ Pastries — C

	Cal	kJ	Fat	Cb
Krispy Kreme:				
Doughnuts: *Per Doughnut*				
Butterscotch Twist, 56g	230	970	12	30
Cinnamon, 46g	205	865	13	20
Strawberries & Creme, 77g	335	1390	20	34
Very Vanilla, 80g	335	1400	17	41
Chocolate Iced: With Sprinkles, 71g	305	1275	12	46
Custard Filled, 86g	325	1365	17	38
Cream Filled, 86g	375	1575	21	43
Glazed: Original, 52g	230	955	13	24
Blueberry, 80g	335	1405	17	43
Chocolate Iced: 66g	285	1185	12	40
Raspberry, 86g	340	1430	15	46
Strawberry: Iced, 68g	300	1255	15	38
Jam, 77g	265	1110	14	30
Lite n' Easy:				
Frozen Desserts: Apple Crumble (1), 165g	190	800	2.5	39
Apricot Pudding (1), 165g	180	745	2.5	36
Raspberry & Apple Crumble (1), 165g	200	840	2.5	39
Rice Pudding (1), 176g	205	845	3.5	36
Little Bites:				
Brownie, Choc Fudge, 40g	195	810	10	24
Muffins: Choc Chip, 32g	145	595	7	18
Little Bites, Cookies & Cream, 2 muffins, 38g	180	755	9	21
McCafe/McDonald's ~ *See pages 197-198*				
Mr Kipling:				
Almond Slice, 32g	130	535	4.5	20
Angel Slice, 33g	135	575	6	20
French Fancies, 24g	90	380	2.5	17
Christmas: Cake Slices, 47g	170	715	4	32
Mince Pies, 60g	240	1010	9	38
Pudding Slices, 47g	150	640	3	29
Melinda's:				
Cakes: *Prepared as Directed*				
Red Velvet, 1 slice, 70g	460	1920	20	60
Muffins: Lemon Curd Delight, 57g	315	1315	15	37
Risotto, 63g	260	1085	6	42
Slices: Chocolate Fudge Brownie, 56g	345	1440	18	41
Chocolate Walnut, 35g	175	740	10	21
Gingerbread, 80g	285	1190	13	39
Lemon Delicious, 35g	150	620	6	22
Passionfruit, 40g	190	790	9	24

	Cal	kJ	Fat	Cb
Mills & Wares:				
Christmas Cake: Iced, 50g	175	740	3	35
Not Iced, 50g	170	710	3.5	33
Fruit Cake, 70% Less-Fat, 50g	150	635	2	30
Plum Pudding: ⅓ can, 100g	325	1350	8.5	56
Microwavable: ¼, 100g	345	1450	8.5	62
Single Serve, 80g	260	1080	7	45
Muffin Bars,				
average all types (1)	160	670	6	23
Muffin Break:				
Cakes: Apple, 135g	510	2120	31	50
Banana, 123g	425	1770	23	48
Banana Bread, 128g	410	1705	17	56
Blueberry, 140g	435	1820	23	51
Carrot, 186g	760	3180	46	78
Cheesecake: Chocolate, 189g	665	2780	41	62
Cool & Creamy, 164g	480	2000	33	37
Chocolate Mousse, 197g	855	3565	61	70
Fruit, 172g	445	1860	5.5	83
Mud, 182g	880	3675	62	70
Sticky Date, 215g	725	3030	26	112
Muffins:				
Bran: Blueberry Apple, 165g	495	2065	3	57
Carrot Apple, 169g	490	2045	23	56
Gluten Free: Apple, 158g	340	1425	6	63
Choc Banana, 158g	395	1645	10	67
Choc Chip, 158g	430	1790	11	71
Orange 158g	320	1325	5	59
Low-Fat: Apple Bran & Sultana	380	1595	3	69
Other varieties, av.	325	1355	2.5	60
Savoury: Sweet Chilli & Corn	355	1490	14	49
Spinach & Feta	365	1515	18	36
Sundried Tomato, Parmesan, & Olives	300	1245	11	36
Soy & Linseed: Banana Nut, 149g	430	1790	14	60
Fruit & Nut, 149g	450	1880	11	73
Mixed Berry, 149g	370	1550	10	56
Traditional: Blueberry, 160g	510	2130	21	67
Choc Chip, 160g	600	2495	27	75
Scones: Plain 86g	220	920	5	37
Date, 100g	265	1110	5	48
Slices: Jelly, 172g	485	2030	20	69
Lemon Coconut, 138g	580	2430	26	81
Mars Bar, 90g	425	1765	27	44
Rocky Road, 149g	665	2770	36	76
Vanilla, 244g	515	2150	20	79
Swirls, Apple/Banana/Berry, average	235	985	7	38

Updated Nutrition Data ~ www.CalorieKing.com.au
Persons with Diabetes ~ See Disclaimer (Page 22)

Cakes ◊ Buns ◊ Donuts ◊ Muffins ◊ Pastries

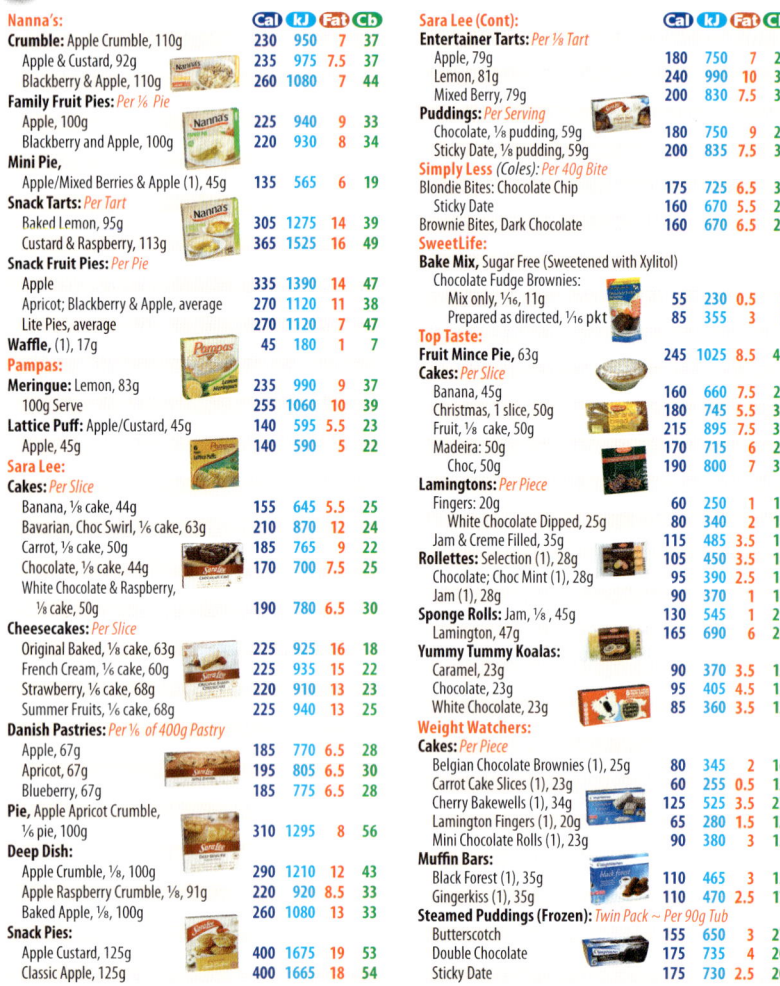

Nanna's:
	Cal	kJ	Fat	Cb
Crumble: Apple Crumble, 110g	230	950	7	37
Apple & Custard, 92g	235	975	7.5	37
Blackberry & Apple, 110g	260	1080	7	44
Family Fruit Pies: *Per ⅙ Pie*				
Apple, 100g	225	940	9	33
Blackberry and Apple, 100g	220	930	8	34
Mini Pie,				
Apple/Mixed Berries & Apple (1), 45g	135	565	6	19
Snack Tarts: *Per Tart*				
Baked Lemon, 95g	305	1275	14	39
Custard & Raspberry, 113g	365	1525	16	49
Snack Fruit Pies: *Per Pie*				
Apple	335	1390	14	47
Apricot; Blackberry & Apple, average	270	1120	11	38
Lite Pies, average	270	1120	7	47
Waffle, (1), 17g	45	180	1	7

Pampas:
	Cal	kJ	Fat	Cb
Meringue: Lemon, 83g	235	990	9	37
100g Serve	255	1060	10	39
Lattice Puff: Apple/Custard, 45g	140	595	5.5	23
Apple, 45g	140	590	5	22

Sara Lee:
	Cal	kJ	Fat	Cb
Cakes: *Per Slice*				
Banana, ⅛ cake, 44g	155	645	5.5	25
Bavarian, Choc Swirl, ⅙ cake, 63g	210	870	12	24
Carrot, ⅛ cake, 50g	185	765	9	22
Chocolate, ⅛ cake, 44g	170	700	7.5	25
White Chocolate & Raspberry, ⅛ cake, 50g	190	780	6.5	30
Cheesecakes: *Per Slice*				
Original Baked, ⅛ cake, 63g	225	925	16	18
French Cream, ⅙ cake, 60g	225	935	15	22
Strawberry, ⅙ cake, 68g	220	910	13	23
Summer Fruits, ⅙ cake, 68g	225	940	13	23
Danish Pastries: *Per ⅙ of 400g Pastry*				
Apple, 67g	185	770	6.5	28
Apricot, 67g	195	805	6.5	30
Blueberry, 67g	185	775	6.5	28
Pie, Apple Apricot Crumble, ⅙ pie, 100g	310	1295	8	56
Deep Dish				
Apple Crumble, ⅛, 100g	290	1210	12	43
Apple Raspberry Crumble, ⅛, 91g	220	920	8.5	33
Baked Apple, ⅛, 100g	260	1080	13	33
Snack Pies:				
Apple Custard, 125g	400	1675	19	53
Classic Apple, 125g	400	1665	18	54

Sara Lee (Cont):
	Cal	kJ	Fat	Cb
Entertainer Tarts: *Per ⅛ Tart*				
Apple, 79g	180	750	7	26
Lemon, 81g	240	990	10	32
Mixed Berry, 79g	200	830	7.5	30
Puddings: *Per Serving*				
Chocolate, ⅛ pudding, 59g	180	750	9	22
Sticky Date, ⅛ pudding, 59g	200	835	7.5	31

Simply Less (Coles): *Per 40g Bite*
	Cal	kJ	Fat	Cb
Blondie Bites: Chocolate Chip	175	725	6.5	35
Sticky Date	160	670	5.5	25
Brownie Bites, Dark Chocolate	160	670	6.5	23

SweetLife:
	Cal	kJ	Fat	Cb
Bake Mix, Sugar Free (Sweetened with Xylitol)				
Chocolate Fudge Brownies:				
Mix only, 1/16, 11g	55	230	0.5	1
Prepared as directed, 1/16 pkt	85	355	3	1

Top Taste:
	Cal	kJ	Fat	Cb
Fruit Mince Pie, 63g	245	1025	8.5	40
Cakes: *Per Slice*				
Banana, 45g	160	660	7.5	21
Christmas, 1 slice, 50g	180	745	5.5	30
Fruit, ⅛ cake, 50g	215	895	7.5	34
Madeira: 50g	170	715	6	27
Choc, 50g	190	800	7	30
Lamingtons: *Per Piece*				
Fingers: 20g	60	250	1	11
White Chocolate Dipped, 25g	80	340	2	14
Jam & Creme Filled, 35g	115	485	3.5	19
Rollettes: Selection (1), 28g	105	450	3.5	18
Chocolate; Choc Mint (1), 28g	95	390	2.5	16
Jam (1), 28g	90	370	1	19
Sponge Rolls: Jam, ⅛, 45g	130	545	1	29
Lamington, 47g	165	690	6	26
Yummy Tummy Koalas:				
Caramel, 23g	90	370	3.5	13
Chocolate, 23g	95	405	4.5	13
White Chocolate, 23g	85	360	3.5	13

Weight Watchers:
	Cal	kJ	Fat	Cb
Cakes: *Per Piece*				
Belgian Chocolate Brownies (1), 25g	80	345	2	16
Carrot Cake Slices (1), 23g	60	255	0.5	13
Cherry Bakewells (1), 34g	125	525	3.5	22
Lamington Fingers (1), 20g	65	280	1.5	12
Mini Chocolate Rolls (1), 23g	90	380	3	15
Muffin Bars:				
Black Forest (1), 35g	110	465	3	15
Gingerkiss (1), 35g	110	470	2.5	17
Steamed Puddings (Frozen): *Twin Pack ~ Per 90g Tub*				
Butterscotch	155	650	3	27
Double Chocolate	170	735	4	20
Sticky Date	175	730	2.5	20

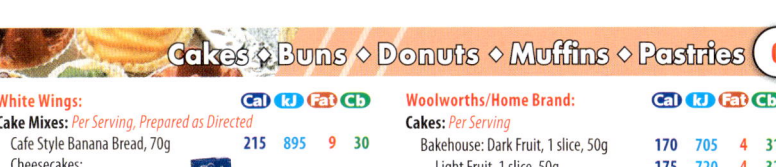

Cakes ◆ Buns ◆ Donuts ◆ Muffins ◆ Pastries

White Wings:

	Cal	kJ	Fat	Cb
Cake Mixes: *Per Serving, Prepared as Directed*				
Cafe Style Banana Bread, 70g	215	895	9	30
Cheesecakes:				
Creamy Lemon, 88g	255	1065	12	34
Smooth Continental, 80g	250	1035	13	30
Chocolate Dream, 1/12 cake, 85g	280	1170	13	36
Chocolate Heaven, slice, 85g	270	1115	12	35
Chocolate Profiteroles, 74g	215	895	16	19
Golden Buttercake, 69g	220	920	8.5	32
Moist: Chocolate, 1/12 cake	190	780	8.5	24
Sultana Buttercake, 1/10	205	860	6	34
Raspberry Swirl, slice, 89g	300	1255	14	39
Red Velvet, slice, 71g	280	1160	3	59
97% Fat Free: Angelic Vanilla, 1 slice, 75g	185	780	2	39
Orange & Poppyseed, 75g	190	805	2	40
Cupcakes:				
Baby Cakes: Angel, 19g	80	325	3	13
Double Choc, 20g	80	340	3	13
Chocolate, 63g	245	1030	13	30
Banana; Chocolate, 63g	245	1020	12	31
Red Velvet, 59g	230	965	2.5	49
Sweetheart Choc-Vanilla, 60g	215	890	10	28
Vanilla, 63g	155	640	3	29
Slice Mixes: *Per Slice, Prepared as Directed*				
Choc Chunk Brownie, 50g	205	850	8	30
Hedgehog, 46g	205	865	10	30
Home-Style,				
Carrot & Walnut, 105g	375	1565	20	43
Muffin Mixes: *Per Muffin*				
Blueberry, 67g	210	885	7.5	32
Milk/Rich Choc Chip, 70g	270	1120	13	35
Triple Choc, 70g	270	1125	13	34
97% Fat Free: Banana, 58g	150	635	1.5	31
Choc Chip, 62g	165	680	1.5	34
Orange & Poppyseed, 55g	155	645	1	33
Mousse Mix,				
Rich Chocolate Royale, 92g serve	195	810	6.5	28
Pancakes Shaker, average (1), 46g	90	375	1	18
Pudding Mixes: *Per 1/4 Packet, Prepared as Directed*				
Butterscotch Sponge	285	1190	4.5	56
Chocolate on Choc Sponge	285	1180	46	54
Classic Creme Caramel, 1/6 pkt	220	930	5.5	37
Chocolate with Choc. Sce,	285	1180	46	54
Lemon Sponge	280	1180	4.5	56

Woolworths/Home Brand:

	Cal	kJ	Fat	Cb
Cakes: *Per Serving*				
Bakehouse: Dark Fruit, 1 slice, 50g	170	705	4	31
Light Fruit, 1 slice, 50g	175	720	4	32
Banana Bread, 1 thick slice, 100g	310	1290	9	51
Bavarian, Chocolate, 1/6 cake	230	955	12	29
Buttercake: Chocolate, 1/8 cake, 56g	180	750	6.5	27
Double Choc, 1/8 cake, 60g	210	865	9	28
Sultana, 1/8 cake, 60g	195	820	7	30
Cheesecakes: Cookies & Cream, 68g	230	955	14	24
Strawberry, 1/6 cake, 68g	210	870	12	23
Ginger Kisses (1), 25g	90	385	4.5	12
Cup Cakes: Chocolate, 33g	125	530	3.5	23
Strawberry, 33g	130	550	4.5	22
Mini, Iced with Sprinkles (1), 38g	145	600	4	25
Danish, Pecan, custard filled, 1/6 whole, 75g	245	1015	11	31
Donuts: Cinnamon (1), 45g	140	575	4	22
Jam Ball (1), 80g	285	1195	14	36
Fruit Cakes: Dark, 50g	195	815	7	31
Light, 50g	195	805	7	31
Lamingtons: Chocolate, 60g	180	745	4	33
Finger, Chocolate, 25g	85	345	2.5	14
Mud Cakes: Choc, 1/8, 75g	255	1070	13	37
Caramel Flavoured, 75g	260	1090	13	37
Muffins: *Per Muffin*				
Blueberry: Large, single, 170g	605	2515	26	87
Medium (4-Pack), 110g	390	1630	17	56
Mini (8-Pack), 22g	80	325	3.5	12
Choc Chip: (4-Pack), 110g	475	1990	25	59
Mini (8-Pack), 22g	95	400	5	12
Double Choc Chip: 4-Pack, each, 110g	520	2180	27	61
Mini (8-Pack), each, 22g	105	435	5.5	12
Pavlova, Shell, 10g	40	170	0	9.5
Pie, Apple, 1/8 pie, 75g	175	725	7.5	25
Slices: Apricot, 88g	395	1655	21	45
Caramel, 88g	380	1585	20	48
Rocky Road, 63g	340	1420	20	37
Sponge, Round, Double, unfilled, 1/8, 29g	85	355	2	15
Sponge Rolls: Double Choc., 1/10 roll, 50g	195	815	8	28
Honey, 1/10 roll, 50g	185	775	8	26
Swiss, 1/10 roll, 50g	175	740	6	29
Tarts: Baked Lemon, 1/8 tart, 76g	235	980	7.5	41
Caramel Macadamia, 1/8 tart, 79g	350	1450	18	42
Neenish, 50g	265	1100	15	31

Updated Nutrition Data ~ www.CalorieKing.com.au
Persons with Diabetes ~ See Disclaimer (Page 22)

Cheese

Cheese Ready Reckoner ~ Cheddar Style

- **C** ~ Calories
- **kJ** ~ Kilojoules
- **F** ~ Fat (grams)
- **Cb** ~ Carbohydrate (Grams)

	FULL FAT 34% Fat / 34% Fat				LIGHT 25% Less Fat / 25% Fat				EXTRA LIGHT 50% Less Fat / 15% Fat			
	Cal	kJ	Fat	Cb	Cal	kJ	Fat	Cb	Cal	kJ	Fat	Cb
Thin Slice, 21g	85	350	7	0	70	295	5	0	55	230	3	0
Thick Slice, 30g	120	500	10	0	100	425	7	0	85	350	4.5	0
3cm Cube, 30g	120	500	10	0	100	425	7	0	85	350	4.5	0
Shredded, ½ cup, 60g	240	1000	20	0	200	850	14	0	170	700	9	0
100g Quanity	400	1670	34	0	330	1380	23	0	270	1130	15	0
Small Block, 250g	1000	4180	84	0	830	3470	58	0	700	2320	38	0

Cheese A-Z

Per 30g, Unless Indicated

	Cal	kJ	Fat	Cb
Babybel: *Each*				
Original, Mini, 21g	70	295	6	0
Light, 21g	50	210	3	0
Tasty Cheddar, 20g	75	305	6.5	0
Bega: Tasty Bar-B-Cubes, 5 pieces, 25g	100	425	8.5	0
Slices: *Per 21g Slice*				
So Light, average	45	180	2	0
So Extra Light	55	230	3	0
Super	70	290	5.5	1.5
Super Lights	35	145	0.5	2
Super Slim	45	180	2	1.5
Thick & Tasty, 30g	100	420	8	2
Sticks, Tasty, 20g	80	340	7	0
Stringers (1), 20g	60	250	4	0
Blue Brie, 30g	110	455	10	0
Blue Vein, average, 30g	110	465	10	0
Boursin, 30g	120	500	13	0.5
Brie, average, 30g	110	470	10	0
Camembert, 30g	90	380	8	0
Caraway, 30g	115	475	8.5	1
Castello: Blue	130	535	13	0
White, 30g	120	495	12	0
Cheddar, average, Mature/Semi-Matured	120	500	10	0
Cheese Dips ~ *See Page 93*				
Cheese Spreads:				
Weight Watchers, Cream Cheese, Light, 25g	50	200	3.5	2
Kraft ~ *See Next Page*				
Chèvre ~ *See Goat Cheese*				
Colby, 30g	115	485	10	0

Coles:

	Cal	kJ	Fat	Cb
Cheddar:				
Extra Tasty, 30g	120	510	10	0
Tasty Cheddar, 30g	125	530	11	0
Tasty Cheddar Lite, 30g	100	425	7	0
Slices: Colby, Tasty, 21g	85	350	7	0
Lite, 21g	50	200	3	0
Coon:				
Blocks: Extra Tasty/Colby, avg				
Slice, 30g	120	500	10	0
100g quantity	400	1670	33	0
Tasty, 30g	120	510	10	0
Light & Tasty, 30g	100	420	7	0
Slices: Tasty, 21g	85	355	7	0
Extra Tasty, 21g	85	355	7	0
Colby, 21g	85	350	7	0
Light & Tasty, 21g	70	295	5	0
Swiss Slices, 21g	75	395	6	0
Shredded: Pizza, 25g	85	345	6.5	0
Light & Tasty, 25g	85	350	6	0
Cottage, Regular/Creamed:				
Plain: 2 Tbsp, 40g	50	205	2.5	1
½ cup, 120g	145	610	7	2.5
With Gherkin, ½ cup, 120g	110	465	2.5	12
With Chives/Onion, ½ cup, 120g	110	460	3	9
Light/ Low-Fat:				
2 Tbsp, 40g	35	150	1	1.5
¼ cup, 60g	55	230	1.5	2.5
100g quantity	90	380	2.5	4

Cheese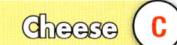

Cheese A-Z (Cont)

Item	Cal	kJ	Fat	Cb
Per 30g Unless Indicated				
Cream Cheese:				
Plain: 1 Tbsp, 20g	65	275	6.5	0.5
100g quantity	330	1380	32	3
With Fruit, 25g piece	85	360	7	3
Philadelphia (Kraft) ~ See next page				
Weight Watchers, Cream Cheese, Light, 25g	50	200	3.5	2
Cream Cheese Spread:				
1 Tablespoon, 20g	65	265	6	0.5
Emmenthal, 30g	130	540	9.5	1
Danish Blue:				
Castello, Extra Creamy, 25g	100	415	9	0.5
Wedges, 25g each	100	415	9	0.5
Devondale: Light 'n Tasty, 30g	100	425	7	0
Cheddar: Mild, 30g	120	500	10	0
Colby, 25g	100	420	8.5	0
Organic Tasty, 25g	105	440	9	0.5
Tasty; Vintage, 30g	120	500	10	0
Shredded, Mild, ½ cup, 60g	245	1030	21	0
Slices: Mild Cheddar, thick slice, 30g	125	515	11	0
Thin slice, 21g	85	350	7.5	0
Sandwich Slice, 21g	65	270	5	0
Seven, 21g	35	150	1.5	0.5
Edam: Average, 30g	100	420	7.5	0
Mainland, 21g	70	290	5.5	0
Farm Cheese, unripened:				
Fresh, moist, 16% fat, 30g	65	270	5	0
Firmer, less moist, 25% fat, 30g	100	425	8.5	0
Farmer's Union: Light Cheddar	105	430	7.5	0.5
Romano/Pepato	100	405	7	0
Tasty Mature Cheddar	120	510	10	0.5
Fetta: *Average all Brands:*				
Regular: 28% fat, 30g	100	380	8.5	0
100g portion	305	1275	28	0
24% fat, 30g	90	370	7	0
Reduced Fat (16% fat)	70	295	5	0
Marinated, drained, 30G	105	440	9	0
Gloucester, 30g	120	508	10	0
Goat/Chèvre Cheese:				
Australian Goats Milk Feta, 25g	60	260	5	0.5
Herb & Garlic *(South Cape)*, 25g	60	260	5	0.5
Gorgonzola, 30g	105	440	8.5	0.5
Gouda, 30g	110	460	9	0
Gjetost, 30g	140	585	9	13
Gruyere, 30g	125	520	10	0
Haloumi: *Lemnos*, 30g	85	355	8	0.5
Pittas, 30g	95	395	7	1
Havarti, 30g	120	510	11	0

Item	Cal	kJ	Fat	Cb
Per 30g Unless Indicated				
Italian Grated Cheese, 25g	100	415	8	0
Jarlsberg: Regular	105	438	8	0
Lite, 30g	80	335	5	0
Kraft: *Per 21g Slice*				
Singles: Original	60	255	4.5	1
Cheddar; Extra Tasty Style	70	295	5.5	0.5
Free	30	135	0.5	2
Light; Light n'Tasty	50	215	3.5	0
Swiss Style	65	280	5	0
Cheese Slices, 21g	70	285	6	0.5
Cheese Spread: *Per 1 Tablespoon, 20g*				
Cheddar	60	240	5	1
Light Cheddar Cheese	50	205	3.5	1.5
Cream Cheese	65	260	6	0.5
Light Cream Cheese	55	230	4.5	1.5
Cheestik: Stick, 20g	70	285	6	1
Wedge, 20g	70	285	6	1
Cheesy Pops, 12g	40	170	3.5	0.5
Fridge Sticks, 20g stick	55	230	4	1
Live Active:				
Light Slices (1), 20.5g	40	175	2.5	1
Cream Cheese, Light, 40g tub	55	235	3	2
Non-Refrigerated Cheese: *Per Serving*				
Cheddar (Kraft), 25g	80	340	6.5	0
(The) Laughing Cow: 18g portion	50	220	5	1
Light, 18g portion	30	120	2	1
Kiri Cream Cheese Spread, 18g	60	255	6	0.5
Mainland: *Per 4 Slices, 45g*				
Extra Tasty	105	425	6.5	0
Tasty	95	400	8	0
Mascarpone (49% fat), 50g	215	900	24	1.5
Wattle Valley, (42% Fat), 50g	200	835	21	1.5
Mozzarella: Pizza, ½ cup, 75g	275	1145	22	0.5
Regular, 30g	95	385	7	0
Shredded, 2 Tbsp, 25g	80	330	6	0
Sliced, 21g	65	270	4.5	0
Reduced Fat/Light *(Mil Lel; Perfect Italiano)*, Shredded, 2 Tbsp, 25g	60	250	3.5	0
Muenster, 30g	110	460	9	0.5
Neufchatel, average, 30g	95	400	9.5	0.5
Nimbin, billy, 30g	115	490	9.5	0
Nut & Fruit Cheese, 30g	105	440	8.5	5
Paneer *(Lemnos)*, ½ packet, 100g	125	530	7.5	0

Updated Nutrition Data ~ www.CalorieKing.com.au
Persons with Diabetes ~ See Disclaimer (Page 22)

Cheese ~ Cream Cheese ◆ Snacks

Cheese A-Z (Cont)

Per 30g Unless Indicated

Item	Cal	kJ	Fat	Cb
Parmesan, Grated, 4 Tbsp	140	580	10	0
Kraft (non-refrigerated): 2 tsp	45	195	3.5	0.3
Cheese Blend, 2 tsp	40	170	2	3
Pasta Cheese, Shredded, 2 Tbsp, 25g	90	385	7.5	0
Pecorino, 30g	105	445	8	0
Pepato, 30g	105	430	7	0.7

Philadelphia Cream Cheese: *Per 30g Unless Indicated*

Item	Cal	kJ	Fat	Cb
Regular Block:				
10g Serve	35	145	3.5	0.5
1 Tbsp, 20g	70	295	7	0.5
½ cup, 125g	440	1840	42	3.5
250g block	880	3675	85	6.5
Light Block:				
2 tsp, 10g	25	100	2.5	0.5
1 Tbsp, 20g	50	200	4.5	0.5
Regular Spreadable:				
2 tsp, 10g	30	115	2.5	0.5
1 Tbsp, 20g	55	230	5	0.5
½ cup, 125g	345	1440	32	4
250g tub	690	2875	64	8.5
Minis, 40g	105	440	10	1.5
Flavours: Chives & Onion, 40g	75	300	5.5	2
Light Spreadable:				
2 tsp, 10g	20	80	1.5	0.5
1 Tbsp, 20g	35	155	3	1
Minis, 40g	70	300	5.5	1.5
Extra Light (5% Fat), 20g	25	110	1	1.5
Pizza Cheese, 2 Tbsp, 25g	80	325	5.5	0
Provolone, Raclette	110	460	9	0
Quark/Quarg: Average, 30g	50	200	3	1
Burra, Skim, ½ cup, 120g	90	380	0.5	3.5

Ricotta Cheese:

Item	Cal	kJ	Fat	Cb
Creamed (10% fat): 1 T., 20g	30	115	2	0.5
¼ cup, 70g	95	395	7	2
100g portion	135	565	10	2.5
Pantalica, Low-Fat, 25g	25	110	1	1
Perfect Italiano, (10% Fat):				
¼ cup, 70g	90	375	7	2
Light (6% Fat):				
1 Tbsp, 20g	15	65	1	0.5
¼ cup, 70g	55	225	3.5	1.5
100g portion	75	320	5	2
Extra Light, 25g	15	50	0.5	0.5
Baked Ricotta: Avg all brands, 30g	90	380	7	1
50g portion	150	630	12	2
Romano, 30g	115	470	8.5	0
Shredded, 2 Tbsp, 20g	75	315	6	0
Roquefort, 30g	110	465	9	0.5
Sheep's Milk Cheese, 30g	85	350	7	0
Shredded Cheese: Average				
25g portion	90	385	7.5	0
½ cup, 60g	221	925	17	0.3
Light, 25g	85	350	6	0
Mozarella: Regular, average, 25g	80	330	6	0
Light (eg. Perfect): 25g	60	250	3.5	0
½ cup, 60g	205	855	15	0.3
St Claire; St Paulin, avg., 30g	110	460	8	0
Stilton, 30g	125	515	11	0
Stracchino, 30g	85	360	6.5	0
Swiss: 30g	115	480	9	0
Slices, 21g	75	315	6	0
Reduced Fat, 30g	100	415	6.5	0
Watsonia, Lite	100	430	7	0.2
Weight Watchers: 21g	70	300	5	0
Grated, Tasty, 30g	100	405	7	0.2
Reduced Fat, Natural Cheddar Slices, 21g	45	190	3	1
Westacre (Aldi):				
Light Cheddar Slices, 21g	75	300	5	0.5

Cheese Snacks ~ Brands

Item	Cal	kJ	Fat	Cb
Coles, Cheese & Crackers, all flavours, 22g	90	360	5.5	7
Damora (Aldi):				
Dippits: Cheddar, 22g pack	90	360	5.5	7
French Onion, 22g pack	85	360	5.5	17
Kraft: *Per Packet*				
Dunkers, av. all flav., 104g	360	1510	19	37
Le Snak:				
Cheese varieties, 22g	90	370	6	6
Deli, average 36.6g	90	365	4	11
On The Go (Mainland):				
Extra Tasty: 30g	130	530	8	7.5
Light, 30g	110	465	6	7.5
Tasty	125	525	11	7.5
Snackabouts:				
Cheese Spread	105	430	6.5	8.5
Chicken Flavour	115	485	7.5	9
Nuts Peanut Butter	145	605	9.5	11
Vegemite	85	350	2	11
Vegemite, Cheesybite	95	400	4.5	10
The Laughing Cow, Cheez Dippers, 35g	100	430	6	9
Weight Watchers, Cheese & Crackers	110	455	6	7

Cheese Substitutes ~ Brands

Item	Cal	kJ	Fat	Cb
Soycheese (Simply Better):				
Mild, 30g	85	360	8	0.5
Chives, 30g	100	410	8.5	0.5
Tofutti: Slices (1), 19g	70	290	5	2
Better Than Cream Cheese, 30g	80	335	8	1

Chicken

Chicken Meat ~ Raw

	Cal	kJ	Fat	Cb
Breast Meat: *Per 100g, Edible Portion Without Bone*				
With skin	165	690	9.5	0
Lean, without skin	105	440	1.5	0
Single Breast:				
Medium size: With skin, 150g	245	1025	14	0
Lean, without skin, 130g	135	565	2	0
Large size, without skin, 240g	360	1505	4	0
Double Breast: *Double the figures of single breast*				
Thigh Meat: *Per 100g, Edible Portion Without Bone*				
With skin	225	940	18	0
Lean, without skin	120	500	5	0
Medium size:				
With skin, 115g	260	1080	21	0
Lean, without skin, 100g	120	500	5	0
Tenderloins, without skin, 100g	120	500	5	0
Drumstick: *Weights with Bone*				
Per 100g: With skin	115	480	7	0
Lean, without skin	90	370	5.5	0
Medium size:				
With skin, 125g	145	600	9	0
Lean, without skin, 115g	105	440	6.5	0
Large size: With skin, 160g	185	770	11	0
Lean, without skin, 140g	125	520	7.5	0
Wing: *Per 100g, Weights with Bone and Skin*				
Medium size, 80g	125	520	10	0
Large size, 125g	195	810	15	0
Chicken Skin: *Raw, 100g*	360	1510	34	0
Baked, 100g	460	1920	47	0

Roasted Chicken

Note: 100g weight is for edible portion only and does not include bone weight.

	Cal	kJ	Fat	Cb
Breast Meat: With Skin	190	790	8.5	0
Lean, without skin	150	635	4	0
Thigh Meat: With skin	225	940	15	0
Lean, without skin	175	735	9	0
Drumstick: With skin	220	920	13	0
Lean, without skin	180	750	7.5	0
Wing: With skin	260	1090	17	0
Lean, without skin	195	810	8	0

Rotisseried Chicken:
If no basting or added fat, use 'roasted' figures.
If basted with fat or oil:
Add per 100g meat ~ 20 calories/85kJ, 2g fat

Updated Nutrition Data ~ www.CalorieKing.com.au
Persons with Diabetes ~ See Disclaimer (Page 22)

Quarter Chicken ~ Roasted

	Cal	kJ	Fat	Cb
Dry Roasted/Rotisseried: *No Added Fat*				
Breast Quarter: *Breast + Wing*				
Small: With skin	380	1590	23	0
Lean, without skin	200	835	6	0
Large: With skin	590	2470	36	0
Lean, without skin	330	1380	11	0
Leg Quarter: *Drumstick + Thigh*				
Small: With skin	290	1210	18	0
Lean, without skin	190	800	9	0
Large: With skin	350	1460	22	0
Lean, without skin	250	1050	12	0

Chicken Portions ~ Roasted

	Cal	kJ	Fat	Cb
Roasted or Rotisseried: *No Added Fat*				
Breast:				
Small: With skin	310	1300	18	0
Lean, without skin	185	770	5	0
Medium: With skin	420	1755	25	0
Lean, without skin	250	1040	8	0
Large: With skin	485	2030	29	0
Lean, without skin	290	1215	9	0
Drumstick:				
Small: With skin	100	420	6	0
Lean, without skin	65	270	3	0
Large: With skin	120	500	8	0
Lean, without skin	85	355	4	0
Thigh:				
Small: With skin	185	775	12	0
Lean, without skin	125	520	6	0
Large: With skin	225	945	14	0
Lean, without skin	165	690	8	0
Wing:				
Small: With skin	70	290	5	0
Lean, without skin	20	85	1	0
Large: With skin	100	420	7	0
Lean, without skin	40	170	2	0

Crumbed & Pan Fried
Add to the above figures for roasted:
Per 100g cooked chicken - 45 cal/190 kJ/5g fat
Battered & Deep-Fried
See KFC ~ *See Page 193*

Chicken Sizes

Small	~	Size 9-11 (0.9-1.1 kg)
Medium	~	Size 12-15 (1.2-1.5 kg)
Large	~	Size 16-21 (1.6-2.1 kg)
Extra Large	~	Size 22-25 (2.2-2.5 kg)

C Chicken Products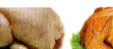

Chicken Offal

	Cal	kJ	Fat	Cb
Giblets, fried, 50g	125	520	6	1.5
Livers: Raw, 100g	115	490	5	0
Floured & Fried, 100g	200	835	11	1.5
Neck, simmered, with skin	100	420	7	0
Stuffing, average all types, ¼ cup, 50g	100	420	4	11

Chicken Products ~ Brands

Ingham: *Per Serving*

	Cal	kJ	Fat	Cb
Crumbed: Breast Kiev, 175g	460	1915	29	27
Breast Schnitzel, 200g	440	1845	19	48
Breast Tenders, 67g	125	515	9	9.5
Thigh Fillets, 100g	215	895	13	15
Free Range: *Per 100g*				
Breast Fillet	110	470	2.5	1
Drumstick	140	580	7.5	2
Thigh Fillet	140	595	7.5	1.5
Marinated:				
Kebabs: Homestyle BBQ / Satay, 180g	290	1215	13	14
BBQ Plum, 180g	280	1155	13	6.5
Honey Soy, 180g	250	1050	10	9
Half Chicken, Chilli & Garlic, 318g	535	2235	38	2
Whole: BBQ, 250g	350	1465	20	3.5
Festive Favourite, 250g	460	1920	29	12
Microwave Roast, 250g	350	1465	18	2.5
Roll, 250g	515	2160	38	17
Frozen:				
Asteroids: Cheese & Bacon, ⅓ pkt, 100g	235	1975	13	15
Tempura	210	880	12	12
Breast Chipees, (10), 100g	255	1060	15	15
Breast Kiev: Cordon Bleu, 175g	295	1230	32	40
Garlic Butter, 175g	455	1915	29	27
Breast Munchies, ¼ packet, 100g	260	1090	13	26
Breast Tenders: Honey & Soy, 67g	130	550	5	12
Original; Sweet Chilli, 67g	135	565	5.5	12
Tempura, 67g	110	460	3.5	8.5
Chicken Strips, Original, 62g	135	555	7.5	7.5
Chicken Twirls: Cheddar, 100g	240	1010	13	19
Southern Style, 100g	240	1000	12	20
Duets: Alfredo, 175g	460	1920	33	24
Broccoli & Cheese, 175g	350	1455	19	23
Cordon Bleu, 175g	400	1665	24	22
Nuggets: Original (4), 100g	245	1015	13	18
Tempura (5), 100g	230	960	12	18
Premium Ribbons:				
Coconut, 100g	150	630	5	10
Southern Style, 100g	155	650	5.5	10
Tempura, 100g	180	760	7.5	12
Schnitzels, Original (1), 200g	490	2060	28	43
Selections, Breast, Sweet Thai Chilli, 118g	210	890	10	8.5

Lenard's:
If frying, add 50 cal/210 kJ/5g fat per 100g serve.
Per Serving, Uncooked

	Cal	kJ	Fat	Cb
Chicken Mince, raw, ⅕ packet, 100g	105	440	2	1
Baguette: Camembert & Bacon	580	2425	38	16
Florentine, 285g	575	2405	39	14
Mild Thai, 285g	570	2370	37	18
Breast Pastelle:				
Malaysian Peanut Sate, 250g	435	1815	15	34
Mushroom & White Wine, 250g	385	1600	11	32
Pumpkin & Cashew, 250g	410	1705	11	36
Smoked Salmon, 250g	405	1695	13	33
Casserole: Chasseur, 250g	430	1785	25	19
Honey Mustard, 250g	460	1910	27	19
Tuscan, 250g	430	1795	27	13
Crumbed: Cordon Bleu Fillet, 200g	365	1535	19	18
Ham & Asparagus Fillet, 200g	310	1290	13	19
Hawaiian Fillet, 196g	310	1295	13	20
Kiev, 192g	375	1560	20	17
Parmigiana Fillet, 204g	360	1505	20	15
Schnitzel: Cajun, 180g	395	1640	12	43
Chicken, 180g	395	1655	12	44
Herb & Garlic, 180g	395	1655	12	44
Wings: Cajun, 100g	220	905	11	13
Southern Style, 100g	230	950	14	10
Easyliving: Bombay Chicken, 250g	370	1545	19	26
Chicken Cacciatore, 250g	240	995	10	15
Chicken Lasagne, 250g	440	1845	22	36
Trad. Italian Meatballs, 250g	415	1730	23	26
Enchilada: Hawaiian Chicken, 270g	540	2260	28	43
Mild Mexican, 270g	505	2100	22	46
Kebabs: BBQ (1), 90g	115	485	4.5	5.5
Chinese Honey (1), 90g	120	505	5	5
Satay (1), 90g	130	545	6	5.5
Sundried Tomato (1), 90g	115	480	4.5	5
Teriyaki & Garlic (1), 90g	115	485	4.5	5
Marinated Breast, on bone,				
Souvlaki, 250g	485	2030	28	5
Portuguese, 250g	490	2040	28	7
Sundried Tomato, 250g	485	2030	28	6
Marinated Cutlets: BBQ, 200g	390	1620	26	8
Cacciatore, 200g	395	1655	28	4.5
Honey Mustard, 200g	395	1650	27	7
Sweet Thai Chilli, 200g	395	1655	26	11
Tandoori, 200g	390	1625	26	6.5

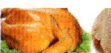

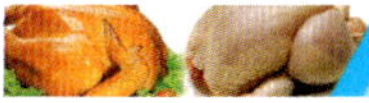

Chicken Products

Lenard's (Cont):	Cal	kJ	Fat	Cb
Marinated Drumsticks: Chinese Honey	290	1210	16	6
Sundried Tomato, 200g	285	1185	15	5.5
Marinated Breast Steaks: Honey Mustd.	305	1280	8	6.5
Sweet Thai Chilli, 250g	310	1285	7	10
Teriyaki & Garlic, 250g	300	1250	7.5	10
Thai Spice, 250g	305	1270	7.5	8.5
Marinated Wings: BBQ, 100g	190	795	12	4.5
Chinese Honey, 100g	190	800	12	5
Satay, 100g	195	820	12	5
Sweet Thai Chilli, 100g	195	810	12	5.5
Peri Peri Grill, 100g	190	790	14	3
Thai King, 100g	190	800	12	5
Mignon, Garlic, 165g	370	1550	30	1.5
Parcels: Sweet Asian, 155g	415	1720	21	41
Thai Curry, 155g	395	1645	22	34
Pillows: Mild Curry, 220g	560	2335	32	46
Mushroom Florentine, 220g	535	2225	33	36
Tandoori, 220g	540	2250	32	40
Pocketed Breast:				
Baby Spinach, Dill & Fennel, 180g	230	960	5	9
Balsamic & Olive, 180g	205	845	3.5	10
Mild Wasabi, 180g	210	865	5.5	6
Roll-Up: Italian, 200g	300	1240	13	19
Swiss, 200g	305	1270	14	20
Rolls: Camembert & Bacon, 250g	385	1610	17	14
Dijon & Garlic, 250g	385	1610	16	17
Florentine, 250g	380	1585	17	12
Honey Macadamia, 250g	430	1805	21	23
Mild Thai, 250g	375	1555	15	15
Moroccan, 250g	390	1615	13	25
Shashlicks: BBQ, 135g	115	480	3.5	7
Portuguese (1), 135g	115	485	3.5	7.5
Stir-Fry: Chinese Honey, 250g	235	970	4.5	18
Curry, 250g	305	1265	8.5	12
Singapore Sizzle, 250g	270	1120	10	17
Sweet Thai Chilli, 250g	245	1015	5.5	13
Thai King, 250g	280	1175	7	10
Strudel: Mini, 95g	275	1150	18	19
Original Recipe, 245g	530	2200	34	32
Spinach Fetta & Pinenut, 245g	570	2390	38	30
Stuffed Quarters: Five Spice Risotto, 369g	755	3150	39	29
Lemon & Garlic Risotto, 369g	740	3095	41	20
Mango & Sweet Chilli Risotto, 378g	755	3155	37	33
Tandoori Risotto, 378g	740	3090	40	22
Wellington, 265g	585	2450	33	34

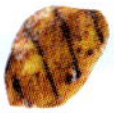

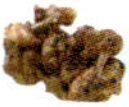

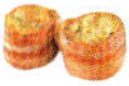

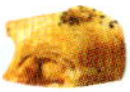

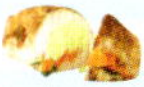

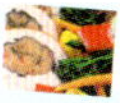

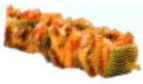

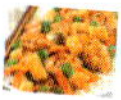

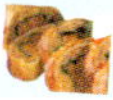

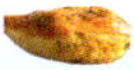

Steggles:	Cal	kJ	Fat	Cb
Frozen:				
Breast Chunks: Mild Spice, ¼ packet	170	700	8	7
Southern, ¼ packet, 100g	165	690	8	6.5
Breast: Kiev, Garlic, 200g	430	1800	24	19
Tenders: Crumbed, ⅓ pkt, 125g	255	1060	11	21
Lemon & Herb, ¼ packet, 100g	190	785	8	14
Burger, Southern (1), 90g	140	590	4.5	14
Crackles: Cheese, ¼ pkt, 100g	260	1090	14	19
Garlic, ¼ packet, 100g	205	855	11	12
Fillets: Mediterranean (1), 150g	145	595	2	16
Premium (1), 145g	255	1065	12	15
Filo, Spinach & Feta (1), 180g	420	1750	23	29
Fingers: Premium, ¼ packet, 100g	210	875	6.5	26
Salt & Vinegar, ¼ packet, 100g	235	980	10	23
Meatballs, Napolitano, 125g	135	570	3	9
Nuggets, Premium, ¼ pkt 100g	245	1020	14	19
Rissoles, Herb & Onion, ⅛ packet, 100g	195	820	9	15
Steak: Original, ¼ pkt, 100g	145	600	3	11
Garlic & Pepper, ½ pkt, 115g	170	700	2	18
Smokey BBQ, ½ pkt, 115g	130	555	0.5	5.5
Strips: Peri Peri, ¼ pkt, 100g	195	815	9	16
Southern, ¼ packet, 100g	200	840	8.5	18
Tenders, Sweet Chilli, 55g	115	480	5	11
Veggie Subs, Crunchy Pot., ¼ pkt	180	760	5	24
Wings, Oven Roasted (3), 115g	310	1290	23	3.5
Fresh/Chilled:				
Breast Fillet: Moroccan (1), 183g	235	985	5	15
Mushroom Risotto (1), 183g	240	1010	5	16
Parmigiana (1), 200g	340	1420	10	29
Breast Topper: Mushroom (1), 200g	310	1285	12	9.5
Red Pesto (1), 200g	265	1105	14	6.5
Chicken Enchilada, 250g	545	2275	34	30
Filo: Chicken & Mushroom (1), 180g	410	1710	20	30
Spinach & Feta (1), 180g	420	1750	23	29
Kebab, all flavours, 90g	135	565	6	5
Kiev, Crumbed, 180g	355	1485	18	21
Nibbles, all flavours, 100g	310	1300	25	6
Patties, crumbed (1), 50g	145	600	10	7.5
Schnitzels, (1) 180g	310	1290	9	29
Wrap, Sweet Chilli Chicken (1), 250g	515	2140	23	42
Whole Chicken:				
Family Feast, ¼, 300g	570	2390	41	1.5
Garlic & Herb, 100g	200	835	14	2.5
Microwaveable, 100g	190	780	13	2

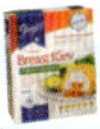

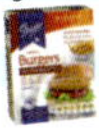

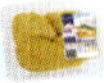

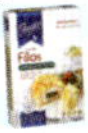

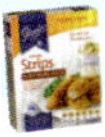

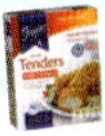

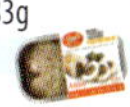

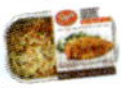

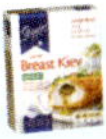

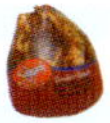

Updated Nutrition Data ~ www.CalorieKing.com.au
Persons with Diabetes ~ See Disclaimer (Page 22)

C Chicken Products ♦ Duck ♦ Turkey

Chicken Products (Cont) | Cal | kJ | Fat | Cb

Butchers & Supermarkets:
Average All Outlets:

	Cal	kJ	Fat	Cb
Baguettes: Apricot & Walnut, (1), 209g	620	2595	41	22
Camembert, Bacon & Spinach (1), 290g	615	2565	44	13
Breast Fillets: With skin, 100g	165	690	9.5	0
Without skin, 100g	105	440	2	0
Crumbed: Cordon Bleu (1), 195g	380	1590	19	22
Kiev (1), 195g	400	1660	19	22
Pamigiana (1), 200G	380	1595	8.5	19
Roma (1), 205g	365	1530	13	23
Schnitzel: Spicy (1), 180g	410	1715	13	44
Herb & Garlic (1), 180g	415	1735	13	45
Drumsticks: Raw, 100g	155	645	9.5	0
Raw, no skin, 100g	120	495	5	0
Kebab Sticks: BBQ (1), 90g	105	445	3.5	5.5
Satay (1), 90g	120	505	5	6
Teriyaki & Galic (1), 90g	105	445	3.5	6
Marinated Drumsticks: Honey Soy, 200g	270	1120	13	5.5
Sundried Tomato, 250g	330	1380	16	6
Marinated Wings: BBQ, 100g	165	685	8.5	4
Honey Soy, 100g	165	690	8.5	6.5
Satay, 100g	170	710	9	6.5
Marinated Steaks: *Per 200g*				
Honey Mustard (1)	270	1130	9.5	5.5
Sweet Thai Chilli (1)	270	1135	8.5	8.5
Teriyaki & Garlic (1)	260	1100	8.5	5
Maryland, (1) 220g	395	1635	23	12
Roast Chicken, Cooked: Whole, 750g	1335	5590	60	42
Half, 375g	670	2795	30	21
Roll Ups: Italian (1), 225g	335	1390	14	26
Mexian (1), 225g	330	1385	13	29
Peking (1), 225g	325	1360	12	30
Swiss (1), 215g	345	1450	16	25
Sausages: Chipolata (1), 60g	155	635	13	3
Bratwurst (1), 120g	320	1335	27	5.5
Curry (1), 120g	320	1335	27	6
Plain (1), 120g	315	1320	27	5.5
Sage & Garlic (1), 120g	320	1335	27	6

Duck & Goose

	Cal	kJ	Fat	Cb
Duck: Roasted, meat only, 100g	190	790	10	0
Meat, fat & skin, 100g	340	1420	29	0
Goose: Roasted, meat only, 100g	240	995	4.5	0
Meat, fat & skin, 100g	305	1275	22	0
Stuffing, average all brands, 100g	200	840	8	22

Turkey Products, Fresh ~ Brands | Cal | kJ | Fat | Cb

	Cal	kJ	Fat	Cb
Raw: Meat + Skin, 100g	160	665	8.5	0
Without Skin, 100g	120	490	3.5	0
Roasted Turkey: *Per 100g*				
Light: With Skin	170	710	7	0
Without Skin	155	650	4	0
Dark: With skin	220	910	13	0
Without Skin	170	710	7	0
Coles: *Per Serving*				
Turkey Breast Classic: Cranberry, 100g	140	585	5	7
Mince, 100g	155	650	10	0.5
Ingham: *Per Serving*				
Breast Fillet, 250g	290	1200	3.5	3
Breast Steak, 200g	200	840	1	0
Classic Breast: Oven Roasted, 100g	125	525	5	1
Smoked, 100g	125	510	4	1.5
Breast: Oven Roasted, 100g	105	445	4	4
Supreme, Ham, 100g	105	445	3	1.5
Drumstick, 250g	405	1685	24	0
Marinated: Breast Buffet, average, 250g	285	1185	11	3
Whole Turkey, 250g	250	1040	6.5	2.5
Mince, 200g	310	1295	19	1
Mini Drumstick, 250g	265	1100	4.5	1.5
Tenderloins, 200g	210	875	2.5	1
Thigh Chops, 250g	410	1705	22	1.5
Thigh Strips, 200g	340	1425	21	1
Turkey Sausages: Bratwurst (1), 80g	130	540	9	2
Spanish Chorizo, (1), 80g	130	545	8	3

Turkey Products, Frozen ~ Brands

Ingham: *Per Serving (Frozen)*

	Cal	kJ	Fat	Cb
Breast: Roast, 200g	170	720	2	3
With Cranberry Apple Stuffing, 200g	265	1110	12	9
With Sweet Herb & Mustard, 200g	175	735	1.5	4.5
Kiev, 175g	420	1750	27	20
Thigh Roast, 200g	295	1240	18	4.5
Whole Turkey: 250g	340	1425	14	1.5

Steggles: *Per Serving*

	Cal	kJ	Fat	Cb
Breast: Buffet Carve, 100g	130	540	4.5	3.5
Roast, 167g	210	875	7.5	4.5
Hindquarter, 100g	130	555	6	0
Steaks, Crumbed, 100g	130	540	2.5	8
Thigh Roast, 167g	205	860	8	4.5
Whole Turkey, 100g	140	575	7	0.5

Chocolate ◆ Confectionery

Chocolate ~ Quick Guide

Chocolate:
Average All Brands

Blocks: Plain/Nuts/Fruit, average

	Cal	kJ	Fat	Cb
1 small square, 5g	27	110	1.5	3
5 squares, 25g	130	550	7.5	15
1 Small block, 100g	530	2215	30	58
1 Large block, 200g	1050	4380	60	116
1 Family block, 250g	1325	5540	75	145

Dark Chocolate:

	Cal	kJ	Fat	Cb
45% Cocoa, 100g	530	2210	30	58
70% Cocoa: Lindt, 100g	520	2180	40	33
Club (Nestle), 100g	555	2320	45	31
85% Cocoa (Lindt), 100g	530	2210	46	19

White Chocolate: 30g

	Cal	kJ	Fat	Cb
White Chocolate: 30g	165	690	10	17
50g Bar	280	1170	17	28
1 large block, 200g	1120	4680	69	112

Other Chocolate ~ Quick Guide

Boxes: *(Milk Tray/Roses)*
Average all brands:

	Cal	kJ	Fat	Cb
1 chocolate	60	250	2	8
1 small box, 225g	1085	4525	52	142

After Dinner Mints, 1 mint — 35 | 150 | 1 | 6

Caramel Centre:

	Cal	kJ	Fat	Cb
Milk Caramel *(Nestle)*, 30g	150	630	7	20
Caramello *(Cadbury)*, 30g	150	615	8	18
Caramel *(Dove)*, 30g	150	630	8	18

Cream/Peppermint filled:

	Cal	kJ	Fat	Cb
4 squares, 30g	145	610	6.5	20
1 medium block, 100g	485	2030	22	65

Chocolate Coated Nuts:

	Cal	kJ	Fat	Cb
Peanuts, Almonds: 30g	180	755	14	8.5
1 packet, 100g	605	2520	45	29

Choc Coated Ginger, (1) 11g — 50 | 215 | 2.5 | 7
Choc Coated Raisins, 30g — 120 | 500 | 4.5 | 17

Chocolate Fudge: 30g

	Cal	kJ	Fat	Cb
Chocolate Fudge: 30g	130	545	4	23
With Nuts, 30g	140	585	5	24

Cooking Choc/Bits/Melts: 100g

	Cal	kJ	Fat	Cb
Cooking Choc/Bits/Melts: 100g	545	2270	32	57
Freddo Buttons, (20), 12.5g	65	280	4	7
M&M's Minis, ⅓ packet, 46g	230	960	10	31

Liqueur Filled, e.g. Liqueur Cherries,
average, 1 piece, 12g — 50 | 210 | 2 | 6

Rocklea Road *(Darrell Lea)*, 50g — 260 | 1085 | 16 | 26
Truffles, 1 medium, 21g — 120 | 505 | 8.5 | 10

Carob: Average, 30g

	Cal	kJ	Fat	Cb
Carob: Average, 30g	130	550	9	14
100g block	440	1830	30	47
Buttons/Bits, 100g	510	2140	30	63

Updated Nutrition Data ~ www.CalorieKing.com.au
Persons with Diabetes ~ See Disclaimer (Page 22)

Chocolate Gift Boxes ~ Brands

	Cal	kJ	Fat	Cb
Cadbury Roses: 150g box	720	3015	35	95
225g box	1085	4525	52	142
450g box	2165	9045	105	285
Cadbury Milk Tray: 200g box	1000	4160	56	117
420g box	2095	8740	117	246
560g box	2790	11650	156	328
Cadbury Favourites: 95g box	475	1985	25	56
300g box	1500	6270	78	177
Darrell Lea, Dark Choc Ginger, 200g box	845	3520	29	137
Ernest Hillier, Delectable Classics, 250g	1190	4970	65	143
Guylian: La Trufflina, 90g box	550	2305	43	38
Seashell Original, 125g box	685	2865	44	66
Lindt: Fioretto, 138g box	760	3180	47	75
Lindola, 180g box	985	4125	67	88
Lindor Hazelnut, 150g box	940	3930	74	63
Petits Desserts, 170g box	960	4015	66	82
Swiss, Thins, 125g box	690	2875	43	69
Toblerone, Tobelle, 160g box	805	3380	45	93

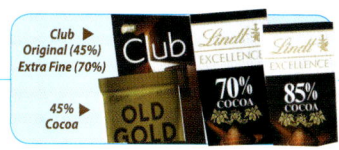

Club ▶ Original (45%) Extra Fine (70%)
45% Cocoa

Dark chocolate may contain beneficial antioxidants – but still limit quantity for weight control.

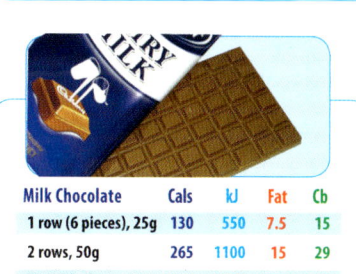

Milk Chocolate	Cals	kJ	Fat	Cb
1 row (6 pieces), 25g	130	550	7.5	15
2 rows, 50g	265	1100	15	29
250g block	1325	5540	75	145

Chocolate ◆ Confectionery

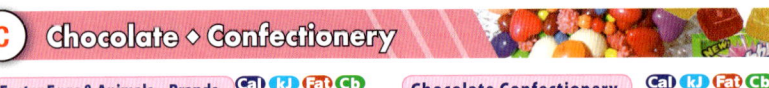

Easter Eggs & Animals ~ Brands

	Cal	kJ	Fat	Cb
Cadbury: *Per Egg*				
Hunting Eggs, 17g	90	380	5	10
Deluxe Bunny, 100g	560	2335	35	54
Egg: Cherry Ripe, 110g	565	2365	34	61
Dairy Milk, 105g	565	2352	31	62
Dream, 110g	760	3160	38	61
Old Gold, 100g	535	2230	33	55
Creme Eggs: Milk Chocolate, 39g	175	720	6	28
Mini: Caramello, 13g	65	265	3	8
Dairy Milk, 6.8g	75	305	4	8
Lindt: Easter Bunny, 100g	565	2365	36	55
Gold Bunny, 100g	535	2240	32	55
Gold Egg, 70% Cocoa, 100g	525	2180	41	33
Mini Egg, Dark Chocolate, 16g	100	410	8	7
Mini Bunny, Milk Chocolate, 10g	55	225	4	4
Red Tulip: *Per Chocolate Egg*				
Size No. 2 (8.5cm long/35g)	180	745	9	22
Size No. 4 (11.5cm long/75g)	385	1600	20	47
Size No. 6 (13cm long/100g)	510	2130	26	62
Size No. 9 (15.5cm long/150g)	765	3195	39	93
Size No. 12 (18.5cm long/200g)	1020	4260	52	124
Easter Rabbit: Classic, 200g	1030	4300	52	125
Carnival Rabbit, 180g	925	3870	46	113
Sweet William:				
Easter Bunnies: Original, 13.5g	75	300	4.5	7
Rice Crackle, 75g pkt	375	1570	22	43
No Added Sugar, 13.5g	65	280	4.5	1.5
Hard Candy Easter Eggs:				
Average: Small, 70g	185	775	0	46
Medium, 100g	265	1105	0	65
Large, 200g	530	2210	0	130

Christmas Novelties ~ Brands

	Cal	kJ	Fat	Cb
Cadbury: Caramello Santa, 20g	100	420	5.5	12
Christmas Baubles, 5 pieces, 25g	125	515	5	18
Marshmallow Santa, 35g	150	615	3.5	27
Magical Elves, 12g	65	265	3.5	7.5
Darrell Lea:				
Jingle Bells (4), 20g	110	445	6	12
Mini Santa, 20g	110	445	6	12
Xmas Puddings, mini (1), 17g	85	350	4.5	9
Xmas Nougat Pudding, 150g	670	2800	25	105
Lindt: Reindeer, 100g	550	2280	33	56
Christmas Santas, Mini, 10g	60	245	4	5
Candy Canes: Giant (20cm), 85g	300	1250	0	74
Medium (13cm), 15g	55	230	0	14
Mini (6cm), 7g	30	120	0	7

Chocolate Confectionery

	Cal	kJ	Fat	Cb
Per Bar/Piece Unless Indicated				
Aero (Nestle):				
Bars: Choc./Mint, average, 40g	215	900	13	23
Fun Size, 12g	65	270	4	7
Block, (118g) 3 pcs, 15g	80	340	5	8.5
Almond Roca, 1 piece	70	290	5	6
Aniseed Rings:				
Choc-coated (1), 11g	50	200	2	8
Darrell Lea (1), 15g	60	245	1.5	12
Anthon Berg, Liqueur Bottle	80	335	4	8.5
Baci (Perugino), 1 piece, 15g	85	355	6	7
Ballantyne:				
Ginger Lovers, 25g	110	450	4	18
Entertainments, 1 sachet	30	135	1	5.5
Roast Hazelnut & Honey Roast Cashew, 25g	140	575	8.5	13
Bertie Beetle, 10g	50	210	2.5	7
Black Forest (Cadbury), 4 pieces, 25g	130	535	6.5	16
Boost Bar (Cadbury):				
60g bar	315	1310	17	36
Twin Pack, 77g	400	1680	22	46
Max Caramel, 60g	295	1220	16	37
Mini/Fun Size, 14g	75	305	4	8.5
Stix, Twin Pack, 55g	280	1160	16	34
Bounty: 45g bar, average	220	910	12	26
Mini/Fun Size, 14g bar	70	285	3.5	8
Brunch Bar (Cadbury):				
Hazelnut, 35g	155	635	7	20
Mixed Berry, 35g	155	640	5.5	23
Peanut, 35g	180	755	11	18
Toasted Coconut, 35g	160	675	7.5	21
Bubbly Chocolate (Cadbury):				
40g bar, avg all types	220	915	13	23
Blocks (155g), avg, 3 pces, 25g	135	560	8	15
Cadbury:				
Bars, 50g bar/roll	265	1110	15	29
75g bar	400	1665	22	43
Mini/Fun Size, 18g bar	95	400	5.5	11
Miniatures, 10g each	50	220	3	6
Blocks:				
135g Block: 4 pieces, 25g	135	560	7.5	15
Whole Block, 135g	725	3025	40	80
220g Block: 4 pieces, 25g	135	560	7.5	15
Whole Block, 220g	1180	4930	65	130
Buttons, 8 pieces, 25g	135	560	7.5	15
Dark Almonds, 7 pieces, 50g	265	1100	17	23

Chocolate ♦ Confectionery

Per Bar/Piece Unless Indicated

	Cal	kJ	Fat	Cb
Caramel Whip, 65g bar	295	1235	11	46
Caramello (Cadbury):				
Bars: 55g	270	1130	14	33
75g	370	1540	19	45
Block (220g), 2 rows, 50g	250	1030	13	30
Nibbles, 8 pieces, 25g	125	520	6	16
Caramello: Creme Egg, 39g	175	720	6	28
Koalas: 20g	100	410	5	12
Twin, 40g	195	820	10	24
Celebrations (MasterFoods), 11g	60	250	3.5	6.5
Cherry Ripe:				
Bars: 52g Bar	240	1010	12	30
Twin Pack, 80g	370	1550	19	46
Fun/Treat Size, 18g	85	350	4.5	11
Double Dipped, 50g	250	1040	16	23
Chocolate Almonds, (7) 50g	270	1125	17	23
Chocolate Eclair (Pascall), 1 piece	30	120	1	4
Chocolate Honeycomb ~ See page 82				
Chocolate Peanuts, 13-14 pces, 50g	240	1170	19	22
Chokito Bars: 55g	260	1085	10	38
Twin Pack, 70g	330	1380	13	49
Club (Nestlé), Blocks (200g):				
Orange, 3 pieces, 22.5g	120	490	7	12
Original, (3), 22.5g	120	505	7	13
Roasted Almond (3), 22.5g	125	525	8	11
Coconut Rough, 50g	250	1035	21	16
Coins: 1 large, 6g	30	130	1.5	3.5
80g bag	410	1720	21	50
Coles, Multi Packs:				
Cherry Bites (1)	85	350	4	11
Chocolate Wafer Breaks (1)	90	375	5	10
Malt Balls, 1 mini pack	80	340	4	11
Nutty Nougat Caramel (1)	100	420	6	11
Blocks: Belgian Dark, 25g	145	595	12	8
Belgian White, 25g	140	585	8.5	15
Fruit & Nut, 5 pieces, 34g	170	720	9.5	20
Mint Chocolate, 50g	265	1110	15	30
Cote d'Or: Bouchee, Milk, 25g	130	555	7.5	15
Milk & Almond, 45g	250	1050	17	23
Nougatti, 30g	145	605	7.5	17
Creme Egg (Cadbury),				
Egg, 39g	175	720	6	28

Chocolate (Cont)

Per Bar/Piece Unless Indicated

	Cal	kJ	Fat	Cb
Crunch (Nestlé):				
45g bar	235	980	13	27
King Size, 80g bar	420	1745	23	48
Crunchie: Original, 50g bar	245	1015	11	35
Mini/Snack, 18g bar	90	380	4	13
Block, 135g	665	2770	34	81
Curly Wurly (Cadbury), 26g	120	490	4.5	18
Daintree Estates:				
Dark Chocolate, 70% Cocoa, ¼ block, 20g	110	468	9	9
Milk Chocolate, 45% Cocoa, ¼ block, 20g	115	480	8	10
Darrell Lea:				
Choc-Coated Bars: Per Bar				
Ginger Fudge, 55g	250	1040	9	40
Peanut Brittle, 45g	215	900	10	29
Nougat: Almond, 45g	205	860	8	31
Peppermint, 40g	170	715	4.5	31
Strawberry, 40g	170	715	4.5	31
Confectionery:				
Aniseed Rings: Milk Chocolate (2), 30g	120	495	2.5	23
Dark Chocolate (2), 30g	115	485	2.5	23
Licorice Bullets:				
Dark Choc Strawberry, 30g	120	490	3	20
Milk Chocolate, 26g	100	430	3.5	11
White Choc Raspberry, 20g	85	360	3	14
Caramel Snows, 18g	80	325	3	13
Choc: Orange Balls (2), 13g	65	265	2.5	9
Peanuts, 25g	160	665	11	12
Peanut Brittle, 45g	215	900	10	29
Peanut Brittle Fingers, 3 pieces, 21g	105	435	5	13
Peanut Clusters, 25g	150	600	10	10
Scorched Almonds, 30g	160	680	10	15
Coconut Ice, 25g	110	465	5	17
Fruit Jubes (4), 28g	100	405	0	24
Ginger Milk Chocolate, 12.5g	55	230	2	9
Honeycomb, Choc-Coated, 2 pcs, 30g	120	495	6	16
Milk Choc, pieces 30g	110	465	3	19
Toasted Marshmallows, 19g	85	350	4	11
Rocklea Road:				
Dark, 145g packet	725	3030	42	75
Milk, 145g packet	755	3150	44	76
White, 145g packet	775	3235	47	76

Updated Nutrition Data ~ www.CalorieKing.com.au
Persons with Diabetes ~ See Disclaimer (Page 22)

Chocolate ◆ Confectionery

Chocolate (Cont)

	Cal	kJ	Fat	Cb
Per Bar/Piece Unless Indicated				
Dove Individuals *(Mars)*				
Caramel, 7.7g	40	160	2	5
Dark Chocolate, 7g	40	160	2.5	4
Milk Chocolate, 7g	40	160	2.5	4
Peppermint, 7.7g	40	160	2	5
Dream *(Cadbury)*:				
Dream, 4 pieces, 25g	140	590	8.5	14
Dream Egg, 38g	260	1090	13	21
Droste Pastilles: 5 pieces, 25g				
Dark	135	570	8.5	15
Extra Dark, 75%	140	595	11	11
Milk & White	140	585	9	14
Empower, Low Carb Choc, 4 squares	80	325	6	1
Favourites *(Cadbury)*, 1 piece	60	255	3	8
Ferrero Rocher: Classic (1)	75	300	5.5	5.5
Rondnoir (1), 10g	55	220	3.5	4.5
Flake *(Cadbury)*: 30g bar	160	670	9	17
Mini Size, 14g	75	315	4.5	8
Bites, 1 piece, 3.6g	20	85	1	2
Freddo *(Cadbury)*:				
Dairy Milk/White, 15g	80	330	4.5	8.5
Giant Freddo, average, 35g	185	775	11	20
Milky Top, 10g	55	230	3	6
100's & 1,000's, 35g	180	750	9	23
Furry Friends *(Cadbury)*,				
1 piece, 15g	80	330	4.5	8.5
Fruit & Nut *(Cadbury)*:				
50g bar	255	1055	14	28
75g bar	380	1590	20	42
220g block, serving, 2 rows, 8 pieces	255	1065	14	29
Fund-Raiser Bars, 100g	550	2300	30	60
Ginger, Choc-Coated, 8g	40	155	1.5	6.5
Gold Choc Coins, (80g Bag)				
10 pieces, 41g	215	900	11	26
Golden Rough *(Nestlé)*, 20g	110	455	6.5	11
Guylian: Seashells, 11g	60	250	4	6
Praline Seashell bar, 40g	230	960	16	20
Hazelnut *(Cadbury)*				
55g bar	310	1285	21	25
75g bar	420	1755	28	35

	Cal	kJ	Fat	Cb
Per Bar/Piece Unless Indicated				
Honeycomb Choc-coated pieces:				
1 small piece, 13g	55	230	2	9
1 large piece, 18g	75	320	3	13
Violet Crumble Pieces (1)	50	210	2	8
Kinder: Surprise, edible part, 20g	115	470	11	11
Bueno, 1 wafer, 21g	125	525	9	12
Chocolate Bar, 20g	120	490	7	11
Kisses *(Hershey's)*, 9 pieces, 41g	200	835	12	25
Kit Kat:				
Bars: Original: 2 fingers, 20g	105	435	5.5	13
4 fingers, 45g	235	980	13	28
King Size, 65g	340	1425	18	40
Mini Fun Size, 17g	90	370	4.5	11
Blocks: Original, 170g	890	3725	48	103
White, 170g	930	3875	54	100
Chunky: Original, 60g bar	315	1315	17	37
King Size, 78g bar	410	1710	22	48
Chunky3: Caramel, 65g	340	1420	19	39
Cookies & Cream, 65g	335	1405	18	40
Caramel Duo, 45g bar	240	990	13	28
Lil' Chocits *(Aldi)*,				
average all types, 1 bar, 18g	105	430	7	9
Lindt: Lindor Balls, average	75	310	5.5	5.5
Blocks, Dark Chocolate:				
50% Cocoa: 1 piece, 10g	55	225	3.5	5.5
100g Block, 10 pieces	540	2250	37	53
70%, 1 piece, 10g	55	220	4	3.5
100g block, 10 pieces	525	2200	41	33
85% Cocoa, 1 piece, 10g	55	220	4.5	2
100g block, 10 pieces	530	2210	46	19
Fioretto, 1 piece, 12g	65	265	4	6
Extra Creamy, 4 pieces, 40g	225	935	15	21
Intense Orange, 4 pieces, 40g	195	815	14	16
Wafer Block, 4 pieces, 40g	210	880	12	23
Swiss Gold:				
Fruit/Nuts, avg, 4 pces, 40g	225	940	15	21
Pieces w. Soft Centre (100g block/18 pieces):				
Extra Dark, 1 piece, 5g	35	150	3	2
Milk, 1 piece, 6g	35	150	2.5	2.5
M&M's:				
Milk Chocolate, 49g packet	240	1005	11	32
Crispy Chocolate, 38g	190	780	8	27
Mini's, 35g tube	175	730	8	23
Mix-Ups, ¼ packet, 40g	200	830	9	28
Peanut, 46g packet	235	985	12	28
Macro *(Woolworths)*,				
Choc Almonds, 30g	170	705	11	15

Chocolate ◆ Confectionery

Chocolate (Cont)

Per Bar/Piece Unless Indicated	Cal	kJ	Fat	Cb
Maltesers: 10 balls, 25g	125	525	6	17
Fun Size packet, 12g	60	255	3	8
40g packet	200	840	9	27
100g box	500	2100	23	67
Maraschino, Choc Coated Cherries, (1)	50	210	2	8
Mars Bar: 53g bar	240	1010	9	38
Fun Size, 18g	85	345	3	13
Snack Size, 40g	185	760	7	28
Twin, 72g	330	1370	13	51
Marvellous Creations:				
Clinkers, average all flavours, 1 piece, 8g	40	175	2	5
Jelly Crunchie Bits, small piece, 8g	40	165	2	5
Peanut Toffee Cookie, small piece, 8 g	40	165	2	4.5
Milk Choc Mallow, 20g	80	340	2.5	14
Milky Bar:				
Original: 50g bar	280	1170	17	28
King Size, 75g bar	420	1755	26	42
Milk and Cookies, 80g	435	1810	26	46
Original, ½ 160g block, 80g	445	1865	28	44
Buttons, 25 buttons, 20g	110	470	7	11
Milky Way: Original, 25g	110	465	4	19
Fun size, 12g	55	225	2	9
Mint Pattie (Nestle), 20g	85	360	2	16
Moro: Bar, 65g	285	1190	10	45
Mega bar, 100g	435	1820	15	70
Snack bar, 50g	220	920	7.5	36
Newman's: Ginger, 1 piece, 11g	50	215	2.5	7
Ginger in Dark Chocolate, 50g bar	220	920	12	31
Nougat Bars (Pantheon), average, 100g	390	1670	4	84
Old Gold (Cadbury), 220g Blocks:				
Original: 1 square, 6g	30	130	2	3.5
1 row, 4 squares, 25g	130	545	7.5	15
Whole Block, 220g	1150	4795	65	127
Roast Almond: 1 square, 6g	35	135	2	3
1 row, 4 squares, 25g	135	565	8.5	12
Whole Block, 220g	1190	4975	76	106
Old Jamaica, 1 row, 4 squares, 25g	125	515	6	16
Peppermint, 220g block, 4 sqs., 25g	115	475	5.5	16
70% Cocoa (220g),				
1 row, 4 sqs., 25g	135	570	11	8.5
1 square, 6g	35	140	2.5	2
Whole Block, 220g	1205	5015	90	74

Per Bar/Piece Unless Indicated	Cal	kJ	Fat	Cb
Ovalteenies, sachet, 15g	60	255	1	13
Peppermint Crisp (Nestlé), 35g bar	175	720	7	26
Picnic:				
46g bar	245	1020	14	26
Twin Pack (2 Bars): 67g	360	1490	20	37
Actual weight, 78g	415	1730	23	41
Fun/Treat Size, 19g bar	100	420	6	11
Cookie Crunch, 46g	220	920	11	28
Pods, average all types:				
5 pods, 22g	115	480	5.5	15
10 pods, 45g	230	960	11	30
Roast Almond (Cadbury), 25g	135	570	8.5	12
Rocky Road, average, 50g	240	1005	14	25
Rolo (Nestle), Rolls:				
1 piece 5g	25	100	1	3.5
50g Roll	240	1005	11	35
Block (200g), 1 row, 29g	145	610	8	18
Scorched Almonds (Nestle), Choc-coated, 50g	270	1125	17	23
Scorched Peanuts, 210g packet	1165	4870	81	94
Simply Less:				
Dark Chocolate: 20g piece	85	360	4.5	2
With Coffee Beans, 20g pce	85	355	4.5	2.5
With Peppermint, 20g piece	85	350	4.5	2
With Sweet Orange Flavour, 20g piece	85	350	4	2
Smarties: 10 Smarties, 10g	50	200	2	7
20g pack	95	400	4	14
50g pack	240	1000	9.5	35
50g bar	260	1095	14	29
Snack (Cadbury):				
55g bar	265	1105	12	35
75g bar	360	1510	17	48
Blocks: 135g	630	2635	30	84
220g Block, 50g piece	235	975	11	31
Snickers: 53g bar	260	1080	13	30
Snack Size, 40g	195	815	10	23
Fun Size, 18g	90	370	4.5	10
Twin Bar, 72g	350	1470	18	41
Sweet William:				
Bars: No Added Sugar, 50g	245	1025	17	5
Not Nuts, 50g	260	1075	15	30
Dairy Free: Orig., 50g	260	1080	16	28
Rice Crackle, 50g	260	1075	15	29
Blocks: Dairy Free, Original, 4 pieces, 17g	90	370	5.5	10
White Delight, 4 pieces, 17g	90	385	5.5	11
Sweet As, No Added Sugar:				
Original, ½ block, 50g	250	1040	18	4.5
Nutty Crunch, ½ block, 50g	245	1030	17	8

Updated Nutrition Data ~ www.CalorieKing.com.au
Persons with Diabetes ~ See Disclaimer (Page 22)

Chocolate ◆ Confectionery

Chocolate (Cont)

Per Bar/Piece Unless Indicated

	Cal	kJ	Fat	Cb
Terry's, Choc Orange Ball:				
Milk Choc: 1 piece	45	190	2.5	5
Whole Ball, 175g	930	3875	51	102
Dark Choc: 1 piece	45	185	2.5	5
Whole Ball, 175g	895	3735	51	100
Tim Tam ~ See Biscuits				
Time Out (Cadbury): 40g bar	215	890	12	25
Twin Pack bar, 60g	320	1340	17	37
Mini/Fun Size, 12g	65	270	3.5	7.5
Toblerone:				
100g bar: 1 piece, 8.5g	45	185	2.5	4.5
12 pieces	500	2090	30	51
50g bar (Dark/Milk)	250	1045	15	26
35g bar (Milk)	185	770	10	21
400g Bar (Xmas/Father's Day)	2000	8360	120	204
Fruit & Nut, 1 piece, 8.3g	40	170	2	5
Honeycomb Crisp, 100g Bar:				
1 piece, 8.4g	45	180	2.5	5.5
12 pieces	520	2175	28	63
Tinys (1), 6g	30	130	2	3.5
Tony Ferguson: No Added Sugar				
Dark Choclette, 16g	75	305	5.5	1
Milk Choclette, 16g	75	320	6	1
Top Deck (Cadbury): 55g bar	300	1250	18	31
220g Block, 50g piece	275	1140	16	29
Turkish Delight (Fry's):				
55g bar	215	895	5	40
Fun/Treat Size, 15g	60	245	1.5	11
Twin Pack (2 x 38g)	295	1225	7	55
Twirl (Cadbury): Twin Finger Bar, 39g	210	875	12	23
Mini/Fun size, 15g	80	335	4.5	8.5
Twix: 55g bar	280	1160	14	36
King Size, 2 pack, 72g	365	1520	18	47
Fun Size, 14.5g bar	75	305	3.5	10
Violet Crumble:				
50g bar	235	985	8.5	38
Pieces, each, 11g	50	215	2	8

Per Bar/Piece Unless Indicated

	Cal	kJ	Fat	Cb
Wagon Wheels (Arnott's):				
Large: Original, 48g	210	865	7.5	32
Double Choc	215	905	9	32
Mini, 25g Biscuit	110	455	4	17
Well, naturally:				
AntiOx, 80g block	380	1575	31	10
Bars, Sugar-Free Dark Chocolate:				
Almond Chip, 45g	220	920	20	2.5
Mint Crisp, 45g	205	855	18	2.5
Rich Dark, 45g	215	895	20	2.5
Whip (Cadbury), 60g bar	270	1115	9.5	42
Whistler's, The Big Freckle, 300g	1200	5020	60	145
Whittaker's:				
Coconut Slab, 50g	300	1250	21	23
Peanut Slab, 50g	285	1185	18	22
Blocks (250g), average all types:				
33% Cocoa, 1 row, 25g	150	615	11	10
62% Cocoa, 1 row, 25g	135	555	7.5	15
72% Cocoa, 1 row, 25g	140	580	8.5	13
White Knight, 25g bar	110	460	3	20
Wonka:				
170g Blocks, average all types:	910	3810	52	98
¼ Block, 45g	240	1010	14	26
1 piece, 7g	40	160	2.5	4
Woolworth:				
200 Gram Blocks, average all types:				
1 row, 4 pces, 20g	110	460	6	12
2 rows, 40g	215	900	13	24
½ block, 100g	540	2260	32	60
Whole block, 200g	1080	4510	64	120

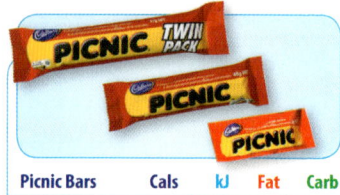

Picnic Bars	Cals	kJ	Fat	Carb
Small, 19g	100	420	6	11
Medium, 46g	245	1020	14	26
Twin Pack, 67g*	415	1730	23	41

*Figures based on actual wt of 78g

MORE 'PORTION WATCH' PHOTOS:
www.CalorieKing.com.au

Confectionery ~ Lollies ♦ Gum

Per Piece Unless Indicated	Cal	kJ	Fat	Cb
Includes: Allens, Cadbury, Pascall, LifeSavers, Mastercraft, Scanlen, Red Tulip				
Anaconda Jelly, Jumbo (30cm), 50g	160	670	0	37
Aniseed Rings: Plain	15	65	0	4
Chocolate coated, 11g	50	200	1.5	7.5
Ball Gum	20	90	0	5
Banana Split Bar	80	335	0	20
Bananas	15	50	0	4
Big Bananas	80	325	0	20
Barley Sugar	25	110	0	6.5
Big Charlie Fruit	65	275	0	16
Black Cats	15	55	0	3.5
Bliss Bombs, 40g packet	170	710	7	27
Boiled Sweets: 100g	295	1240	0	81
1 small, 5g	15	65	0	4
1 medium, 8g	25	105	0	6.5
Bols Hard Jubes (K-Mart), 10 pieces, 20g	70	295	0	18
Bon Bons (1)	20	75	0	5
Bubble Gum: Hubba Bubba, regular	20	85	0	5
Hubba Bubba Tape	15	70	0	4
Butter Menthol: Roll (1)	10	40	0	2.5
Square (1)	15	65	0	4
Butterscotch	25	105	0.5	6
Candy Canes ~See page 80				
Cannonballs	30	125	1.5	4
Caramels: Average	25	100	0	5
Jersey, 1 piece	40	170	2	6
Milk Chocolate (Pascall)	45	190	2.5	6
Chewing Gum: Per Piece				
Wrigley:				
P.K; Juicyfruit	5	25	0	1
Doublemint	5	20	0	0
Spearmint	10	30	0	0
Sugar Free:				
Eclipse, 1 piece	10	30	0	0
Mentos: Aqua Kiss	5	15	0	0
Blast, all flavours	5	20	0	0
SweetLife, Dental	2	10	0	0
Wrigleys, all flav., 5 pcs	5	20	0	0
Chews (Nat'l Conf. Co), 1 piece	25	100	0	5.5
Chicos (Allens), each	15	65	0	3
Choc Bullets, small, 10 pcs, 20g	85	345	3	13
Choc Mint Crunch, 8g	35	140	0.5	7.5
Chocolate Caramels (Pascall), 3 pcs, 25g	130	540	7	16
Chocolate Eclairs (Pascall):				
Average, 2 pieces, 13g	60	250	2.5	9
200g Packet	920	3840	37	135

Per Piece Unless Indicated	Cal	kJ	Fat	Cb
Chupa Chups, all flavours	50	220	0	12
Clinkers	15	70	0.5	2
Coconut Ice, 25g	110	465	4.5	17
Coffee Confectionery: Coffee bean (chips):				
Choc-coated, 30g	140	585	8	20
Kopiko, each	20	75	0	3.5
Coffee Creams	40	170	1	8
Columbines (Pascall):				
(1) 5g	25	90	1	4
(10) 50g	215	905	7.5	37
Coke Bottles	10	40	0	2.5
Country Mints	25	110	0	4.5
Crown Mints (Menz), 2 mints	25	105	0	6.5
Crown Musks, (4), 12g	45	190	0	12
Double Dips	80	340	4.5	10
Eclairs (Jubilee): 1 eclair	15	65	0	4
Chocolate, average (1)	30	125	1	5
Eclipse Mints, (1), 2g	5	30	0	0
E.S. Mints	10	45	0	2.5
Eucalyptus & Honey	20	90	0	5
Fairy Floss, 35g	130	545	0	34
Fantales, 1 piece, 7g	30	125	1	5.5
Fizzy Colas (Haribo), 5 pieces, 20g	65	275	0	15
Freckles (Allen's): 10 pieces, 33g	155	650	5.5	25
Large (loose), 25g each	120	500	4.5	19
Frogs Alive	25	100	0	5.5
Fruit & Nut Truffle	40	175	1.5	7
Fruit Bars (IXL), Strawberry, 1 bar	75	315	1	16
Fruitang, all flavours	15	65	0.5	2.5
Fruit Bon Bons	25	105	0	6
Fruit Gums (Rowntrees): 1 gum, 3g	10	45	0	2.5
48g roll (17 gums)	170	710	0	43
Fruit Jellies, average (1), 5g	15	65	0	4
Fruit Jubes	20	85	0	4.5
Fruit Leather, average	55	230	0	13
Fruit 'n Cream, 25g	85	360	0	21
Fruit Rings	20	85	0	5
Fruit Roll-Ups (Uncle Tobys), (1)	50	215	0	11
Fruit Tingles, each	10	35	0	2.5
Fudge, 1 piece (2cm x 2cm)	80	320	1.5	17
Ginger Bears (Buderim), 50g packet	155	640	0.5	37
Goaties, Mini Milkshakes, 1 packet, 11g	40	175	1	7
Gob Stoppers (Wonka), 50g	190	800	0	47
Gold Bears (Haribo), 10 pieces, 25g	85	355	0	20
Gummi Fruits, 25g	80	335	0	18

Updated Nutrition Data ~ www.CalorieKing.com.au
Persons with Diabetes ~ See Disclaimer (Page 22)

85

Confectionery ~ Licorice ◆ Lollies

Per Piece, Unless Indicated	Cal	kJ	Fat	Cb
Halva, average, 30g	140	585	5	18
Honeycomb: Plain, 30g	120	500	0	29
Choc-coated pieces:				
1 small piece, 13g	65	270	3	9
1 large piece, 18g	95	400	4	13
Humbugs	25	105	0	6
Ice Cream Cones	10	50	0	2.5
Ice Mint (Snow's), (1)	15	60	0	4
Jaffas: 1 Jaffa	15	60	0.5	2.5
110g packet	515	2150	19	83
Jaw Breaker Ball Gum	35	155	0	9
Jellea: Babies, 4 pces, 21g	70	285	0	17
Beans (10), 30g	110	460	0	27
Jellies (Pascall)	20	85	0	5
Jelly Babies: Regular	15	65	0	4
Giant	75	315	0	18
Jelly Beans: Medium size (1)	10	40	0	2.5
10 medium beans, 25g	95	400	0	25
Large, average, 1 bean	20	85	0	5
Jelly Belly: 1 bean	5	20	0	1
40g serve (approx 35 beans)	145	600	0	37
100g packet	360	1500	0	92
Jersey Caramels, (1)	40	170	2	6
Jols, avg, 25g box	55	235	0	0
Jubes: (Allen's), Marella	15	60	0	3.5
Pascall	15	60	0	3.5
Killer Pythons, 44g each	145	615	0	34
King Frogs, 10g	50	215	2.5	12
Kool Fruits (Allens), (1), 40g	15	65	0	3.5
Kool Mints (Allen's), !1), 4g	15	65	0	3.5
Lifesavers: Average, each	10	35	0	2.5
Whole packet, 34g	135	560	0	33
Licorice:				
Allsorts: Average, 10g	30	135	0	8
Darrel Lea, 1 pce, 21g	70	300	0.5	17
Bites: Original, 25g	80	340	0.5	18
Strawberry, 25g	90	370	1	19
Big Stick/Twist, 50g	115	480	0.5	26
Big Strap, 88g	200	840	1	46
Bullets: (Choc-coated), each	10	45	0	2
200g packet	840	3520	27	141
Chew (Pascall), each	25	105	0.5	4.5
Carob-coated sticks (Lewis) (1), 50g	145	605	4.5	25
Fruit flavours (1), 9g	30	130	0	7
Licorice Yards (Pascall) (1), 50g	165	690	1	37
Soft Black (1), 12g	35	145	0	8
Twists: Red, 5 pieces, 50g	170	710	1.5	38
Black, 4 pieces, 60g	190	790	1	43

Per Piece, Unless Indicated	Cal	kJ	Fat	Cb
Lollipops: Mini, 8g each	30	135	0	8
Medium, 16g each	65	270	0	16
Large (10cm diam.), 100g	400	1680	0	98
Allen's, (1)	30	125	0	7.5
Artisse, (1)	25	100	0	6
Chupa Chups, (1)	50	200	0	12
Mackintosh's Toffee	35	145	1	6
Mallow Bites Chocs (Pascall),				
5 balls, 25g	100	425	2.5	19
Mallow Rolls, 35g Roll	140	580	4	25
Mallows: Toasted (1), 9g	35	145	1.5	4
Small/Drinking, 4g (1)	10	50	0	3.5
Miniature, 1g (1)	5	15	0	1
150g packet	505	2115	1	125
Choc Mallow Bites, all flavours, 1 pce, 5g	20	85	0.5	4
Swirls, all flavours, 5g	20	70	0	4
Marella Jubes (Allen's)	15	60	0	3.5
Marshmallows: Small, 5g	15	70	0	4
Large, 10g	30	125	0	8.5
Pink/White	35	140	0	8
Mentos: Rolls, 38g pack	145	615	0	35
Fruit/Mint/Tropical, each	10	45	0	2.5
Blast Chewing Gum (1)	5	15	0	0
Mini,, 10g roll	40	165	0	9
Milk Bottles/Milko: Small	15	55	0	3.5
Large, 10g	40	170	0	9
Milk Chocolate Caramel, 10g	50	215	3	6.5
Mint Leaves, large	15	60	0	3.5
Mint Patties (Nestlé), 20g	85	360	2	16
Minties, (8),	30	125	0	7
Mints, XXX (2), 5.5g	20	90	0	5.5
Musk	10	40	0	4
Musk Stick, (1), 10g	40	160	0	9
(The) Natural Confectionery Co:				
Average all types: 3 pieces, 25g	85	355	0	20
6-9 pieces, 50g	170	710	0	40
180g bag	610	2550	0	143
Chews (Fruity Mix), 4 pieces, 25g	95	400	0.5	22
Forbidden Fruit, 5 pieces, 32g	110	450	0	25
Jungle Jellies, 5 pieces, 30g	100	420	0	24
Mini Bearables, 25g	85	360	0	20
Party Mix, 5 pieces, 25g	85	355	0	20
Snakes, 4 pieces, 36g	120	510	0	29
Squirms, 6 pieces, 40g	135	555	0	32
Tropical Bliss: 5 pieces, 27g	90	385	0	22
Nerds (Wonka), 45g Box	170	710	0	42
Nougat:				
Choc-coated, 30g	125	525	4	23
Plain, 1 small piece, 8g	35	150	1	6
100g bar	430	1790	10	73

Confectionery ◆ Lollies

Per Piece, Unless Indicated	Cal	kJ	Fat	Cb
Party Mix, 5 pieces	75	300	0	18
Peppermint Choc Drops, 25g	100	415	0	25
Peppermints: Small	10	35	0	2.5
Medium	15	60	0	4
Large	20	85	0	4.5
Pez, 1 packet, 8.5g	30	125	0	8.5
Pineapple Lumps (*Pascall*), 6 pcs, 25g	110	450	3.5	19
Push Pop Lollipop, 15g	60	250	0	14
Python, giant, 44g	145	615	0	34
Raspberries	15	70	0	4
Raspberry Twister, 28g	100	415	0	22
Redskin, Stick, 15g	60	255	0	14
Roll-Ups (*Uncle Tobys*), Fruit flav., av.	50	220	0	11
Sherbet: Cone, with Mallow Top	60	245	0	14
Sherbet, powder, 14g	55	230	0	13
Sherbies (*Allen's*), (1)	30	120	0.5	7
Skittles:				
Citrus, 55g	220	920	2.5	49
Crazy Cores, 25g	100	410	1	22
Fruit, 55g pack	225	935	2.5	12
Littles: Tube, 35g	140	595	1.5	32
Sours, 50g	195	815	2	43
Smarties: 1 Smartie, 1g	5	25	0	0.5
50g Carton	240	1000	9.5	36
Bar, 50g	265	1095	15	30
Block, 180g	945	3945	51	107
Snakes, (Jelly): Small, 6g	20	85	0	4.5
Medium, 10g	30	130	0	7
Giant (30cm), 50g	165	690	0	39
Snakes Alive (*Allens*), (1), 13g	45	185	0	10
Snowballs (*Eskimo*), Choc-coated, *25g*	110	460	4.5	16
Sour Worms	15	60	0	4
Sparkles, 25g	85	350	0	20
Toasted Marshmallow, 19g	85	345	4	11

Per Piece, Unless Indicated	Cal	kJ	Fat	Cb
Starburst: Average all types: 20g	65	275	0	15
100g quantity	315	1320	0	74
180g bag	570	2375	0	135
Babies (10), 25g	80	330	0	19
Bananas & Cream (3), 25g	80	330	0	18
Fruit Chews: 5 pieces, 25g	95	400	2	20
58g pack, 12 pieces	220	925	5	48
Fruitmix Mix (180g pack), 10 pcs, 40g	125	530	0	30
Gummi Fruits, 5 pieces, 25g	75	320	0	18
Party Mix, 25g	80	325	0	19
Rattlesnakes, 3 pieces, 30g	95	390	0	22
Squirts, 5 pieces, 25g	80	335	0	18
Sucks Lollipops, 1 pop, 13g	45	190	0	12
Strawberries & Cream (Allens),	35	145	0	8
Chocolate Coated Strawberry Creams	60	250	1.5	8
Teeth, 25g serving	85	350	0	20
Tic Tacs: All flavours, 5 pieces	10	40	0	2
Whole Container, 24g	95	390	0	24
Toffee Apple, medium, 1, 170g	225	950	3.5	50
Toffees: Small, 5g	20	85	0	4
Large, 9g	35	145	0	6.5
Turkish Delight:				
Plain/Rose/Flavoured: 1 cube, 20g	70	290	0	17
With nuts/coconut, 20g	80	335	1	17
Pantheon, 50g bar	195	810	2	42
Fry's, Choc-coated, 55g bar	215	895	5	40
Werther's: Toffees, 1 piece	20	90	0.5	4.5
Caramel Creme (1), 6.2g	25	110	0.5	5
Chewy toffee, 1 piece	25	110	1	4.5
Eclair, 1 piece	30	115	1	4
White Frogs, 10g	55	235	3	6
Wine Gums (*Pascalls*), 1	15	60	0	4
Wizz Fizz, 1 sachet, 14g	55	230	0	13
Wonka:				
Fabulicious Raspb. Twister (5), 28g	110	450	1	24
60g packet				
Fruit Tingles, 13g	50	205	0	12
Gobstopper (1), 1.7g	5	30	0	1.5
Nerdalicious, 1 stick	115	475	1	26
Nerds, 45g box	170	710	0	42
Sherbert Fizz, 1 stick, 60g	115	470	1.5	24
XXX Mints: 1 piece	10	50	0	2.5
1 packet, 45g	185	765	0	45

CALORIE KING TIP!

Don't take promotion of 'No Artificial Colours or Flavours' to mean such confectionery is healthy; or can be eaten often in extra amounts.

The sugar content is still high and the 99% Fat Free claim means it is 99% sugar!

Confectionery ~ Carob ◆ Cough & Cold

Sugar-Free Confectionery

	Cal	kJ	Fat	Cb
Per Piece, Unless Indicated				
Darrell Lea, Choc Bar, 50g	255	1055	19	1.5
Double 'D', Chews (1), 6g	15	70	0	0
Butter Candy Drops: Reg. 6g	20	70	0	0
With Choc Creme Centre, 5g	15	65	0.5	0
Eucalyptus Drops, 3.5g	10	40	0	0
Flavoured Drops (1), average, 3.5g	10	40	0	0
Summer Mints (1)	10	40	0	0
Extra Professional, each	5	25	0	0
Jols, Pastilles/Licorette: (1)	1	5	0	0
1 Box, 25g	55	235	0	0
Sugar Free Gum: Glean (1)	5	20	0	1
Jila (1)	2	10	0	1
Lido, Glace; Lion Mints, each	10	35	0	0
Ricci, Sugar Free, all types	5	20	0	0
Ricola, Sugar Free	1	5	0	0
Slim Fruits, Pastilles, all flavours (1), 1g	2	10	0	0
Sulá Natura, Sugar Free Candies, avg., (1)	10	40	0	0
The Sugarless Co: Chews, 7g	20	80	0.5	0
Bliss, all flav.	10	25	0	0
Fruit Jellies, Cool Jac (1), all flav.	15	50	0.5	0
Aura, all flavours, 5g	15	65	0	0
Lollipops, all flavours (1), 10g	30	110	0	0
Tony Ferguson:				
Sugarless Chews (1)	20	80	0.5	0
Sugarless Hard Candy (1)	12	50	0	0
Well, Naturally: Fruit Mix, 3.2g	10	30	0	0
Caramel Cream, 3.2g	10	40	0	0
Werthers, Sugar-Free Toffee (1)	10	45	0.5	0
Wrigley's, Sugar-Free Eclipse Mints (1), 2g	10	30	0	0

Carob Confectionery

	Cal	kJ	Fat	Cb
Carob Blocks, average, 75g	385	1615	25	33
100g block	515	2155	33	44
Carrobean: Apricot, 75g	340	1425	21	34
Coconut; Malt, 75g	400	1680	29	26
Carob Rice Cake, 35g	160	675	9.5	20
Lewis, No Added Sugar				
Carob Almond: 110g block	500	2085	36	46
1 row, 4 pieces, 16g	70	305	5.5	7
Carob Rocky Road, 40g	185	770	9.5	20

Yoghurt Confectionery

	Cal	kJ	Fat	Cb
Yoghurt Apricot/Berry Pieces (Go Natural), 10 pieces, 30g	150	615	7.5	19
Yoghurt Buds (Plain/Sugar Free), 50g	260	1090	15	33
Yoghurt Gum, ⅓ packet, 20g	65	270	0	15
Yoghurt-coated: Nuts, 50g	265	1110	17	26
Apricots, 18g each	60	240	2.5	10
Sultanas, 50g	210	870	12	28
Yoghurt Cluster, 22g	100	405	5.5	11
Ginger, 50g	210	875	8	37

Cough & Cold

	Cal	kJ	Fat	Cb
Per Piece				
Anticol, Lozengers	15	60	0	3.5
Butter Menthol	10	40	0	4
Double 'D':				
Eucalyptus (1), average	25	90	0	6.5
Butter Menthol (1), average	25	90	0	6
Fisherman's Friend: Original (1)	5	20	0	1
Sugar Free, average (1)	5	20	0	1.5
Super Strong Mints (1)	5	20	0	1.5
Honey & Eucalyptus	15	70	0	4
Kaiser, Bio Menthol; Mentha Fresh	5	20	0	2
Lemsip, Lozenges	10	40	0	2
Listerine, Throat	10	40	0	4
Soothers	15	65	0	4
Throaties: Gums	5	25	0	1
Drops	18	75	0	4

Medicated Lozenges

	Cal	kJ	Fat	Cb
Difflam; Duro-Tuss, 1 lozenge	5	20	0	1
Cepacol, 1 lozenge	15	60	0	2
Strepsils Plus, 1 lozenge	10	40	0	2
Vicks, Throat Lozenges	5	25	0	1

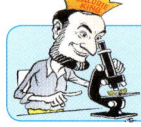

For Full Nutritional Data
~ See Author's Website
www.CalorieKing.com.au

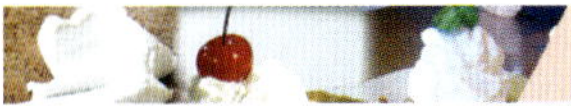

Cream ◇ Custard

Cream

Item	Cal	kJ	Fat	Cb
Sour Cream:				
Regular (35% Fat): 1 Tbsp, 20ml	70	300	7.5	0.5
300ml bottle/carton	1005	4200	105	9
Extra Light (12.5% Fat), 1 Tbsp, 20ml	30	115	2.5	1.5
Light (18% Fat), 1 Tbsp, 20ml	40	165	4	1
200ml carton	375	1565	36	8
Thickened Cream:				
Regular/Pure (35% fat): Avg. all brands				
1 Tbsp, 20ml	65	280	7	0.5
300ml container	1040	4340	110	9
Double/Thick Cream (55% fat):				
Average all brands: 1 Tbsp	90	380	10	0.5
½ cup, 125ml	580	2425	60	4.5
Light Thickened, 1 Tbsp, 20ml	45	185	4	1.5
Whipping Cream *(40% fat):*				
Unwhipped: 1 Tbsp, 20g	80	330	8.5	0.5
300ml bottle/carton	1045	4360	110	6
Whipped: ¼ cup, 30g	105	435	12	1
1 heaped Tbsp, 15g	50	215	6	0.5
½ cup, 60g	210	865	24	2
Scalded/Clotted Cream *(48% fat)*, 1 T., 20g	90	375	10	0.5
Bulla, Crème Fraiche, 50ml	165	700	18	1
Coles, Light Sour Cream, 50g	95	400	9	2
Nestle:				
Reduced Fat Cream *(38% fat):*				
25ml	55	225	5.5	1
250ml can	550	2250	55	5
Pauls:				
Lactose Free *(22% fat),* Zymil, Light, 100ml	230	950	22	5
Pure Cream *(35% fat):*				
1 Tbsp	75	315	8	0.5
300ml carton	995	4150	105	10
Philadelphia:				
Cooking Cream *(30% less fat):*				
Original, 25ml	65	265	6	1
60% less fat, 25ml	45	190	3	3
Dessert Cream *(50% less fat)*, 25ml	70	285	6	1
Simply Less *(Coles):*				
Light Thickened Cream, 1 Tbsp, 20ml	40	165	4	1

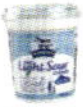

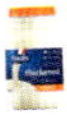

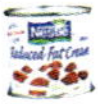

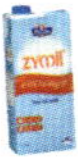

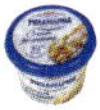

Whipped Cream

Item	Cal	kJ	Fat	Cb
Pressure Pak: *Per ⅓ Cup, 80ml*				
Dairy Whip:				
Whipped Cream: Regular, ⅓ cup	50	205	4.5	1.5
Lite, ⅓ cup, 17g	40	165	3	2.5
Dream Whip:				
Regular, ⅓ cup, 20g	55	240	5.5	2
Light, ⅓ cup, 20g	45	180	3.5	2.5
Woolworths, Select:				
Regular, ⅓ cup, 20g	60	245	5.5	2
Light, ⅓ cup, 20g	45	190	3.5	2.5

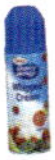

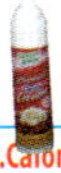

Custard ~ Bands

Item	Cal	kJ	Fat	Cb
Custards, Carton: *Average:*				
Chocolate, 100g	125	530	3.5	20
Vanilla, 100g	100	410	2	15
Ambrosia, Devon, 1 Tub, 150g	150	630	4.5	23
Birds, with Skim Milk, 125g	85	360	0.5	18
Brownes,				
Vanilla, ½ cup, 125ml	160	655	3.5	25
Coles: Chocolate, 1 Cup, 150g	145	600	5	20
Simply Less, ⅓ cup, 90g	70	285	1	12
Dairy Farmers: Chocolate, 1 tub, 100g	125	530	3.5	20
Vanilla, Thick, ⅕ tetra pak, 100g	100	410	2	15
Pouring: ⅕ Tetra Pak, 100g	90	375	2	15
Lite, ⅕ Tetra Pak, 100g	75	315	1	14
Foster Clark's:				
500ml Ctn, ½ cup, 125ml	125	515	4	18
Cups: Chocolate, 140g	125	525	4	18
Vanilla, 140g	130	550	3.5	20
Snak Pack, 140g	160	670	5	24
Harvey Fresh, ½ cup, 125ml	120	500	4	17
Pauls: *Per ½ Cup, 125g*				
Banana; Vanilla	130	540	3.5	20
Chocolate	140	590	3.5	23
Double Thick: Chocolate	180	810	7.5	26
Vanilla	150	615	5	21
Premium: Brandy	170	750	7.5	21
Vanilla	179	715	7.5	21
Low Fat: Vanilla	105	430	1	15
Simply Less *(Coles):*				
Vanilla, Low-Fat, ½ cup, 125g	95	395	1	17

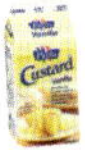

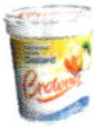

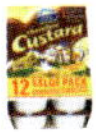

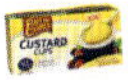

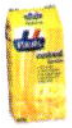

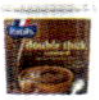

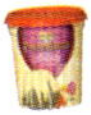

Custard Powder

Item	Cal	kJ	Fat	Cb
Custard Powder: *Average All Brands*				
3 level T., 30g, makes 600ml	110	460	0	25
Made-Up: ½ cup, 125ml				
With sugar + whole milk	115	480	5	14
W. artificial sweetener + skim milk	65	270	0	7
Egg Custard, avg., ½ cup, 125ml	155	640	6.5	19
Homemade Custard:				
Boiled/Baked: ½ cup, 125g	125	520	6	14
With egg & whole milk, ½ cup	150	620	7	14
W/ skim milk/artificial sweetener, ½ cup	60	250	0	7
Bird's Lowfat Instant,				
½ cup prepared, 125g	85	360	0.5	18
Foster Clark's, Egg Custard Mix, made up, ½ cup, 125ml	155	640	6.5	19
White Wings, Vanilla, ⅓ cup, 102g	95	390	4	11

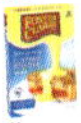

Updated Nutrition Data ~ www.CalorieKing.com.au
Persons with Diabetes ~ See Disclaimer (Page 22)

D Desserts ◆ Dairy Desserts

Dairy Desserts ~ Brands

	Cal	kJ	Fat	Cb
Aeroplane: *Per ¼ of 85g packet, 125g Prepared*				
Wobble, average all flavours	125	520	3	21
Blue Cow Mousse: *Per 120g Tub*				
Chocolate	450	1870	38	15
White Chocolate	410	1705	37	15
Brownes (W.A.):				
Classic Creme, Caramel, 150g	200	825	4.5	33
YoGo: Original Chocolate, 200g	270	1130	6	43
98% Fat Free, Chocolate, 200g	190	800	3	33
CalciYum, average all flavours, 100g tub	95	390	1.5	14
Coles: Choc Snack, 100g tub	130	530	4	18
Mousse, avg., all flavours	115	470	6	12
Divine Classics,				
Creme Caramel, 1 tub	200	825	6	29
Foster Clark's, Snack Pack	160	670	5	24
Vanilla Custard Cups, 140g	130	550	3.5	20
Fruche: *Per 150g Tub*				
Tropical Mango	175	730	4.5	26
Strawberry Fields	170	715	4.5	25
Vanilla Bean	170	710	4.5	25
Vanilla Bean w. Berry Layer	165	675	3.5	26
Heinz:				
Creamed Rice:				
Chocolate (97% Fat Free), 220g	265	1100	6	45
Vanilla (99% Fat Free), 220g	210	870	1	41
Nestle:				
Aero: *Per Tub*				
Chocolate Mousse, 62g	70	290	1.5	10
Choc Peppermint, 70g	105	440	3.5	15
Club Classic, Chocolate, 125g	240	1010	12	27
Soleil Diet Desserts: *Per Tub*				
Cheesecake, 125g	100	410	0	16
Chocolate Mousse, 62g	70	290	1.5	10
Creme Caramel, 125g	75	320	1	13
Dark Chocolate, 125g	125	520	2.5	18
Milky Bar, 90g tub	150	625	7.5	16
Milo: Energy, 100g Tub	130	540	4.5	17
Mousse, 70g	100	420	4	13
Mousse: Chocolate, 62g	130	545	7.5	13
Chocolate Mud, 62g	130	545	7.5	13
Milo Combo Mousse, 70g	100	420	4	13
Rolo, 125g tub	240	1000	11	31

Dairy Desserts (Cont)

	Cal	kJ	Fat	Cb
Pauls:				
Choc Shock, 100g	155	645	6	21
Banana Custard, 100g	105	440	2.5	17
Custard Snack Pack, 150g	230	965	9	31
Double Thick: Chocolate, 100g	155	650	6	21
Vanilla, 100g	120	490	4	16
Petit Miam:				
Fromage Frais,				
average all varieties, 60g tub	70	300	3	8
Simply Less *(Coles): Per 90g Tub*				
Mousse, Dark Chocolate	170	700	2.5	25
Tiramisu	170	690	2	27
YoGo:				
Choc Crispy M&M's, 150g	250	1045	9	38
Choc Rock, 100g	105	445	3	17
Banana Split; Berry; Chocolate Rock, 150g	155	655	4.5	24
Triple Trek, 100g	105	440	3	16
YoGo Mix: Chocolate & M&M's Minis, 150g	250	1055	9	38
Chocolate & Choc Chips, 150g	265	1100	11	35
Chocolate & Honeycomb Chunks, 150g	275	1140	12	36
YoGo Swirl, Choc. Vanilla, 150g	160	660	4.5	25
Yalla:				
Chocolate Mousse,				
⅓ of 300g tub, 100g	385	1600	29	24
Chocolate Mousse & Yoghurt, 120g tub	390	1630	30	25
Raspberry, Chocolate Mousse, 120g tub	375	1560	26	27

Other Desserts

	Cal	kJ	Fat	Cb
Apple Crumble, ¾ cup, 200g	335	1395	11	55
Apple Pie, 1 slice, 150g	365	1525	16	53
Banana Split: 1 banana,				
3 scoops Ice Cream & topping	470	1965	17	74
Blancmange, 1 serve, 120g	175	740	9	24
Cheesecake:				
Small, Buffet slice, 75g	260	1075	17	23
Large serve, 125g	430	1790	28	38
with extra cream	535	2225	40	39
Sara Lee Cheesecakes *~ See Page 70*				
Chocolate Dessert Cups, 150g	190	805	5.5	27
Chocolate Mousse, 125g	395	1650	35	17
Creme Brulee, 250g	370	1545	31	26
Creme Caramel *(Divine),* 150g	200	825	6	29
Jelly Cup, all flavours, 150g	110	450	0	27
Lemon Meringue Pie, 150g	270	1120	8.5	46
Panna Cotta: Chocolate, 200g	730	3060	57	50
Vanilla, 200g	630	2635	56	28
Pavlova: With fruit/cream, 120g	270	1140	15	33
Erica's Kitchen: Plain, Whole, 300g	870	3635	1.5	200
⅙ Pavlova, 50g	145	605	0.5	34
Pavlova Magic/Pavlova Mix, ⅙ serve	185	770	0	43

Desserts ♦ Dairy Desserts

Other Desserts (Cont)

	Cal	kJ	Fat	Cb
Souffle, average, 1 serve	235	985	9	32
Tiramisu, 100g serve	365	1530	25	32
Trifle, average, 1 serve, 120g	200	840	8	27
Zabaglione, ½ cup	160	670	7	11

Desserts ~ Brands

	Cal	kJ	Fat	Cb
Ambrosia, Rice Cream, ½ of 200g can	200	835	4.5	33
Coles Smart Buy, Vanilla, 210g	235	980	6	39
Heinz, Creamed Rice: Chocolate, 97% Fat Free, ½ of 420g can, 210g	245	1030	5.5	42
Small 220g can	265	1100	6	45
Lite n' Easy, Rice Pudding, 176g	200	850	3.5	36
Parsons, Vanilla 215g	215	905	3.5	37
Tom Piper, Vanilla, 215g	215	905	3.5	37
Wicked Sister,				
97% Fat Free:				
Luscious Vanilla: With Blueberry, 1 tub	170	700	3	34
With Caramel, 1 tub	190	800	4	35
With Cinnamon, 1 tub	165	695	4	31

Jelly

	Cal	kJ	Fat	Cb
Jelly: Regular; Sweetened				
1 serve, ½ cup, 120g	65	275	0	16
1 sachet (makes 500ml)	275	1150	0	66
Gelatine, dry, 7g sachet	25	105	0	0
Junket tablet, each	1	5	0	0.5
Aeroplane, Jelly Cups, 150g	115	475	0	28
Reduced Sugar, ½ cup, 125g	70	290	0	15
Light, all flav., 1/4 pkt prepared	10	40	0	4
Ready to Eat, all flav., 1 cup, 150g	115	470	0	25
Brookdale (Aldi), Avg., all flav, ¼ pkt	80	340	0	17
Jelly Lite: ½ cup, 125g	10	35	0	0
1 cup serve, 250ml	15	70	0	0
1 sachet (makes 500ml)	35	145	0	0.5
Weight Watchers, 125ml	10	35	0	0.5

Pancakes

	Cal	kJ	Fat	Cb
Pancakes: *Average all Types:*				
Small, 8cm diameter, 25g	60	240	2	8
Medium, 10cm diameter, 40g	90	385	3	12
Large, 12cm diameter, 83g	190	795	6.5	26
Basco, Pancake Shake, Buttermilk (1), 43g	100	415	1	21
Creative Gourmet,				
French Style, Frozen (1), 50g	100	425	3	17
Golden: Original (1), 60g	135	570	3.5	21
Chocolate (1), 60g	135	560	2.5	24

Pancakes (Cont)

	Cal	kJ	Fat	Cb
Green's: *Per 3 Pancakes, Prepared*				
Shake: Banana, 150g	300	1245	2	64
Buttermilk, 150g	305	1275	3	60
Chocolate, 150g	300	1250	3	60
Low-Fat, 150g	300	1240	3	57
Maple; Vanilla, 150g	305	1265	2.5	63
Macro: *Per Pancake*				
Buttermilk, Gluten Free (1), 40g	90	370	1	18
White Wings: *Prepared as Directed*				
Buttermilk (1), 46g	90	375	1.5	17
(3), 139g	270	1130	4	51
Shaker: Original (1), 45g	85	350	0.5	17
3 Pancakes, 135g	250	1055	2	51
Golden Syrup (1), 45g	95	400	1	19
3 Pancakes	290	1195	3	57
Crepes: Plain, each	110	460	5	15
Crepes Suzette (2)	380	1590	18	42
Seafood Crepes (2)	540	2260	37	29

Pikelets

	Cal	kJ	Fat	Cb
Pikelets: 1 only, 12g	30	130	1	6
Tip Top: Golden Pikelets, 25g ea	60	240	1.5	9
Bites; Chocolate Bites (4), 35g	80	340	2	14
White Wings, Pikelet Mix Shaker, Orig. (4)	180	750	1.5	37
Woolworths Pikelets, (1), 25g	60	255	1.5	10

Waffles

	Cal	kJ	Fat	Cb
Waffles: Plain, 33g	125	520	8.5	19
W. Syrup, Ice Cream, Cream	315	1320	8	54
Nanna's, Original (1), 17g	45	180	1	7

Toppings

	Cal	kJ	Fat	Cb
Toppings: *Per Tbsp, 20g, Average All Brands*				
Caramel, Raspberry/Strawberry	35	150	0	9.5
Chocolate	40	165	0	10
Golden Syrup, 1 Tbsp, 20ml	85	360	0	21
Maple Syrup	45	190	0	12
Brookdale (Aldi): Caramel	50	210	0	12
Chocolate	45	190	0	12
Strawberry	40	165	0	10
Coles, Caramel	45	190	0	11
Cottees, Thick & Rich Choc, 30g	60	240	0	14
Diet Topping, 26ml	10	35	0	1.5
SPC, Fruit Sauce, Cranberry; Plum	50	215	0	12

Updated Nutrition Data ~ www.CalorieKing.com.au
Persons with Diabetes ~ See Disclaimer (Page 22)

D Dips

Dips ~ Brands

	Cal	kJ	Fat	Cb
Black Swan: *Per 1 Tbsp, 20g*				
Chunky: Basil w. Cashews & Parm.	105	430	8.5	4.5
Pumpkin w. Cashews & Parm.	75	305	5.5	4
Tomato w. Cashews & Parm.	85	345	7	3.5
Classic: Avocado w. Sea Salt	65	275	6	2.5
Caviar	75	305	6.5	3
Cheese & Chives/Spring Onion	60	255	6	1.5
Corn Relish	45	195	3.5	2.5
Eggplant	40	165	3	2.5
French Onion	55	225	5	2
Guacamole	55	235	5.5	1.5
Hommus	55	225	5	1.5
Olive	70	285	7	1
Spicy Capsicum	65	270	6	1.5
Spinach & Pinenuts	60	245	5.5	2
Tzatziki	25	100	1.5	2
Farmer's Best: Aioli	65	260	6	1.5
Baby Spinach & Feta	60	255	6	1.5
Beetroot Tzatziki	30	125	2	2.5
Capsicum & Feta; Guacamole	25	105	2	1
Caramelised French Onion	55	220	5	2
White Hommus	50	215	3	5
Skinny: French Onion	45	180	3	2
Hommus	35	155	2.5	3
Roasted Capsicum	40	175	2.5	3.5
Tzatziki	20	75	0.5	2
Chris' Dips: *Per 1 Tbsp, 20g*				
Delicatessen: Creamy Basil	65	270	6	1.5
Hommus & Dukkah	50	215	4	3
Roasted Capsicum	30	115	2.5	1.5
Spicy Yellow Pepper	55	230	5	1.5
Spinach, Pinenut, Pecorino & Chilli	65	260	5.5	1.5
White Caviar & Almond Meal	80	325	7.5	2
Lite & Fresh: Hommus	35	145	2	3.5
Spicy Capsicum	35	135	3	1
Tzatziki	15	60	0.5	1.5
Traditional: Avocado	60	240	5.5	1
Caviar	65	260	5.5	3
Corn Relish	50	2010	4	2.5
Creamy Basil	65	270	6	1.5
Eggplant	30	125	2	2.5
Egyptian Beetroot	20	90	0.5	3.5
French Onion	55	220	4.5	2
Hommus	40	155	3	2
Kalamata Olive	50	195	4.5	0.5
Semi-dried Tomato	50	205	4.5	1.5
Spicy Capsicum	50	200	4.5	1
Three Olive	80	330	8.5	0.5
Tzatziki	20	90	1.5	1
Coles: *Per 1 Tbsp, 20g*				
Avocado	50	200	4.5	1
Beetroot & Mint	25	105	1	3.5
Caviar	65	265	6	2
Chunky Basil w. Pinenuts & Parmesan	105	440	10	2
French Onion	45	175	3.5	1.5
Hommus w. Lemon & Garlic	40	170	3	2.5
Tzatziki	20	70	1	2
Copperpot: *Per 1 Tbsp, 20g*				
Chunky: Guacamole w. Cashews	50	210	3.5	3.5
Basil w. Cashew & Parmesan	100	425	10	1.5
Spinach & Feta w. Cashews	70	295	6.5	2
Classic: Avocado	50	205	4.5	1.5
Corn Relish	40	165	3	2.5
French Onion	45	185	4	1.5
Hommus	55	220	4	3.5
Roasted Capsicum	50	195	4	2
Layered: Basil & Caps. w. Cream Cheese	55	235	4.5	2.5
Chilli Crab & Spring Onion	30	115	2	1
Guacamole & Spicy Salsa	40	170	3	1.5
Sundried Tomato w. Cream Cheese	60	245	5.5	2
Kraft: *Per 1 Tbsp, 20g*				
French Onion	45	190	3.5	2.5
Gherkin	45	180	3.5	2
Onion & Bacon	45	195	4	2
Prawn & Crab	50	200	4	2.5
Smoked Salmon & Dill	50	200	4	2
Philadelphia Spreadable ~ *See Page 74*				
Poseidon: *Per 1 Tbsp, 20g*				
Caviar Salad	75	305	6.5	3
Hommus	55	225	5	1.5
Tzatziki	25	100	1.5	2
Simply Less *(Coles): Per 1 Tablespoon, 20g*				
Hommus: Light	35	140	2	3
Spicy Roast Pumpkin & Harissa	20	85	0.5	3
Tzatziki, Light	15	65	0.5	2
Yumi's: *Per 1 Tbsp, 20g*				
Blue Range: Tuna w. Caramelised Onion	65	275	6	1.5
Tuna w. Cracked Black Pepper	90	370	8.5	1
Tuna w. Tomato & Basil	80	320	7.5	0.5
Tuna w. Tomato & Olives	75	315	7	1
Classic: Baba Ganoosh	45	1780	4.5	1
Creamed Beetroot	40	155	3	1.5
Eggplant & Garlic	60	255	6.5	0.5
Kalamata Olive	75	320	10	0.5
Middle Eastern Hommus	50	200	4.5	1.5
Middle Eastern Tahini	70	280	6.5	0.5
Spicy Pumpkin	35	140	2.5	2
Fish: Gourmet Tuna Mousse	85	350	7.5	0.5
Smoked Trout Mousse	85	355	8.5	0.5
Gold Chunky: Cashews & Coriander	100	405	9	3
Macadamia & Sundried Tomato	95	400	7.5	4.5
Pumpkin & Pepitas	55	220	4.5	2

Egg ~ Egg Dishes

Chicken Eggs
Cal | kJ | Fat | Cb

Note: Egg weight is minimum weight of category.

Boiled/Poached: *Per Egg*

	Cal	kJ	Fat	Cb
Jumbo, 67g	100	420	7.5	0.2
Extra Large, 60g	90	375	7	0.2
Large, 53g	80	335	6	0.2
Medium, 48g	70	290	5	0.1
Egg Yolk, large	65	270	6	0
Egg White, large	15	60	0	0.1

Omega-3 Enriched Eggs:
1 Extra Large Egg, 60g	80	335	6	1

Other Eggs

	Cal	kJ	Fat	Cb
Duck; Turkey, 1 egg, 70g-80g	130	545	10	0.5
Goose, 1 egg, 145g	270	1130	19	2
Quail, 1 egg, 10g	15	60	1	0

Egg Whites

	Cal	kJ	Fat	Cb
100% Albumen, dry, 5g	20	75	0	0.4
The Cutting Edge, *(Golden Eggs)*, 100g	50	210	0	0.5

Egg Substitutes

Frozen Mixes (Cholesterol-Free):
	Cal	kJ	Fat	Cb
1 sachet, 100g	165	680	9	3

Egg Replacement Powder:
Egg-Like (Country Harvest)
1 heaped tsp (= 1 egg)	10	40	0	2.5

EGGS ~ IDEAL FOR WEIGHT CONTROL

Eggs are an excellent calorie-controlled unit of food.
They are nutritious and satisfy hunger.

Nutritional features include:
- High in protein, vitamins, and iron.
- Rich in lutein ~ protects vision as we age.
- Rich in choline ~ enhances brain development in foetus and newborns. Choline may also enhance memory function through life.

EGGS & CHOLESTEROL ~ *See Page 216*

Updated Nutrition Data ~ www.CalorieKing.com.au
Persons with Diabetes ~ See Disclaimer (Page 22)

Cooked Egg Dishes

Fried Eggs:
	Cal	kJ	Fat	Cb
Plain, 2 large eggs	265	1100	22	0.5
With bacon, 2 slices	300	1255	23	1
With sausage, 2 thin, fried	460	1920	32	8

Scrambled Eggs:
	Cal	kJ	Fat	Cb
Plain, 1 large egg (53g)	125	520	11	1
With 1 Tbsp milk & 1 tsp fat				
With skim milk, no fat	85	355	6	1
Scrambled eggs, 2 large	250	1045	22	2
With 2 slices bacon	550	2300	45	3
With 1 slice toast (+ 3 tsp fat)	390	1620	13	12

Omelettes:
Plain, with minimal fat:
	Cal	kJ	Fat	Cb
1 large egg (53g)	115	475	10	0.5
2 large eggs	225	945	19	1
With cheese, 20g	310	1285	26	1
With ham, 30g	260	1080	20	1

Restaurant Style:
3 eggs/cheese/ham/ tomato/butter	500	2090	30	18

Egg & Cheese Dishes:
	Cal	kJ	Fat	Cb
Cauliflower Cheese, 200g	245	1020	18	8.5
Cheese Soufflé, 120g	300	1255	22	25
Devilled Eggs, 2 halves	130	535	11	0.5
Eggs Benedict, 1 egg, cheese & ham	365	1515	10	41

Quiche: *Average:*
1 serve, 150g	470	1950	33	27

Scotch Egg, 125g | 300 | 1240 | 21 | 13 |

Eggnogs & Egg Flips

Eggnogs/ Egg Flips:
Brownes (WA)
	Cal	kJ	Fat	Cb
Eggnog, 300ml	230	960	5	33
Pauls (Qld), 300ml	235	950	5	33
Homemade Eggnog, 250ml cup	250	1045	9	20
Xmas Eggnog (with Rum), 250ml	300	1255	9	20

F. Fats ◆ Spreads ◆ Oils

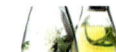

Butter

	Cal	kJ	Fat	Cb
Butter: 1 tsp, 5g	35	150	4	0
1 Tbsp, 20g	145	605	16	0
½ cup, 125g	910	3800	100	1
100g quantity	740	3100	83	1
Single Serve, Butter Pat, 7g	50	210	6	0
Garlic/Herb Butter ~ Same as butter				
Ghee/Clarified Butter, 100% fat, 1 T., 20g	175	735	20	0

Margarine Spreads

Average All Brands
Regular: *65% Fat, Includes Canola, Dairy Free, Olive, Sterols*

	Cal	kJ	Fat	Cb
1 tsp, 5g	30	120	3	0
1 Tbsp, 20g	115	480	13	0
½ cup, 125g	725	3030	81	0
100g quantity	580	2420	65	0

Reduced Fat Spreads

Per 5g Teaspoon

	Cal	kJ	Fat	Cb
Avo, Avocado Oil	20	80	2	0
Bertolli, Light	25	100	3	0
Eta, 5 Star	25	90	2.5	0
Flora: Light	20	90	2.5	0
Ultra Light	10	50	1.5	0
Flora Pro-Activ:				
Buttery	30	120	3.5	0
Light	20	75	2	0
Olive	20	90	2.5	0
Ultra Light	10	45	1	0
Gold 'N Canola, Lite	25	100	2.5	0
Logicol: Extra Light	10	45	1	0
Light	20	90	2.5	0
Meadow Lea: Light	20	90	2.5	0
Extra Light	15	60	1.5	0
Nuttelex: Lite	20	95	2.5	0
Pulse	25	110	3	0
Pure Vita *(Aldi)*: Canola	25	105	3	0
Sunnyvale *(Aldi)*: Canola	30	125	3	0
Olive Oil, Light	25	105	3	0
Light & Salt Reduced	20	90	2.5	0
Weight Watchers, Canola	20	85	2.5	0

Dairy Blends & Other Spreads

	Cal	kJ	Fat	Cb
Dairy Blends: *(Devondale/Country Gold)*, Average, 1 tsp., 5g	35	150	4	0
Alfa One, Rice Bran Oil:				
Regular, 1 tsp, 5g	35	150	4	0
Light, 1 tsp, 5g	25	95	3	0
Flora, Buttery, 5g	30	130	3.5	0
Cocoa Butter, 1 Tbsp	125	525	14	0

Copha, Lard, Animal Fats

	Cal	kJ	Fat	Cb
Chicken/Goose Fat:				
1 Tbsp, 20g	175	740	20	0
½ cup, 125g	1100	4600	20	0
Copha:				
1 Tbsp, 20g	175	740	20	0
100g quantity	885	3700	100	0
200g block	1770	7400	200	0
Dripping, Lard:				
1 Tbsp, 20g	175	740	20	0
½ cup, 125g	1100	4600	125	0
200g block	1770	7400	200	0
Duck Fat (Luv-A-Duck),				
1 Tbsp, 20g	185	740	20	0
½ cup, 125g	1155	4620	125	0
Shortening, Suet:				
1 Tbsp, 20g	175	740	20	0
½ cup, 125g	1100	4600	125	0

Vegetable Oils

Includes Canola, Carotino, Corn, Cottonseed, Flaxseed, Palm, Grapeseed, Olive, Light Olive, Peanut, Sesame, Soybean, Sunflower, Sunola.

	Cal	kJ	Fat	Cb
1 tsp, 5ml	45	185	5	0
1 Tbsp, 20ml	175	735	20	0
½ cup, 125ml	1100	4600	125	0

Fish Oil

	Cal	kJ	Fat	Cb
Fish Oil, All types:				
1 tsp, 5ml	30	125	3.5	0
1 Tbsp, 20 ml	125	530	14	0
Capsules: 500 mg, (1)	5	20	0.5	0
1000 mg, (1)	10	40	1	0

Oil Sprays

Alfa One:

	Cal	kJ	Fat	Cb
Rice Bran: 2-3 second spray, 5g	45	185	5	0
5-6 second spray, 10g	90	370	10	0
Always Fresh, Spanish Olive Oil, Average all varieties, 5g	30	120	3.5	0
Gold'n Canola, Pure & Simple:				
2-3 second spray, 5g	35	140	4	0
5-6 second spray, 2 tsp.,10g	65	280	7.5	0
ProChef: *Per 2-3 second Spray, 5g*				
Canola	45	185	5	0
Olive Oil: Classic	50	200	5	0
Garlic Lovers	45	185	5	0

Fish ~ Fresh ◆ Shellfish F

Fish, Fresh ~ Quick Guide

	Cal	kJ	Fat	Cb
Fresh Fish: *Per 100g Edible Portion*				
Low-Fat White Fish:				
Examples: Barramundi, Bream, Cod, Dhufish, Flounder, John Dory, Kingfish, Ling, Perch, Pike, Schnapper, Shark, Sole, Whiting:				
Raw, average, 100g	90	375	1.5	0
Steamed/Poached/Grilled	100	420	2	0
Baked: *Minimal Fat*				
Flesh only, 100g	110	460	2	0
Fried, no batter, 100g	175	730	7	0
Lightly floured, 100g	200	840	7	3
Crumbed, 100g	225	940	11	1.5
In batter, 100g	275	1150	15	2
Higher Fat:				
Per 100g Edible Portion				
Atlantic Herring, raw	160	660	9	0
Bream, raw	120	500	5	0
Gemfish, raw	175	735	11	0
Milkfish, raw	190	795	11	0
Mullet, raw	120	500	5.5	0
Pacific Herring, raw	195	815	14	0
Rainbow Trout, raw	155	650	8.5	0
Salmon (Atlantic), raw	200	840	13	0
Yellowtail, raw	145	610	5	0

Other Fish & Shellfish

	Cal	kJ	Fat	Cb
Abalone (Mutton Fish) raw, 100g	105	440	0.5	6
Barramundi: raw, 100g	90	375	1.5	0
Aquaculture, raw, 100g	100	420	2	0
Basa, raw, 100g	80	345	2	0
Black Tip Shark, raw, 100g	115	480	0.5	0
Blue Granadier/Hake, raw, 100g	80	345	0.5	0
Calamari (Squid): Plain, 100g	80	335	1	0
Deep fried, 1 cup, 100g	205	860	9.5	7
Catfish, raw, 100g	80	335	0.5	0
Clams: Meat only				
4 large/9 small, 100g	80	335	1	0.5
Cockles, boiled, 100g	50	200	0.5	0
Coral Trout, raw, 100g	90	375	1	0
Crab, cooked, flesh only, 100g	60	250	0.5	0
Crayfish/Lobster:				
1 small, 350g				
Flesh only, cooked, 100g	90	375	1	0
Cuttlefish: Fresh, 100g	80	335	1	0
Dried, 30g	90	375	0.5	1
Dhufish/Jewfish, raw, 100g	90	375	1.5	0
Diamond Scale Mullet, 100g	95	390	1	0
Eel: Raw, 100g	185	775	12	0
Smoked, 100g	330	1380	28	0
Golden Snapper/Hoki, raw, 100g	90	375	0.5	0

Other Fish & Shellfish (Cont)

	Cal	kJ	Fat	Cb
Herring Rollmop, with filling (2), 40g	100	420	7	3
Jewfish/Dhufish, 100g	90	375	1.5	0
Mackerel, raw, 100g	100	420	1	0
Moreton Bay Bug: Average, 230g				
Flesh only, 70g	65	270	0.5	0
Mussels: Shelled, raw, 100g	90	375	2	4
Boiled, shelled, 100g	105	445	3	4
Weighed with shell, 100g	30	135	1	1
Octopus, raw, 100g	80	345	1	2
Orange Roughy/Sea Perch,				
raw, fillets, 100g	125	525	7	0
Oysters: Shelled, raw, 6 medium, 60g	45	185	1.5	0.5
In batter, fried, 6, 140g	370	1555	18	41
Kilpatrick, ½ dozen	160	670	11	2.5
Natural, ½ dozen	45	185	1.5	0.5
Prawns/Shrimp: Boiled, shelled, 100g	80	320	1	0
Weighed with shell, 100g	30	120	0.5	0
In batter, deep fried, 100g	250	1050	15	12
King Prawn, raw, each, 30g	25	110	0	0
Garlic Prawns, 100g serve	265	1110	20	0
Queenfish, (NT) raw, 100g	85	360	0.5	0
Red Emperor, raw, 100g	95	390	0.5	0
Salmon (Atlantic), raw, medium fillet, 70g	140	590	9.5	0
Salmon/Tuna Patty:				
Small, baked, average, 35g	100	410	5.5	7
Medium, baked, average, 50g	140	585	8	9
Scallops: Raw, 80g	70	290	1	1.5
Battered & fried, 100g	215	900	11	10
Scampies/Yabbies:				
Raw in shell, 1 only, 65g	30	125	0.5	0
In breadcrumbs, fried, 100g	315	1315	18	20
Smoked Fish: *Per 100g*				
Cod, 100g	100	420	1.5	0
Salmon, 1 slice (8 x 6cm) 12g	15	70	0.5	0
South African Fillets, 100g	150	630	1	0
Tuna; Trout, 100g	130	545	3.5	0
Schnapper, avg., raw, 100g	95	400	1.5	0
Shrimps ~ *See Prawns*				
Spanish Mackerel, raw, 100g	140	585	6	0
Sweet Lip, (Nthn Terr.), raw, 100g	95	395	1	0
Swordfish, raw, 100g	120	505	4	0
Trevally, raw, 100g	100	420	1	0
Trout, Rainbow, raw, 100g	155	650	8.5	0
Tuna, Sushi, 1 piece, 2.5cm x 2.5cm	60	255	0.5	0
Whitebait, floured, fried, 100g	525	2195	48	30

Adjustment for Frying
*Frying: Add 50 cal/210 kj/5 fat
Per 100g serving.*

Updated Nutrition Data ~ www.CalorieKing.com.au
Persons with Diabetes ~ See Disclaimer (Page 22)

95

Fish ~ Frozen

Fish, Frozen ~ Quick Guide

Item	Cal	kJ	Fat	Cb
Frozen Fish:				
Average All Brands				
Fish Fingers: 1 finger, 25g	50	210	3	3.5
Fried, 1 finger	65	275	4	4.5
Fish Cakes: 1 cake, 50g	120	495	6.5	9
Fried, 1 cake	140	585	8	13
Fish Fillets (White):				
Plain, uncoated, 1 fillet, 100g	80	335	0.5	0
Crumbed/Breaded, 70g fillet	150	630	8	12
Fried	190	795	8.5	7
Battered, 1 fillet, 70g	150	630	7.5	8
Fried, 70g fillet	200	835	12	10
Fried, 100g fillet	275	1150	18	14
Prawns: Cooked, peeled, 100g	80	320	1	0
Cutlet, fried, 4 large, 30g	75	315	4.5	3.5
Crab/Seafood Sticks, plain, 1 stick, 67g	105	430	3.5	13
Seafood Extender, 5-6 pces, 50g	75	320	2.5	8
Austrimi Seafoods: *Per Serving, Uncooked*				
Crumbed Kal-Rings (4-5), 100g	235	980	11	24
Natural Squid Rings (4-5), 50g	40	165	0.5	0.5
Seafood Balls, Plain, 50g	50	195	0.5	6
Seafood Bites, 4 pieces, 80g	160	660	7	16
Seafood Sticks (1), 67g	105	430	3.5	13
Seafood Highlighters (5-6), 50g	80	335	3.5	8
Birds Eye:				
Fish Cakes: 1 cake, 50g	115	485	6.5	9
Salmon with Vege & Herbs, 1 cake, 80g	160	670	7.5	15
Tuna with Potato & Herbs, 80g	155	650	5.5	18
Fish Fingers, (3), 75g	155	655	6.5	14
Crumbed Fillets: *Per Fillet, 70g*				
Deep Sea Dory	150	630	8.5	12
Hoki	150	615	6.5	14
Ocean Select Salmon Fillets: *Per 135g*				
Herb Provencale, 135g	250	1035	16	1
Lemon Pepper, 135g	345	1444	27	1
Oven Bake (6 Portions): *Per Portion, 70g*				
Barramundi, 67g	150	630	8	10
Herb & Garlic	150	615	6.5	14
Lemon Pepper	160	675	7	15
Lightly Battered	160	675	10	9
Original	150	615	6.5	14
Steam Fish Fillets, avg, 1 fillet, 180g	145	610	5	3
Coles:				
Fish Cakes: (1), 80g	165	685	7.5	15
Tuna w. Sweet Corn (1), 80g	175	740	7.5	19
Fish Fillets:				
In Cheese Sauce, 200g packet	245	1030	14	8
In Parsley Sauce, 200g packet	215	900	12	9
Crumbed: *Per Fillet*				
Hake, 165g	345	1450	17	28
Herb & Garlic, 71g	155	645	7.5	13
Lemon, 71g	155	635	7	14
Reduced Salt, 71g	150	630	7	15
Battered (1), 71g	140	590	9	9
Hoki, Beer Battered, 100g	190	785	10	14
Fish Fingers, (3), 75g	155	635	7	14
Fish Portions, Crumbed (1), 83g	185	765	9	15
I&J:				
Crispy Fish Bites (3), 60g	155	645	11	9
Crumbed Calamari Rings, 88g	215	895	11	20
Sea Shantys (1)	75	305	4	6.5
Seafood Platter, 1 piece, 20g	55	235	3	6
Tasty Fish Fingers (3), 75g	155	655	7.5	15
Flame Grills: *Per Fillet*				
Garlic & Parmesan, 100g	90	365	3	1.5
Lemon Pepper & Garlic, 100g	90	370	3	2
Light & Crispy: *Per Fillet*				
Crumbed: Italian Herb/Lemon	150	630	6	16
Lightly Seasoned	150	635	6	15
Original	150	625	6	16
Snacks: Seafood Basket, ½ pkt, 190g	560	2340	26	61
Seafood Platter, 1 pce, 20g	60	235	3	5.5
IGA Seapoint: *Per Fillet*				
Lemon Crumbed Fish, 71g	185	770	9	16
Ocean Royal *(Aldi):*				
Fillets: Beer Battered, 100g	190	790	9	15
Hoki: Skin On, 100g	90	385	3.5	6.5
Skinless, 100g	35	140	0.5	0.5
Salmon: Atlantic, Natural, 2 pieces, 250g	525	2180	34	16
Atlantic, Lemon Pepper, 2 pieces, 250g	565	2350	40	12
Sealord:				
Dory Fillet, Classic Crumb, 80g	170	700	9	12
Fish Fingers, 25g	60	245	3	6
Fish Tapas, Kumara Crumb, 100g	190	780	8.5	15
Hoki: Beer Batter (1), 75g	170	715	12	8.5
Classic Crumb (1), 80g	130	540	6.5	7
Lemon Pepper Crumb (1), 80g	150	610	7	12
Potato Crumb (1), 80g	150	635	7	12
Tempura Batter (1), 75g	160	675	8.5	9
Simply Crumbed:				
With Wholemeal (1), 120g	225	940	10	19
With Seeds (1), 120g	205	860	8.5	17
With Toasted Oats (1), 120g	235	985	13	16
The Fishmonger *(Aldi),* Prawns, 100g	85	352	0	0

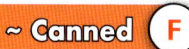

Fish ~ Canned F

Canned Fish ~ Quick Guide

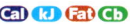
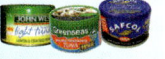

Canned Fish:
Average All Brands
Note:
Canned fish e.g. tuna and salmon, vary in fat content and hence Cal/kJ. Variable factors include fish species, location and season.

	Cal	kJ	Fat	Cb
Anchovies, drained, 6 thin fillets, 30g	55	230	3	0
Caviar: Black, 1 Tbsp, 15g	15	60	1	0
Lumpfish, Red, 1 Tbsp, 15g	25	95	1	0
Clams, baby, 100g	85	355	2	0.5
Crab Meat, 100g	60	250	0.5	1
Herrings in Tomato Sauce, 100g	190	795	14	1.5
Kipper Fillets in Brine, 100g	165	690	10	0.5
Oysters/Mussels, smoked, in oil				
100g, drained	180	740	12	7
Prawns, peeled, 100g	100	420	1	1.5
Salmon:				
Pink: 105g can, drained	120	505	6	0.5
210g can, drained	250	1050	12	1
Red: 105g can, drained	135	575	7.5	0.5
210g can, drained	270	1150	15	1
'Australian' (Ocean Perch),				
100g serve (90g drained)	155	645	8.5	0.5
Sardines: In Oil, 100g	310	1290	26	0
Drained of oil, 100g	220	915	15	0
In Tomato Sauce, 100g	160	680	10	1.5
In Water, 100g	155	645	8	0
Shrimps, drained, 100g	100	420	1	1.5
Tuna: In Brine/Water, 100g	105	445	2	0
100g, drained	125	515	3	0
In Oil, 100g	290	1215	23	0
100g, drained of oil	215	890	13	0
Fish Spreads/Pastes *(John West):*				
1 Tbsp, 25g	50	210	3.5	1

Always Fresh:

	Cal	kJ	Fat	Cb
Anchovies, Flat, 45g can, drained, 27g	55	235	3	0.5
Crabmeat, ¼ of 170g can, 30g drained	20	75	0	0
Herring Fillets in Sauce, 190g can,				
average all varieties, ½ can, 95g	195	815	15	5.5
Peeled Prawns, ¼ of 200g can, 30g drained	30	125	0.5	0.5
Smoked Mussels, ¼ of 85g can, 16g drained	35	150	2	1
Smoked Oysters, ¼ of 85g can, 16g drained	40	160	2.5	1.5

Updated Nutrition Data ~ www.CalorieKing.com.au
Persons with Diabetes ~ See Disclaimer (Page 22)

Ally:

	Cal	kJ	Fat	Cb
Pink Salmon (210g can), ½ can, dr., 79g	115	485	4.5	1

Brunswick:
Sardines: *Per 106g Can, Drained*

In Soy Oil, 84g	175	730	12	0
In Spring Water: 84g	130	540	7	0
No Added Salt, 84g	130	540	7	0
In Tomato Sauce, 106g	140	590	7.5	2.5
With Hot Peppers, 84g	170	720	11	0

Seafood Snacks: *Per 100g Can, Drained*

Kippered, 90g	155	645	9	0

Captain:

Pink Salmon, 105g	135	570	6	0
Red Salmon, 105g	190	760	11	0

Coles:

Prawns, peeled, ½ can, 60g	55	235	0.5	0.5
Crab Meat, ½ can, 60g	40	170	0.5	1

Salmon: *Per Can, Drained*

Pink: 105g can	135	565	6	0
210g can	270	1125	12	0
No Added Salt, 105g can	135	565	6	0
Red: 105g can	160	670	8.5	0
No Added Salt, 105g can	160	670	8.5	0

Sardines: *Per 125g Can, Drained*

In Vegetable Oil, 90g	160	665	8.5	0
In Tomato Sauce, 125g	110	470	3	0.5

Smart Buy,

Tuna with Tomato & Onion, 95g can	90	375	3	4.5

Tuna Chunks: *Per 95g Can, Drained*

In Brine: 70g	75	305	0.5	0
Pole & Line,				
in Brine/Springwater, 70g	80	335	0.5	0
In Olive Oil: 70g	160	655	10	1
Pole & Line, 70g	105	435	3	0
In Springwater, 70g	70	295	0.5	0

Tuna Flavoured: *Per 95g Can*

Italian Style	60	250	1	2
Japanese	85	355	0.5	3
Mexican	75	315	0.5	6
Mild Indian Curry	120	495	5.5	6.5
Moroccan Style	70	280	0.5	1
Spanish	65	280	1	1.5
Sweet Chilli	130	540	0.5	14
Tomato & Basil	130	535	6	2
Tomato & Chilli	80	330	0.5	4

Tuna, Sandwich: *Per 95g Can, Drained*

In Brine, 70g	60	250	1	0
In Olive Oil, 70g	185	770	15	1

97

Fish ~ Canned

Greenseas:

	Cal	kJ	Fat	Cb
Salmon: *Per 95g Can*				
Alaskan: Natural Smoked Flavour	150	620	9.5	1
In Springwater, drained, 65g	75	315	1.5	0
Seasalt & Cracked Pepper	160	665	11	0
Sundried Tomato & Basil	170	705	11	3
Balsamic Vinegar & Cracked Pepper	170	700	12	3
Lemon & Sea Salt	160	670	11	1.5
Tuna: *Per 95g Can*				
Cracked Pepper & Balsamic Vinegar	160	680	11	3
Herb & Garlic	145	595	9	0
In Mayonnaise	190	790	15	5
98% fat free	85	355	1.5	5.5
Lemon Pepper	110	455	5.5	0.5
Lime & Cracked Black Pepper, 99% fat free	70	300	1	1
Natural Smoke Flavour	160	665	11	0.5
Red Curry	130	540	7	4.5
Salsa	125	515	8	2.5
Sandwich Flakes, drained, 65g	160	670	13	0
Sea Salt & Cracked Pepper	145	610	9	0
Spicy Chilli, 98% fat free	90	380	1.5	4.5
Sundried Tomato & Basil	140	570	8.5	3.5
Sundried Tomato & Onion, 98% fat free	95	395	2	6.5
Sweet Chilli	160	675	8.5	7
Tomato & Capsicum, 97% fat free	95	395	2.5	4
Tomato & Caramelised Onion	140	585	7	5
Tomato & Chilli	130	545	7.5	4.5
Tomato & Onion	140	590	9	3.5
Tuna, Not Drain: *Per 75g Can*				
Extra Virgin Olive Oil Blend	140	585	8	0
In Springwater	80	325	1	0
Chunks: *Per 95g Can, Drained*				
In Brine, 65g	75	310	1	0
In Extra Virgin Olive Oil, 95g can drained, 70g	110	450	4.5	0
½ of 180g can drained, 65g	100	415	4	0
In Springwater, 65g	75	310	1	0
Sandwich Spread: *Per 95g Can*				
Mayonnaise & Sweetcorn	185	770	13	7
Seeded Mustard Mayonnaise	215	900	16	8.5

IGA:

	Cal	kJ	Fat	Cb
Sea Point Salmon: *Per ½ 210g Can, Drained*				
Red Sockeye, 80g	130	545	8	0
Sea Point Tuna: *Per ½ 185g Can, Drained*				
Chunks in Brine, 67g	80	330	1	0
Chunks in Canola Oil, 67g	145	610	5.5	0

John West: *Per Serving, Drained*

	Cal	kJ	Fat	Cb
Anchovies Fillets, 45g can, 27g	50	210	3	0
Herring Fillets, in Tomato Sauce, 200g can, 100g	185	775	14	1.5
Kipper Fillets, Smoked in Brine, ½ of 200g can, 75g	125	520	7	0.5
Salmon: *Per Can, Drained*				
Pink: 105g can, 79g	120	500	5	0.5
210g can, 158g	240	1000	11	1
Red: 105g can, 79g	130	550	6.5	0.5
210g can, 158g	260	1095	13	1
Salmon Slices: *Per 125g Can, Drained*				
In Springwater, 75g	80	330	1	0.5
Lemon & Cracked Pepper, 76g	130	540	6	0.5
Salmon Tempters: *Per 95g Can*				
Lemon & Cracked Pepper	155	650	10	0.5
Mayonnaise	130	545	5.5	4.5
Smoke Flavour	130	545	6.5	0
Springwater	55	225	1	0.5
Sweet Chilli & Lime	100	425	2	6.5
Sardines: *Per 110g Can*				
In Springwater, 75g	170	710	13	0.5
In Tomato Sauce, 110g	150	635	9	2.5
In Vegetable Oil, 75g, (drained)	200	830	16	0.5
Tuna:				
Chunk Style: Olive Oil Blend, ½ of 185g can	120	500	5	0.5
In Brine, ¼ of 425g can	85	360	1	0.5
In Springwater, ½ of 185g can	75	310	0.5	0.5
No Drain Tuna: ½ of 130g can				
In Brine/Springwater, 65g	85	360	1	0.5
In Olive Oil, 65g	115	470	4.5	0.5
Tuna & Beans: *Per 185g Tub*				
Capsicum, Sweet Corn, Red Kidney Beans & Chilli	285	1195	14	14
Three Beans	300	1240	14	15
Tuna Chunks In Oil: *Per 95g Can, Drained*				
Chilli, Lime & Ginger; Garlic & Soy, 70g	115	485	4.5	1
Seasalt & Cracked Pepper, 70g	110	455	3.5	1
Tuna Slices: *Per 125g Can, Drained*				
Olive Oil Blend, 83g	160	670	7.5	0.5
Smoked, 83g	160	665	7.5	0.5
Sweet Chilli, 106g	155	640	2.5	8.5
In Springwater, 82g	95	400	1	0.5

Fish ~ Canned F

John West (Cont):	Cal	kJ	Fat	Cb
Tuna Tempters: *Per 95g Can, Drained*				
Mango Chilli, 95g	125	515	5	7
Mild Indian Curry, 86g	110	445	5	3
Oven Dried Capsicum & Chilli, 90g	155	650	10	1.5
Oven Dried Tomato & Basil, 81g	130	530	6.5	2.5
Light Tuna Tempters: *Per 95g Can, Drained*				
Lemon & Cracked Pepper, 82g	65	270	1	1
Onion & Tomato, 87g	70	300	0.5	4
Springwater, 66g	55	230	0.5	0.5
Sweet Chilli, 88g	90	370	1	7
Pole & Line Skipjack: *Half of 185g Can, Drained*				
Chunk Style: In Olive Oil Blend, 136g	80	330	1	0.5
In Springwater, 128g	75	310	1	0.5
Tuna To Go: *Per 61g Snack Pack*				
Plain	140	590	6	14
Sweet Chilli	145	595	6	14
Tomato & Basil	145	595	6	14
King Oscar:				
Sardines: *Per ½ 105g Can, Drained*				
In Oil, 40g	70	290	5	0
In Olive Oil with Lemon Juice, 40g	140	570	12	0
In Pure Spring Water, 40g	70	288	5	0.5
In soybean Oil, 80g	70	290	5	0.5
In Tomato Sauce, 40g	75	305	4	1.5
Ocean Rise *(Aldi):*				
Herring Fillets, in Curry Sce, ½ can, 100g	195	820	14	7
Mackerel Fillets, in Tomato Sce, 125g can	200	845	13	6
Mussels, Danish in Oil, 75g drained	125	510	7	1
Salmon: Flavoured, avg. 95g can	105	440	3	6
Pink, ¼ can, 95g	120	500	3	1
Sprats, in Garlic/Oil, drained, 75g	125	510	7	1.5
Tuna Slices: In Olive Oil, drained, 84g	125	525	4	0
In Springwater, 125g can	100	415	0.5	0
Tuna, Yellowfin in Oil, drained, 70g	155	650	9	2
Paramount:				
Salmon: *Per Serving, Drained*				
Pink, Cleaned, Filleted & Boned, 60g	40	160	1	1
Pink, Wild Alaskan, 80g	120	505	6	0.5
Smoked Fillets in Oil, 85g	180	745	11	0.5
Red, Wild Alaskan, 80g	135	565	7	0.5
Safcol:				
Salmon: *Per Serving, Drained*				
Skinless & Boneless	95	400	3	0
Premium, Atlantic Salmon,				
In Springwater, 68g	120	510	7.5	0.5
Lemon & Pepper, 68g	65	270	2.5	0.5
Mild Red Chilli, drained, 60g	110	455	7.5	1
Skinless & Boneless, ½ can, 70g	90	375	3	0.5

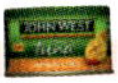

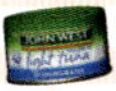

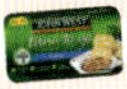

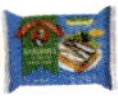

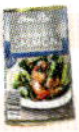

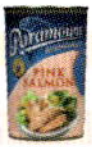

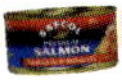

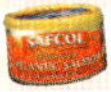

Safcol (Cont):	Cal	kJ	Fat	Cb
Salmon, Pieces: *Per 100g Pouch*				
Mediterranean, 100g	145	610	9	2.5
With Lemon & Dill, 100g	105	435	2.5	1
With Mild Red Chilli, 100g	185	760	12	3
Tuna: *Per 95g Can, Drained*				
In Brine, 70g	60	255	0.5	0.5
In Canola Oil, 70g	160	675	12	0.5
In Extra virgin Olive Oil, 74g	160	660	8	0.5
In Springwater, 70g	70	285	0.5	0.5
Fresh Tomato & Onion, 95g	100	410	2.5	5
Lemon Pepper, 64g	95	390	5	1
Mild Chilli & Rstd Garlic in Springwater, 85g	70	290	0.5	3
Penang Curry, 95g	140	575	7	2
Premium, In Extra Virgin Olive Oil, 95g	145	605	8.5	0.5
Sandwich Style, 70g	165	690	12	1
Sweet Chilli Sauce, 95g	95	385	1	7
Tangy Lem. & Oregano in Springwater, 65g	80	320	1	1
Thai Green Curry, 95g	120	500	5.5	5
Thai Red Curry, 95g	130	550	6.5	4.5
Tuna Pouches: *Per Single Serve, 100g*				
With Lemon & Black Pepper	125	530	1.5	3.5
With Oven Dried Tom. & Herb	140	580	6.5	1.5
With Sweet Chilli Sauce	125	525	1	7

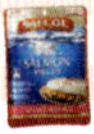

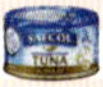

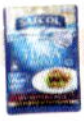

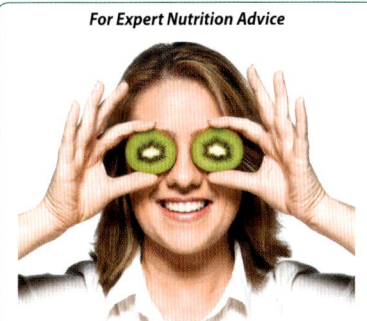

For Expert Nutrition Advice

look no further than an **Accredited Practising Dietitian**

For expert information to help you eat healthier and feel better, you can find an Accredited Practising Dietitian (APD) at www.daa.asn.au, or call toll free on 1800 812 942

Updated Nutrition Data ~ www.CalorieKing.com.au
Persons with Diabetes ~ See Disclaimer (Page 22)

Fish ~ Canned

Sealord:		Cal	kJ	Fat	Cb
Salmon: *Per 100g, Drained*					
Alaskan/Canadian Pink		135	570	7.5	0.5
Red		165	685	10	0.5
Salmon Sensations,					
Cracked Pepper & Lemon; Smoked, 85g can		145	600	9	2
Tuna, Chunky, In Springwater, 62g		75	305	1	0.5
Tuna Sensations: *Per 95g Can*					
Lemon Pepper		210	885	14	5
Savoury Onion		110	455	3.5	6
Smoked		240	1000	18	5
Sundried Tomato & Olive		120	500	5	5.5
Sweet Thai Chilli		105	440	1	6.5
Tomato & Basil		115	480	4.5	2.5
Tuna Lite, 98% Fat-Free: *Per 85g Can*					
Lemon & Cracked Pepper		90	365	0.5	3
Mexican Salsa		65	275	0.5	5
Sundried Tom. & Basil		80	325	0.5	4
Tuna Lite w. Rice Crackers: *Per Packet*					
Lemon & Cracked Pepper		145	600	0.5	16
Sundried Tomato & Basil		135	560	0.5	17
Seakist:					
Tuna: *Per ¼ 425g Can, Drained*					
Chunks in Brine, 64g		65	270	0.5	0.5
Chunks in Springwater, 64g		65	270	0.5	0.5
Tuna Lunch Kit, with Crackers:					
Mayonnaise with Sweetcorn		275	1145	19	12
Sweet Chilli Mayo		240	1000	15	13
Thousand Island Dressing		195	815	10	13
Sirena:					
Tuna in Oil, Italian Style: *Drained*					
95g Can, 70g		115	470	5	1
185g Can, 140g		225	9.5	10	1.5
100g quantity		160	675	7	1
Lite Tuna in Oil (La Vita): *Drained*					
95g Can, 70g		90	370	2.5	0
185g Can, 140g		180	740	4.5	0
Tuna in Springwater: *Drained*					
95g Can		75	320	0.5	0
185g Can		155	640	1.5	0
100g quantity		110	460	1	0
Tuna Slices: *Per 125g Can, Drained*					
Chilli & Oil, 75g		120	505	5.5	1
Italian Style, 75g		120	505	5.5	1

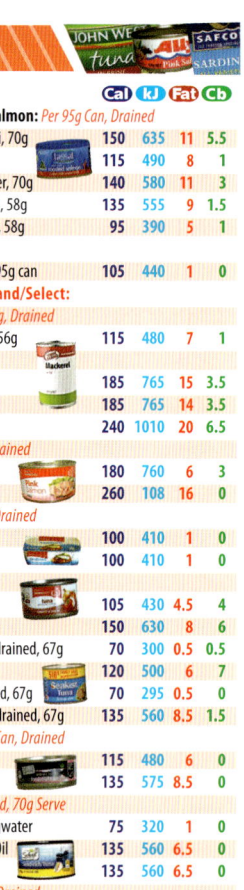

Tassal:		Cal	kJ	Fat	Cb
Premium Tasmanian Salmon: *Per 95g Can, Drained*					
Asian Style, Sweet Chilli, 70g		150	635	11	5.5
In Brine, 63g		115	490	8	1
Lemon & Cracked Pepper, 70g		140	580	11	3
Roasted with Canola Oil, 58g		135	555	9	1.5
Roasted in Springwater, 58g		95	390	5	1
Weight Watchers,					
Tuna, in Springwater, 95g can		105	440	1	0
Woolworths/Home Brand/Select:					
Home Brand: *Per Serving, Drained*					
Mackerel, in Natural Oil, 56g		115	480	7	1
Mussels:					
Smoked: 70g		185	765	15	3.5
In Vegetable Oil, 70g		185	765	14	3.5
Oysters, Smoked, 70g		240	1010	20	6.5
Salmon: *Per 210g Can, Drained*					
Pink, 160g		180	760	6	3
Red, 160g		260	108	16	0
Sardines: *Per 125g Can, Drained*					
In Oil, 94g		100	410	1	0
In Spring Water, 90g		100	410	1	0
Tuna: *Per 95g Can*					
In Salsa		105	430	4.5	4
In Tomato and Onion		150	630	8	6
Tuna Chunks: In Brine, drained, 67g		70	300	0.5	0.5
In Oil, drained, 70g		120	500	6	7
In Springwater, drained, 67g		70	295	0.5	0
Sandwich Tuna in Oil, drained, 67g		135	560	8.5	1.5
Select Brand: *Per 105g Can, Drained*					
Salmon: Pink, 84g		115	480	6	0
Red, 84g		135	575	8.5	0
Tuna: *Per 95g Can, Drained, 70g Serve*					
Chunks: In Brine; Springwater		75	320	1	0
In Extra Virgin Olive Oil		135	560	6.5	0
In Pure Olive Oil		135	560	6.5	0
Flaked: *Per 95g Can, Not Drained*					
Lightly Smoked Flavour		150	635	8.5	1
In Chilli		135	560	6.5	1.5
In Lemon & Cracked Pepper		75	315	0.5	1
In Sweet Chilli		135	560	6.5	1.5
In Sweet Mustard		140	580	5.5	5
In Tomato Salsa		140	580	6.5	5
In Tomato with Basil		120	495	5	1

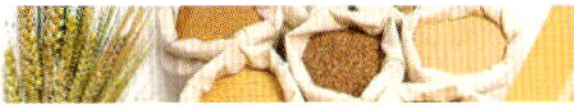

Flours

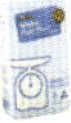
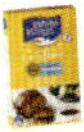
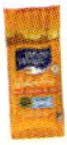

	Cal	kJ	Fat	Cb
Plain/Self Raising: 2 Tbsp, 25g	90	380	0	19
1 cup unsifted, 155g	555	2325	2	113
1 cup sifted, 140g	500	2095	1.5	102
Stoneground, Plain, 1 cup, 140g	280	1170	2	53
Wholemeal, Plain, 1 cup, sifted, 140g	490	2040	3	92
Biscuit/Cake/Pasta Flour, *White Wings*, 100g	355	1490	1.5	70
Cornflour, 2½ Tbsp, 30g	110	470	1	25
Gluten Free Flour, 100g	335	1400	0	81
Greewheat Freekeh, 100g dry	350	1470	2.5	72
Potato Flour, ½ cup, 80g	285	1195	0	67
Rye/Rice, average, 2 Tbsp, 30g	100	420	0.5	24
Soybean: Defatted, 30g	100	420	0.5	12
Full Fat, 30g	130	550	6	11

Grains

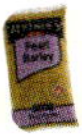
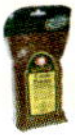
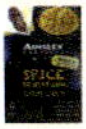
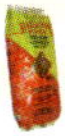
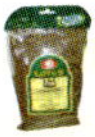
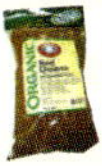

	Cal	kJ	Fat	Cb
Amaranth, dry, ½ cup, 100g	375	1565	6.5	65
Arrowroot, dry, ½ cup, 65g	230	955	0	55
Barley: Pearl, dry, 2 Tbps, 30g	100	410	0.5	19
Cooked, ½ cup, 80g	80	335	0.5	15
Bulgar, (Cracked Wheat):				
Dry, ½ cup, 70g	225	945	1	42
Cooked, ½ cup, 90g	75	310	0.5	14
Carob Flour/Meal/Powder, ¼ cup, 25g	55	230	0	22
Cornmeal, dry, 1 cup, 140g	465	1940	3	97
Cous Cous ~ *See Sago/Semolina*				
Flax/Linseed: 1 Tbsp, 14g	70	290	5	5
¼ cup, 45g	220	925	15	15
Meal: 1 Tbsp, 10g	55	230	4	3
½ cup, 60g	310	1295	24	17
L.S.A., 1 Tbsp, 12g	60	260	5	3.5
Matzo Meal, Coarse, 1 cup, 90g	330	1370	1	69
Millet/Maize Meal/Manioc, ¼ cup, 30g	115	475	1.5	19
Pearl Barley ~*See Barley*				
Polenta/Cornmeal:				
Dry, 1 cup, 138g	465	1940	3	97
Cooked, 1 cup, 270g	290	1215	1.5	59
Fried, 2-3 pieces, 150g	180	755	12	15
Psyllium Husks, 1 Tbsp, 6g	10	50	0	0
Quinoa: Raw, ½ cup, 85g	315	1310	5	55
100g quantity	370	1540	6	64
Cooked, ½ cup, 90g	110	465	2	20
Sago/Semolina, raw, ½ cup, 85g	305	1280	1	80
Tapioca: Pearl: Raw, ½ cup, 75g	260	1095	0	64
Cooked, ½ cup, 125g	50	200	0	12
Tapioca Cream, ½ cup, 90g	120	500	7	30

Rice ~ Quick Guide

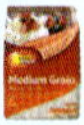
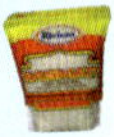
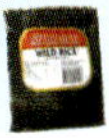

	Cal	kJ	Fat	Cb
Average All Brands				
White Rice: Average all grains/lengths				
Raw, ½ cup, 100g	350	1470	0.5	79
Cooked, ½ cup, 80g	130	540	0.5	29
1 cup, 160g	260	1075	0.5	58
Fried, 1 cup, 150g	340	1420	13	44
Brown Rice:				
Raw, ½ cup, 100g	370	1535	2.5	77
Cooked, ½ cup, 80g	120	510	1	26
Basmati Rice:				
½ cup, cooked, 80g	85	360	0.5	18
Riviana Ezi-Cook, 80g cooked	90	375	0.5	19
Wild Rice:				
Raw, ½ cup, 100g	360	1500	1	69
Cooked, ½ cup, 75g	80	320	0.5	15

SunRice:

Per 100 Dry (Uncooked) Unless Indicated

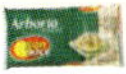
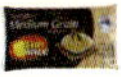
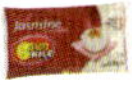
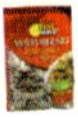

	Cal	kJ	Fat	Cb
Arborio Mediterranean	350	1470	0.5	78
Basmati Indian Aromatic	365	1520	1	78
Brown Calrose Medium Grain	350	1460	3	71
Brown Long Grain	350	1460	3	71
Doongara CleverRice	350	1470	0.5	78
Japanese Style Sushi	345	1440	0.5	77
Jasmine	355	1480	0.5	78
Organic White Medium Grain	350	1470	0.5	79
Vita-Rice, Parboiled Long Grain	360	1500	0.5	78
Wild Blend Entertainer	355	1480	0.5	78
White Long Grain	350	1470	0.5	78
90 Seconds Rice:				
Long Grain White, ½ package, 125g	250	1050	4	49
Medium Grain Brown, ½ package, 125g	235	975	4	43
Mexican, ½ pack, 125g	200	830	4.5	31
Heat & Serve, average all flavours, 300g	440	1830	2	92
Quick Cups: Egg Fried Rice, 125g	185	775	4.5	30
Jasmine Rice, 125g	215	895	3	42
Teriyaki Rice	195	810	2.5	37

Rice Dishes

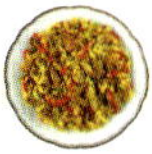

	Cal	kJ	Fat	Cb
Nasi Goreng, 250g	395	1650	13	62
Paella, Chicken/Prawn	340	1425	12	32
Rice Pilaf with butter, plain, 160g	270	1110	6.5	45
Rice Porridge, 1 cup	90	380	0.2	21
Rice Pudding, 1 cup, 240g	350	1460	9.5	57
Risotto, Seafood, 300g	545	2285	14	76

Updated Nutrition Data ~ www.CalorieKing.com.au
Persons with Diabetes ~ See Disclaimer (Page 22)

NO MORE EXCUSES!!

Now... 3 Easy Ways to Track Your Calories
A Must! For Serious Weight Control

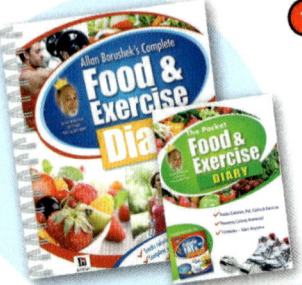

1) *FOOD & EXERCISE DIARIES*

- Choose between Pocket Size (10 weeks) or Larger Size (12 months)
- Not Dated ~ Start Anytime!

FROM NEWSAGENTS AND BOOKSTORES

www.hinkler.com.au

2) ONLINE

- Food & Exercise Diary
- Easy to Use
- Database ~ over 20,000 foods

www.CalorieKing.com.au

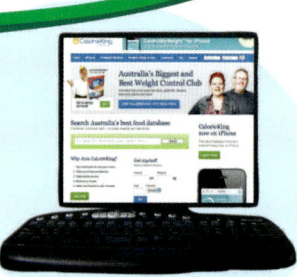

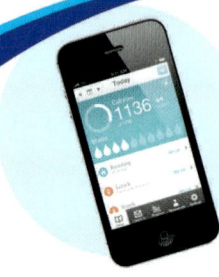

3) *ControlMyWeight™ App*
Food & Exercise Diary (By CalorieKing)

- For on-the-go people
- Australia's best food database

Available for iPhone

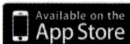

Fruit ~ Fresh F

Fruit ~ Fresh

	Cal	kJ	Fat	Cb
Weights As Purchased				
Achacha, 1 medium, 50g	5	25	0	1
Apple, average all types:				
Weights with core & skin:				
Small, (5 per ½ kg), 100g	50	210	0	11
Medium (3 per ½ kg), 150g	75	310	0	16
Large, 235g	120	485	0	25
Flesh only (without core or skin),				
100g quantity	50	210	0	11
Toffee Apple, 1 medium	225	950	3.5	50
Apricots:				
Small (16 per ½ kg), 30g	10	40	0	2
1 medium (12 per ½ kg), 40g	15	60	0	2.5
1 large (8 per ½ kg), 60g	20	85	0	4
Avocado, average all types, ripe:				
1 small, 180g (110g flesh)	225	940	24	1
½ small avocado	115	470	12	0.5
1 medium, 240g (160g flesh)	330	1370	34	1
½ medium avocado	165	685	17	0.5
1 large, 300g (200g flesh)	410	1710	43	1.5
½ large avocado	205	855	22	0.5
1 extra large, 400g, (300g flesh)	620	2570	64	2
½ extra large	310	1285	32	1
Cocktail: 1 small, 20g	40	170	4	0.1
1 large, 40g	80	340	8.5	0.2
Other:				
Salad Slice, 12.5g	20	85	2	0.1
Mashed, 1 Tbsp, 20g	30	135	3	0.1
100g quantity, flesh only, no stone	205	855	22	0.5

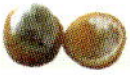

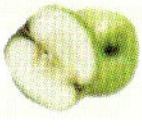

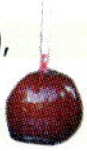

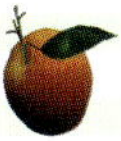

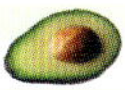

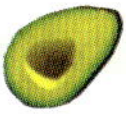

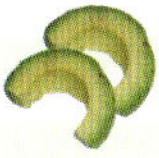

Note: Avocados contain no cholesterol. The fat of avocados is mainly mono-unsaturated which has a beneficial effect on blood cholesterol. Not all avocado fat is absorbed.

	Cal	kJ	Fat	Cb
Babaco, ⅛ medium,120g	40	165	0	7
Banana: (Weights are with skin),				
1 mini/Sugar Finger/Lady Finger, 90g	55	225	0	12
1 small (13cm/5"), 130g	75	315	0	17
1 medium (16cm/6"), 170g	100	420	0	22
1 large (18cm/7"), 210g	120	500	0	27
1 extra large (20cm/8"), 250g	150	630	0	33
Flesh only (no skin), 100g	90	375	0	20
½ cup mashed, 120g	115	480	0	25

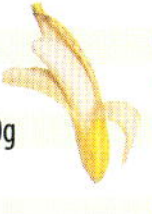

Note: Flesh weighs approx 65% of total weight.

	Cal	kJ	Fat	Cb
Blueberries: ½ cup, 75g	35	155	0	8.5
Small punnet, 150g	70	305	0	17

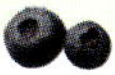

Weights As Purchased	Cal	kJ	Fat	Cb
Blackberries, ½ cup, 80g	40	165	0	6
Brambleberries, 100g	50	210	0	8
Breadfruit, ¼ small, 100g	95	395	0	27
Cantaloupes ~ See Rockmelon				
Cape Gooseberries: 5 med., 20g	10	45	0	2
¾ cup, no husk, 100g	55	220	0	11
Carambola, (Starfruit) 1 medium, 100g	35	150	0	7
Cherries, average all types:				
1 medium, 6g	5	15	0	0.5
16 medium or 25 small, 100g	55	225	0	10
Chinese Jujube, flesh, 100g	80	345	0	20
Coconut, ⅛ average, 100g	310	1290	30	4
Coconut water, 250ml	50	210	0	12
Crabapples, ½ cup slices, 110g	85	355	0	22
Cranberries, ½ cup, 50g	25	95	0	6
Cumquats: 6 small, 50g	30	125	0	7
5-6 large, 100g	70	295	1	16
Custard Apple:				
1 slice (⅛ whole), 50g	30	120	0	6
½ medium, 200g	110	470	1	23
Dragon Pearl,				
1 medium, 330g,	90	380	0.5	22
Durian, flesh, 100g	145	615	5.5	27
Elderberries, 145g	105	440	1	27
Feijoa, (Pineapple Guava),				
1 medium, 100g	40	165	0.5	8
Figs, green/black:				
1 large or 2 small, 85g	40	165	0.5	7
1 medium, 50g	25	100	0	4
Fruit Salad, fresh, ½ cup, 100g	45	190	0	8
Grapefruit, white/pink:				
½ medium, 100g	30	110	0	6
½ large, 140g	45	190	0	8
Grapes, average all types,				
1 small bunch (22 medium), 120g	75	315	0	19
1 medium bunch, 200g	125	525	0	30
1 large bunch, 500g	300	1280	0	78
Globe grapes, 10 large, 180g	110	460	0	28
Guava, 1 small, 90g	30	125	0.5	3
Granadilla, 1 med. (45g), edible portion, 18g	20	75	0	1
Honeydew Melon:				
White Skin ¼ small, 200g	50	210	0.5	10
1 cup cubes, 150g	55	225	0.5	11
Yellow skin, ¼ small, 200g	60	240	0	12
1 cup cubes, 150g	45	180	0	8
Honey Murcots, 1 medium, 120g	40	165	0	8
Jaboticaba flesh, 100g	65	275	0	13
Jackfruit, flesh, ⅛ average, 100g	80	325	0	17
Keriberries, 100g	50	210	0	7.5

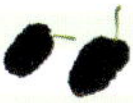

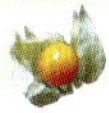

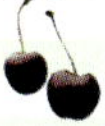

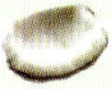

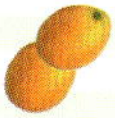

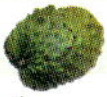

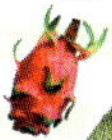

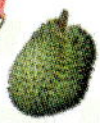

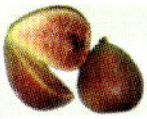

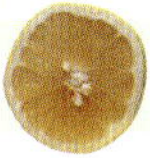

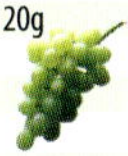

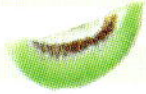

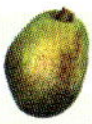

Updated Nutrition Data ~ www.CalorieKing.com.au
Persons with Diabetes ~ See Disclaimer (Page 22)

103

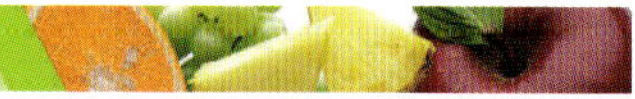

Fruit ~ Fresh

Fruit (Cont)

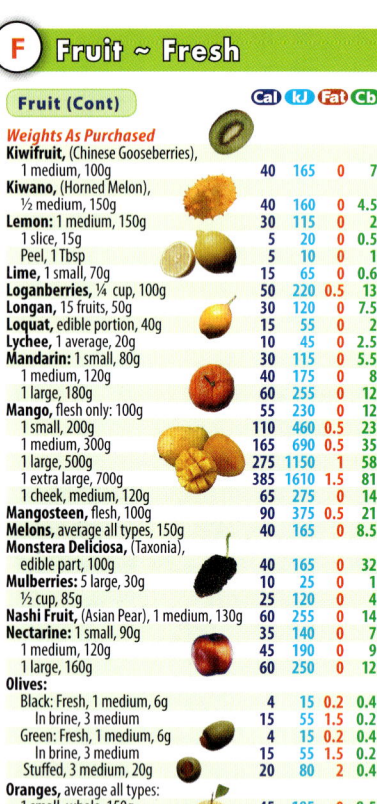

Weights As Purchased — Cal | kJ | Fat | Cb

Item	Cal	kJ	Fat	Cb
Kiwifruit, (Chinese Gooseberries), 1 medium, 100g	40	165	0	7
Kiwano, (Horned Melon), ½ medium, 150g	40	160	0	4.5
Lemon: 1 medium, 150g	30	115	0	2
1 slice, 15g	5	20	0	0.5
Peel, 1 Tbsp	5	10	0	1
Lime, 1 small, 70g	15	65	0	0.6
Loganberries, ¼ cup, 100g	50	220	0.5	13
Longan, 15 fruits, 50g	30	120	0	7.5
Loquat, edible portion, 40g	15	55	0	2
Lychee, 1 average, 20g	10	45	0	2.5
Mandarin: 1 small, 80g	30	115	0	5.5
1 medium, 120g	40	175	0	8
1 large, 180g	60	255	0	12
Mango, flesh only: 100g	55	230	0	12
1 small, 200g	110	460	0.5	23
1 medium, 300g	165	690	0.5	35
1 large, 500g	275	1150	1	58
1 extra large, 700g	385	1610	1.5	81
1 cheek, medium, 120g	65	275	0	14
Mangosteen, flesh, 100g	90	375	0.5	21
Melons, average all types, 150g	40	165	0	8.5
Monstera Deliciosa, (Taxonia), edible part, 100g	40	165	0	32
Mulberries: 5 large, 30g	10	25	0	1
½ cup, 85g	25	120	0	4
Nashi Fruit, (Asian Pear), 1 medium, 130g	60	255	0	14
Nectarine: 1 small, 90g	35	140	0	7
1 medium, 120g	45	190	0	9
1 large, 160g	60	250	0	12
Olives:				
Black: Fresh, 1 medium, 6g	4	15	0.2	0.4
In brine, 3 medium	15	55	1.5	0.2
Green: Fresh, 1 medium, 6g	4	15	0.2	0.4
In brine, 3 medium	15	55	1.5	0.2
Stuffed, 3 medium, 20g	20	80	2	0.4
Oranges, average all types:				
1 small, whole, 150g	45	185	0	8.5
1 medium, whole, 230g	70	285	0	13
1 large, whole, 300g	90	375	0	17
1 extra large, whole, 400g	120	500	0	23
Flesh only, 100g	40	175	0	8
Passionfruit, average:				
1 small, 50g	15	60	0	1
1 medium, 80g	25	100	0	2
Pawpaw (Papaya):				
100g (No skin/seeds)	35	145	0	7
1 medium (460g), 300g, (No skin/Seeds)	100	420	0	21
Peach: 1 small/Donut, 85g	35	150	0	6.5
1 medium, 120g	50	210	0	9.5
1 large, 170g	70	300	0	14
1 extra large, 250g	105	440	0	20

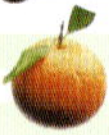

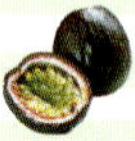

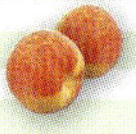

Weights As Purchased — Cal | kJ | Fat | Cb

Item	Cal	kJ	Fat	Cb
Pears, average all varieties:				
1 small, 115g	65	275	0	11
1 medium, 150g	85	355	0	14
1 large, 200g	110	470	0	18
1 extra large, 280g	155	665	0	26
Pepino, ½ medium, 105g	25	100	0	5
Persimmon, 1 medium, 150g	75	310	0	17
Pineapple:				
1 cup cubes, 140g	60	250	0	12
1 thin slice (1.2 cm), 50g (no skin)	20	90	0	4
1 thick slice (2.5cm), 85g (no skin)	40	150	0	7
Whole: Mini (500g) 250g peeled	110	445	0.5	21
Medium (1kg) 500g peeled	215	890	1	41
Large (1.4kg) 700g peeled	300	1245	1.5	58
Note: Edible portion is approximately 50% of whole weight				
Plantain, raw, ½ only, 100g	120	510	0.5	32
Plums, average all varieties:				
1 small, (4cm diam.), 70g	25	110	0	5
1 medium (5cm), 100g	35	155	0	7
1 large, (6cm diam.), 150g	55	235	0	10
Pomegranate, whole (8cm diam.), 154g	70	290	0	12
Pomelo, flesh only, 100g	40	160	0	9
Prickly Pear, 1 medium, 140g	40	160	0	9
Quince, 1 medium, 100g	50	220	0	9
Rambutan, 1 medium, 40g	30	115	0	7
Raspberries, 1 cup, 100g	55	225	0	7.5
Rhubarb, raw, ¾ cup, cube, 100g	20	75	0	1
Rockmelon/Cantaloupe:				
½ small, 400g	115	480	0	23
½ medium, 550g	160	660	0.5	32
½ large, 750g	220	900	1	43
1 cup cubed, 160g	45	190	0	9
1 buffet slice, 75g	20	90	0	4.5
Sapodilla (Chico), 1 medium, 170g	140	590	2	34
Sapotes, 1 medium, 130g	175	730	1	44
Starfruit (Carambola), 1 medium, 100g	35	150	0	7
Strawberries: 5 small, 75g	20	80	0	3
5 medium or 3 large, 100g	25	105	0	4
1 Extra Large, 50g	15	55	0	2
1 Jumbo, 70g	20	75	0	3
1 cup, no stems, 150g	40	165	0	6
1 Punnet: Small, 250g	65	265	0	10
Large, 500g	125	525	0	19
Sugar Cane, peeled, 100g	30	120	0	7
Tamarind, ½ cup, 60g	145	600	0	23
Tangelo: 1 small, 110g	30	135	0	6
1 medium, 140g	40	175	0	8
Tangerine, 1 small, 85g	35	140	0	8

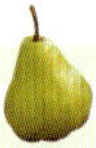

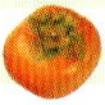

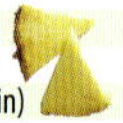

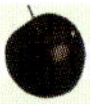

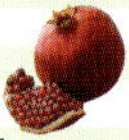

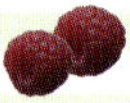

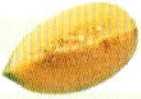

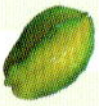

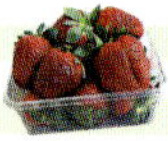

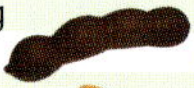

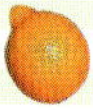

Fruit (Cont)

Weights As Purchased

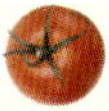

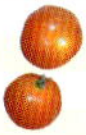

	Cal	kJ	Fat	Cb
Tomatoes, Ripe:				
1 small, 100g	20	75	0	3
1 medium, 150g	30	115	0	4
1 large, 200g	35	150	0	5
Chopped, 1 cup, 200g	35	150	0	5
Slices: 1 medium, 20g	4	15	0	0.5
1 large slice, 27g	5	15	0	0.6
Wedges (4), 70g	15	60	0	2
Cherry, (Tom Thumb):				
1 large or 4 small, 70g	10	50	0	2
¾ cup, 110g	20	80	0	2.5
Grapes, (4-5), 60g	10	45	0	1.5
Tear-drop, (Yellow), 3 med., 75g	5	20	0	1
Tree, (Tamarillo), 1 medium, 80g	25	110	0	2.5
Yellow, Acid-free, 100g	20	75	0	2.5
Sundried Tomatoes ~ *See Page 146*				
Watermelon: *Without Skin or Rind*				
Thin Slice, ½ circle, 150g	45	190	0.5	9.5
Buffet Slice, 40g	10	50	0	2.5
Thick Slice (3cm), ½ circle, 300g	90	380	1	19
¼ circle, 150g	45	190	0.5	9.5
1 cup balls/cubes, 150g	45	190	0.5	9.5
Wedge, ⅛ whole, 375g, with rind/skin	115	475	1	24
Round Seedless:				
Medium Size, 8kg (23cm diam.)				
⅛ whole, with rind/skin, 500g, without rind/skin	150	635	1.5	32
Wedge, 1/16 whole, 250g	75	320	1	16
Mini Size, 3kg (16cm diam.):				
¼ whole, 750g, with rind/skin) 375g , without rind/skin	115	475	1	24

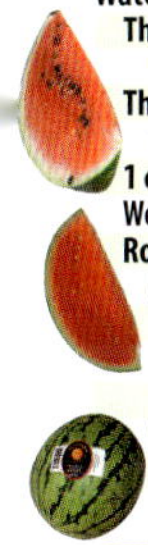

Frozen Fruit ~ Brands

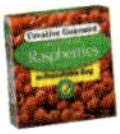
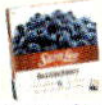

	Cal	kJ	Fat	Cb
Creative Gourmet: Blackberries	80	335	1	16
Blueberries, 100g	50	210	0	12
Cherries, 100g	60	250	0	11
Forest Fruits, 100g	65	270	0	14
Mixed Berries, 100g	45	190	0.5	7
Raspberries, 100g	55	225	0.5	7.5
Strawberries, 100g	25	90	0.5	3
Smoothie Cubes: Berry Antioxidant (2)	80	335	1	15
Breakfast, 2 cubes, 60g	95	385	1.5	17
Strawberry; Tropical, 2 cubes, 60g	55	230	0.5	12
Sara Lee: Blueberries, 100g	55	215	0	12
Mixed Berries, 100g	50	210	0.5	9.5
Raspberries, 100g	45	190	0.5	6
Sweethaven *(Aldi)*: Blueberries, ⅕ pkt	65	260	0.5	13
Mixed Berries, ⅕ pkt	50	200	0.5	8.5
Raspberries, ⅕ pkt	55	230	0.5	10

Updated Nutrition Data ~ www.CalorieKing.com.au
Persons with Diabetes ~ See Disclaimer (Page 22)

Dried Fruit

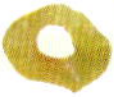
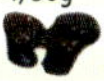
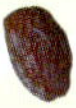
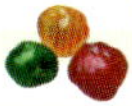
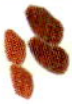
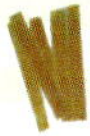
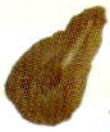
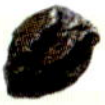
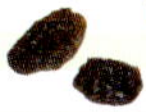

	Cal	kJ	Fat	Cb
Apple Rings, 10 rings, 30g	85	350	0	19
Apricots, dried: Aust'n, 5-6 pces, 30g	60	245	0	14
Turkish, 3-4 pieces, 30g	60	250	0	15
Banana Chips, ¼ cup, 30g	155	650	9	18
Banana, whole (12cm), 30g	90	375	0	18
Craisins, *(Ocean Spray)*, ¼ cup, 35g	115	480	0	30
Cranberries *(Craisins)*,				
[1]Sweetened· ¼ cup 35g	115	480	0	30
Crystallised Fruit, average, 30g	100	420	0	24
Currants, 2½ Tbsp, 30g	80	335	0	20
Dates, (Medium): With stones, 3-4, 30g	85	365	0	20
Pitted, 4-5 dates, 30g	85	345	0	21
½ cup chopped, 90g	260	1090	0	61
Large/Californian, Medjool (1), 24g	65	280	0	16
Figs, 2 medium, 30g	70	290	0	17
Ginger: Crystallised, 30g	100	420	0	24
Sucrose Free *(Buderin)* 5g pieces	15	65	0	4
Glace Fruit, average: 30g	100	420	0	23
Cherries (Maraschino), (2)	15	60	0	2
Fig, 1 medium, 45g	120	490	0	25
Ginger, 30g	90	375	0	23
Pineapple Ring, 1 medium, 45g	145	605	0	34
Goji Berries, 3 Tbsp, 30g	100	420	1	20
Mango, 4 strips, 30g	110	450	0	27
Mixed Fruit, ½ cup (loose), 65g	170	730	0	43
Nectarines, 3 pieces, 30g	60	255	0	14
Papaya, Spears, 30g	75	315	0	20
Paw Paw, Spears, 1 medium, 30g	75	315	0	20
Peach, 2 pieces, 30g	70	300	0	19
Pear, 2 small or 1 large piece, 30g	70	280	0	16
Peel, mixed, ¼ cup, 30g	30	120	0	7.5
Pineapple, 1 ring, 33g	115	480	0	25
Prunes: Dried, without stone (Pitted):				
Moist, 3-4 prunes, 30g	70	290	0	10
1 medium (13/100g)	15	65	0	2.5
1 large (11/100g)	20	90	0	3
Stewed, 4 prunes + 30g syrup				
Stewed with sugar	100	420	0	25
Stewed without sugar	80	335	0	20
Raisins, seedless, 30g	85	355	0	24
Sultanas: 2 Tbsp, 30g	90	385	0	23
School Snack Pack, 40g	130	535	0	30

Fruit Straps & Rolls ~ Brands

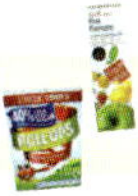

	Cal	kJ	Fat	Cb
Fruit Wise Straps,				
average all fruits, 1 strap, 14g	50	210	0	11
Uncle Toby's Roll-Ups,				
(40% Less Sugar), 1 roll, 16g	50	210	0	11

Fruit ~ Cans ◆ Jars ◆ Snacks

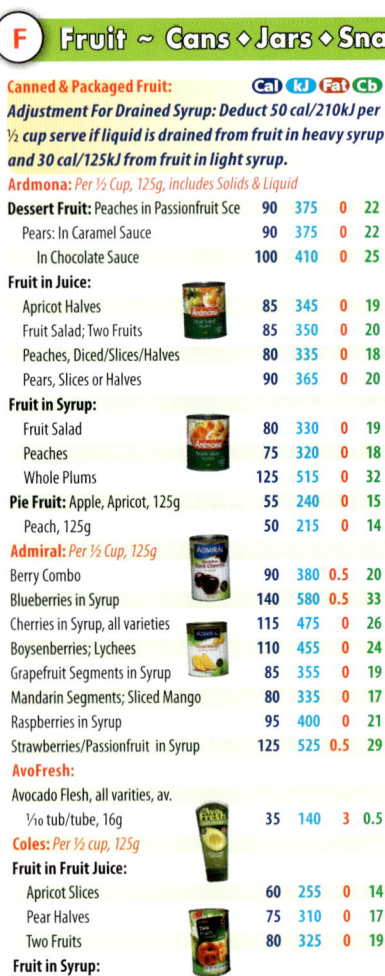

Canned & Packaged Fruit: **Cal** **kJ** **Fat** **Cb**

Adjustment For Drained Syrup: Deduct 50 cal/210kJ per ½ cup serve if liquid is drained from fruit in heavy syrup and 30 cal/125kJ from fruit in light syrup.

Ardmona: *Per ½ Cup, 125g, includes Solids & Liquid*

	Cal	kJ	Fat	Cb
Dessert Fruit: Peaches in Passionfruit Sce	90	375	0	22
Pears: In Caramel Sauce	90	375	0	22
In Chocolate Sauce	100	410	0	25
Fruit in Juice:				
Apricot Halves	85	345	0	19
Fruit Salad; Two Fruits	85	350	0	20
Peaches, Diced/Slices/Halves	80	335	0	18
Pears, Slices or Halves	90	365	0	20
Fruit in Syrup:				
Fruit Salad	80	330	0	19
Peaches	75	320	0	18
Whole Plums	125	515	0	32
Pie Fruit: Apple, Apricot, 125g	55	240	0	15
Peach, 125g	50	215	0	14

Admiral: *Per ½ Cup, 125g*

	Cal	kJ	Fat	Cb
Berry Combo	90	380	0.5	20
Blueberries in Syrup	140	580	0.5	33
Cherries in Syrup, all varieties	115	475	0	26
Boysenberries; Lychees	110	455	0	24
Grapefruit Segments in Syrup	85	355	0	19
Mandarin Segments; Sliced Mango	80	335	0	17
Raspberries in Syrup	95	400	0	21
Strawberries/Passionfruit in Syrup	125	525	0.5	29

AvoFresh:

	Cal	kJ	Fat	Cb
Avocado Flesh, all varieties, av.				
¹⁄₁₀ tub/tube, 16g	35	140	3	0.5

Coles: *Per ½ cup, 125g*

	Cal	kJ	Fat	Cb
Fruit in Fruit Juice:				
Apricot Slices	60	255	0	14
Pear Halves	75	310	0	17
Two Fruits	80	325	0	19
Fruit in Syrup:				
Blueberries	120	500	0	29
Mango	125	515	0	31
Lychees	80	325	0	19

Golden Circle: *Per ½ Cup, 125g*

	Cal	kJ	Fat	Cb
Fruit Salad: Traditional in Natural Juice	70	295	0	16
Chunky/Traditional in Syrup	105	435	0	24
Chunky in Natural Juice	70	295	0	16
Pineapple: Thins, 1 slice	25	100	0	5
Pieces/Crushed/Sliced in Syrup	100	430	0	24
In Natural Juice	70	300	0	16

Fresh Packs ~ *Same as fresh fruit*

Goulburn Valley: *Per ½ Cup, 125g*

	Cal	kJ	Fat	Cb
Fruit in Juice: Apricot Halves, 125g	85	345	0	20
Fruit Salad, 125g	65	265	0	16
Peaches, Slices/Halves	65	270	0	16
Pears, Slices/Halves	65	260	0	16
Two Fruits	65	275	0	16
Whole Plums	85	345	0	20
Fruit in Juice Cups: Diced Peaches, 220g	135	570	0	33
Fruit Salad, 220g	135	555	0	33
Two Fruits, 220g	135	570	0	33
Fruit Snacks: *Per 140g Tub*				
Harvest: Apple with Guava Puree	85	345	0	19
Fruit Salad in Juice	80	335	0	18
Peach with Banana & Mango Puree	75	305	0	15
Pear: With Cranberry Juice	80	325	0	17
With Grapefruit Juice	75	300	0	15
With Pomegranate & Blueberry Juice	70	290	0	15
Fruit Snack Tubs in Juice: *Per 140g Carton*				
Apricots	90	365	0	21
Peaches/Two Fruits	85	350	0	21
Pear	80	340	0	20
Puree: *Per 140g Tub*				
Apple	90	375	0	22
Apple Pear	85	360	0	22
Apple Mixed Berry	90	375	0	22
Apple Strawberry/Blackcurrant	90	380	0	22

Heinz:

	Cal	kJ	Fat	Cb
Fruit Snacks: *Per 120g Cup*				
Fruit Cups, average	75	315	0	17
Fruit Wobblers, av.	80	325	0	18
Splats, 120g Pouch	80	325	0	18
Stewed Fruit: *Per 100g Tub*				
Apple & Apricot with Mixed Spice	85	355	0	20
Apple & Rhubarb with Vanilla Bean	100	410	0	23
Pear & Plum with Cinnamon	70	285	0	15

IGA: *Per ½ Cup, 125g*	Cal	kJ	Fat	Cb
Fruit Salad	85	360	0	20
Two Fruits in Juice	80	325	0	18
John West,				
Passionfruit in Syrup (170g), ¼ can, 42g	40	165	0	9
SPC:				
Fruit in Juice: *Per ½ Cup, 125g*				
Apricot Halves	75	320	0	18
Fruit Salad	80	335	0	18
Peaches	60	260	0	15
Pears	65	275	0	17
Two Fruits	65	275	0	16
Fruit in Light Syrup: *Per ½ Cup, 125g*				
Apricot Halves; Fruit Salad	80	330	0	19
Peaches: Sliced	55	240	0	14
With Vitamin C	75	315	0	17
In Mango Puree	95	400	0	23
Fruit Snacks: *Per 120g Tub*				
Diced Peaches in Juice with Vitamin C	60	250	0	14
Pears & Peaches with Fibre	65	265	0	15
Peaches with Honey	60	250	0	13
Pears with Citrus & Echinacea	60	245	0	13
Fruit Squeezies: *Per 50g Tube*				
Apple & Banana Puree	40	160	0	8.5
Apple Puree with Raspberry Juice	45	180	0	10
Banana & Pear Puree w. Passionfruit Juice	50	200	0	11
Squeezie, Fruit Crush-ups:				
Strawberry, 90g Pouch	60	250	0	15
Tropical, 90g Pouch	65	265	0	16
Squeezie, Power Pulp:				
Mixed Berry, 150g Pouch	100	425	0.5	26
Tropical, 150g Pouch	105	445	0.5	27
Jelly & Fruit: *Per 120g Tub*				
Grape Jelly with Apples	90	375	0	21
Lime Jelly with Pears	90	370	0	23
Mango Jelly with Peaches	85	365	0	23
Orange & Raspb. Jelly with Peaches	90	370	0	21
Peaches in Mango	90	370	0	23
Pineapple flav. Jelly w. Peaches	90	370	0	21
Raspberry Jelly with Pears	90	385	0	24
Jelly n' Fruit Splits, average, 120g tub	95	405	0	23

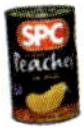
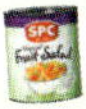
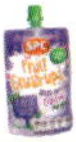
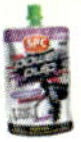
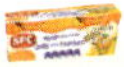
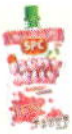

Updated Nutrition Data ~ www.CalorieKing.com.au
Persons with Diabetes ~ See Disclaimer (Page 22)

Sweet Valley:	Cal	kJ	Fat	Cb
Tubs: Mandarin in Juice, 125g	60	245	0	14
Peaches, Diced, in Juice: 125g	55	225	0	12
220g	105	430	0	24
Two Fruit, 220g	95	405	0	21
Canned: Apricot Halves, ⅕ can, 165g	100	430	0	22
Fruit Salad in Juice, ⅛ can, 103g	70	280	0.5	13
Peach Slices:				
In Juice, ⅕ can, 165g	85	350	0.5	19
In Syrup, ⅕ can, 165g	115	470	0.5	26
Pineapple:				
Chunks in Juice, ¼ can, 108g	70	280	0	15
Slices in Juice, ¼ can, 108g	65	270	0	15
Two Fruits in Juice, ⅛ can, 103g	65	265	0	15
Weight Watchers: *Per ½ Cup, 125g*				
Apricot Halves	35	140	0	7
Fruit Salad	45	180	0	9
Peach Slices; Peaches in Mango	40	170	0	9
Snack Pack: *Per 135g Container*				
Apricots	40	160	0	9
Fruit Salad	35	145	0	9
Peaches	30	115	0	5.5
Low-Joule Fruit in Jelly: *Per 120g Tub*				
Pears/Peach/Two Fruits in Jelly	10	45	0	2
Woolworths: *Per ½ Cup, 125g*				
Diced Two Fruits in Fruit Juice	70	285	0	16
Fruit Salad Portion in Fruit Juice	70	290	0	16
Peach Slices in Fruit Juice	65	280	0	15
Pineapple Pieces/Slices in Fruit Juice	55	235	0	14

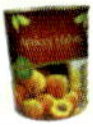
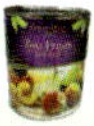
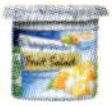
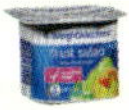

Miscellaneous

	Cal	kJ	Fat	Cb
Lychees, canned, ½ cup, 125g	105	445	0	24
Cherries: Maraschino, 5, 30g	80	325	0	20
Sour Pitted, drained, 30g	25	105	0	5.5
Prunes, in Liqueur, ½ cup, 125g	280	1170	0	40

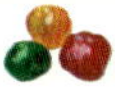

Stewed Fruit

Average All Fruits: Apple, Apricot, Pears, Plums, Peaches	Cal	kJ	Fat	Cb
Stewed with sugar, ½ cup, 125g	100	420	0	25
Stewed without sugar, with fluid, ½ cup, 120g	60	250	0	11

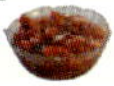

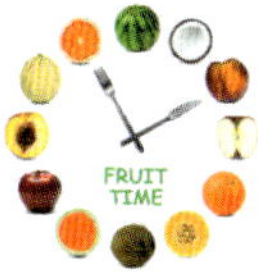

Ice Cream & Frozen Yogurt

Ice Cream ~ Quick Guide

	Cal	kJ	Fat	Cb
Regular Ice Cream: 10% fat				
Vanilla; Flavoured, average:				
1 small scoop, 50ml, 25g	50	210	3	5.5
1 regular scoop, 100ml, 50g	100	420	5.5	11
1 litre container, 500g	1005	4200	55	110
Reduced-Fat Ice Cream: Less than 6.5% fat				
Average, 1 scoop, 100ml, 50g	85	355	3	14
1 litre container, 500g	850	3550	30	138
Low-Fat Ice Cream: Less than 4% fat				
(e.g. Peter's Light & Creamy)				
100ml scoop, 50g	70	290	2	14
1 litre container	690	2885	22	140
Super Premium/Rich Ice Cream:				
More dense, higher fat (e.g. Connoisseur, Sara Lee)				
10% Fat, 100ml, 100g	180	750	10	24
15% Fat, 100ml, 100g	250	1045	15	23

Deli's/Milk Bars

	Cal	kJ	Fat	Cb
Per 100ml Scoop (50g)				
Choc Top/Bomb, each, 105g	320	1335	18	36
Fried Ice Cream Balls, each	170	710	10	21
Frozen Yoghurt, all flavours	90	365	2	15
Gelati, all flavours, average	70	280	1.5	14
Ice Cream: *Per 100ml Scoop (50g)*				
Baileys	115	490	7.5	11
Banana; Bubblegum; Pineapple	110	470	7	12
Butterscotch; Cappuccino; Chocolate	115	490	7.5	11
Caramel	120	500	7	12
Chocolate Choc Chip; Crazy Cone	120	500	8	13
Chocolae Fantasy; Cookies & Cream	125	525	8	12
English Toffee; Boysenberry	120	505	7	13
Honeycomb; Rum & Raisin	120	490	7	12
Jaffa; Mango; Passionfruit Swirl	115	480	7.5	11
Macadamia Nut	120	500	8	10
Pistachio	125	530	8.5	11
Toblerone	120	500	7.5	12
Triple Chocolate	125	510	8	11
Average other flavours	125	520	7	12
Premium: Milo; My Macadamia	130	535	7.5	13
Butterscotch; Dble Choc Chip	120	500	7.5	12
Mango	115	480	7.5	10
Average other flavours	110	470	7	11
Sorbet: Lemon	55	230	0	14
Mango	55	230	0	14

Soft Serve Ice Cream

	Cal	kJ	Fat	Cb
Frosty Boy: *Per Serving (100g)*				
D'Lite: Chocolate	115	490	0.5	23
Frosty	120	495	1	23
Soft Serve: Chocolate	135	560	4	20
Vanilla	135	570	4.5	19
Mr Whippy, Dairy Queen, 1 serve	85	355	1	18
Mr Whippy Lite, with Yoghurt, 100ml	95	400	1.5	19
New Zealand Natural:				
Choco'Lite: Kids Cup, 60g	75	315	0.5	15
Large Cup, 180	230	950	1	45

Soft Serve Yogurt

	Cal	kJ	Fat	Cb
Average All Brands				
SingleServe: 100ml/50g	75	320	1.5	13
with cone	85	370	1.5	15
120ml cup (80g)	120	510	2.5	21
200ml cup (100g)	150	635	3	26
New Zealand Natural ~ See Page 111				
YoFrost (Frosty Boy), 100g serve	120	500	2	21

Italian Confections

	Cal	kJ	Fat	Cb
Cassata, 1 portion	180	755	7.5	22
Gelati: Water-base, with cone	90	375	0	20
Milk-base, 1 serve, with cone	120	500	3.5	15
Chocolate, Nougat, Pistachio	120	500	3.5	15
Tartufo, 1 portion, 100g	200	835	7	30

Sorbet

	Cal	kJ	Fat	Cb
Non-milk/Nonfat, 100ml/50g	55	230	0	15
Milk-base (8% fat), 100ml/50g	100	420	4	14

Ice Cream Cones

	Cal	kJ	Fat	Cb
Cone Only: *No Ice Cream Included*				
Single Cone	15	60	0	3
Double Cone; Cup	25	100	0	5.5
Party Cone	15	60	0	3
Square Cone/Cup	10	50	0	3
Sugar Cone	40	167	0	8
Wafer Cone	10	40	0	3
Waffle (large)	120	495	2	23

 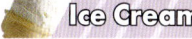

Ice Cream & Frozen Yogurt ~ Brands

Baskin Robbins:

Classic Ice Cream: *Per 114g Scoop*

	Cal	kJ	Fat	Cb
Caramel Chocolate Crunch	310	1290	17	35
Choc Chip Cookie Dough	285	1195	15	33
Chocolate	250	1035	14	27
Chocolate Trilogy	280	1180	16	30
Cookies 'n Cream	280	1165	17	27
Cotton Candy	250	1045	12	32
Hokey Pokey	265	1100	13	34
Jamoca Almond Fudge	275	1135	15	30
Love Potion #31	270	1115	14	30
Mango Mania	220	910	10	28
Mint Chocolate Chip	260	1075	16	25
Peanut Butter 'n Chocolate	310	1300	20	26
Pistachio Almond	280	1170	19	22
Pralines 'n' Cream	295	1220	14	37
Rocky Road	295	1225	15	35
Tiramisu	270	1130	13	34
Vanilla	230	970	14	22
Very Berry Strawberry	210	880	11	25
World Class Chocolate	275	1140	16	27

No Sugar Added Ice Cream: *Per 114g Scoop*

	Cal	kJ	Fat	Cb
Caramel Turtle Truffle	250	1035	8.5	39
Pineapple Coconut	215	890	6.5	19

Ice Confections: *Per 114g Scoop*

	Cal	kJ	Fat	Cb
Sherbet, Rainbow	145	600	2	29
Sorbet: Citrus Twist Ice	115	470	0	28
Wild 'n Reckless	140	580	2	28

Frozen Yoghurt: *Per 114g Scoop*

	Cal	kJ	Fat	Cb
Maui Brownie Madness	250	1040	11	33
Strawberry; Wildberry	190	795	6	30

Note: *Cone & Topping are extra*

Extras, Sugar Cone | 45 | 190 | 0.5 | 9 |

Smoothies/Shakes ~ *See Page 186*

Ben & Jerry's:

Ice Cream Tubs: *Per Scoop from 1 Pint Tub*

	Cal	kJ	Fat	Cb
Chocolate Chip Cookie Dough, 105g	270	1135	14	33
Chocolate Fudge Brownie, 102g	250	1040	11	33
Chunky Monkey, 107g	290	1210	18	29
Half Baked, 106g	270	1130	13	35
Maple Tree Hugger, 105g	245	1020	12	32
New York Super Fudge Chunk, 107g	305	1265	18	31
Phish Food, 107g	250	1035	13	40
Strawberry Cheesecake, 105g	265	1105	15	28
Sweet Cream & Cookies, 107g	255	1070	13	29
Triple Caramel Chunk, 107g	230	975	13	32

Ben & Jerry's (Cont):

Scoop Shop: *Per Single Scoop*

	Cal	kJ	Fat	Cb
A Cookie Affair, 92g	255	1060	15	28
Butter Pecan, 90g	270	1130	21	18
Chocolate Chip, 92g	230	970	13	25
Chocolate Fudge Brownie, 92g	225	945	10	30
Clusterfluff, 94g	290	1220	18	29
Maple Tree Hugger, 92g	255	1060	10	29
Peanut Butter Cookie Dough, 91g	270	1115	16	26
Vanilla, 92g	200	840	12	20

Bulla:

Creamy Classics: *Per 200g Cup*

	Cal	kJ	Fat	Cb
Caramel Fudge Sundae	240	1000	11	33
Choc Fudge Sundae	240	1005	11	33
Choc Mint Sundae	255	1060	11	34
Chocolate Hazelnut Sundae	250	1030	12	31
Cookies & Cream	225	940	12	26
Rich Choc Chip	225	940	10	24
Strawberry Sundae	210	885	10	29

Creamy Classics: *Per 47g Scoop from 2Lt Tubs*

	Cal	kJ	Fat	Cb
Chocolate Chip	110	461	6.5	13
Other flavours, average	95	395	5	11
Light 98% Fat-Free, Vanilla	60	240	1	11
Real Dairy, average all flavours	90	385	5	11

Bars: *Per Bar*

	Cal	kJ	Fat	Cb
Creamy Classics, average	210	880	13	19
Light, 98% Fat-Free, avg. all flav.	80	320	1.5	14
Crunch, average all flavours	180	755	12	16
Mini Splits, all flavours	55	230	2	8
Splits, average all flavours	95	390	3.5	15

Frozen Yoghurts:

Crunch: *Per Serving*

	Cal	kJ	Fat	Cb
Passionfruit with Honey Oat, 225g	330	1370	5	57
Summer Berries with Honey Oat, 225g	320	1340	5	55
Vanilla with Berry Oat, 225g	320	1335	5	54

Fruit 'n Yogurt, 2L Tubs,

	Cal	kJ	Fat	Cb
average all flavours, 70g scoop	100	415	2	18

Fruit 'n Yogurt Bars:

	Cal	kJ	Fat	Cb
Average all flavours, 59g	80	330	2	13
Minis, 34g	50	200	1	8.5

Fruit 'n Yogurt Cups,

	Cal	kJ	Fat	Cb
average all flavours, 100g cup	135	560	3	23

Gourmet Cups,

	Cal	kJ	Fat	Cb
average all flavours, 100g cup	160	665	3	31

Updated Nutrition Data ~ www.CalorieKing.com.au
Persons with Diabetes ~ See Disclaimer (Page 22)

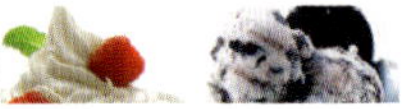

Ice Cream & Frozen Yogurt ~ Brands

	Cal	kJ	Fat	Cb
Cadbury:				
Ice Cream: *Per Scoop, 100ml*				
Caramello	105	430	5	13
Triple Chocolate	100	415	5.5	11
Creamy Vanilla	100	415	5.5	11
Dairy Milk Chip	115	470	6.5	12
Honeycomb & Chocolate with Crunchie	105	435	5.5	13
Light: Chocolate Vanilla	75	305	1	14
Turkish Delight	85	355	1	17
Vanilla	75	310	1	14
4-Pack,				
Creamy Vanilla, 100ml cup	125	520	7	14
Ice Cream Bars: *Per Bar*				
Caramello	195	810	11	21
Creamy Vanilla	270	1120	16	29
Crunchie	170	715	10	13
Flake	250	1035	13	30
Picnic	285	1195	15	32
Rocky Road	260	1095	13	33
Triple Chocolate	250	1050	13	32
Yowie: Choc Shake	250	1040	8	38
Pops, Chocolate	95	400	3	15
Coles:				
Coles Tubs: *Per 100ml Scoop, Unless Indicated*				
Bubblegum, 47g	86	360	1.5	17
Chocolate Choc Chip, 47g	115	480	6.5	13
Cookies & Cream, 47g	110	470	5.5	14
HokeyPokey, 47g	85	365	1.5	17
Neapolitan, 47g	95	395	5	11
Rocky Road, 47g	115	485	6	13
Rum & Raisin, 47g	115	480	6.5	13
Vanilla: Regular, 47g	100	410	5	13
Light, 47g	70	295	1.5	13
Finest: Caramel Date & Pecan, 47g	120	500	7.5	11
Fig, Ginger & Honey, 47g	110	455	6	12
Madagascan Vanilla Ban, 47g	120	505	9	9.5
Premium: Caramel & Macadamia, 72g	190	790	12	18
Chocolate Fudge, 72g	175	730	9	21
Rich & Creamy Vanilla, 72g	170	720	11	16
97% Fat Free: English Toffee	75	325	1.5	14
Vanilla	80	335	1.5	15
Ice Cream Bars: *Per Bar*				
Classic, Vanilla, 114g	375	1555	24	36
Minis: Almond, 60g	205	860	14	19
Vanilla, 60g	200	830	13	19
Connoisseur:				
Cafe Grande, 71g	195	820	11	21
Caramel Honey Macadamia, 69g	190	790	12	19
Choc Honey Nougat, 69g	180	745	10	21
Chocolate Obsession, 73g	195	820	14	19
Classic Vanilla, 91g	225	940	14	23
Cookies & Cream, 65g	180	755	9.5	21

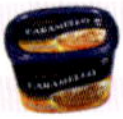

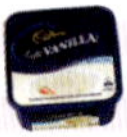

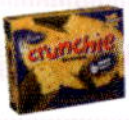

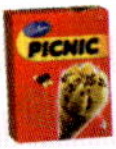

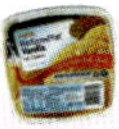

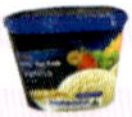

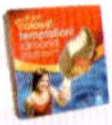

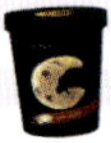

	Cal	kJ	Fat	Cb
Everest:				
Indulgent Desserts: Baci, 100g	290	1210	19	26
After Dinner Mint, 100g	300	1260	22	24
Cassata, 80g	165	700	.05	25
Giandiotto, 100g	250	1040	14	25
Murray Mud Cake, 100g	310	1290	20	30
Tartufo, 100g	210	870	9	30
Gelativo: *Per 125ml Cup*				
Gelato: Coffee	140	585	6	18
Hazelnut	170	710	8	20
Vanilla Bean	155	650	6	21
Sorbet, Strawberry; Tropical Fruits	95	395	0	22
Golden North:				
Ice Cream: Average all flavours, 100ml	95	400	6	9.5
Low-Fat, 100ml	75	330	1.5	14
Giant Twin Bars	270	1130	20	21
Swings, Vanilla Cups	130	550	8	13
Maggie Beer:				
Ice Cream: *Per 120ml Tub*				
Burnt Fig Jam Caramel & Honeycomb	195	810	11	22
Strawberries & Cream, 92g	200	825	12	19
Passionfruit, 89g	220	910	15	19
Quince & Bitter Almond, 92g	225	945	14	23
Vanilla Bean & Elderflower	220	925	16	17
Magnum ~ *See Streets*				
Mini Melts: *Per 70g Cup*				
Banana Split; Buble Gum	165	690	11	15
Chocolate	170	700	11	15
Choc Mint	165	695	11	15
Cookie Dough	170	700	11	15
Strawberry & Cream	165	685	11	14
Nestle/Peters: *Per Scoop, 100ml*				
Entice: Caramel Choc Mudslide, 48g	90	370	3	14
Chocolate Trio, 49g	90	385	3.5	14
Cookies n' Cream, 46g	90	375	3	14
Light & Creamy:				
Chocolate Vanilla Swirl, 46g	75	310	1.5	14
Classic/FrenchVanilla, 46g	70	300	1	14
Creme Brulee, 46g	75	310	1.5	14
Raspberry Ripple, 48g	75	320	1	14
Slice, Vanilla, 46g	75	310	1.5	14
No Added Sugar, Vanilla, 50g	60	260	1.5	5
Original: Chocopolitan, 47g	90	370	3.5	13
Neapolitan; Triple Treat, Van., 46g	80	340	3	14
Overload: Rolo, 54g	130	545	5	19
Violet Crumble, 51g	115	480	4	19
Caramel Cookie Madness, 51g	120	500	3.5	20

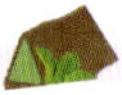

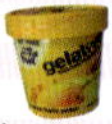

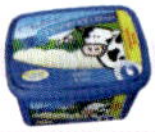

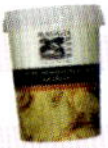

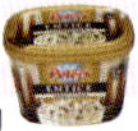

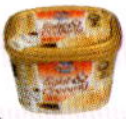

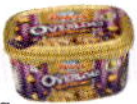

110

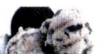

Ice Cream & Frozen Yogurt ~ Brands

	Cal	kJ	Fat	Cb
Nestle/Peters (Cont):				
Billabong:				
Bars: Chocolate, 60g	80	340	1.5	14
Caramel, 60g	80	330	1.5	14
Rainbow, 48g	125	510	4.5	19
Vanilla, 61g	90	370	1.5	16
Bar, Triple Swirl, 68g	90	375	1.5	16
Cups: Choc Vanilla, 50g	75	310	1.5	1
Strawberry Vanilla, 50 g	75	305	1.5	14
Choc Wedge:				
Choc Ripple, 55g	170	705	11	17
Vanilla, 59g	165	690	10	17
Dixie Cup, Vanilla, 51g	105	440	5.5	14
Drumsticks:				
Boysenberry, 85g	235	980	10	35
Chocolate Mint, 80g	230	960	10	33
Honey Macadamia, 86g	295	1225	16	34
Kit Kat, Vanilla Choc, 76g	230	965	12	30
Mocha, 83g	275	1145	15	31
Super Choc, 78g	275	1145	16	30
Vanilla, 74g	225	945	12	29
Twister, White Choc. & Raspb., 78g	205	855	7.5	32
Minis, Vanilla, 52g	175	735	10	20
Eskimo Pie, 64g	200	830	14	19
Frosty Fruits: 83g bar	85	370	0	21
Sorbet, cup 104g	100	420	0	23
Giant Sandwich, 62g	170	710	5	29
Heaven:				
Chocolate Truffle, 88g	310	1285	20	29
Extra Chunky Cookie, 83g	320	1320	19	33
Rich Vanilla, 89g	300	1255	20	28
Vanilla Bean, 87g	295	1230	19	27
Vanilla Macadamia, 87g	315	1315	21	28
Icy Pole, avg. all flavours	50	200	0	12
Maxibon:				
Honeycomb	315	1320	16	40
Vanilla	320	1325	16	40
Milo: Scoop Shake, cup	235	975	8	38
Smooth Stick, 66g	100	410	2	17

	Cal	kJ	Fat	Cb
New Zealand Natural:				
Supermarket Ice Cream: *Per 946ml Tubs*				
Chocolate Ecstacy, 66g	145	610	7.5	17
Classic Vanilla, 71g	140	580	8	15
Cookies 7 Cream, 60g	150	635	8.5	18
Fruits Of The Forrest, 70g	120	515	2.5	24
Macadamia Supreme, 62g	155	650	10	14
White Chocolate & Raspberry, 66g	160	670	8.5	19
Zilch *(No Added Sugar):*				
Vanilla Bean: 1 small scoop, 45g (75ml)	65	280	2	4
1 medium scoop, 65g (100ml)	95	395	3	5.5
Ice Cream Shops: *NZ Natural Franchise*				
Cones: *Does not Include Ice Cream*				
Kid's, Plain, 3.6g	15	60	0	3
Waffle Cone, Small, 13g	55	220	0.5	11
Waffle Cone, Large 17g	70	285	1	14
Ice Cream: *Per Regular Scoop, 130g*				
Boysenberry	285	1195	14	36
Cafe Espresso	305	1270	18	30
Choc Fudge Brownie	365	1520	19	41
Choco'lite: Hard Serve	200	840	3.5	35
Soft Serve	150	630	0.5	30
Chocolate Ecstacy	285	1200	15	32
Classic Vanilla	285	1190	17	28
Cookies & Cream	315	1315	18	34
Creme de Coconut	295	1240	18	28
Hokey Pokey Butterscotch Candy	305	1270	16	35
Mint Choc Kisses; Orange Choc Chip	300	1260	18	30
Rum & Raisin; Strawberry Surprise	280	1175	15	32
Tiramisu	305	1275	17	34
Toffee Caramel Cup	315	1325	18	34
Walnut Butterscotch	360	1510	23	32
Fruit Flo Ice Cream: *Per Regular Cup, 235g*				
Cool Bananas D'Lite with Banana	320	1340	5.5	57
Natural D'Lite, avg. all flavours	300	1255	5.5	53
Sorbet, regular, avg. all flavours, 130g	170	715	0	41
Frozen Yoghurt: *Per Regular Cup*				
Low-Fat, avg. all flav., 130g	235	985	4	45
Soft Serve, all flavours, 120g	180	760	3.5	31
Fruit Flo Frozen Yogurt: *Per Regular Cup, 235g*				
Forest Berry: With Blueberry	360	1500	4	67
With Strawberry	340	1410	4	62
Mango Passion: With Banana	425	1770	7.5	79
With Mango	340	1425	4.5	63
Soft Serve Yogurt, avg. regular cup, 120g	180	760	3.5	31

Updated Nutrition Data ~ www.CalorieKing.com.au
Persons with Diabetes ~ See Disclaimer (Page 22)

Ice Cream & Frozen Yogurt ~ Brands

Norgen Vaaz:	Cal	kJ	Fat	Cb
Ice Cream: *Per 58g Scoop*				
Banana Bongo	120	495	6.5	13
Boysenberry Twist; Bubblegum	125	515	7	14
Chocolate Obsession; Honeycomb	140	590	7.5	16
Cookies N Cream	140	590	7.5	16
Hokey Pokey	130	545	6.5	16
Licorice Licks; Vanilla Supreme	120	510	7	12
Milk Chocolate	130	545	7.5	14
Peppermint Choc Chip	135	565	8	14
Vienna Coffee	120	505	7	12
Whipshake	100	410	2.5	15
Low-Fat, average all flavours	80	330	1.5	15
Gourmet: *Per 61g Scoop*				
Classic Ferraro	160	675	10	17
Double Swiss Chocolate	145	600	9	14
Ginger Megs	135	565	7	17
Green Tea	125	515	7	12
Irish Creams & Scorched Almond	160	675	10	16
Mint Cookie Slice	150	635	9	17
Stairway to Heaven	170	720	9	21
Vanilla Bean	140	580	9	13
White Chocolate & Raspberry Swirl	145	605	7.5	15
Sorbet: *Per 68g Scoop*				
Green Apple	80	330	0	19
Lemon	75	320	0	19
Mango	70	300	0	17
Sara Lee:				
Ice Cream: *Per Scoop*				
Cookies & Cream, 63g	165	690	9	19
French Vanilla, 73g	165	695	11	16
Hazelnut Fudge, 73g	165	695	10	18
Honeycomb & Butterscotch, 72g	170	790	9	20
Rocky Road, 66g	170	705	10	19
Rum & Raisin, 62g	140	580	7.5	15
Ultra Chocolate, 73g	170	710	11	16
Simply Less *(Coles):*				
Bars, Choc. Raspberry; Van. Caramel, 36g	60	250	1	11
Ice Cream, Chocolate; Vanilla, 45g scoop	75	310	1.5	12
Skinny Cow:				
Ice Cream Cookies, average	125	520	1.5	24
Sundae Cups, averave	110	460	2.5	8
Sticks/Bars, average	80	340	2	6
Smooze:				
Fruit Ice: Mango, Pink Guava & Coconut, 65ml	65	275	2	11
Pineapple & Coconut, 65ml	70	285	2	12
Simply Coconut, 65ml	105	440	5	14
So Good Bliss:				
Ice Cream: *Per 2 Scoops, 63g*				
Chocolate Bliss	90	380	2	17
Vanilla Bliss	95	390	2	18

Soylait:	Cal	kJ	Fat	Cb
Ice Confection: *Per Scoop, 70g*				
Baci; Creme Caramel	95	400	2.5	18
Mocha; Vanilla Mango	95	400	2.5	18
SPC, Frostbite Stix (1), all flavours	45	185	0	11
Streets:				
Blue Ribbon Ice Cream Tubs: *Per Scoop*				
Choc Banana Chip, 46g	85	345	2	15
Chocolate 45g	75	320	2	13
Goody Drops, 46g	80	330	1.5	15
Hokey Pokey, 46g	80	340	1.5	16
Neapolitan Twist, 47g	80	330	1.5	15
Vanilla, 45g	85	355	3.5	13
Light: Cookies & Cream, 46g	80	340	2	15
Vanilla, 45g	75	310	1	14
3 in 1: Fruit Basket, 49g	85	350	2	15
Peppermint Cream, 45g	80	320	2	13
Triple Chocolate, 45g	80	330	2	13
Viennetta, Choc. Cream; Vanilla, 45g	140	590	10	13
Bars: Bubble O'Bill, 65g	150	630	8	18
Cornetto Classic:				
Caramel Toffee Twist, 68g	215	890	11	25
Peppermint Cream, 68g	210	865	10	26
Supreme Milk Chocolate, 68g	210	865	10	25
Vanilla & Choc Nut, 68g	215	890	11	25
Cornetto Enigma, Hazelnut & Choc., 80g	265	1095	13	33
Golden Gaytime: 77g Bar	235	975	15	22
Vanilla & Chocolate, 80g	265	1100	15	30
Vanilla & Raspberry, 78g	235	985	10	32
Magnum: Almond	330	1370	23	27
Black Espresso	255	1065	16	23
Classic	285	1185	19	25
Ego Caramel	340	1425	21	35
Gold	380	1590	26	34
Peppermint	275	1150	18	25
Pink Marc de Champagne	290	1210	20	34
Strawberry White Crumble	320	1340	21	30
White	300	1240	20	27
Mini: Almond	180	740	12	15
Classic	155	650	11	13
Ecuador Dark	180	735	13	14
White	160	670	11	14
Sandwich, with Almonds, 98g	290	1200	16	33

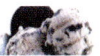
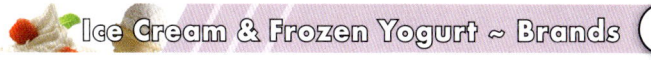

Ice Cream & Frozen Yogurt ~ Brands

Streets (Cont):	Cal	kJ	Fat	Cb
Splice:				
Pine Lime, 61g	80	320	1	15
Real Fruits: Orange, 70g	70	285	0	16
Passionfruit, 70g	80	320	0	18
Pineapple, 70g	70	280	0	16
Strawberry, 70g	60	260	0	15
Calippo: Lemon; Raspb. Pineapple, 105g	90	380	0	22
Mini: Lemon; Raspberry Pineapple, 62g	55	225	0	12
Tropical Fruit, 62g	55	225	0	13
Paddle Pop: Banana; Chocolate, 68g	110	450	3.5	17
Bubblegum Berry Lava, 67g	110	460	3	19
Caramel, 68g	115	470	4	17
Choc Orange Hero/Villian, 53g	85	360	3	13
Cyclone, 92g	90	380	0	24
Icy Twist, Lemonade, 71g	65	270	0	16
Rainbow, 68g	110	450	3	17
Scribbler, 35g	30	130	0	8
Thickshake, Chocolate, 104g	165	685	3	30
Tofutti:				
1 L Container: *Per ½ cup, 80g*				
Chocolate	240	1005	15	23
Cookie Crunch; Better Pecan, avg.	280	1170	16	26
Weight Watchers:				
Mini Cups: *Per 145ml*				
Berry Mudslide	125	525	1.5	24
Cookies & Cream	115	475	1.5	22
Creamy Chocolate	110	470	1	21
Creamy Vanilla	100	425	0.5	20
White Choc & Raspberry	130	545	2	25
Sundaes: *Per 125ml Cup*				
Choc Berry Bliss	125	530	1.5	25
Double Chocolate	145	615	3	26
Rich Caramel	135	565	1	29
Toffee Pecan	140	585	2	27
Weis:				
Ice Cream: *(1 L Tub), Per Scoop*				
Coffee with Cream, 68g	155	660	10	16
Homestyle Caramel w. Butterscotch Brittle	140	590	8	16
Macadamia Mango & Cream, 70g	140	585	8.5	14
Mango & Cream, 70g	110	465	10	18
Vanilla Bean, 78g	185	765	11	20
Vanilla & Raspberries	140	580	5	20
Ice Cream Bars: *Per 80g Bar*				
Banana Passionfruit Pineple	115	480	3.5	20
Mango & Cream	60	240	2	10
Strawberry with Choc Nut	170	700	9	19
Mini:				
Mango & Cream, 40g	60	240	2	10
Roasted Hazelnut & Cream	95	390	5.5	9

Weis (Cont):	Cal	kJ	Fat	Cb
Sorbet (1 L Tub):				
Mango, 75g scoop	85	350	0	20
Other flavours, average, 75g scoop	90	375	0	22
Wendy's:				
Ice Cream: *Per Junior Scoop, 80g*				
Bailey's Scorched Almond	190	790	11	20
Banana Rhapsody	180	755	10	19
Bubblegum	170	700	10	16
Chocollo	100	425	0.5	16
Cookies & Cream	190	785	10	21
Honeycomb Smash	190	800	10	23
Macadamia Dream	190	795	13	17
Mango-A-Go-Go	160	670	8.5	19
Moccaccino	175	730	10	20
Rainbow; Vanilla Dream	170	700	10	17
Rum & Raisin	170	715	9	21
Wicked Chocolate	185	765	10	20
Wild Boysenberry	170	705	9	20
SupaSoft: *Ice Cream & Small Cone*				
Bitz, Wendy's, 300g	370	1550	6	69
Cone, Vanilla, 109g	150	615	2.5	28
Fun Cones: Choc Dip, 109g	195	815	7	29
Clown, 109g	180	740	3.5	33
Monster, 112g	165	695	2	33
Teddy Cone, 127g	255	1070	5.5	46
Supa Choc Cones:				
Freckle, 119g	235	985	7.5	38
Rocket, 124g	280	1160	12	38
Sherbet, 119g	235	975	7	38
Cones: *Without Ice Cream*				
Plain, 3.6g	15	60	0	3
Waffle, 13.5g	60	240	1	11
Sundaes: *Per Small Cup*				
Flake, 235g	490	2055	16	81
Fundae, 106g	205	845	6.5	35
Fudge, 220g	410	1715	11	72
Frozen Yoghurt, small cup, 95g	110	465	1	23
Woolworths Home Brand:				
2 Litre Tubs: Vanilla, 42g Scoop	85	360	4.5	13
Light Vanilla, 47g	70	295	1.5	13
Bars, Chocolate Coated, 59g	185	770	13	16
Select, Creamy Pops, avg. all flavours, 51g	100	410	5	12

Updated Nutrition Data ~ www.CalorieKing.com.au
Persons with Diabetes ~ See Disclaimer (Page 22)

"Join Australia's Biggest & Best Online Weight Control Club"

The CalorieKing Program is simple and effective. Enjoy peace of mind with a safe, practical program that has been developed by Allan Borushek and his team. ➤

For more info visit
www.CalorieKing.com.au

Personalised diet plans
A realistic, achievable plan based on your body's needs, goals and lifestyle.

Easy-to-use tools
Includes a food & exercise log with reports; and CalorieKing's food database of Australian foods – everything you need to track your progress, set goals and stay motivated.

Online community
24/7 support from our friendly online community. Discuss problems, make new friends and stay motivated.

Meal plans & recipes
Let us suggest menus that fit perfectly in our plan. Find healthy recipes in our extensive database.

Meals ~ Canned & Packaged

Meals ~ Quick Guide

	Cal	kJ	Fat	Cb
Pies, Sausage Rolls, Patties:				
Average All Brands				
Pies: Family, ¼ pie, 125g	295	1225	17	26
Meat/Pork, single, 175g	450	1880	27	41
Party Pies, each, 43g	110	460	5.5	12
Sausage Roll: Small/Party, 30g	110	470	6	11
Medium/Party, 75g	215	910	14	14
Large, 120g	350	1450	22	29
Jumbo, 175g	505	2120	32	42
Beef/Hamburger Patty, average				
1 patty (50g raw), grilled	140	590	9.5	4
Fried	150	625	11	3.5
Crumbed, fried	170	710	13	7.5

Baked Beans ~ Quick Guide

	Cal	kJ	Fat	Cb
Canned Baked Beans:				
Average All Brands				
In Tomato Sauce: 100g	85	345	0.5	12
¼ cup, 3 Tbsp, 70g	60	255	0	9
½ cup, 140g	120	505	0	19
½ large can (420g), 210g	175	725	1	29
1 large can, 420g	350	1450	2	49

Note: Baked Beans are a nutritious vegetarian food.
The tomato sauce contains no fat.

2 Minute Chef: *Per Packet, Prepared*

	Cal	kJ	Fat	Cb
Black Pepper Beef with Rice	410	1700	5	69
Chicken Korma with Rice	480	2000	14	69
Honey Beef with Rice	445	1860	8	76
Spaghetti Bolognese	465	1930	14	67

Ainsley Harriott:
Cous Cous: *Per ½ Sachet, Prepared*

	Cal	kJ	Fat	Cb
Lemon, Mint & Parsley	195	810	2	36
Moroccan Medley	180	755	2	33
Mushroom	190	790	2	36
Roasted Vegetable	190	800	1.5	36
Spice Sensation	170	700	2	31
Sundried Tomato & Garlic	200	830	2	36
World Kitchen: Aromatic Thai Style	180	740	2.1	32
Chilli	200	820	2	38
Wild Mushroom	190	790	1.5	36

Allied Chefs: *Per Packet (Sold in School Canteens)*

	Cal	kJ	Fat	Cb
Nacho Dippers	260	1090	13	22
School Range, Hotcakes, 60g	150	630	4	23
Spaghetti/Twista Bolognese	255	1060	6.5	29
Lasagne: Traditional	235	990	10	24
Vegetable	285	1185	6.5	45

Australian Eatwell:
Vegetable Burger: *Per 125g Patty*

	Cal	kJ	Fat	Cb
Chickpea & Sunflower	175	740	2	26
Exotic Satay	190	790	1.5	29
Red Lentil	150	625	1.5	22

Organic Vegie Burger: *Per 100g Patty*

	Cal	kJ	Fat	Cb
Chickpea, Cumin & Coriander	105	440	2	20
Jasmine Rice, Lime Leaf & Lemon Grass	140	590	7	14
Mixed Grain, Parsley & Thyme	110	450	1.5	18

Bakewell:

	Cal	kJ	Fat	Cb
Pastie, 155g	380	1600	20	40
Pies: Meat Pie, 175g	430	1785	22	41
Party Pie, 60g	165	685	8.5	18
Sausage Roll: 72g	195	800	10	19
Party Sausage Roll, 38g	105	425	5.5	10

Bean Supreme:

	Cal	kJ	Fat	Cb
Gourmet Burgers, 1 pattie, 75g	165	690	9	8
Vegetarian Sausages:				
Rosemary, Sage, Parsley, (2)	170	710	8	9
Sundried Tomato & Olive (2)	145	610	6	9

Big Ben:

	Cal	kJ	Fat	Cb
Pies: Extra Tasty Meat, 175g	460	1925	24	45
Traditional, Meat, 175g	425	1770	22	41

Birds Eye:

	Cal	kJ	Fat	Cb
Bubble 'n Squeak Patties (1)	160	670	10	15
Corn Fritters (1), 55.6g	115	490	5.5	14
Lasagne, Bechamal, ¼ pkt, 225g	320	1345	12	39
Pommes, ¼ pkt, 87g	155	650	6.5	20
Special Fried Rice, ¼ pkt, 125g	150	625	2	27
Vegetable Fingers (3), 90g	175	730	7.5	21
Simply Kids Patties, Chicken & Vege., 60g	115	485	4.5	13

WOK Ready: *Per ½ of 750g Packet*

	Cal	kJ	Fat	Cb
Pad Thai with Chicken & Prawns, 375g	375	1575	3.8	59
Teriyaki Beef Noodles, 375g	415	1730	8	53
Thai Green Chicken Curry, 375g	430	1785	15	52
Thai Red Beef Curry, 375g	435	1810	14	53

Borg's:
Appetizers: *Per Piece*

	Cal	kJ	Fat	Cb
Feta Cheese Triangles, 30g	80	340	3	12
Ricotta Cheese Triangles, 30g	80	325	3.5	10
Spinach & Ricotta Triangles, 30g	85	350	4	10
Vegetarian Triangles, 30g	70	285	3	8

Pastizzi: Chicken & Vegetable, 60g | 145 | 600 | 7.5 | 15 |
| Pizza Supreme, 60g | 140 | 575 | 8 | 12 |
| Spinach & Ricotta Cheese, 60g | 135 | 570 | 7 | 15 |

Savoury Pastrie, Ricotta Cheese, 60g | 160 | 655 | 8.5 | 16 |

Updated Nutrition Data ~ www.CalorieKing.com.au
Persons with Diabetes ~ See Disclaimer (Page 22)

115

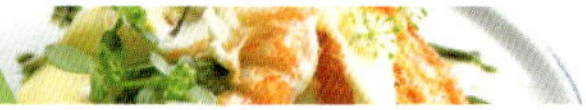

Meals ~ Canned & Packaged

	Cal	kJ	Fat	Cb
Campbell's:				
Spaghetti Sauce: *Per ⅓ of 415g Can*				
Bolognese, 140g	90	380	3	11
With Beef, 140g	155	650	6.5	14
Chiko, Roll, 163g	300	1255	10	42
Chop Chop!: *Per 85g Can*				
Chicken Chunks: Italian Tomato	90	375	2.5	3
Smoked in Springwater, drained	70	280	1.5	1
Sweet Chilli	120	490	4.5	6.5
Teriyaki	95	395	1	6.5
Chicken Shredded: Chilli with Lite Mayo	135	550	6	2.5
Cracked Pepper with Lite Mayo	140	570	7	3.5
Lite Mayo	130	550	6	2
Springwater with Sea Salt, drained	70	280	1	1
Sundried Tomato with Lite Mayo	135	570	7	3
Wholegrain Mustard with Lite Mayo	140	580	7.5	3
Coles:				
Canned/Packaged:				
Baked Beans:				
In Tomato Sauce: 140g can	125	510	1	25
Organic (400g can), ½ can, 200g	160	680	3.5	28
In Ham Sauce, ½ Cup, 140g	130	545	1.5	26
2-Minute Noodles: *Per 85g Pkt*				
Beef	245	1015	2	47
Chicken	255	1050	2.5	47
Smart Buy: Beef	415	1740	18	54
Chicken	400	1665	17	53
Oriental	415	1740	18	56
Spaghetti:				
In Tomato & Cheese Sauce, 140g can	110	450	1	20
Smart Buy, Spaghetti, ¼ 420g can	65	275	0.5	14
Meals: *Per ½ of 410g Can*				
Beef Curry, 205g	250	1030	11	19
Chicken Curry, 205g	170	710	7.5	15
Vegetables & Steak, 205g	150	640	5.5	14
Frozen:				
Bechamel Beef Lasagne, 400g	580	2430	27	55
Butter Chicken, 375g	560	2340	21	71
Beef Satay, 375g	570	2380	21	69
Chicken: Breast Tenders, 100g	215	895	9	15
Kiev (1), 175g	460	1915	29	27
Korma, 375g	520	2160	20	64
Mini Kiev (1), 40g	120	490	8.5	5
Nugget (1), 20g	50	200	3	3.5
Dim Sims, Mini (1), 16g	35	145	2	4
Hamburger Patty (1), 50g	115	470	8	3.5

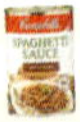

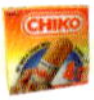

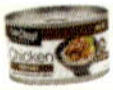

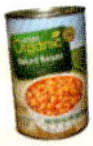

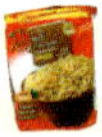

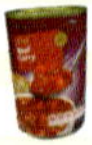

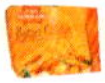

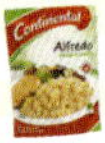

	Cal	kJ	Fat	Cb
Coles (Cont):				
Frozen (Cont):				
Macaroni Cheese, 400g	700	2930	40	60
Sheperd's Pie, 400g	310	1280	9	38
Spaghetti Bolognese, 400g	445	1850	16	50
Tuna Bake, 400g	615	2560	33	51
Light Meals: Beef Lasagne, 350g	360	1510	8.5	48
Chicken Fettuccine, 320g	300	1240	7.5	41
Chicken Rissotto, 320g	310	1285	7.5	41
Pies (Multi-Pack): *Per Pie*				
Beef Pie, 175g	400	1660	21	37
Chicken & Vegetable, 175g	380	1600	18	39
Chunky Beef, 175g	390	1615	21	35
Single Pies: Beef, 175g	400	1670	21	37
Chunky Beef, 175g	390	1615	21	35
Party Pies, each, 46g	115	475	6.5	10
Sausage Rolls, each, 42g	115	470	6	11
Smart Buy (6 Pack):				
Meat Pies (1), 150g	360	1520	20	33
Continental				
Asian Rices: *Per ¼ of 120g Packet*				
Chinese	115	485	2	24
Oriental Fried Rice	115	490	1.5	24
Satay	140	580	2	27
Couscous, average all flavours, ¼ of 130g packet, 32.5g	145	600	2.5	25
Rices of the World, average all flavours, ¼ pkt	130	535	1.5	26
Hot Pot Casserole: *Per ¼ of 80g Packet*				
Curry	435	1820	13	46
French Onion	290	1215	10	20
Savoury	275	1155	11	16
Sweet & Sour	400	1670	16	37
Pasta & Sauce: *Per ¼ of 80-100g Packet*				
Alfredo	125	525	2.5	20
Bacon Carbonara	120	490	2	19
Cheese & Black Pepper	100	430	2.5	18
Chicken & Mushroom	130	535	2.5	21
Chicken Curry	110	465	2.5	19
Creamy Mushroom & Bacon	115	475	2	19
Four Cheeses	140	580	3	22
Macaroni Cheese	140	580	2.5	24
Mushroom, Garlic & Pepper	130	545	3	20
Savoury Tomato & Onion	95	390	1.5	17
Sour Cream & Chives	125	515	3.5	18
Sour Cream & Mushrooms	105	435	2.5	17
Pasta & Sauce Lite: *Per ¼ of 85g Packet*				
Alfredo	100	425	2	17
Bacon Carbonara	105	440	2	17
Chicken Curry	90	380	2	15

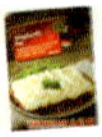

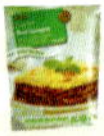

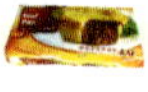

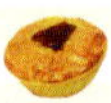

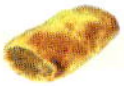

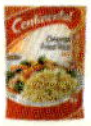

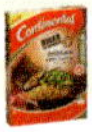

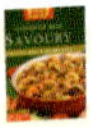

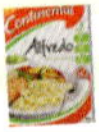

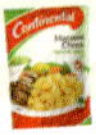

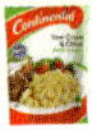

Meals ~ Canned & Packaged — M

Continental (Cont):

	Cal	kJ	Fat	Cb
Rices: *Per ¼ of 120-135g Pkt*				
Cheesy	140	575	3	25
Chicken	125	525	1.5	26
Chicken & Sweet Corn	130	535	2	25
Chicken & Vegetables	130	540	1.5	26
Rich Beef & Mushroom	135	555	2.5	25
Risotto: *Per ¼ Packet*				
Cheese & Bacon	135	560	1	27
Classic Cheese	135	560	1.5	27
Mushroom & Garlic	135	560	1	27
Other Side Dishes: *Per ¼ Pkt, Prepared as Directed*				
Macaroni Cheese: & Bacon	160	675	3.5	24
Nacho Cheese	155	650	3.5	24
Super Saucy	160	670	3.5	25
Potato Mash: Cheese	150	620	4	22
Homestyle	145	600	4	21
Pumpkin	145	610	4	21
Smooth & Creamy	150	615	4.5	21
Sour Cream & Herbs	145	610	4	22

Colonial Farm:

	Cal	kJ	Fat	Cb
Burgers: Chicken Burger, 85g	360	1500	16	14
Cocktail Spring Roll (1), 17g	40	160	1.5	5
Chicken: Garlic Balls (1), 40g	120	490	8.5	5.5
Parcel: With Cheese & Broccoli, (1), 120g	210	875	10	10
With Cheese & Herb Sauce (1), 120g	260	1090	12	10
Peri Peri Chicken Sticks (1), 20g	55	225	3.5	3
Meatballs, Flamegrilled (1), 15g	30	130	2	0.5
Mini Dim Sims: Beef (1), 12g	30	120	1.5	3
Chicken/Vegetable (1), 12g	20	90	0.5	4
Nuggets, Chicken (1), 20g	55	225	3	4.5
Samosas, Vegeteable (1), 17g	40	170	2	4.5
Schnitzel: Chicken (1), 125g	235	970	12	14
With Cheese (1), 120g	320	1335	21	20
Vienna (1), 135g	365	1515	22	27
Veal: Cordon Bleu (1), 140g	275	1150	14	17
Parmigiana Balls (1), 40g	95	390	6	5
Parcel, with Parmigiana Sce (1), 120g	260	1085	15	14

Elmsbury (Aldi):

	Cal	kJ	Fat	Cb
Pie Slices: Chicken & Vege, 2 sl., 350g	925	3860	50	86
Steak & Gravy, 2 slices, 350g	915	3820	54	74
Pies: Chicken & Veg. (1), 175g	400	1670	18	41
Meat, Party (1), 46g	115	480	6	12
Premium Grain Fed Beef (1), 225g	475	1980	19	54
Quiche, Party (1), 44g	115	470	6	12
Sausage Roll, Party (1), 36g	100	410	6	10
Tempters, Spinach & Ricotta, 1 piece, 30g	70	285	3.5	7

Fantastic Noodles:

	Cal	kJ	Fat	Cb
Bowls: *Per 85g Bowl*				
Beef	390	1630	17	52
Chicken	395	1655	17	53
Oriental	390	1645	17	53
Gluten Free: *Per 40g Cup*				
Beef	140	580	0.5	33
Chicken	155	650	0.5	37
Instant 2 Minute Noodles: *Per 85g dry cake, Prep'd as Directed*				
Beef	380	1595	16	52
Chicken	380	1580	16	53
Mighty Meal: *Per 105g Bowl*				
Beef	470	1945	23	58
Chicken	475	1995	22	62
Noodle Cup: *Per 70g Cup*				
Beef	325	1365	14	43
Chicken	330	1385	14	44
Chicken & Corn	325	1365	14	44
Chicken Chow Mein	380	1580	15	49
Crispy Bacon	325	1370	14	44
Oriental	330	1380	14	45
Xtra Saucy Noodle Cup, Mi Goreng, 75g cup	375	1565	14	51

Farmwood (Aldi): *Per Serving*

	Cal	kJ	Fat	Cb
Chicken Breast:				
Nuggets, Tempura Style, 100g	230	960	12	18
Schnitzel, 100g	230	960	12	117
Infusions, Alfredo, 1 piece, 175g	380	1590	18	26
Jugglers, 100g	230	970	14	15
Kiev, 175g	455	1890	27	31
Nuggets, 100g	240	990	12	20
Patties: Hamburger (1), 50G	130	540	8.5	5
Tenders, 100g	1175	725	7	12

Corale (Aldi): *Per 210g, ½ 420g Can*

	Cal	kJ	Fat	Cb
Short Cut Spaghetti in Tomato Sauce	125	510	0.5	26
Spaghetti in Tomato & Cheese Sauce	145	600	1	27

Fray Bentos:

	Cal	kJ	Fat	Cb
Pie: *Per ½ of 425g Pie*				
Steak & Kidney, 210g	375	1570	20	31

Four'N Twenty:

	Cal	kJ	Fat	Cb
Jaffle: *Per Jaffle, 110g*				
Baked Bean	225	945	5	37
Egg & Bacon	340	1430	13	38
Ham & Cheese	255	1060	9	33
Pizza Jaffle	230	965	8	32
Pastie, Aussie, 175g	465	1945	23	55

Updated Nutrition Data ~ www.CalorieKing.com.au
Persons with Diabetes ~ See Disclaimer (Page 22)

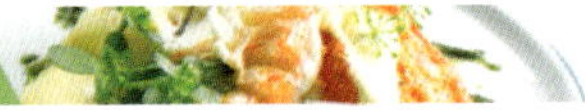

Meals ~ Canned & Packaged

	Cal	kJ	Fat	Cb
Four'N Twenty (Cont):				
Pies: Beef & Cheese, 175g	415	1730	22	35
Beef & Mushy Pea, 175g	440	1840	22	46
Chicken & Vegetable, 175g	405	1695	21	43
Chunky Pepper Steak, 175g	415	1725	21	38
Football, 175g	400	1680	20	38
Hungry Man, 280g	650	2730	35	61
Meat: Pie, 175g	400	1680	20	38
Lite Pie, 175g	335	1405	13	39
King Size, 220g	520	2170	30	44
Microwave, 175g	400	1680	20	38
Traditional, 175g	400	1680	20	38
Traditional Family, 150g	380	1590	23	33
Party Pie, 50g	125	515	7	13
Shepherds Pie, 200g	410	1710	20	43
Steak & Bacon, 175g	395	1660	21	38
Steak & Onion, 175g	435	1820	23	44
Traveller: Beef, 160g	330	1380	14	36
Egg & Bacon, 140g	310	1310	17	33
Pepper Steak, 160g	380	1600	17	42
Sausage Roll: Jumbo, 117g	300	1265	16	31
King Size: 180g	515	2160	31	43
Microwave, 180g	500	2090	28	47
Party, 42g	120	490	6.5	12
Griff's:				
Chicken Mornay, 400g	510	2130	21	62
Curried Prawns, 400g	350	1460	7	58
Fried Rice, 350g	500	2095	21	63
Sweet & Sour Pork, 400g	475	1990	8	76
Hamper: *Per ¼ of 340g Can*				
Camp Pie, 85g	140	580	8	7
Corned Beef: Orig., 85g	200	830	14	0
Easy Slice, 85g	200	830	14	0
Lite, 85g	170	710	11	1
Harvest:				
Canned: *Per 213g, ½ of 425g Can*				
Beef & Red Wine Casserole	130	545	3.5	16
Hearty Irish Stew	145	605	5.5	15
Lamb Hot Pot	130	550	3	17
Mild Curry	150	630	3	17
Ravioli Bolognese	195	810	6	24
Tortellini Bolognese	190	800	6	22
Vegetables & Sausages	165	690	7.5	17
Vegetables & Steak	130	550	4.5	15

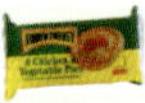

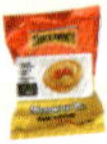

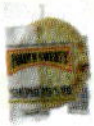

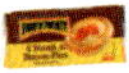

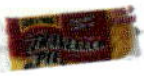

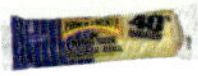

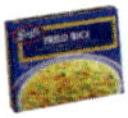

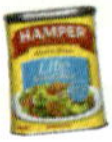

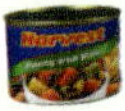

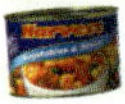

	Cal	kJ	Fat	Cb
Heinz:				
Canned/Packaged				
2 Snap Pots, in Tomato Sauce, 200g can	185	760	1	28
Baked Beanz: *Per 210g, ½ of 420g Can*				
Barbeque	215	905	2	33
Cheesy Tomato Sauce	195	810	2	28
English Recipe	195	810	1	29
Five	195	810	0.5	3
Ham Sauce	205	860	2	31
Tomato Sauce	190	800	1	29
No Added Salt	180	745	0	26
Salt Reduced	190	800	1	29
Sweet Chilli Sauce	205	850	1.5	32
Beans of the Day: *Per 200g, ½ of 400g Pouch*				
Chunky Tomato & Onion	260	1080	1	39
Curried Pumpkin	260	1090	2	38
Fiery Mexican	240	1010	2	31
Spanish with Chorizo	270	1110	3	34
Beanz: *Per 210g, ½ of 420g Can*				
& Bacon	210	880	3	28
& Sausages	250	1030	6.5	30
Kidz, 200g Can	190	805	1	30
Chilli Beans: *Per 200g, ½ of 400g Pouch*				
Hot	220	915	1.5	35
Medium Salsa	190	780	1.5	30
Big Eat: *Per 410g Can*				
All Day Breakfast	450	1885	15	49
Big 'n' Beefy Casserole	220	925	4	27
Chicken & Bacon Casserole	260	1090	8	32
Peppered Steak & Onion	250	1050	4.5	30
Ravioli Bolognese	375	1560	11	51
Spaghetti Bolognese	380	1495	13	41
Shredded Chicken: *Per 85g Can*				
Caesar	140	590	8.5	4.5
Lite Mayo	135	565	6	2
Mustard Mayo	150	635	9	4.5
Natural Smoke	75	305	1	1.5
Spicy Chilli	90	385	2	6
Springwater & Seasalt	65	275	1	0.5
Sweetcorn & Mayo	135	570	8	3.5
Sweet Chilli	145	605	7	8
Tandoori	100	410	2.5	7
Teriyaki	90	370	0.5	8.5
Tomato & Onion	125	510	7	4.5

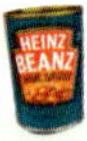

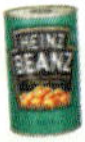

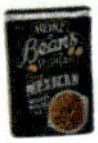

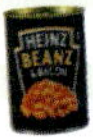

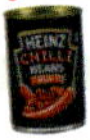

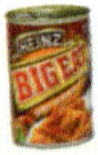

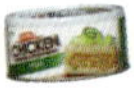

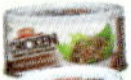

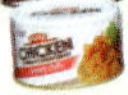

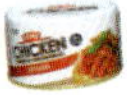

Meals ~ Canned & Packaged

Heinz (Cont):

Canned

Spaghetti:

Item	Cal	kJ	Fat	Cb
& Meatballs, 210g	230	945	9	28
& Sausages, 210g	200	840	6.5	28
Alphaghetti in Tomato Sauce, 220g	135	560	1	26
Bolognese, 220g	145	595	2	25
Extra Cheese, 210g	130	535	1	24
Tomato Sauce, 210g	125	525	0.5	25
Salt Reduced, 210g	125	525	0.5	25
2 Snap Pots, in Tomato Sauce, 200g can	120	500	0.5	25
Kids: OOPS, in Tomato Sauce & Cheese, 220g can	125	520	1	24
Pasta Shapes, 220g can	155	640	1	31

Herbert Adams:

Pasties:

Item	Cal	kJ	Fat	Cb
Cornish, 210g	480	2010	24	51
Traditional, pastie, 175g	385	1615	18	48
Vegetable, pastie, 175g	380	1575	18	44
Pies: Chunky Chicken & Vegetable, 210g	470	1960	22	52
Chunky Pepper Steak, 210g	465	1955	21	51
Chilli con Carne Beef, 210g	510	2120	29	39
Creamy Chicken & Leek	495	2070	26	45
King Island, 210g	500	2075	26	45
King Island Beef with Vegetables, 210g	470	1960	24	50
Party Pie: (1), 50g	135	570	7.5	13
Beef & Burgundy, 22g	60	250	3	6
Pepper Steak, 22g	55	230	3	6
Traditional Shepherd's, 240g	480	1990	26	45
Quiche Lorraine, snack, 160g	430	1790	25	31
Sausage Roll: Party	100	415	5	11
Cheese & Spinach	580	2420	34	53
Vol Au Vents, (1), av., 17g	45	190	3	3.5

Ho Mai:

Yum Cha:

Item	Cal	kJ	Fat	Cb
Mini Dim Sim, 17g	35	145	2	5.5
Cocktail Spring Roll, 17g	40	160	1.5	5.5
Pork & Chive Dumpling, 15g	40	170	1.5	5.5
Sesame Prawn (1), 13g	30	125	1.5	3
Spring Roll (1), 42g	105	430	5.5	11

I & J:

Item	Cal	kJ	Fat	Cb
Beefers: Big Beefer, 80g	215	900	18	0.5
Lean Beefer, 55g	80	340	4	2
Burgers, Bacon, 168g	430	1800	21	39

IGA:

Item	Cal	kJ	Fat	Cb
Baked Beans, ½ cup, 140g	135	555	1	25
Spaghetti in Tomato Sauce, 150g	100	420	1	20

International Cuisine (Aldi):

Item	Cal	kJ	Fat	Cb
Beef Lasagne, 400g	545	2280	25	53
Beef Stroganoff, 350g	285	1200	5.5	37
Beef in Red Wine Sce with Mash, 350g	250	1055	3	36
Butter Chicken, 375g	475	1975	17	53
Chicken Risotto, 350g	295	1230	4	46
Chicken Tikka Masala, 375g	470	1960	18	50
Dim Sims, 50g	110	465	5	14
Lamb Rogan Josh, 375g	505	2100	18	57
Macaroni & Cheese, 375g	425	1780	16	54
Malaysian Satay Beef, 375g	485	2020	18	47
Mushroom Tortellini, 400g	400	1680	7.5	63
Supreme Pizza, ½ Pizza, 250g	575	2400	19	70
Spaghetti Bolognese, 375g	375	1570	11	50
Spring Rolls, Mini (1), 50g	110	450	5	13
Sundried Tomato, Chicken & Pasta, 350g	335	1395	6	48
Thai Green Chicken Curry, 375g	520	2160	22	46
Vegetable Cannelloni, 400g	300	1250	10	47
Yum Cha Selection, 2 pieces, 32g	80	340	4.5	8.5

Kraft:

Mac & Cheese: *Per Serving, Prepared*

Item	Cal	kJ	Fat	Cb
Original, 150g	260	1090	10	34
Deluxe, 226g	410	1710	14	50

Easy Mac: *Per 73g Bowl, Prep'd*

Item	Cal	kJ	Fat	Cb
Bacon Carbonara	300	1260	7	50
Cheese	310	1290	8	50
Chicken	290	1200	6	50
Nacho Cheese	300	1265	7	50

Easy Mac: *Per 70g Sachet*

Item	Cal	kJ	Fat	Cb
Bacon Carbonara	280	1160	6.5	45
Cheese	280	1175	7.5	44
Chicken	265	1100	6	44
Chilli Cheese	280	1160	6.5	45
Nacho Cheese	280	1180	7	45

Latina Fresh:

Agnolotti: *Per ½ Packet, Prepared as Directed*

Item	Cal	kJ	Fat	Cb
Basil, Pesto & Parmesan	470	1960	13	71
Ricotta & Spinach	490	2040	9.5	76

Kids Mini Ravioli:

Item	Cal	kJ	Fat	Cb
Beef & Vegetable	385	1620	11	52
Cheese & Vegetable	385	1620	11	52
Fettuccine, Egg, ½ packet	520	2180	7	92
Gnocchi, Potato, ½ packet	415	1730	14	64

Updated Nutrition Data ~ www.CalorieKing.com.au
Persons with Diabetes ~ See Disclaimer (Page 22)

Meals ~ Canned & Packaged

	Cal	kJ	Fat	Cb
Latina Fresh (Cont):				
Meals for One: *Per Meal*				
Canelloni	448	1875	25	37
Lasagne	540	2240	26	49
Penne Carbonara	560	2330	24	64
Ricotta & Spinach Agnolotti	490	2030	17	69
Spaghetti Bolognese	400	1650	12	53
Ravioli: *Per ½ Packet, Prepared*				
Beef	665	2760	19	97
Beef & Rosemary	530	2205	15	72
Chicken & Mushroom	460	1915	6.5	73
Chicken & Garlic	570	2380	7.5	94
Tortellini: *Per ½ Packet, Prepared as Directed*				
Ham & Cheese	615	2565	15	88
Mixed Veal	635	2660	18	89
Three Cheese	510	2140	12	74
Veal	575	2400	17	79
Lean Cuisine:				
Balanced Serve: *Per Serve*				
Beef in Red Wine Sauce w. Mash	260	1080	5	36
Chicken & Vegetable Risotto	300	1260	4.5	47
Chicken Florentine w. Linguine	280	1185	5	39
Classic Beef Stroganoff w. Pasta	315	1315	8.5	39
Creamy Salmon & Dill Pasta	320	1335	7.5	42
Honey Soy Beef with Noodles	235	965	3	35
Lamb & Rosemary Hot Pot	250	1060	6.5	32
Malaysian Chicken Curry w. Rice	285	1190	4.5	49
Satay Chicken Noodles	335	1395	8	46
Spaghetti Bolognese	300	1245	6	43
Thai Green Chicken Curry w. Rice	290	1220	5	48
Classic:				
Chicken & Spinach Risotto	290	1210	4.5	44
Creamy Chicken Pasta Bake	335	1400	7	47
Pumpkin, Spinach & Ricotta Lasagne	415	1740	8	61
Rich Beef Lasagne	410	1700	10	57
Spaghetti Carbonara	365	1520	10	49
Vegetable Cannelloni	365	1520	9	52
Steam: *Per Packet*				
Agnolotti with Spinach & Ricotta	390	1630	10	59
Atlantic Salmon with Pasta	350	1465	8	45
Cheese & Pepper Chkn w. Pasta	375	1580	7.5	50
Chicken Tikka Masala	370	1530	8	53
Lean Cuisine (Cont):				
Steam (Cont): *Per Packet*				
Chilli Con Carne with Rice	340	1410	4	52
Indian Beef Korma	405	1680	11	51
Indian Style Butter Chicken with Rice	365	1515	9.5	52
Meatball Arrabbiata	310	1295	6	38
Mexican Beef & Rice w. Tortilla Wraps	385	1610	7.5	56
Ravioli with Ricotta & Capsicum	370	1540	10	47
Satay Beef with Rice	420	1755	10	59
Slow Cooked Beef	380	1590	8	51
Slow Cooked Chicken	350	1450	7.5	49
Sundried Tomato Chicken with Pasta	405	1685	9.5	56
Thai Red Chicken Curry w. Rice	345	1425	6	53
Tortellini with Beef & Parmesan	340	1425	9	49
Leggo's:				
Fresh Pasta: *Per ½ of 360g Packet, Cooked*				
Agnolotti, Spinach & Ricotta	500	2090	11	78
Beef Ravioli	490	2045	14	67
Ricotta & Rstd Veg. Tortellini	475	1985	7	82
Fresh Agnolotti: *Per ¼ of 630g Packag*				
Chicken Mozzarella & Napoli	430	1810	12	61
Ricotta, Spin. Cracked Pepper	420	1750	10	64
Fresh Large Agnolotti: *Per ¼ of 320g Package*				
Classic Mozzarella & Prosciutto	420	1740	16	47
Herb Chicken with Leek & Garlic	410	1720	15	47
Semi-Dried Tomato w. Basil & Mozzarella	430	1795	15	57
Veal & Caramelised Onion	400	1660	14	50
Lenard's:				
Easyliving Meals: *Per 250g Serving*				
Bombay Chicken	370	1545	19	26
Chicken Dumplings with Vegetables	280	1175	11	37
Chicken Lasagne	470	1965	25	37
Chicken Cacciatore	240	1010	10	14
Satay Chicken	580	2420	40	25
Teriyaki Chicken	265	1095	10	17
Traditional Italian Meatballs	420	1750	24	28
Tender Gold Meals:				
Seasoned Breast Fillet, 150g	150	635	2.5	1
Shashlick Sun-Dried Tomato, 70g	70	285	1	2.5

Meals ~ Canned & Packaged

Linda McCartney:

	Cal	kJ	Fat	Cb
Vegetarian:				
Pies: Country (1), 166g	415	1725	24	42
Farmhouse (1), 146g	380	1585	24	34
Sausage (1), 50g	100	425	4.5	4.5
Sausage Roll (1), 57g	160	670	8	15

Lite n' Easy:

	Cal	kJ	Fat	Cb
Frozen Meals: Apricot Chicken with Rice	420	1760	10	54
Baked Turkey	325	1360	5	44
Beef Korma	345	1450	6	34
Beef n' Black Bean	360	1500	4	46
Beef Stroganoff with Pasta	410	1710	9	49
Beef with Red Wine & Mushroom	360	1500	10	30
Braised Asian Lamb Shanks	395	1650	9	41
Braised Chicken & Almonds	460	1920	15	55
Braised Lamb Shanks	330	1395	7	26
Butter Chicken	415	1730	7.5	47
Chicken Dijon	470	1970	13	55
Chicken Enchilada	390	1635	12	45
Chicken Parmigiana	415	1730	11	41
Chicken Schnitzel	395	1640	9	47
Chicken Tikka Masala	425	1770	5	48
Chicken with Satay Sauce	415	1740	5	64
Chilli Con Carne with Rice	405	1700	7	55
Corned Beef	355	1480	11	28
Crumbed Chicken Breast with Wedges	345	1430	7	37
Crumbed Fillet of Fish	395	1640	11	53
Curried Beef Sausages	380	1590	12	41
Fettuccine Provencale	420	1750	8	64
Fisherman's Pie	460	1910	12	39
Fragrant Thai Chicken	385	1600	5.5	50
Hearty Beef Casserole	370	1545	10	25
Homestyle Macaroni Cheese	465	1950	13	58
Honey Soy Chicken	395	1650	9	52
Malay Beef Curry	380	1590	5.5	44
Meatloaf, Mash & Gravy	400	1680	7.5	46
Pepper Steak	410	1720	10	38
Porcupines in Tomato Sauce	350	1445	8	34
Rigatoni	395	1650	7.5	50
Roast Beef	375	1560	5	40
Roast Chicken	400	1680	10	47
Roast Chicken in Mushroom Sauce	365	1520	6	38
Roast Lamb	340	1410	6.5	39
Roghan Josh	425	1770	11	52

Lite n' Easy (Cont):

	Cal	kJ	Fat	Cb
Frozen Meals: (Cont): Salt & Pepper Chicken	425	1780	12	50
Sausage & Onion Gravy	370	1545	10	36
Savoury Beef Rissoles	330	1385	8	32
Shepherd's Pie	370	1540	8	47
Spaghetti Bolognaise	420	1750	6.5	60
Spaghetti Marinara	415	1740	9	48
Special Lasagne	385	1610	9	40
Spinach & Ricotta Tortelloni	430	1795	10	58
Steak with Mushroom Sauce	335	1400	10	22
Sweet & Sour Chicken	430	1800	9	53
Tandoori Chicken	400	1660	11	39
Tasmanian Salmon Pasta	440	1840	8	61
Tortilla Stack	455	1900	11	64
Soups: Chicken Noodle	105	440	2.5	10
Pea & Ham	165	680	2.5	20
Tomato	120	495	4	15
Meals in a Bowl: Aromatic Chicken Curry	245	1030	6	30
Asian Rice Bowl	235	980	4	36
Baked Potato Bolognaise	225	930	3.5	29
Chicken & Chorizo Rice Pot	235	985	3	34
Chicken & Vegetable Risotto	235	990	5.5	25
Chicken Alfredo Pasta	260	1080	4	31
Chicken Spaghetti	275	1150	4.5	44
Fettuccini Bolognaise	270	1120	5	35
Hokkien Stir Fry	215	890	6	25
Pasta Carbonara	290	1220	4	45
Peri Peri Chicken	230	955	1.5	28
Roast Chicken Linguine	250	1050	8	28
Sesame Beef Noodle	225	945	5.5	26

McCain:

	Cal	kJ	Fat	Cb
Attack A Snack: *Per 200g Meal*				
Bacon & Mushroom Spirals	255	1065	12	27
Bechamel Lasagnese	230	945	8	28
Beef Chow Mein	200	825	6.5	15
Macaroni Cheese	290	1200	13	32
Sausage & Herb Potato	220	910	10	23
Spaghetti Bolognese	220	900	4.5	32
Healthy Choice: *Per Meal*				
Apricot Chicken, 350g	350	1445	3.5	65
Beef Florentine, 320g	285	1190	8	36
Beef Goulash, 370g	405	1680	10	62
Beef Lasagne, Large, 400g	465	1940	8	72
Beef Stroganoff, 300g	315	1320	9	41
Chinese BBQ Chicken, 350g	355	1480	8	55
Chinese Chicken & Cashews, 280g	275	1135	7	40
Creamy Chicken Carbonara, 300g	310	1300	7.5	44

Updated Nutrition Data ~ www.CalorieKing.com.au
Persons with Diabetes ~ See Disclaimer (Page 22)

Meals ~ Canned & Packaged

McCain (Cont):

	Cal	kJ	Fat	Cb
Healthy Choice (Cont): *Per Meal*				
Fillet of Lamb, 310g	255	1065	7	31
Honey Mustard Chicken, 300g	310	1295	7.5	49
Lemon Chicken, 350g	440	1840	9	72
Mexican Chicken, 280g	260	1085	3	45
Singapore Noodles w. Chicken	265	1100	7	37
Spaghetti Bolognese, 400g	380	1570	6.5	56
Tender Beef in Seeded Mustard Sce, 310g	290	1210	10	34
Healthy Choice Plus: *Per Meal*				
Beef Hot Pot, 420g	270	1120	6	35
Creamy Chicken Pasta, 420g	420	1750	11	55
Honey Stirfry Chicken, 420g	380	1585	6.5	63
Hearty Meals: *Per Meal*				
Bangers & Mash, 400g	555	2305	30	52
Beef & Bacon Pasta Bake, 400g	500	2090	20	52
Chicken Parmagiana, 320g	490	2035	26	39
Fettucine Carbonara	605	2515	26	72
Lamb Cutlet w. Gravy	380	1595	17	40
Pork Riblets, 320g	390	1625	16	42
Roast Beef, 320g	285	1195	8.5	32
Roast Chicken, 320g	270	1105	6.5	26
Roast Lamb, 320g	305	1275	10	31
Shepherd's Pie, 400g	420	1760	20	40
Spaghetti Bolognese, 400g	470	1950	16	56
Steak Diane, 320g	305	1270	13	28
Sweet Chilli Chicken Parm.	450	1885	21	39
Tuna Mornay, 400g	640	2680	32	62
Veal Cordon Bleu, 320g	495	2080	26	42
Stir & Serve: *Per ½ of 620g Pkt*				
Beef, Rigatoni & Mushroom	275	1140	9	33
Braised Beef & Golden Potatoes	295	1230	9	37
Chicken w. Veg. & Farfalle Pasta	290	1220	9	35
Rigatoni & Broccoli	305	1270	9	37
Made For You: *Per Meal*				
Beef Lasagne, 390g	395	1650	8.5	55
Cottage Pie w. Sweet Pot., 340g	235	980	7	31
Supreme Pizza, 215g	330	1375	5.5	46
Thai Green Chicken Curry	275	1140	6.5	33
Vegetable Lasagne, 380g	380	1590	10	52

Maggi:

	Cal	kJ	Fat	Cb
2-Minute Noodles: *Per 74g Pkt*				
Beef	330	1390	13	46
Chicken	325	1370	13	46
Original	330	1370	13	46
99% Fat Free: *Per 76g Pkt*				
Beef	280	1180	2	57
Chicken	280	1160	2	56

Maggi (Cont):

	Cal	kJ	Fat	Cb
Fusian Noodles: *Per Cup*				
Hot & Spicy	320	1320	16	39
Mi Goreng Singapore	315	1310	16	39
Satay	320	1340	16	40
Soy & Mild Spice	315	1305	15	38
Noodle Cup: *Per Cup, Prepared as Directed*				
Asian Beef	270	1120	10	38
Beef	265	1110	11	38
Chicken	265	1115	11	38
Indian Curry	270	1115	11	37
Laksa	270	1135	11	39
Oriental	270	1135	11	38
98% Fat-Free:				
Beef	265	1105	1	55
Chicken	265	1105	2.5	54
Fusian Block: *Per 72g Block, Prepared*				
2-Minute Noodle, Mi Goreng Singapore	355	1480	17	44
Hot & Spicy	360	1500	17	45
Satay	360	1500	17	45
Soy & Mild Spice	350	1470	17	44
Marathon:				
Dim Sims: (1), 50g	95	400	2.5	14
Mini: Beef (1), 17g	30	135	1	4
Chicken (1), 17g	25	105	0	3.5
Puffy Dog (1), 33g	95	395	4	10
Spring Roll (1), 160g	240	1010	7.5	35
Mini (1), 50g	60	260	1	11

Michelina's:

	Cal	kJ	Fat	Cb
Classics: *Per Packet*				
Beef Burgundy, 255g	225	935	7	28
Beef Ravioli, 255g	300	1245	12	36
Beef Teriyaki, 284g	340	1410	3.5	58
Cheese Cannelloni, 255g	260	1075	8	37
Cheese Stuffed Rigatoni, 284g	300	1260	8.5	43
Cheese Tortellini, 255g	375	1570	17	42
Fettuccine Pesto, 284g	290	1200	7	46
Lasagne with Meat Sauce, 255g	295	1230	7.5	41
Pepper Steak & Rice, 255g	290	1220	4	49
Prawns & Veg. Alfredo, 255g	300	1255	7.5	43
Spaghetti Bolognese, 284g	320	1340	4.5	54
Budget Gourmet:				
Creamy Parmesan Spirals, 115g	140	590	2	24
Fettuccine Alfredo, 115g	135	560	3	22
Rotini Arrabbiata, 115g	140	580	1.5	27
Wild Rice Pilaf, 115g	165	690	3	32

Meals ~ Canned & Packaged

Mrs Mac's (WA):	Cal	kJ	Fat	Cb
Pastie: Microwave	425	1765	23	43
Old Style Vegetable	450	1875	23	51
Traditional	510	2120	27	52
Pies: Angus Beef	765	3195	40	72
Beef	515	2160	27	50
Beef & Mushroom	480	2000	24	52
Beef, Cheese & Bacon	550	2300	30	51
Big Country	725	3025	36	72
Big Minced Beef & Cheese	790	3300	42	74
Chilli Beef & Cheese	535	2240	28	53
Choice Steak	485	2020	22	52
Curry	480	2000	23	54
Pepper Steak	490	2040	22	52
Pizza	515	2160	27	54
Roast Style, Chicken & Vegetable	445	1850	19	54
Shepherd's	505	2095	23	56
Steak & Cheese	510	2120	25	51
Cruizer Pie: Premiem Steak	445	1850	20	47
Beef, Cheese & Onion	485	2015	25	47
Chicken, Bacon & Cheese	475	1995	24	51
Microwave Pie: Beef	515	2160	27	50
Beef & Cheese	525	2200	28	49
Beef & Mushroom	480	2000	24	52
Beef & Pepper	515	2140	26	51
Quiche: Egg, Cheese & Bacon	470	1960	28	37
Ricotta & Spinach	425	1770	23	39
The Good Eating Pie:				
Beef: 200g	420	1755	15	49
Beef, 120g	420	1755	15	49
Beef, 50g	115	480	4	14
Cruizer: Beef	380	1585	16	40
Beef & Cheese	350	1450	13	42
Mini Beef, 55g	100	425	3.5	12
Potato Top: Beef, 180g	295	1225	7.5	38
Sausage Roll	275	1155	11	34
Sausage Roll: Angus Beef	410	1710	24	37
Bacon & Cheese	435	1805	26	39
Beef	355	1480	21	33
Giant Sausage Roll	445	1855	24	44
Homestyle	330	1370	18	32
Microwave Roll	480	2015	26	47
Spinach & Ricotta	400	1665	23	39
Sweetreats: Apple & Custard	285	1190	14	37
Spiced Apple	280	1170	13	38

Nissin:	Cal	kJ	Fat	Cb
Cup Noodles: *Per Cup*				
Chicken	325	1360	13	43
Chilli Crab	340	1415	14	45
Laksa	360	1510	19	39
Seafood	340	1420	16	40
Spicy Seafood	315	1320	12	43
Tom Yam Seafood	350	1455	18	39
Old El Paso:				
Salsa Dips: *Per 1 Tablespoon, 25g*				
Chunky; Thick & Chunky	10	40	0	1.5
Nachos Supreme	20	80	0	3.5
Spicy Bean	20	85	0	3.5
Roasted Capsicum	20	80	0	4
Seasoning Mix, avg. all varieties, 1 tsp, 5g	15	60	0	2.5
Recipe Kit: *Per Serving, Prepared*				
Beef Fajitas, 146g	280	1170	8.5	30
Beef Jumbo Taco, 134g	250	1040	13	16
Chicken Burritos, 191g	310	1290	14	25
Chicken Enchiladas, 192g	305	1275	13	20
Chilli Con Carne Burrito, 165g	300	1245	15	22
Hard n Soft: Beef Hard Tacos, 141g	230	950	12	13
Beef Soft Tacos, 163g	250	1040	15	11
Healthy Fiesta, Chicken, 176g	225	950	4.5	25
Quesadilla, Cheesy Chicken, 156g	310	1300	12	20
Soft Taco, Crispy Chicken, 93.5g	215	905	9	19
Taco Shell: Jumbo Shell, 19g	85	360	4	11
Regular Shell, 11g	50	210	2.5	6
Stand 'n Stuff Shell, 14g	65	265	3	8
Tortilla Wraps: Burrito, 40g	135	570	4	22
Enchilada: 28g	90	360	2	14
Minis, 25g	85	355	2.5	14
Light, 40g	115	475	2	19
Wholegrain, 40g	120	510	3	18
Sauce, average all varieties 1 Tbsp, 25g	15	55	0	2
Vegetables, canned: *Per ¼ Can*				
Jalapeno Chilies, 62.5g	10	40	0	2
Mexe Beans, 106g	65	275	0.5	8
Refried Beans, 109g	85	345	0.5	11
Refried Beans with Chilli, 109g	80	335	0.5	11
OptiSlim:				
Heat & Serve:				
Beef Stroganoff, 300g	235	990	6	25
Chilli Con Carne, 300g	260	1080	7	26
Chunky Beef & Potato, 300g	225	945	2.5	28
Spinach & Ricotta Tortellini, 300g	230	970	4.5	40
Vegetarian Tikka Masala, 300g	175	735	1	34

Updated Nutrition Data ~ www.CalorieKing.com.au
Persons with Diabetes ~ See Disclaimer (Page 22)

Meals ~ Canned & Packaged

	Cal	kJ	Fat	Cb
Orgran:				
Falafel Mix, dry, 40g	140	575	0.5	27
Spaghetti in Tomato Sauce, 220g	140	580	01	27
Pappa Nutal: *Per Pattie, 125g*				
Chick Pea	290	1220	10	37
Hot Mexicana	290	1220	10	37
Mediterranean	290	1220	10	37
Patties:				
Pasties, Party, 42g	110	460	5	14
Pies: Mini Party Pies, 22g	60	245	3.5	5.5
Party Pies, Regular, 47g	120	500	6	12
Party Quiche, Quiche Lorraine, 40g	100	430	5.5	9.5
Sausage Rolls, Party (1), 38g	105	430	6	10
Vegetable Roll (1), 175g	360	1495	17	43
Gluten Free: Meat Pie, 175g	385	1600	16	45
Party Pies, 50g	110	465	5	14
Sausage Rolls, 100g	255	1070	10	34
Vegie Rolls, 93g	195	815	6.5	30
Quorn:				
Frozen:				
Burgers: Chicken-Style (1), 70g	85	355	3	3
Southern Burger, 62g	125	515	7	8
Dippers, 80g	135	560	6.5	9
Fillets, Crispy (1), 100g	190	795	8.5	14
Meat-Style Balls, 70g	70	300	1	6
Sausages (2), 100g	130	545	4	10
Sausage Roll, 50g	160	655	11	9.5
Schnitzel, 120g	270	1125	15	23
Chilled Meals:				
Mince, 75g	75	305	1.5	1
Sausages, BBQ, 50g	90	370	5	1
Strips: Fajita, ½ pkt, 100g	110	465	2.5	4.5
Sweet Chilli, ½ pkt, 100g	145	610	4	13
Red Embers Bakery:				
Pies: Beef Stroganoff	500	2080	25	51
Chicken Leek & Mushroom	535	2240	28	53
Premium Steak	490	2040	22	51
Roast Vegetable	435	1825	20	55
Steak, Cheese & Onion	720	3000	36	69
Sausage Roll, Premium	520	2170	31	47
Rice A Riso:				
Chicken, cooked, ¼ packet	160	655	0.5	34
Sanitarium:				
Canned:				
Vegie Delights:				
Casserole Mince, ⅓ can, 138g	115	470	0.5	6.5
Nutmeat, 2 slices (10mm thick), 85g	175	725	8	3.5
Nutolene, 2 slices (10mm thick), 85g	220	910	18	3
Sausage, Vegetarian (1) 40g	65	275	3	2.5
Savoury Lentils, ⅓ can, 138g	85	365	0.5	13
Tender Pieces, ⅓ can, 138g	130	545	1	10

	Cal	kJ	Fat	Cb
Sanitarium (Cont.):				
Frozen:				
Vegie Delights:				
Lentil Patties (1), 75g	135	555	6	9
Not Burgers (1), 94g	195	820	7	19
Tender Crumbed Schnitzels (1), 75g	140	595	6	11
Chilled:				
Vegie Delights:				
Bacon Style Rashers, 4 rashers, 58g	135	570	7.5	6.5
Burger, Thai Sweet Chilli & Lime (1), 75g	130	550	7	8
Hot Dogs (2) 100g	200	840	8.5	12
Vegie Roast, ¼ packet, 120g	255	1055	6.5	24
Deli Luncheon: *Per 375g*				
Henchen, 6 slices, 62g	115	485	5	8
Smoked, 6 slices, 62g	120	490	5	8
Deli Slices, smoked, 2 slices, 42g	70	300	4	3
Soy Sausages: BBQ (2), 100g	205	855	8	10
Original (2), 100g	200	825	9	8.5
Curried (2), 100g	220	915	11	12
Rosemary, Sage (2), 120g	190	800	9	7.5
Sundried Tomato & Olive (2), 120g	160	660	7	8.5
Vegie (2), 100g	220	915	11	11
San Remo				
Fresh Pasta: *Per ½ of 375g Packet, Prepared as Directed*				
Agnolotti with Spinach & Ricotta	535	2235	12	88
Gnocci, with Cheese & Spinach	385	1600	7	70
Ravioli: With Beef	555	2320	14	85
W. Chargrilled Vegetables	520	2170	8.5	92
W. Chicken & Mushrooms	600	2500	16	91
Tortellini: W. Beef/Veal	555	2320	14	85
With Cheese & Spinach	490	2050	11	78
With Ham & Cheese	500	2085	10	80
With Spinach & Ricotta	445	1860	10	73
La Pasta: *Per ¼ of 120g Packet, Prepared as Directed*				
Alfredo	130	545	3	21
Chicken Curry	110	470	2	20
Creamy Mushroom & On.	125	525	2	22
Four Cheeses	130	550	3	21
Macaroni Cheese	130	550	3	21
Mushroom & Herb	130	545	3	21
La Pasta Single Snack: *Per 80g Packet, Prepared as Directed*				
Creamy Bacon	355	1480	10	53
Creamy Cheese	345	1440	8	54
Macaroni Cheese	350	1460	8.5	55
Sour Cream & Chives	345	1440	7.5	56
Lite: Alfredo	320	1330	5.5	52
Carbonara	305	1275	4.5	52

Meals ~ Canned & Packaged   M

San Remo (Cont):
Potato Mash,

	Cal	kJ	Fat	Cb
Creamy Mash, ¼ pkt, 25g	105	440	2.5	18

Ready Meal: *Per ½ of Packet*

	Cal	kJ	Fat	Cb
Cannelloni, Spinach & Ricotta, 237g	300	1250	18	27
Lasagna: Bolognese, 237g	300	1255	13	31
Spinach & Ricotta, 237g	370	1550	24	30
Penne w. Napoletana Sce, 175g	215	890	5.5	34
Ravioli Beef with Bolognese Sauce, 175g	200	840	9	20

Sauces ~ See Page 157

Sara Lee:

	Cal	kJ	Fat	Cb
Lasagna, Beef, 200g	265	1110	13	26
Quiche Lorraine: Snack Size (1), 119g	350	1455	22	28
Lorraine, ⅙ quiche, 100g	280	1160	18	21

Sargents:
Pies:

	Cal	kJ	Fat	Cb
Aussie Angus: Beef, 190g	490	2035	28	42
Beef & Onion, 190g	470	1960	26	44
Chunky Beef, 175g	420	1741	21	40
Extra Special: Grain Fed Beef	505	2120	25	49
Wagyu Beef	460	1910	25	40
Party Range:				
Meat Pie, 38g	95	405	5	11
Sausage Roll, 30g	80	340	4.5	8
Premium: Chunky, Beef Royale	410	1715	21	41
Chunky: Chicken Supreme	415	1740	21	43
Family, ¼ pie, 137g	300	1245	15	29
Traditional:				
Chicken & Vegetable	400	1660	20	42
Meat	450	1880	26	41
Steak & Onion	435	1825	25	42
Slow Cooked, Angus Beef & Veges	495	2070	25	51

Silly Yaks:
Individual Pies:

	Cal	kJ	Fat	Cb
Meat, 190g	385	1610	19	27
Pumpkin & Basil, 180g	275	1145	13	31
Steak & Mushroom, 190g	380	1590	18	30

Simply Less (Coles): *Per Meal*
Frozen:

	Cal	kJ	Fat	Cb
Beef & Vegetable Lasagne, 400g	430	1795	11	63
Chicken & Veg. Thai Green Curry, 370g	385	1600	11	48
Chicken, Chorizo & Prawn Paella, 370g	345	1435	7.5	51
Rstd Pumpkin, Pea & Fetta Risotto, 370g	420	1750	10	65
Sundried Tom. & Basil Chicken Penne, 370g	355	1485	8	49
Sweet Chilli Prawn Noodles, 370g	300	1260	4	56

Snowy River:

	Cal	kJ	Fat	Cb
Pasties, 150g	315	1320	14	40
Pies: Meat, 150g	340	1420	18	31
Party, 42g	90	385	4	12
Sausage Rolls: 100g	255	1070	13	27
Party, 25g	65	270	3	7

Spam ~ *See page 139*

SPC:
Baked Beans: *Per ½ cup, 140g*

	Cal	kJ	Fat	Cb
BBQ Sauce	135	555	1	22
Cheesy Cheddar	120	500	1	17
Ham Flavoured	145	605	0.5	28
Rich Tomato	125	525	1	19
Salt Reduced	120	500	1	17
Man Beans: Hot Chilli, 220g	155	650	2.5	30
Steakhouse, 220g	200	820	1.5	41

Spaghetti: *Per ½ cup, 140g*

	Cal	kJ	Fat	Cb
Cheesy Cheddar	110	465	1	22
Rich Tomato Sauce	105	440	0.5	21
Tomato & Cheese	155	655	2	29
Salt Reduced	105	440	1	20

Pasta Shapes: *Per 220g Can*

	Cal	kJ	Fat	Cb
Numberghetti				
Tomato & Cheese; Secret Vegies	155	655	2	29

Spagasaurus: *Per 220g Can*

	Cal	kJ	Fat	Cb
Secret Vegies	145	610	1	30
Tomato Sauce	145	610	1	30

St. Dalfour: *Per 175g Can*
French Bistro (Gourmet to Go):

	Cal	kJ	Fat	Cb
Chicken with Vegetables	155	655	4	18
Couscous	310	1295	9	46
Three Beans w/ Sweetcorn	185	770	7	21
Tuna & Pasta	180	745	6.5	14
Wild Pink Salmon with Vegetables	160	670	3	18

Stagg:
Chilli with Beans: *Per ½ of 425g can*

	Cal	kJ	Fat	Cb
Chunky Beef	275	1155	15	25
Classic	280	1175	15	25
Dynamite Hot	290	1210	15	26
Lean Beef	215	905	6	26

Suimin:
Taste of the Orient: *Per 70g Cup*

	Cal	kJ	Fat	Cb
Braised Beef	335	1400	14	46
Chicken & Sweet Corn	340	1420	14	47
Chicken	335	1400	14	46
Curried Prawn	340	1435	14	47
Hot & Spicy	335	1390	13	43
Oriental Chicken	340	1415	14	47
Prawn & Chicken	340	1430	14	46
Spicy Thai	330	1385	14	45

Updated Nutrition Data ~ www.CalorieKing.com.au
Persons with Diabetes ~ See Disclaimer (Page 22)

125

Meals ~ Canned & Packaged

	Cal	kJ	Fat	Cb
SunRice				
90 Seconds: *Per ½ Packet, Prepared as Directed*				
Brown Basmati	230	960	3	44
Chicken Rice	250	1050	3.5	50
Egg Fried Rice	240	990	4	45
Jasmine	250	1050	4	49
Long Grain White	250	1050	4	49
Mexican Style	200	830	4.5	32
Roasted Vegeable	205	860	2.5	38
Singapore Fried Rice	200	835	5.5	32
Thai Coconut	245	1030	6	40
White Basmati	190	790	2	37
Meals: *Per 320g Packet*				
Chinese: Beef & Black Bean	370	1550	7	60
Sweet & Sour	415	1730	3.5	77
Chinese Style Mongolian Beef	374	1570	8	62
Indian: Butter Chicken Curry	480	2010	18	60
Korma Curry	470	1965	20	52
Tikka Masala	480	2010	19	55
Thai: Chicken Satay	550	2305	23	63
Green Curry	435	1825	8	74
Mussaman Curry	485	2020	19	58
Red Curry	475	1985	11	77
Vegetable Curry	475	1980	20	61
Quick Cups: *Per Cup*				
Basmati Rice	215	895	3	35
Brown Rice	210	885	4.5	36
Chicken Rice	190	800	4	33
Egg Fried Rice	185	775	4.5	30
Jasmine Rice	215	895	3	42
Teriyaki Rice	195	810	2.5	37
White Rice	175	725	3.5	31
Tandaco:				
One Pan Dinner,				
¼ packet, average all varieties, 50g	170	715	1	33
Tasty Bite:				
Asian Meals: *Per ½ of 285g Packet*				
Green Curry Chicken & Jasmine Rice	130	530	8	12
Massaman Vegetables	130	530	6	14
Red Curry Vegetables & Jasmine Rice	150	640	9	16
Satay Vegetables	150	630	8	16
Yellow Curry Veg. & Jasmine Rice	150	625	11	14
Tasty Bite (Cont.)				
Indian Meals: *Per ½ of 285g Packet*				
Agra Peas & Greens	140	590	10	9
Bengal Lentils	160	665	8	16
Bombay Potatoes	100	420	4	13
Jaipur Vegetables	170	715	11	10
Jodhpur Yellow Dal	105	445	4	12
Kashmir Spinach	130	545	8	8
Madras Lentils	120	505	5	14
Mumbai Mushrooms	220	905	6	34
Punjab Eggplant	145	605	9	13
Indian Meals: *Per 342g Packet*				
Peas Paneer & Basmati Rice	105	425	15	54
Spinach Dal & Basmati Rice	375	1555	9	62
Taste of India: *Per 200g, ½ of 400g Bowl*				
Dhal: Chana	300	1255	14	31
Kabuli Dhal	230	960	8	29
Green Matar	245	1010	11	27
Makhani	270	1125	12	28
Moong Dhal	205	850	8	24
Rajma Dhal	235	975	7	31
Meat Curry: Balti Chicken	245	1025	15	7.5
Beef Vindaloo	240	1000	13	7
Butter Chicken	365	1510	27	8
Chicken Korma	310	1280	21	5
Lamb Rogan Josh	234	980	13	5
Mango Chicken	270	1120	16	12
Vegetarian: Aloo Baigan	190	785	12	17
Gujarati Aloo	200	840	11	21
Kashmiri Dum Aloo	260	1090	19	18
Mattar Paneer	335	1400	25	11
Palak Paneer	325	1345	25	9
Pav Bhaji	270	1230	19	18
Taste of Rice: *Per ½ of 250g Packet*				
Bombay Vegetable Biryani	260	1075	13	29
Brown Jasmine	285	1190	5.5	51
Cajun Style Fried Rice	190	790	5	32
Classic Prawn Fried Rice	250	1035	8	38
Farmhouse Cheese & Mushroom	200	840	6	32
Indonesian Nasi Goreng	200	825	6.5	31
Mexican Chilli & Tomato	240	1000	8.5	37
Peking Egg Fried Rice	215	890	7	31
South Seas Tuna & Coconut	280	1170	10	38
Spanish Saffron & Vegetable	190	800	5	33
Thai Style Sweet Mango	250	1050	7	42
Vegetable Fried Rice	160	655	4	26
White Basmati	220	915	3.5	41

Meals ~ Canned & Packaged

	Cal	kJ	Fat	Cb
Temptation:				
Quiche: 4 Cheese & Bacon, 140g	415	1725	28	28
4 Pumpkin, Leek & Feta, 140g	385	1610	25	44
Lorraine, ⅙ whole, 150g	370	1545	25	24
Petite Quiches: Lorraine 17g	50	215	3	4
Cheese & Spinach	65	265	4	5.5
The Biggest Loser: *Per 420g Packet*				
Beef Bolognese with Cheese Tortellini	400	1660	10	50
Beef Ragu with Pasta	355	1480	3	54
Lamb Korma with Rice	375	1560	6	62
Meatballs with Pasta	350	1450	4.5	51
Satay Beef Sausages with Rice	405	1680	12	56
Tilda:				
Steamed Basmati Rice: *Per ½ of 250g Packet*				
Brown	175	720	2.5	32
Lime & Coriander	160	665	2.5	31
Mushroom	150	630	3.5	26
Pure	205	850	3.5	39
Tom Piper:				
Per ½ or 400g can, 200g				
Braised Steak & Onions	160	670	5.5	13
Braised Steak & Veg.	150	620	4.5	16
Homestyle Stew	130	540	3.5	15
Sausages and Vegetables	150	620	5.5	14
Savoury Mince & Veg.	150	630	6	14
Sweet Curry	175	720	5.5	19
Tony Ferguson: *Per 200g Packet*				
Basil/Capsicum Italian Chicken	190	785	7.5	11
Coconut Chicken Curry	190	790	8	10
Homestyle Beef Casserole	175	735	5	2.5
Spicy Tomato Beef Curry	170	700	55	8
Trident:				
2 Minute Noodles,				
85g packet prepared	365	1530	14	49
Hotbox: *Per 65g Packet*				
Bangkok Heat, Hot & Spicy Thai	324	1350	15	42
Hong Kong, BBQ Beef	300	1260	12	42
Shanghai Sizzle, Chilli Beef	335	1390	14	46
Mega Cup Saucey Noodles: *Per 115g Cup*				
BBQ Spare Rib	640	2650	26	86
Beef Szechuan	570	2375	22	77
Honey Soy	570	2390	22	81
Mongolian Lamb	540	2255	20	69
Satay Chicken	580	2415	24	78
Migs: *Per 85g Cake, Prepared*				
Mi Goreng: Barbecue	410	1720	18	55
Original	355	1480	15	48
Satay	365	1520	15	48

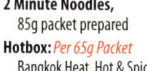

	Cal	kJ	Fat	Cb
Trident (Cont.)				
Noodleman Bowl: *Per Bowl*				
BBQ Chicken	295	1220	13	36
Beef	385	1615	18	45
Chicken	375	1560	15	49
Hot & Spicy	305	1255	12	42
Tukka Tubz:				
BBQ Beef Fried Rice w. Smokey Beef Bitz, 260g	340	1410	9	47
Couch Potato, 260g	235	975	6	32
Italian Chicken with Pasta, 260g	340	1410	9	47
Kickin' Chicken, Honey Soy Chicken w. Rice	260	1075	5	39
Uncle Bens:				
Express: *Per ½ Packet, 125g*				
Chinese Style Rice	200	825	3.5	37
Egg Fried Rice	220	920	3.5	37
Golden Vegetable Rice	190	795	3	37
Mexican Style	200	840	3	37
Mushroom Rice	195	815	3	37
Savoury Chicken Rice	190	790	3	36
Special Fried Rice	215	890	4	35
Thai Sweet Chilli Rice	180	745	2.5	36
Tomato & Basil Rice	220	915	4.5	37
Wholegrain Rice w. Mediterranean Veg.	220	915	6	35
Risotto: *Per 250g Packet*				
Chicken & Mushroom	460	1920	8.5	82
Grilled Mediterranean Vege.	420	1745	6	80
Tomato & Italian Herbs	455	1890	10	80
Watties:				
Baked Beans: *Per ½ Cup, 140g*				
In Tomato Sauce	140	590	1	22
With Sausages, 150g	175	720	4	22
With Steak & Bacon	150	625	1.5	21
Spaghetti: *Per ½ Cup, 140g*				
In Tomato Sauce	95	390	0.5	19
With Cheesy Meatballs	115	480	2	17
With Extra Cheese	100	430	2	17
With Meatballs	125	525	3.5	18
With Sausages	120	510	3.5	18
Weight Watchers:				
Canned/Packaged:				
Baked Beans in Tomato Sauce, 130g	115	470	0.5	17
Frozen:				
Meals: *Per Packet*				
Beef Burgundy	145	600	3	14
Beef Cannelloni	305	1280	8	43
Beef Hot Pot	205	850	4.5	27
Butter Chicken	355	1490	9	52
Chicken Fettuccine	325	1360	5	54

Updated Nutrition Data ~ www.CalorieKing.com.au
Persons with Diabetes ~ See Disclaimer (Page 22)

Meals ~ Canned & Packaged

Weight Watchers (Cont):	Cal	kJ	Fat	Cb
Meals (Cont): *Per Packet*				
Chicken Fried Rice	335	1410	2	66
Chicken Hot Pot	250	1040	9	31
Chicken Pesto Spaghettini	345	1425	7	50
Chicken Risotto	315	1315	6	51
Cottage Pie	260	1090	8	35
Creamy Chicken & Mushroom Fettuccine	300	1250	7	41
Creamy Mushroom Agnolotti	320	1345	10	46
Creamy Tomato Gnocchi	315	1320	6	54
Creamy Vegetable Lasagne	270	1120	5.5	44
Lasagne Beef	355	1480	6.5	49
Satay Chicken	355	1490	6.5	58
Thai Chicken Curry	335	1410	7	57
Tuna Bake	310	1295	6.5	46
Wraps:				
Spinach & Ricotta Cheese	240	1000	3.5	38
Sweet Chilli Chicken	235	975	3	38
White Wings:				
Hamburger Helper, dry, 110g	370	1550	2	60
Stuffing Mix, dry, 100g	485	2030	31	48
Woolworths/Select:				
Canned/Packaged:				
Pasta & Sauce:				
Alfredo: ¼ pkt, 31g dry	120	490	1.5	21
Prepared, ⅔ cup, 165g	210	875	3	35
Four Cheeses: ¼ pkt, 31g	120	500	2	21
Prepared, ⅓ cup, 110g	130	550	2	22
Macaroni Cheese (180g): ¼ pkt, 31g dry	120	500	1.5	21
Prepared as directed, ⅔ cup, 170g	220	910	3	36
Chicken Breast,				
Chunks In Brine,				
½ 345g can, 100g (drained)	135	565	2	0.5
Chicken Breast: *Single Serve, 85g Cans*				
Shredded Chicken Breast:				
In Mayonnaise	115	480	6	1
In Mustard Mayonnaise	125	515	6	2
In Sweet Chilli	160	660	7.5	5
In Springwater	50	215	1	0.5
In Tomato & Onion	135	560	8	2
Smoked Flavour	70	295	1	2.5
Quick Mac, Macaroni & Cheese, 70g sachet, prepared	275	1150	4	50

Woolworths/Home Brand:	Cal	kJ	Fat	Cb
2" Noodles: *Per 85g Packet*				
Beef	400	1685	17	52
Chicken	420	1750	18	54
Oriental	405	1700	18	52
Noodle Cups: *Per Cup*				
Beef	325	1340	15	40
Chicken	330	1360	14	42
Chicken & Corn	315	1320	13	40
Oriental	340	1420	14	44
Frozen:				
Bakehouse:				
Family Pie (500g), Meat, ¼, 125g	265	1115	12	28
Individual Pies: Beef, 180g	440	1835	25	41
Chicken & Vegetable, 180g	415	1735	22	43
Gourmet: Family Pies (500g), avg., ¼, 125g	275	1150	13	28
Individual Pies: Angus Beef, 200g	435	1825	19	44
Beef & Guiness, 200g	420	1755	19	42
Party Pie, Angus Beef, 35g	90	365	4	10
Home Brand:				
Family Pie (500g), ¼, 125g				
Meat	325	1340	18	28
Individual Pie, Meat, 150g	310	1285	13	34
Party Pie, Meat, 42g	95	390	5	10
Dim Sims, 30g	95	400	2.5	15
Lasagne, Beef, 400g packet	555	2320	24	56
Mini Spring Rolls: Beef (1), 50g	115	480	5	15
Vegetable (1), 50g	105	430	4	16
Patties, 100% Aust.Beef, 1 pattie, 125g	275	1140	20	0
Sausage Roll, Jumbo, 150g	430	1800	23	41
Zoglo's:				
Vegetarian Burgers (1)	120	500	5	4.5
Vegetarian Links (1)	50	220	2.5	2
Vegetarian Meatballs (1)	65	270	2.5	2
Vegetarian Schnitzel, 100g	200	845	10	11

Meals ~ CalorieKing Recipes

Recipes

See www.calorieking.com.au for all recipes & serving sizes

	Cal	kJ	Fat	Cb
Appetizers & Snacks:				
Cheesey Grape Balls (4)	160	675	10	11
Stuffed Mushrooms (2)	115	470	3	15
Vietnamese Rice Paper Rolls (1)	180	735	3	24
Beef Dishes:				
Beef Casserole	475	1985	14	28
Beef Stroganoff	285	1185	10	11
Beef & Mushroom Burger	475	1980	12	57
Beef & Snowpea Stir-Fry	195	830	6	7
Chilli Con Carne	305	1265	12	16
Cottage Pie with Mushrooms	340	1435	7	31
Crumbed Veal Steaks	400	1465	8	30
Chicken Dishes:				
Chicken & Avocado Tortillas	410	1715	12	38
Chicken & Mushroom Loaf	490	2050	13	41
Chicken Cacciatore Casserole	400	1665	8	33
Chicken Kiev	205	865	9	9
Lemon Chicken Casserole with Rice	365	1520	7.5	45
San Choy Bow	215	900	10	8
Satay Chicken Skewers	220	930	8.5	5.5
Spaghetti Bolognese with Chicken	435	1815	5.5	57
Fish Dishes:				
Baked Fish	250	1250	6	25
Chilli Octopus Stir-Fry	405	1685	12	42
Curried Fish	165	680	2.5	9
Paella	320	1335	9	23
Tuna Mornay, low-fat	430	1800	5.5	24
Tuna & Corn Patties	165	685	4	18
Lamb Dishes:				
Crumbed Lamb Cutlets with Apple & Glazed Carrots	410	1715	12	42
Italian Style Lamb Shanks	480	2000	6	18
Lamb Curry	330	1385	14	11
Lamb Pilaf	485	2030	5	77
Mongolian Lamb	234	980	8	7.5
Shepherd's Pie	335	1400	11	36
Pork Dishes:				
BBQ Pork Wrap	355	1475	3	46
Pork Spare Ribs with Ginger Soy Glaze	235	965	5	14
Pork Steaks with Apple Sauce	305	1275	6	28
Pork Stir-fry with Snowpea	285	1200	12	11
Sweet Chilli Pork	304	1240	12	23

	Cal	kJ	Fat	Cb
Salads:				
Asian Chicken	335	1420	4.5	53
Asparagus, Avocado & Prawn	230	950	9	9
Broccoli & Tabbouleh	220	920	10	29
Chicken Thai Noodle	475	1985	8.5	80
Chickpea, Ricotta & Rocket	245	1015	13	20
Nicoise	340	1410	12	31
Warm Beef & Pasta	380	1595	6	49
Soups: *Per 250ml Cup*				
Chicken & Vegetable				
Chicken w. Rice Dumplings	110	450	1	22
Corn Chowder	225	940	4	41
Kumera (Sweet Potato)	120	500	4	16
Lentil & Vegetable	105	440	3	15
Minestrone:				
Minestrone (with Beans)	260	1090	8.5	29
Minestrone (w/out Beans)	215	880	8	23
Pea & Ham	415	1740	13	43
Potato & Leek	200	830	4	32
Pumpkin	205	885	5	29
Split Green Pea	325	1365	5	43
Spring Vegetable	80	330	3.5	11
Sweet Potato (Kumera)	120	500	4	16
Tomato (Mediterranean)	110	460	6	10
Vegetarian Dishes:				
Avocado Tacos (1)	170	710	6	28
Capsicum & Mushroom Risotto	360	1495	11	43
Chickpeas, Vegetables & Couscous	405	1700	9	66
Eggplant and Tofu	320	1320	6	50
Felafel Wrap	500	2080	12	77
Greek Vegetable Wrap	150	640	1	29
Spinach & Rice Pie	260	1095	8	32
Desserts:				
Apple & Raspberry Custard Crumble	200	830	1	44
Apple Strudel	105	420	4	18
Baked Stuffed Apples	180	755	2.5	41
Berry Coulis	225	930	6	39
Chocolate Mousse	450	1875	10	80
Christmas Ice Cream Pudding, frozen	225	930	6	39
Low-Fat Sticky Date Pudding	175	730	3	35
Mango Sorbet	60	250	0	15

Updated Nutrition Data ~ www.CalorieKing.com.au
Persons with Diabetes ~ See Disclaimer (Page 22)

Meat ~ Beef

Raw & Cooked Weights

Cooking reduces the weight of meat by 10-30% due to water and fat losses. Actual losses depend on cooking method and cooking time.

Average Cooking Weight Losses:

Steaks & Chops:
- Medium cooked - 20% loss
- Well done - 30% loss
- Roasts - 25% loss
- Stir fry - 10% loss

Examples:
100g raw steak:
 = approximately 80g cooked, medium or 70g cooked, well done
100g cooked steak, medium
 = approximately 125g raw
100g cooked steak, well done
 = approximately 140g raw

What 100g Meat Looks Like (Cooked Weight):

- Half the size of this book
- Palm of a lady's hand • Pack of cards

Terminology

For the purposes of this section, lean meat has all visible fat removed.

Lean plus fat refers to untrimmed meat with a maximum of 6 mm (¼ inch) of border fat, plus intramuscular fat, depending on the cut of meat. Retail meats have become leaner over the years and many cuts have as little as 1-2 mm of border fat. Consumers are also requesting all border fat to be removed.

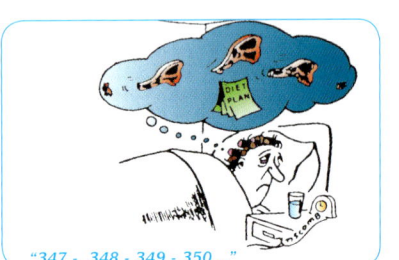

"347 - 348 - 349 - 350..."

Steak ~ Quick Guide

Cal | kJ | Fat | Cb

100 Gram Portion (no bone):

Raw:
	Cal	kJ	Fat	Cb
Lean + fat, 100g	150	630	7	0
Lean only, 100g	120	500	3	0

Grilled (Medium):
	Cal	kJ	Fat	Cb
Lean + fat, 100g	220	920	10	0
Lean only, 100g	190	795	7	0

Grilled Steak: *Average All Cuts*

Rump/Sirloin/Fillet/Porterhouse
Grilled or BBQ'd, Medium
Figures for lean + fat assume trimmed meat with only a think layer of border fat.

Small Serving: ⅓ size this book

Cal | kJ | Fat | Cb

80g cooked (100g raw)
	Cal	kJ	Fat	Cb
Lean + fat, 80g	175	730	8	0
Lean only, 70g	135	565	5	0

Medium Serving: ½ size this book

120g cooked (150g raw)
	Cal	kJ	Fat	Cb
Lean + fat, 120g	265	1110	12	0
Lean only, 105g	200	835	7	0

Large Serving: ¾ size this book

175 cooked (220g raw)
	Cal	kJ	Fat	Cb
Lean + fat, 175g	385	1610	18	0
Lean only, 155g	300	1255	11	0

Extra Large Serving:

240g cooked (300g raw)
	Cal	kJ	Fat	Cb
Lean + fat, 240g	530	2215	24	0
Lean only, 210g	400	1670	15	0

Jumbo (Steakhouse):

400g cooked (500g raw)
	Cal	kJ	Fat	Cb
Lean + fat, 400g	875	3660	40	0
Lean only, 350g	675	2820	25	0

Beef Fat:
	Cal	kJ	Fat	Cb
Raw, 50g	270	1130	27	0
Cooked, 50g	290	1210	30	0

Pan Frying (with Oil/Fat)

For each 100 grams of pan-fried meat, add to the above figures for grilled meat:
Add Per 100g: *50 cal, 210 kJ, 5g fat.*

Meat ~ Beef

Beef – Individual Cuts | Cal | kJ | Fat | Cb

Note: Revised figures in this section represent the trend to leaner cuts of meat at the retail level, and the extra trimming of fat in the home.

Per 100 Grams Edible, Without Bone

Blade Steak: *Without bone:*
Raw: Lean + fat, 100g	140	580	6	0
Lean only, 100g	130	545	5	0
Grilled, lean only, 100g	175	730	7	0

Corned Beef/Brisket:
Raw: Lean + fat	125	525	5.5	0
Lean only	95	400	1.5	0
Cooked, lean + fat, 100g	245	1020	14	0
Lean only, 100g	210	880	9.5	0

Chuck Steak:
Raw: Lean + fat, 100g	120	510	4.5	0
Lean only, 100g	110	455	3	0

Eye Fillet Roast:
Lean, raw 100g	145	605	7	0
Roasted, lean, 100g	210	880	10	0

Fillet Steak:
Raw: Lean + fat	140	580	6	0
Lean only	125	520	4	0
Grilled: Lean + fat, 100g	205	865	10	0
Lean only, 100g	195	820	8.5	0
1 steak (120g raw),				
Grilled, lean + fat, 95g	195	815	9	0
Lean only, 80g	155	650	7	0

Gravy Beef, raw:
Lean + fat, 100g	160	670	9	0
Lean, 100g	120	500	4	0

Rib Steak: *Edible meat only*
Raw: Lean + fat, 100g	165	685	9	0
Lean only, 100g	120	510	4	0
Grilled: Lean + fat, 100g	215	900	11	0
Lean only, 100g	175	735	6	0
1 steak (250g raw, w. bone)				
Lean + fat	325	1360	16	0

Ribeye Steak (Scotch):
Raw: Lean + fat, 100g	150	625	6.5	0
Lean only	130	555	4.5	0
Grilled: Lean + fat	215	900	10	0
Lean only	195	830	8	0

Round Steak:
Raw: Lean + fat	130	540	5	0
Lean only	115	495	4	0
Grilled: Lean + fat	185	770	7	0
Lean only	175	740	6	0

Beef – Individual Cuts | Cal | kJ | Fat | Cb

Per 100 Grams Edible Portion

Rump Steak:
Raw: Lean + fat	150	630	7	0
Lean only	115	495	3	0
Grilled: Lean + fat	215	895	10	0
Lean only	190	800	7	0

Rib Roast:
Lean + fat	165	685	9	0
Lean only	120	510	4	0

Roast Beef, Topside:
Raw: Lean + fat	130	540	4.5	0
Lean only	115	485	3.5	0
Roasted: Lean + fat, 100g	160	680	6.5	0
Lean only, 100g	150	635	5	0
2 small slices, + fat, 80g	130	540	5	0
Lean only, 70g	105	440	3.5	0
2 large slices, + fat, 120g	190	790	8	0
Lean only, 100g	150	635	5	0
Gravy: Add per Tbsp (20 ml)	20	85	1	0

Silverside, Roast:
Raw: Lean + fat, 100g	130	550	5	0
Lean only, 100g	110	460	2.5	0
Baked: Lean + fat	190	810	6.5	0
Lean only	175	745	4.5	0

Silverside, Corned:
Raw: Lean + fat	130	545	8	0
Lean only	90	375	3	0
Cooked: Lean + fat	205	855	13	0
Lean only	140	585	5	0

Sirloin Steak: *Without bone*
Raw: Lean + fat	165	690	9	0
Lean only	140	580	6	0
Grilled: Lean + fat	215	905	12	0
Lean only	190	805	9	0

T-Bone Steak: *Weights include bone*
Raw: Lean + fat, 100g	115	480	5.5	0
Lean only, 100g	85	355	2	0
Grilled: Lean + fat, 100g	165	690	8	0
Lean only, 100g	135	565	5.5	0
1 medium (250g raw):				
Grilled: Lean+fat, 185g	300	1255	14	0
Lean only, 170g	230	960	9	0
1 large (380g raw):				
Grilled, lean + fat, 290g	460	1925	22	0
Lean only, 265g	360	1505	14	0

Topside Cubes, (lean): Raw | 115 | 485 | 4 | 0
Stir fried | 165 | 680 | 6.5 | 0

Updated Nutrition Data ~ www.CalorieKing.com.au
Persons with Diabetes ~ See Disclaimer (Page 22)

131

Meat ~ Beef

Pan Fried Adjustment
With Fat/Oil:
Add to meat figures for grilled:
Per 100g of panfried meat:
50 cal, 210 kJ, 5g fat
Note: Oil spray coating of pan adds insignificant fat per serving

Beef Stir-Fry

	Cal	kJ	Fat	Cb
Beef Stir-Fry Strips:				
Raw: Lean, 100g	130	545	4	0
Lean, 200g	260	1090	8	0

Hamburger Beef Patties

Home-made Patties are based on raw weight of 100g per patty (8.5 cm diam x 1.5cm thick)

	Cal	kJ	Fat	Cb
100% Meat - Per Patty:				
From Hamburger Mince (20% fat):				
Raw, 100g	250	1040	20	0
Grilled	215	900	14	0
Pan-fried/BBQ'd	230	960	15	0
With Egg/Breadcrumbs/Onion:				
Raw, 100g	240	990	18	3.5
Grilled	205	850	13	3.5
Pan-fried/BBQ'd	220	920	14	3.5
From Lean Mince (10% Fat):				
100% Meat - Per Patty:				
Raw, 100g	170	710	10	0
Grilled	145	605	8	0
Pan-fried/BBQ'd	155	650	9	0
With Egg/Breadcrumbs/Onion:				
Raw, 100g	165	690	9	3.5
Grilled	145	605	7	3.5
Pan-fried/BBQ'd	150	630	8	3.5

Note: Above recipe for meat patties is based on: 500g mince, 1 egg, ½ cup breadcrumbs, ½ onion, seasoning. (Makes 6 x 100g patties).

Frozen Brands ~*See Page 59-65*
Vegetarian Burgers ~*Sanitarium: See Page 124*
Zoglo's: See Page 128

Beef Mince

	Cal	kJ	Fat	Cb
Per 100g (Raw Weight)				
Hamburger Mince: *Per 100g*				
Lean (25% fat)	295	1230	25	0
Lean fat-free (20% fat)	250	1040	20	0
Steak Mince: *Per 100g*				
Lean fat-free (15% fat)	210	880	15	0
Lean fat-free (10% fat)	170	710	10	0
Low Fat/Lean: *Per 100g*				
(Diet Mince/Extra Trim, Weight Watchers):				
90% fat-free (10% fat)	170	710	10	0
93-95% fat-free (5-7% fat)	150	630	7	0
Cooked Mince:				
Steak Mince, 90% fat-free				
Boiled, drained, 100g	170	710	9	0

Mince Descriptions

Descriptions such as 'fine grade', 'premium' or '100% Beef' do not generally reflect the fat content. Unless the actual percentage of fat is stated, assume:
- **Lean ~ 90% lean (10% fat)**
- **Extra Lean ~ 93% lean (7% fat)**
- **25% Less Fat ~ 85% lean (15% fat)**

Meat Balls

	Cal	kJ	Fat	Cb
Basic Recipe: Mince, Egg, Onion, Bread Crumbs				
Using Average Grade Mince (20% Fat/80% Lean)				
Raw (Uncooked Weights):				
1 Mini/Cocktain (20 cent coin), 15g	35	145	3	1
1 Medium (golf ball), 40g	95	400	7	3
1 Large, 80g	190	800	14	6
Using Lean Mince (10% Fat/90% Lean)				
Raw (Uncooked Weights):				
1 Mini/Cocktain (20 cent coin), 15g	25	105	1.5	1
1 Medium (golf ball), 40g	65	270	3.5	3
1 Large, 80g	130	540	7	6

Meat & Lamb

Casseroles & Stews — Cal kJ Fat Cb

To calculate calories, kilojoules and fat per serve:
1. Add up total cal/kJ/fat of all raw ingredients.
2. Divide by the number of serves.

Example For Standard Meat & Vegetable Casserole:
Ingredients (4 serves):

	Cal	kJ	Fat	Cb
500g lean meat, (Chuck Steak/Gravy Beef)	600	2510	20	0
1 cup water	0	0	0	0
2 Tablespoons Oil (40ml)	325	1360	36	0
2 Tablespoons Flour	85	355	0	19
2 cups diced vegetables	90	375	0	13
Totals	1100	4600	56	32
Per Serve (Divide by 4)	275	1150	14	8
Oil Variation				
If 1 Tbsp oil used ~ Per Serve	235	980	10	0
If no oil used ~ Per Serve	200	835	5	0

Lamb — Cal kJ Fat Cb

Weights - As Purchased with Bone
Cooked weights are approximate only

Leg Cuts:
Leg of Lamb Roast:

	Cal	kJ	Fat	Cb
Roasted: Lean + fat, 100g	190	795	7.5	0
Lean only, 100g	175	730	5.5	0
2 slices, 90g	170	710	6.5	0
Lean only, 85g	150	625	4.5	0

Easy Carve Leg - As for Leg of Lamb:
Chump Chop:

	Cal	kJ	Fat	Cb
Raw: Lean + fat, 100g	220	930	17	0
Lean only, 100g	140	585	6.5	0
Grilled: 1 chop, 120g raw with bone				
Lean + fat, 85g cooked, with bone	160	670	9	0
Lean only, 75g, with bone	100	420	4	0
Pan fried: 1 chop, 90g	200	835	13	0
Lean only, 80g	120	500	6	0

Trim Lamb Leg Cuts:

	Cal	kJ	Fat	Cb
Diced Trim Lamb, 100g	130	540	5.5	0
Mince, 100g	145	605	7	0
Lamb Strips, 100g	135	565	6	0
Lamb Steak, Round, 100g	130	550	6	0
Lamb Steak, Topside, 100g	125	530	4.5	0
Mini Roast, Round, 100g	120	505	4.5	0
Mini Roast, Topside, 100g	130	535	5.5	0
Schnitzel, Round, 100g	125	525	5.5	0
Schnitzel, Topside, 100g	125	520	4.5	0

Lamb (Cont) — Cal kJ Fat Cb

Cutlet (Rib-Loin)
1 medium cutlet, 70g raw:

	Cal	kJ	Fat	Cb
Raw, 70g	210	880	20	0
Lean only, frenched	80	335	4	0
Grilled: 1 cutlet	140	585	12	0
Lean only, frenched	60	250	3	0
Pan fried: 1 cutlet	160	670	14	0
Crumbed	200	835	16	0
1 large cutlet, 90g raw:				
Grilled, lean + fat, 70g	170	610	14	0
Lean only, frenched	75	210	4	0

Note: Large size crumbed lamb cutlets (170g) in retail outlets are usually forequarter lamb chops.

	Cal	kJ	Fat	Cb
Loin Chop: Raw, 1 chop, 100g	200	835	14	0
Grilled: 1 chop, 70g	170	710	10	0
Lean only, 60g	90	375	4	0
Pan fried: 1 chop, 75g	200	835	13	0
Lean only	100	420	7	0

Rack of Lamb/Crown Roast ~ See Cutlet, Grilled
Multiply figures by number of cutlets:

Trim Lamb Loin Cuts:

	Cal	kJ	Fat	Cb
Butterfly Steak, raw, 100g	170	720	10	0
Eye of Loin, raw, 100g	130	540	6	0
Lamb Fillet, raw, 100g	135	575	7	0

Forequarter Cuts:
Raw - Per 100g Edible Weight

	Cal	kJ	Fat	Cb
Diced Lamb	155	650	9	0
Easy Carve Shoulder	165	680	10	0
Four Rib Roast	270	1130	23	0
Forequarter Chop: Lean + fat	155	660	9	0
Lean only,	115	480	4	0
Lamb Drumstick	110	465	3.5	0
Lamb Shank, 1 shank, 300g	270	1130	15	0
Lean only, raw, edible weight, 100g	200	835	8	0
Neck Chop: Lean + fat	185	785	12	0
Lean only	130	545	5.5	0
Party Rack	195	810	14	0
Party Ribs	400	1670	39	0

Trim Lamb Cuts

Trim Lamb cuts are special lower fat retail cuts that have been trimmed of all border fat and all bone. Fat should not exceed 5 grams of fat per 100 grams raw meat.

Updated Nutrition Data ~ www.CalorieKing.com.au
Persons with Diabetes ~ See Disclaimer (Page 22)

Meat ~ Veal

Veal

Weights include bone and gristle, unless otherwise stated

	Cal	kJ	Fat	Cb
Forequarter:				
Raw: Lean + fat, 100 g	130	545	5	0
Lean only, 100g	90	375	2	0
Cooked: Lean + fat, 100g	155	650	4.5	0
Lean only, 100g	135	560	2.5	0
Leg Roast: *boneless*				
Raw, lean + fat, 100g	100	420	1.5	0
Roasted: 2 slices, 100g	140	585	1.5	0
Lean only, 100g	130	550	1	0
Loin Chop:				
Raw: Lean + fat, 100g	90	375	3	0
Lean only, 100g	65	270	1	0
Grilled: *1 chop, 115g raw*				
Lean + fat, 85g	85	365	2.5	0
Lean only, 83g	70	300	1.5	0
Pan fried, 1 chop	120	500	6.0	0
Osso Bucco:				
Raw: 100g	50	210	1	0
500g quantity	250	1045	5	0
Schnitzel Steak:				
Raw: Lean + fat, 100g	115	480	3	0
Fried: 1 piece, 110g raw, 77g (cooked wt)	75	315	2	0
Crumbed and pan fried:				
Small serve, 120g	260	1090	17	12
Medium serve, 180g	390	1630	25	18
Large serve, 250g	540	2260	35	25
Veal Leg Steak:				
Raw, 100g	110	460	2.5	0
Pan fried:				
1 small steak, 75g raw, 50g	75	315	2	0
1 steak, 130g raw, 100g	150	630	4	0
Lean only, 95g	135	565	4	0
Veal Shoulder Steak:				
Raw: Lean + fat, 100g	125	525	4	0
Grilled: lean + fat, 100g	135	565	4	0
1 piece, 90g raw, 60g	80	335	2.5	0

Meat Products

Butchers Supermarkets
Ready To Cook
Figures are averages only. Products from different outlets will vary.

	Cal	kJ	Fat	Cb
Beef Olives: Raw, 2 rolls, 180g	250	1045	10	9
Pan-fried in oil/fat	300	1255	15	9
Crumbed Lamb Chops: Raw, 170g	430	1785	31	17
Pan-fried, in oil/fat	520	2170	41	17
Crumbed Steak, pan-fried in oil/fat, 1 medium piece, 180g	390	1630	25	18
Marinated Chops: Raw, 160g	345	1445	30	2
BBQ'd/Grilled	225	940	15	2
Marinated Steak: Raw, 150g	215	905	10	2
Grilled	145	605	7	2
Satay Sticks:				
Beef, grilled/bbq'd., 70g	110	460	5	5
Lamb: Grilled/bbq'd., 70g	125	530	3.5	5
Pan-fried	155	650	10	5
Shishkebabs:				
Meat + Vegetables, grilled/bbq'd., 170g	135	565	6	5

Other Meat Dishes ~ *See International Foods Section, Pages 180-184*

Beef Jerky

Average all Brands:

	Cal	kJ	Fat	Cb
Dried Meat Strips/Jerky/Biltong:				
1 piece, 30g	120	510	8	3.5
50g packet	205	855	13	5.5
Beef Jerky:				
D.Jays, Original, ½ pkt, 25g	80	330	1.5	0.5
Jack Links: Original, ½ pkt, 25g	70	295	1	5
1 packet, 50g	140	590	1.5	10
Peppered, ½ packet, 25g	73	305	1	4.5
Biltong:				
D.Jays: Dry/Moist, 25g	90	365	2	0.5
100g	350	1450	9	2

For Full Nutritional Data
~ See Author's Website
www.CalorieKing.com.au

Meat & Pork

Pork ~ Regular Cuts

	Cal	kJ	Fat	Cb

'Lean + fat' refers to meat as purchased (weight includes bone)

Forequarter Chop:
Item	Cal	kJ	Fat	Cb
Raw: Lean + fat, 100g	190	795	13	0
Lean only, 100g	115	475	4	0
Grilled: Lean + fat, 100g	225	940	16	0
Lean only, 100g	160	680	6.5	0
1 chop, 300g raw, grilled,				
Lean + fat	550	2230	37	0
Lean only, 195g	300	1255	13	0

Forequarter Roast:
Item	Cal	kJ	Fat	Cb
Raw: Lean + fat, 100g	180	760	13	0
Lean only, 100g	105	445	3	0
Roasted: Lean + fat, 100g	215	900	14	0
Lean only, 100g	155	660	6.5	0
2 slices, Lean + fat, 90g	195	810	13	0

Loin/Midloin Chop:
Item	Cal	kJ	Fat	Cb
Raw: Lean + fat, 100g	230	960	18	0
Lean only, 100g	105	440	2	0
Grilled: Lean + fat, 100g	280	1170	19	0
Lean only, 100g	170	710	5	0
1 chop, 200g raw wt, grilled,				
Lean + fat, 140g	390	1630	27	0
Lean only, 125g	210	880	6	0

Leg:
Item	Cal	kJ	Fat	Cb
Raw: Lean + fat, 100g	190	795	13	0
Lean only, 100g	105	440	2	0
Roasted, no added fat:				
Lean + fat, 100g	230	960	14	0
Lean only, 100g	145	600	3.5	0
2 slices, Lean + fat, 90g	205	860	13	0

Neck:
Item	Cal	kJ	Fat	Cb
Lean + fat, 100g	170	710	11	0
Lean only, 100g	110	460	3.5	0
Baked, no added fat:				
Lean + fat, 100g	225	950	15	0
Lean only, 100g	170	710	8	0
2 slices, Lean + fat, 90g	205	855	14	0

Spare Ribs: Lean + fat, 100g   115   480   9   0
BBQ, no added fat,
  Lean + fat, 100g   140   580   10   0
Pork Mince, raw, 100g   315   1315   28   0

New Fashioned Pork

NHF Approved Cuts have less than 5g fat/100g raw

Loin Chop:
Item	Cal	kJ	Fat	Cb
Lean + fat, 100g	165	680	9	0
Lean only, 100g	115	480	2	0
Pan fried, no added fat,				
Lean + fat, 100g	190	795	10	0
Lean only, 100g	145	605	4	0

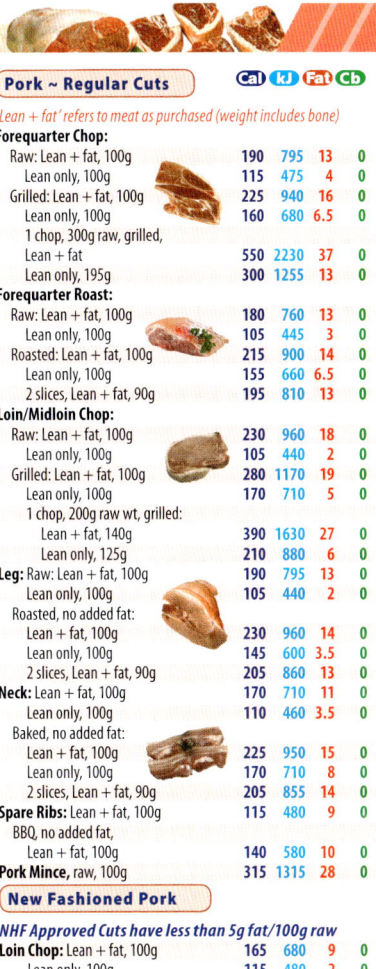

New Fashioned Pork (Cont)

Loin Chop (Cont):
Item	Cal	kJ	Fat	Cb
1 chop, raw, 160g	260	1090	14	0
Pan fried, lean + fat	240	1000	12	0

Leg Steak:
Item	Cal	kJ	Fat	Cb
Lean + fat, 100g	105	440	2	0
Lean only, 100g	100	420	1.5	0
Grilled: Lean + fat, 100g	140	585	3	0
Lean only, 100g	125	525	1.5	0

Leg Steak Chop: *125g raw weight*
Grilled, Lean only   135   565   3   0

Leg Schnitzel:
Item	Cal	kJ	Fat	Cb
Raw: Lean + fat, 100g	105	440	2	0
Lean only, 100g	100	420	1.5	0
Pan Fried, no added fat				
Lean + fat, 100g	145	615	3.5	0
Lean only, 100g	135	560	1.5	0

Leg Strips:
Item	Cal	kJ	Fat	Cb
Raw: Lean + fat, 100g	110	460	2.5	0
Lean only, 100g	100	420	1.5	0
Stir Fried, no added fat				
Lean + fat, 100g	140	595	3	0
Lean only, 100g	135	560	1.5	0

Leg Diced:
Item	Cal	kJ	Fat	Cb
Raw: Lean + fat, 100g	120	500	4	0
Lean only, 100g	100	420	1.5	0
Casseroled, no added fat				
Lean + fat, 100g	170	720	4.5	0
Lean only, 100g	160	660	3	0

Butterfly Steak:
Item	Cal	kJ	Fat	Cb
Raw: Lean + fat, 100g	140	585	6	0
Lean only, 100g	105	430	1.5	0
Grilled, no added fat:				
Lean + fat, 100g	190	800	7.5	0
Lean only, 100g	155	655	3	0
1 steak, 160g raw weight,				
Grilled, Lean + fat	215	900	8.5	0

Pork Belly, raw, 100g   520   2170   53   0

Pork Fillet:
Item	Cal	kJ	Fat	Cb
Raw: Lean + fat, 100g	110	660	2.5	0
Lean only, 100g	100	420	1	0
Pan fried, no added fat				
Lean + fat, 100g	135	560	3	0
Lean only, 100g	120	510	2	0

Pork Mince: *Low Fat*
Item	Cal	kJ	Fat	Cb
Raw, 100g	145	600	7	0
Stir fried, no added fat, 100g	185	775	9	0

Pan/Stir-fried Adjustment
Oil Added:
Per 100g cooked meat ~ Add 50 cal/210 kJ/5g fat

Updated Nutrition Data ~ www.CalorieKing.com.au
Persons with Diabetes ~ See Disclaimer (Page 22)

Meat ~ Pork ◆ Bacon ◆ Game ◆ Offal

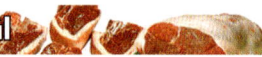

Pork Variety Cuts

	Cal	kJ	Fat	Cb
Brains, braised, 100g	140	585	10	0
Chitterlings, cooked, 100g	300	1255	29	0
Crackling, 30g	145	605	8.5	0
Ears, 1 ear, cooked, 110g	180	750	12	0
Feet, cooked 100g	200	835	13	0
Jowl, raw, 100g	650	2720	70	0
Pork Fat: Raw, 100g	755	3155	82	0
Cooked, 100g	740	3095	78	0
Tail, simmered, 100g	400	1675	36	0
Tongue, stewed, 100g	270	1130	20	0

Bacon

Rib/Middle Cut/Premium:
Thin: *20 slices/kg*

	Cal	kJ	Fat	Cb
1 rasher, raw, 50g	160	660	14	0
Grilled	95	405	7	0
Fried (minimal fat added)	110	470	9	0
Trimmed of Fat: Raw, 40g	80	330	5	0
Grilled/Fried	40	165	2	0

Thick: *12-13 slices/kg*

	Cal	kJ	Fat	Cb
1 rasher: Raw, 80g	255	1055	23	0
Grilled	155	650	11	0
Fried, minimal fat added	180	755	15	0
Eye of Rib, 1 thin rasher, 15g raw, cooked no added fat	20	85	1	0
Bacon Fat, raw, 20g	145	605	16	0

Rindless Rib, Same as 'with rind'. Made from fattier pork so fat content is similar.

	Cal	kJ	Fat	Cb
Shoulder Rashers: 50g raw, each	100	420	7	0
Cooked, no added fat	80	335	4.5	0
All-Eye/Breakfast Rashers, 1 rasher, cooked (40g raw)	55	230	2	0
97% Fat-Free *(Hans; Don)*, 50g	50	210	1.5	0
Weight Watchers Bacon, 125g pkt				
3 slices, 42g	40	170	1	0.5

Ham Steaks

Ham Steaks: *Cooked, no added fat*

	Cal	kJ	Fat	Cb
Small, 65g raw weight	80	340	4	2
Medium, 100g weight	125	520	6	3.5
Large, 130g raw weight	210	885	8	5

Game Kangaroo

	Cal	kJ	Fat	Cb
Buffalo, leg/shoulder,				
Lean meat, cooked, 100g	155	650	1	0
Camel, raw, 100g	100	420	2	0
Crocodile, raw:				
Body; Leg, Tenderloin, 100g	110	460	3	0
Croc Ball Patty, fried, 60g	125	520	6	0
Tail, 100g	120	500	4	0
Emu, lean, grilled, 100g	150	625	3	0
Goat: Raw, 100g	110	460	2.5	0
Roasted, 100g	150	625	3	0
Kangaroo, raw, 100g	120	500	2.5	0
Pigeon,				
Roast, meat only, 100g	230	960	13	0
Quail, 1 whole, roast, 180g	180	755	6	0
Rabbit/Lapin: Raw, meat, 100g	125	525	4	0
Stewed, meat only, 100g	180	755	8	0
Weighed with bones, 100g	90	375	4	0
Snake, raw, 100g	160	670	2	0
Venison/Deer, roasted:				
Lean meat, 100g	150	625	3	0
Lean + fat, 100g	200	835	6	0

Offal & Variety Meats

	Cal	kJ	Fat	Cb
Brains, Lamb, 1 set, raw 145g	160	670	11	0
Haggis, boiled, 100g	310	1295	11	0
Heart, boiled, 100g	110	460	4	0
Kidneys: Raw (2), 100g	80	335	2	0
Fried, 100g	150	630	6	0
Liver:				
Chicken Livers: Raw, 100g	120	490	5	0
Fried, flour coated, 100g	160	660	6.5	0
Lamb: Raw, 100g	155	640	7.5	2.5
Fried, flour coated, 100g	240	1005	14	3
Veal Calf: Raw, 100g	125	515	5.5	3
Fried, 100g	180	760	8	1.5
Liver Paté, average, 2 Tbsp, 50g	140	580	12	0.5
Sweetbread, Lamb,				
Raw, 100g	130	545	8	0
Boiled, 100g	260	1080	17	0
Tongue: Lamb's/Ox, without Fat/Skin,				
Raw, 100g	200	835	15	0
Stewed/boiled: 100g	290	1210	24	0
1 slice, 20g	60	250	5	0
Tripe: Dressed, raw, 100g	70	300	2	0
Simmered, 100g	85	355	3	0
In White Sce, ½ cup, 150g	170	710	6	21

Meat ~ Sausages ◆ Franks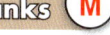

Cooking Methods & Fat Loss
Grilled, fried or barbequed sausages have similar fat content. Average fat loss with cooking is 20-25% of total fat of raw sausage. The leaner the sausage, the less fat that is lost on cooking.

Sausage ~ Quick Guide

Cal | kJ | Fat | Cb

Standard Sausages (Full Fat):
Average All Meats
Beef, Pork, Mutton:
Average fat content of 22%

Thin Sausages: *8-10 per 500g raw weight*

	Cal	kJ	Fat	Cb
50g raw wt: Raw	130	545	11	1
Cooked	110	460	8	2
60g raw wt: Raw	155	650	13	1
Cooked	135	565	10	2.5
70g raw wt: Raw	180	750	15	1.5
Cooked	155	650	12	3

Thick Sausages: *5-7 per 500g raw weight*

	Cal	kJ	Fat	Cb
80g raw wt: Raw	210	875	18	1.5
Cooked	180	750	13	3
90g raw wt: Raw	235	980	20	2
Cooked	200	835	15	3.5
100g raw wt: Raw	260	1085	22	2
Cooked	225	940	16	4
110g raw wt: Raw	285	1190	24	2.5
Cooked	250	1045	18	4.5

Small Links: *Approx 20 per 500g raw weight*

	Cal	kJ	Fat	Cb
1 link, 25g, raw	65	270	5.5	0.5
Cooked	55	230	4	1

Reduced-Fat Sausages: *15% Fat Content (85% Lean)*

	Cal	kJ	Fat	Cb
50g raw wt: Raw	100	420	7.5	1
Cooked	85	355	6	2
60g raw wt: Raw	120	500	9	1
Cooked	100	420	7	2.5
70g raw wt: Raw	140	585	11	1.5
Cooked	120	500	9	3

Low-Fat Sausages: *8% Fat Content (92% Lean)*

	Cal	kJ	Fat	Cb
50g raw wt: Raw	75	315	4	1
Cooked	70	295	3	2
60g raw wt: Raw	90	375	5	1
Cooked	80	335	4	2.5
70g raw wt: Raw	105	440	6	1.5
Cooked	95	400	5	3

Other Sausages

Cal | kJ | Fat | Cb

BBQ/Breakfast/Butchers/Picnic: *Same as standard sausages*

Chicken Sausages, cooked:

	Cal	kJ	Fat	Cb
Standard (16% fat), 50g raw wt	90	375	6	1
Low-fat (8% fat), 50g raw wt	70	295	3	1

Chipolatas: *Small Links*

	Cal	kJ	Fat	Cb
25g link, cooked	55	230	4	0.5
40g link, cooked	90	375	7	1

Chorizo, 1 link, 60g — 230 | 970 | 19 | 3

Frankfurts: *Fat varies (17-25% fat) Frankfurts are precooked and only require heating. Little fat is lost.*

Packaged/Brand: *17% fat average*

	Cal	kJ	Fat	Cb
1 Frankfurt, 50g	100	420	8.5	1
95% Fat Free, 62g	75	315	2	1
Don Footy Franks:				
Skin-On (1), 63g	195	820	17	4
Skin-Less (1), 63g	195	820	17	4
Hans: Lil Frankies, 80g	180	760	13	6
American (1), 63g	145	595	10	5
Cheerios, 63g	140	570	9	8
97% Fat-Free, 63g	90	370	6	2

Deli/Butcher Franks: *22% average*

	Cal	kJ	Fat	Cb
1 Frankfurt, 50g	125	525	10	2.5
Large, raw/cooked, 70g	190	795	15	3.5

Cocktail Frankfurt, 25g each — 80 | 330 | 7 | 1

Canned Frankfurts *(Plumrose):*

	Cal	kJ	Fat	Cb
Skinless Hot Dogs (1), 48g	90	380	7	2
Cocktail, each	30	130	2.5	1

Gourmet/Flavoured Sausages: *8-22% fat*

Brannans (Aldi):

	Cal	kJ	Fat	Cb
Beef, Onion & Bell Pepper (1), 84g	180	745	13	5
Italian Pork (1), 70g	150	615	11	3.5
Coles: Herb & Garlic (1), 70g	160	670	14	2.5
Angus Beef & Pepper, 100g	235	985	20	4
Pork & Cider Apple, 100g	225	945	19	5

Down Under, Low-Fat:

	Cal	kJ	Fat	Cb
Beef with Cheese, 75g	85	355	5	2
Boerwors, 140g	235	980	22	1.5
Hans: BBQ Sizzlers, 50g	120	495	8	7.5
Mini: Smoked Kabana, 25g	55	230	4	2
Chorizo, 25g	90	380	8	0.5
IGA: BBQ Sausage, 80g	160	670	12	4
Sun-Dried Tomato, 60g	145	605	11	2.5
Beef, Honey & Rosemary, 55g	135	560	10	4
Sweet Chilli & Plum, 60g	150	635	12	4
Skinless, Beef, 45g	90	370	5.5	2

Updated Nutrition Data ~ www.CalorieKing.com.au
Persons with Diabetes ~ See Disclaimer (Page 22)

Meat ~ Sausages ◆ Franks ◆ Gourmet

Other Sausages (Cont) | Cal | kJ | Fat | Cb

Italian Sausages:
	Cal	kJ	Fat	Cb
Raw, 75g	190	795	16	5
Cooked, 50g	165	685	11	5

Kangaroo Meat Sausages:
Macro Meats,
Kanga Banga, (98% Fat Free),
raw, 1 sausage, 100g	110	455	1	4.5

Saveloy: Raw, 75g — 210 | 880 | 17 | 2
Cooked — 170 | 710 | 13 | 2
Battered & deep fried, 100g — 310 | 1280 | 21 | 3.5

Skinless Sausages: *Per 50g Raw*
Don's, Regular Fat (22%)	125	525	10	1

Reduced-Fat: Per Sausage
Gourmet Chevups: Chicken, 50g	90	370	5.5	1
Beef; Chilli Beef, 50g	90	375	4	1
Chilli Pork; Pork, 50g	110	460	8	1
The Chevap Co: Pepper, 45g	100	420	6.5	3
Mild; Steak Dianne, 42g	80	340	6.5	3
Woolworths, Chevap Beef, 50g	85	355	6	1

Vienna Sausage: *Precooked:*
1 medium, 75g, raw/cooked	240	995	21	2.5
1 large, 100g, raw/cooked	315	1325	28	3.5

Woolworths Deli:
	Cal	kJ	Fat	Cb
Gourmet Sausages: Lean Beef, 85g	140	575	8.5	1.5
Lamb Rosemary & Garlic, 70g	170	705	14	1
Average other varieties, 85g	210	870	18	1.5
Sausages: Beef Herb & Garlic, 60g	155	650	13	3
Chicken, 90g	145	600	9	5.5
Average other varieties	205	855	17	6
Chipolatas: Beef, Herb & Garlic, 60g	155	650	1.5	2
Beef, 40g	105	435	8.5	2.5
Chicken, 40g	65	265	8	2.5
Beef Gluten Free, 95g	250	1035	20	6
Beef Heart Smart, 75g	125	515	7.5	5
Chevap, Skinless, all varieties, 50g	85	350	6	1

Sanitarium/Vegie Delights:
BBQ Soy Sausages (1), 50g	105	425	4	5
Original Soy Sausages (1), 50g	100	410	4.5	4.5
Vegie-Sausages (1), 50g	110	455	5.5	5.5

Also See Sanitarium ~ Page 124

Liverwurst & Paté | Cal | kJ | Fat | Cb

Liverwurst: *average all types*
1 Tbsp, 25g	80	335	7	0
50g portion	160	660	14	0

Paté, Liver: *average all varieties,*
1 Tbsp, 25g	70	290	6	0.5
1 slice (9 x 7 x ½ cm), 35g	95	405	8	0.5
60g portion	165	690	14	1
Low-Fat (Pork/Liver based), 20g	40	170	4	0
Smoked Salmon, 20g	40	155	3	0.5
Soy, average, 20g	50	195	12	2.5

Fried Onions

	Cal	kJ	Fat	Cb
Lightly oiled pan/BBQ, 100g	100	420	7	8
Heavily oiled pan/BBQ, 100g	140	585	12	8

Gourmet & Indigenous Foods

Ants: | Cal | kJ | Fat | Cb
Honeypot, whole, 100g	15	60	1	0
Choc-coated, 1 Tbsp, 15g	70	290	6	3
Eggs/Larvae, 1 Tbsp, 15g	20	85	1	0
Bee Maggots, canned 2 Tbsp, 30g	70	290	2	0
Blood (Coagulated), Black Pudding,				
Grilled/Fried, 50g patty	80	335	3.5	8
Bogong Moths, whole, 30g	85	355	6	0
Bush Tomato, (Aust.), 100g	10	45	0	1
Caviar, (Sturgeon Roe), 1 T, 15g	40	165	3	0
Caterpillars, canned, 60g	70	290	2	0
Davidson Plums, 100g	20	85	1	1
Eel, smoked, 30g	70	295	4.5	0
Frogs Legs, fried,				
2 medium pairs	200	835	10	5
Goanna/Lizard, BBQ'd, 100g	190	790	7	0
Grasshoppers, chocolate coated, 4, 30g	100	670	9	18
Haggis, boiled, 100g	205	860	12	14
Locusts, Australian Plague,				
1 bowl, 100g	140	580	2	0
Note: Locusts are high in protein, 25g per 100g				
Mangrove Worms, 3 small, 30g	20	85	0.5	0
Silkworms, 30g serve	60	250	2	0
Snake, 100g	110	450	2	0
Snails (Escargots): 2 med., 30g	30	120	0.5	0
In Garlic Butter, 6 only	200	835	10	0
Snail Eggs, 1 tsp	20	85	0.5	0
Witchetty Grubs/Bardies,				
1 large, 30g	95	400	9	0

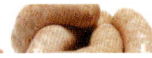

Meat ~ Ham ◇ Deli ◇ Spam

Ham

	Cal	kJ	Fat	Cb
Ham: *Fresh, On-the-Bone:*				
Leg: 2 thin/1 thick slice, 50g	70	290	4	1
Lean only, 45g	50	205	2	1
Virginia/Shoulder, 50g	50	200	1.5	3.5
Pressed/Packaged Ham:				
English Ham, 50g	50	200	1.5	1.5
Leg, 2 slices (10 x 10cm), 50g	50	200	1.5	0.5
Sandwich Ham, 2 slices 50g	65	270	3	4
Shoulder, 2 slices (10 x 10cm), 50g	55	230	3	0.5
Hans, 97% Fat-Free Honey Leg, 50g	55	220	1.5	4.5
97% Fat-Free Traditional; Champagne, 50g	50	195	1	1
Country Fresh, Prem. Smokehouse Leg Ham	25	95	1	0.5
Canned Ham: *Average All Brands*				
Leg, 2 slices (8 x 4 x 0.5cm), 35g	40	165	1.5	0
Shoulder, 2 slices, 35g	40	175	2.5	0
Coles, Leg Ham on Bone, 50g	95	385	6	0.5
Plumrose: Leg Ham, 30g	40	175	2.5	0.5
Deli Ham, 30g	45	180	2.5	0.5
Luncheon Meat, 30g	70	300	6	0.5
Ham & Chicken Roll, 30g	70	290	5.5	1.5
Ham Steaks, medium, 100g	125	520	6	3
Don: Honey Rstd Leg Ham, 25g, 97% fat-free, 25g	25	110	0.5	1
Lite Leg Ham, 25g	25	110	1	0.5

Other Luncheon Meats

	Cal	kJ	Fat	Cb
Brawn, 50g slice	110	460	8.5	0
Camp Pie, canned, 30g	50	200	3	2
Chicken Breast, 97% Fat-Free, 25g	25	95	0.5	1.5
Chicken Devon, 30g	60	240	4	2
Chicken Loaf/Pressed, 30g	40	155	0.5	1
Corned Beef *(Hamper)*,				
Canned, 85g serve	200	830	14	0
Lite, 85g, serve	170	710	11	1
Devon, regular, 30g	70	295	5.5	2
Frankfurter/Fritz/Garlic Roll, 30g	75	310	5.5	1.5
Fritz *(Chapmans, SA)*, 30g	60	250	4	3
Lambs' Tongues *(Hamper)*, 110g	230	945	18	0
Luncheon Beef *(Don)*, 25g	25	110	1	0
Pancetta, 1 slice, 20g	40	155	1.5	0
Polony, average, 30g	65	275	5	2
Roast Beef: 2 slices, 50g	55	225	1.5	1
Shaved *(Don)*, 30g	30	130	1	1.5
Silverside: Packet, 2 slices, 60g	65	270	2	1
97% Fat-Free, 50g	55	225	1	1
Turkey, average, 30g	35	140	1	0

Salami

	Cal	kJ	Fat	Cb
Per 30g Unless Indicated				
Cooked/Moist, average	90	375	7.5	0
Dry: Average all types	120	500	10	0
Cabana/Kabana	85	350	7.5	0
5 pieces, 40g	115	470	10	0
100g portion	280	1170	25	0
Danish Salami	130	540	12	0.5
Hungarian Salami	125	520	11	0.5
Kransky	75	310	5.5	1
Mettwurst	125	530	11	0
Milano	130	535	11	0.5
Pepperoni	125	520	11	0.5
5 pieces, 40g	165	690	14	0.5
Snack Sticks, mini (1), 15g	65	275	5.5	0

Other Continental Meats

Average all Brands
Per 30g Unless Indicated

	Cal	kJ	Fat	Cb
Black Pudding; Bologna	80	335	6	1.5
Cabanossi	110	460	9	1.5
Hungarian	75	310	6	2
Liverwurst	95	390	8	1
Mortadella	95	390	8	0.5
Pancetta, 2 slices, 30g	50	205	2	0.5
Pastrami, 2 slices, 40g	45	165	1.5	0.5
Prosciutto, 2 slices, 25g	65	260	4	0
55% Reduced Fat (Hans)	40	170	2	1
KR Castlemaine:				
Bred Free Range: *Per 40g*				
Chicken	35	150	0.5	1.5
Ham: Honey	40	170	1	1.5
Leg	40	160	1	1
Kabana, 40g	90	360	6.5	1
Salami, Mild	160	675	14	0.5
Slim Stix: Hot	150	630	9	7
Mild	150	615	7.5	9

Spam

	Cal	kJ	Fat	Cb
Spam: 1 thin slice, 42g	130	540	12	1.5
200g can	615	2570	54	7
340g can	1050	4375	91	13
Lite Spam: 1 thin slice, 42g	85	355	5.5	1.5
340g can	690	2875	46	13
Hot & Spicy: 1 slice, 42g	130	540	11	1.5
340g can	1035	4330	91	12
Turkey Spam: 1 slice, 42g	60	250	3.5	1
340g can	485	2030	28	6
Spam with Bacon: 1 sl. 42g	135	565	12	1
340g can	1095	4565	97	6

Updated Nutrition Data ~ www.CalorieKing.com.au
Persons with Diabetes ~ See Disclaimer (Page 22)

Noodles

Quick Guide ~ Noodles

	Cal	kJ	Fat	Cb
Plain Noodles:				
Average All Brands				
Dry, 100g	350	1465	1	74
Cooked, 1 cup, 150g	180	750	0.5	36
Stir-fried, 1 cup, 150g	220	920	7	36
Fried *(Crispy)*, 50g	250	1045	14	30

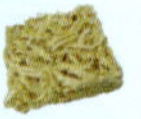

Plain Noodles

	Cal	kJ	Fat	Cb
Ayam, cooked, 40g	140	580	0.5	29
Fantastic, Long Life, 1 serve, 62.5g	225	930	0.5	46
Trident, Pad Thai Noodles, ½ packet, cooked, 150g	200	840	3	43
Wokka: Egg Chow Mein, 220g	325	1350	2.5	60
Thin Egg Style, 220g	290	1200	3	49

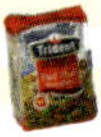

2-Minute Noodles

	Cal	kJ	Fat	Cb
Changs, Beef, dry, 65g packet	240	1010	4	52
Coles: Smart Buy Noodle Block, 370g prepared				
Beef; Oriental	415	1740	18	54
Chicken	400	1665	17	53
Indo Mie, Mi Goreng, 85g	420	1750	17	59
Maggi: Beef/Chicken, avg., 85g	330	1370	13	45
99% Fat-Free, 75g	280	1180	2	57
Nissin, average all flavours, cup	325	1360	14	43
Pandaroo, Mi Goreng, 85g	385	1600	16	51
Trident: Laksa, 85g packet	665	2775	26	91
Hot & Spicy Thai, 80g packet	465	1935	21	55
Woolworths: *Per 85g Packet*				
Homebrand: Beef, prepared	400	1680	17	53
Chicken, prepared	420	1750	18	54

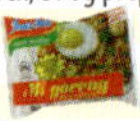

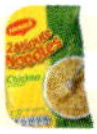

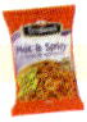

Chinese Rice, Vermicelli Noodles

	Cal	kJ	Fat	Cb
Average: Dry 30g	110	460	0.5	25
Cooked, 1 cup, 170g	150	620	0.5	33
Chang's: *250g Packet*				
¼ packet, 62g	220	925	0.5	49
Bean Vermicelli, 50g portion	175	730	0.5	39
Eskal's, 62g	235	980	1	53
Pandaroo, ¼ pkt. 62g	210	870	0.5	47

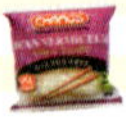

Chow Mein

	Cal	kJ	Fat	Cb
Fantastic, prepared, 117g	325	1365	3.5	62
Trident, prepared, 185g	313	1310	14	40

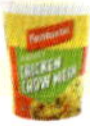

Egg Noodles

	Cal	kJ	Fat	Cb
Average: Dry, 100g	300	1255	2	70
Fresh, thin, 100g	130	545	1.5	22
Chang's, ⅓ of 200g Packet, 70g	195	825	1	39
HealthyBake, Spelt, 50g	190	795	1	36

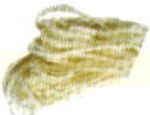

Cup Noodles

	Cal	kJ	Fat	Cb
Fantastic, Xtra Saucy Noodles, Mi Goreng, 75g cup	375	1560	14	51

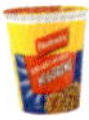

Fried/Crispy Noodles

	Cal	kJ	Fat	Cb
Chang's, average, ¼ packet, 25g	125	520	7	15
Stirling Foods, BBQ; Chilli, avg., 100g	540	2250	34	45

Hokkien Noodles

	Cal	kJ	Fat	Cb
Fantastic, ½ of 450g pkt, 225g	425	1780	4.5	81
Kan Tong, ½ sachet, 110g	175	740	0.5	35
Wokka: Golden, ½ packet, 220g	260	1090	1	51
Thin Style, ½ packet, 220g	275	1150	1.5	55

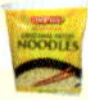

Singapore Noodles

	Cal	kJ	Fat	Cb
Fantastic, ½ packet, 175g	280	1160	3.5	49
Kan Tong, ¼ packet, 100g	160	665	1	27
Trident, 85g packet, prepared	330	1390	13	47
Wokka, 220g pouch	285	1190	1	49

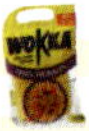

Thai Rice Noodles

	Cal	kJ	Fat	Cb
Chang's, 80g serving	290	1210	0.5	64
Pandaroo, 50g	90	375	0.5	20

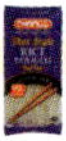

Udon Noodles

	Cal	kJ	Fat	Cb
Hakubaku, dry, ⅓ pkt, 90g	305	1280	1	65
Kan Tong, ½ sachet, 110g	185	785	0.5	32
Trident, 200g packet	390	1610	1	85
Wokka, Udon, 220g packet	290	1215	2	56
Chang's, Wok-Ready Noodles, 150g sachet	210	875	0.5	43

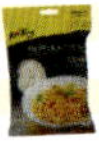

Other Noodles

	Cal	kJ	Fat	Cb
Japanese, Soba/Somen, average, 30g	110	460	0.5	21
Long Life *(Fantasic),*¼ packet, 63g	225	930	0.5	46
Pad Thai Noodles *(Trident)*, 80g	110	450	2	23
Ramen Noodles *(Obento)*, 150g package	220	920	3	38
Rice Flakes Sheet, ⅓ pkt, 75g	265	1105	0	62
Rice Stick *(Chef's Choice)*, 56g	200	835	0	46
Soba Noodles *(Obento)*, 180g pack	260	1090	4	44
Also See Japanese Foods ~ *See Page 182*				
Stir Fry Noodles, *Wokka,* Hokkien, 220g	275	1150	1.5	56

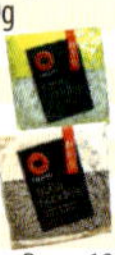

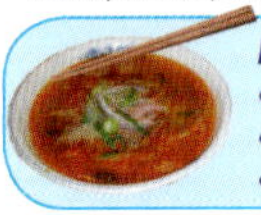

For Noodle Dishes, See:
- Asian Meals ~ Page 180
- Wok-In-A-Box ~ Page 208
- Wok Me ~ Page 208

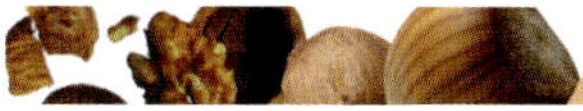

Nuts

Nuts

	Cal	kJ	Fat	Cb
Per 30g Unless Shown				
Acorns, raw, shelled, 30g	115	485	7	12.5
Almonds, shelled:				
Chocolate-coated, 5-6 pieces, 30g	165	690	12	9
Honey Roasted, 30g	180	745	15	8.5
Sugar coated/Vanilla, 30g	140	595	5.5	11
Whole, 25-30 nuts, 30g	175	730	16	1.5
Beer Nuts, 30 nuts, 30g	175	730	15	2.6
Brazil, shelled,				
7-8 medium nuts, 30g	210	865	20	1
Cashews, roasted:				
10 medium, 15g	90	375	7.5	7.1
20 medium, 30g	175	720	15	15
Honey Roasted, 30g	170	720	14	5
Chestnuts: 4 large/6 small, raw, 120g	195	815	1	36
Roasted, 30g	50	220	0.2	11
Canned, water chestnuts,				
sliced/whole, drained, 30g	10	45	0	2
Coconut, fresh, no shell:				
1 piece (3 x 3 x 2cm), 30g	95	390	9	1
½ medium (12cm diam)	615	2570	60	7
Desiccated, 4 Tbsp, 30g	190	795	20	2.2
Hazelnuts, ¼ cup, 30g	190	795	18	1.5
Japanese Nuts, 10 nuts, 20g	100	405	4.5	12
Macadamia Nuts, raw, shelled:				
7 medium/14 small, 30g	220	920	23	1.5
Dry roasted, 30g	215	900	23	1.5
Dark Chocolate-coated, 30g	175	735	13	13
Mixed Nuts, shelled, 20 nuts	190	795	17	2.6
Peanuts: Raw, Unshelled, 30g	120	500	11	2
Shelled, 40 nuts, 30g	170	710	15	2.7
Dry roasted: 30g	190	795	16	4
50g packet	320	1330	27	7
½ cup, 70g	445	1865	37	10
Oil Roasted, shelled, 30g	190	795	16	4.5
Unsalted *(Charlesworth)*, 30g	175	730	15	3.5
Chocolate Coated: ¼ cup, 30g	180	755	14	8.5
100g packet	605	2520	45	29
Honey Roasted *(Charlesworth)*,				
¼ cup, 30g	170	710	13	7.5
Sugar-coated, 30g	225	940	10	23
Pecans: 5-8 halves, 15g	105	435	11	0.7
¼ cup, 30g	210	880	22	1.5
Pine Nuts, shelled, 4 Tbsp, 30g	200	845	21	1.3

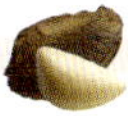

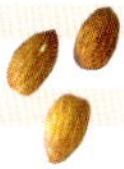

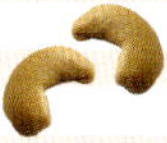

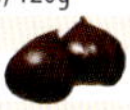

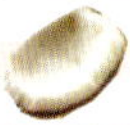

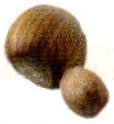

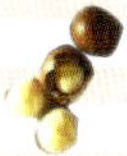

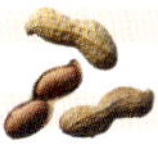

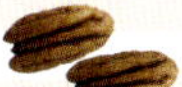

Nuts (Cont)

	Cal	kJ	Fat	Cb
Pistachio: Shelled, 30g, 60 nuts	170	710	15	2
Unshelled, ¼ cup; 23 nuts	85	355	7	1
Savoury Nut Mix, ¼ cup, 25g	165	695	16	1.5
Soybean Nuts, dry roasted, 30g	135	565	7	10
Walnuts, shelled:				
15-20 halves, ¼ cup, 30g	210	870	21	1
Chopped, 1 Tbsp, 8g	55	230	5.5	0.2

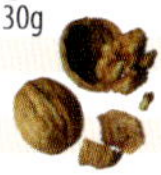

Seeds, Tahini

	Cal	kJ	Fat	Cb
Per 30g Unless Shown				
Caraway/Fennel, 1 tsp, 5g	15	90	0.5	0.2
Coriander, whole, 1 tsp, 5g	15	55	0.2	4
Cumin/Celery Seeds, 1 tsp, 5g	25	95	1	2.3
Fenugreek Seeds, 1 tsp	10	50	0.2	2
Flax Seed/Linseed, 1 Tbsp, 12g	65	250	4	4
Pepitas/Pumpkin Seeds:				
Hulled, dried, 30g	160	670	14	5.3
1 Tbsp, 15g	80	335	7	3
Poppy Seeds, 1 tsp, 2.8g	15	60	1	1
Sesame Seeds: Dried, 1 Tbsp, 11g	70	290	6	2.5
¼ cup, 35g	220	925	21	8
Sunflower Kernels: Dried, 30g	175	735	16	1
1 Tbsp, 11g	65	270	6	0.5
½ cup, 70g	410	1710	36	1.5
Tahini, *(Sesame Seed Paste)*:				
1 rounded tsp, 10g	65	270	6	0.5
1 Tbsp, 25g	160	655	15	0.5
¼ cup, 80g	510	2130	48	1.6

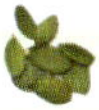

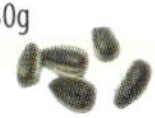

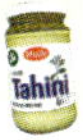

Nut eaters are healthier and live longer say scientists.

Nuts are a nutritious source of protein, vitamins, minerals, fibre, healthy fats, and antioxidants.

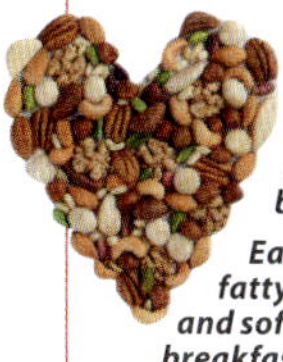

Their fat and fibre help reduce blood cholesterol; and their protein and fibre promote meal satiety (fullness) and reduces hunger levels – of benefit in weight control.

Eat nuts instead of high-sugar or fatty snacks, biscuits, confectionery and soft drinks. Add chopped nuts to breakfast cereals.

More Info: www.nutsforlife.com.au

Updated Nutrition Data ~ www.CalorieKing.com.au
Persons with Diabetes ~ See Disclaimer (Page 22)

Pasta & Spaghetti

Pasta ~ Quick Guide

	Cal	kJ	Fat	Cb

Pasta, Spaghetti, Macaroni
*Pasta includes all shapes and sizes.
(Examples: elbows, shells, tubes, twists, sheets, cannelloni, manicotti, spaghetti, ziti.)
All plain pasta products have similar cal/kJ/Fat on a weight basis (dry).*
(35g Dry = 100g cooked)

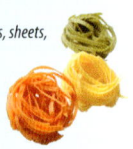

Dry: *Average all types:*

	Cal	kJ	Fat	Cb
35g dry weight	135	555	1	25
100g dry weight	380	1585	3	72
Cannelloni, 1 tube, 10g	40	160	0.5	7
Elbows, 1 cup, 115g	435	1820	3.5	83
Lasagne Sheets (e.g. Leggo's/Vetta):				
Average, 1 small sheet, 16g	60	255	0.5	12
Shells/Spirals, 1 cup, 100g	380	1585	3	72
Guzzis, all types, 100g	365	1530	2.5	70
Wholemeal, Vegetable, 100g	335	1390	2.5	57

Cooked:
Spaghetti: *Plain (No Added Fat):*

	Cal	kJ	Fat	Cb
Small serve, ½ cup,	105	440	0.5	22
Medium serve, 1 cup, 150g	210	85	1	44
Large (restaurant) 2 cups, 300g	420	1755	1.5	86
Extra Large, 3 cups, 450g	630	2630	1.5	128
Macaroni, cooked, 1 cup, 150g	210	875	1	44

Pasta Sauces ~ See Page 150

Restaurant Pasta Dishes

	Cal	kJ	Fat	Cb

Per Whole Dish, Average

	Cal	kJ	Fat	Cb
Baked Spaghetti Parmesan	640	2675	44	160
Cannelloni, 2 tubes	385	1615	14	38
Chicken Cacciatore w. 1 cup pasta, cooked	635	2670	68	49
Chicken Parmigiana w. 1 cup pasta, cooked	610	2555	69	49
Fettuccine Alfredo	480	2000	14	67
Fettuccine Carbonara	485	2020	14	57
Fettuccine with Sausage, Mushroom	460	1925	14	86
Lasagne with Meat, 400g	575	2395	25	56
Ravioli with Meat	340	1430	14	33
Spaghetti with Meatballs	435	1820	14	59
Tortellini, 200g	395	1645	9	58
Veal Parmigiana, 300g	590	2465	38	18

Wheat/Gluten Free

	Cal	kJ	Fat	Cb

Orgran: *Based on Corn, Rice, Vegetables*
Average all types,

	Cal	kJ	Fat	Cb
¼ packet (dry), 63g	220	920	1	50

San Remo,

	Cal	kJ	Fat	Cb
Pasta, all varieties, 50g dry	180	760	1	37

Fresh Pasta (Refrigerated)

Average All Brands

	Cal	kJ	Fat	Cb
Fettuccine: Plain/Vegetable,				
Uncooked, 100g	360	1515	1.5	75
Cooked, 1 cup, 150g	250	1050	3.5	45
Gnocchi, Potato/Pumpkin,				
Uncooked, 1 cup, 145g	260	1085	0.5	60
Lasagna: 1 sheet, raw, 50g	150	630	1	24
Cooked: With meat, small, 220g	315	1325	14	31
Main Meal size, 400g	575	2410	25	56
Ravioli, *Per Medium Serving, 150g*				
Beef, cooked	265	1105	8	40
Chicken & Mushr., cooked	290	1215	5	46
Spinach & Ricotta, cooked	295	1235	8	40
Tagliatelle ~ *Similar to Fettuccine*				
Tortellini: *Per Medium Serving, 150g*				
Beef, cooked	260	1085	6	40
Cheese & Spinach, cooked	280	1175	5	45
Ham & Cheese, cooked	250	1045	5.5	37

Latina Fresh Pasta ~ See Page 120
San Remo ~ See Page 124

Macaroni & Cheese

Home-made/Restaurant:
Average:

	Cal	kJ	Fat	Cb
Small serve, ½cup, 140g	205	860	10	22
Medium serve, 1 cup, 280g	410	1720	20	45
Large serve, 2 cups, 560g	825	3445	40	90

Packaged:

	Cal	kJ	Fat	Cb
Fantastic, Pasta Mac & Cheese,				
80g cup or packet	350	1465	8.5	57
Heinz, ½ 400g can, 200g	170	700	9	18

Noodles ~ See Page 140

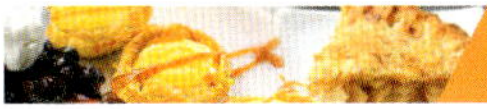

Pastry ◆ Puddings

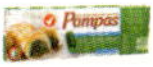

Pastry

	Cal	kJ	Fat	Cb
Choux, 150g	320	1330	20	28
Filo *(Pampas)*, 5 sheets, 85g	280	1175	3	54
Multimix *(Orgran)*, 40g	125	530	0	32
Pie Flan *(Pampas)*: Savoury, ¼ Flan, 55g	250	1035	15	26
Sweet, ¼ Flan, 55g	245	1020	13	30
Puff Pastry: Block, ½, 188g	655	2745	31	82
Roll, ½ roll, 250g	875	3650	42	109
Sheet: ½ sheet, 84g	270	1130	13	33
½ sheet, 168g	540	2260	26	66
Butter, ¼ sheet, 41g	150	625	9	16
Canola, ¼ sheet, 41g	135	560	6.5	16
Reduced Fat *(Pampas)*: 1 sheet	500	2085	20	69
¼ sheet, 41g	125	520	5	17
Quiche *(Pampas)*, ¼ sheet, 100g	370	1550	20	43
Savoury Boats *(Erica)*, 4.16g	20	85	1	2
Savoury Tarts *(Erica)*, 3g	15	55	0.5	1.5
Shortcrust: ½ sheet, 100g	395	1650	22	43
Reduced Fat, ½ sheet, 100g	355	1480	16	47
Sorj, each, 70g	195	810	1	39
Spring Roll, 1 sheet, 13g	40	170	1	7.5
Tart Cases, (Pampas), 23g each	100	425	5	13
Vol au Vent/Oyster Case:				
Small, 3cm, 5g	30	125	2	2.5
Medium, 5cm, 12g	70	300	5	6
Large, 10cm, 25g	135	565	10	12
Pie Case, 60g, 15cm	325	1355	22	28

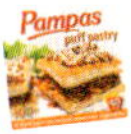

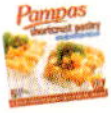

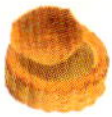

Pizza Bases

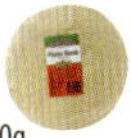

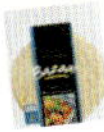

	Cal	kJ	Fat	Cb
Average All Brands:				
Plain, 100g quantity/piece	250	1045	2	49
Small Base, whole, 110g	275	1220	3	74
Regular/Medium, whole, 300g	750	3135	6	147
Large, whole, 550g	1375	5750	11	270
Bazaar: Small, whole, 110g	305	1275	8.5	47
Medium, whole, 166g	460	1925	13	71
Wholemeal, whole, 110g	280	1165	5	44
Boboli, Small, whole, 112g	280	1165	3.5	50
HealthyBake, Organic Spelt,				
Small, whole, 60g	175	735	3	29
Macro, Pizza Dough Mix, 1 base, 135g	490	2050	19	74
McCain, 1 whole, 233g	660	2750	7	126
Simply Wize, Pizza Crust w. Herbs, 70g	200	825	8	32

Updated Nutrition Data ~ www.CalorieKing.com.au
Persons with Diabetes ~ See Disclaimer (Page 22)

Puddings

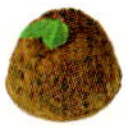

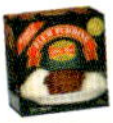

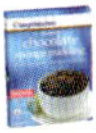

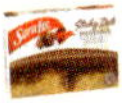

	Cal	kJ	Fat	Cb
Bread Pudding, 100g	160	665	5	22
Christmas Pudding: 100g	280	1170	7	50
Gluten Free, 80g	240	1010	8	38
Spelt, 100g	405	1680	19	45
Instant Pudding:				
Average all brands, ⅙ whole, 115g	120	510	4	117
Cottees, average all varieties, prepared, ⅙ packet, 1/2 cup	150	625	5	21
Plum Pudding:				
Big Sister, 80g	225	940	7	37
Mills & Ware, ¼ whole, 100g	325	1350	8.5	56
Rice Pudding, 100g	150	615	4	24
Sponge Pudding, 100g	160	675	3	31
Green's, average, prepared, ⅙ packet	190	790	3	37
Weight Watchers, avg. all flav., prepared, 200g	300	1265	3	69
Sticky Date Pudding:				
Brumby's, ⅛ pudding, 90g	190	800	4	48
Ferguson Plarre Bakehouse, ⅒ pudding, 90g	340	1430	17	48
Sara Lee, w. sauce ⅙ Pudding, 79g	340	1430	17	48
Weight Watchers, Frozen, (1), 80g	175	730	2.5	20
Yorkshire Pudding: Small piece, avg., 30g	75	320	4	8.5
Aunt Betty's, (1), 16g	50	205	2.5	6
Other Puddings ~ See Cakes Section				

CALORIE KING TIP!

To quench your thirst, drink water rather than sweetened drinks.

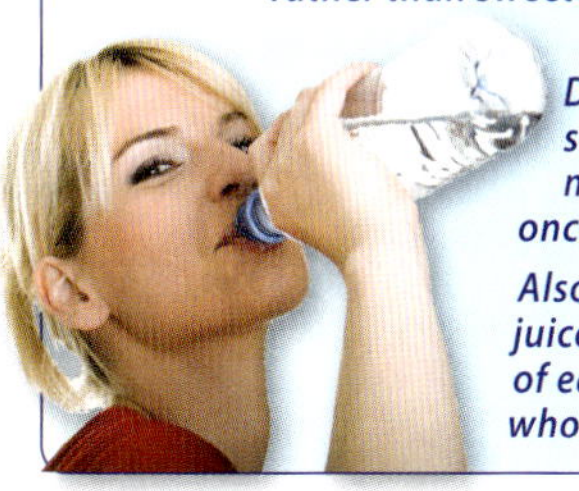

Don't drink soft drinks more than once weekly.

Also limit fruit juice in favour of eating the whole fruit.

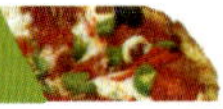

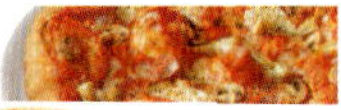

Pizza ~ Ready-to-Eat

Average all Pizza Outlets ~ Figures based on Large Pizza

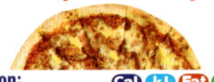

BBQ Chicken & Bacon:

	Cal	kJ	Fat	Cb
Thin N Crispy Crust:				
1 slice (⅛ Pizza), 75g	180	750	7	20
½ Pizza (4 slices), 300g	720	3000	28	80
Whole Pizza (8 slices), 600g	1440	6000	56	160
Classic Crust: ⅛ Pizza (1 slice), 75g	180	750	7	20
½ Pizza (4 slices), 300g	720	3000	28	80
Whole Pizza (8 slices), 600g	1440	6000	56	160
Deep Pan: ⅛ Pizza (1 slice), 85g	210	880	7	26
¼ Pizza (4 slices), 340g	840	3520	28	104
Whole Pizza (8 slices), 680g	1680	7040	56	208

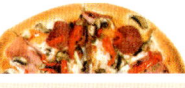

BBQ Meat Lovers:

Thin N Crispy Crust:				
1 slice (⅛ Pizza), 70g	190	795	8	21
½ Pizza (4 slices), 280g	760	3180	32	84
Whole Pizza (8 slices), 560g	1520	6360	64	168
Classic Crust: ⅛ Pizza (1 slice), 75g	200	835	8	22
½ Pizza (4 slices), 300g	800	3340	32	88
Whole Pizza (8 slices), 600g	1600	6680	64	176
Deep Pan:				
1 slice (⅛ Pizza), 85g	230	960	9	27
½ Pizza (4 slices), 340g	920	3840	36	108
Whole Pizza (8 slices), 680g	1840	7680	72	216

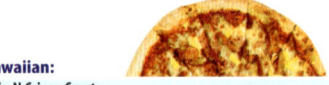

Hawaiian:

Thin N Crispy Crust:				
1 slice (⅛ Pizza), 70g	150	625	5	20
½ Pizza (4 slices), 280g	600	2500	20	80
Whole Pizza (8 slices), 560g	1200	5000	40	160
Classic Crust: ⅛ Pizza (1 slice), 75g	170	710	5	21
½ Pizza (4 slices), 300g	680	2840	20	84
Whole Pizza (8 slices), 600g	1360	5680	40	168
Deep Pan:				
1 slice (⅛ Pizza), 85g	200	835	7	25
½ Pizza (4 slices), 340g	800	3340	28	100
Whole Pizza (8 slices), 680g	1600	6680	56	200

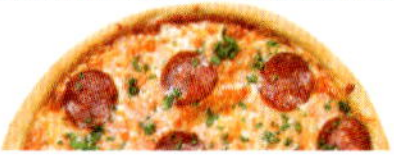

Pepperoni:

Thin N Crispy Crust:				
1 slice (⅛ Pizza), 55g	170	710	8	16
½ Pizza (4 slices), 220g	680	2840	32	64
Whole Pizza (8 slices), 440g	1360	5680	64	128
Classic Crust: 1 slice (⅛ Pizza), 55g	180	750	8	18
½ Pizza (4 slices), 220g	720	3000	32	72
Whole Pizza (8 slices), 440g	1440	6000	64	144
Deep Pan: 1 slice (⅛ Pizza), 70g	210	880	9	22
½ Pizza (4 slices), 280g	840	3520	36	88
Whole Pizza (8 slices), 560g	1680	7040	72	176

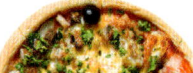

Supreme:

Thin N Crispy Crust: 1 slice (⅛ Pizza), 70g	160	670	7	17
½ Pizza (4 slices), 280g	640	2680	28	68
Whole Pizza (8 slices), 560g	1280	5360	56	136
Classic Crust: 1 slice (⅛ Pizza), 75g	180	750	7	19
½ Pizza (4 slices), 300g	720	3000	28	76
Whole Pizza (8 slices), 600g	1440	6000	56	152
Deep Pan: ⅛ Pizza (1 slice), 80g	200	835	8	23
½ Pizza (4 slices), 320g	800	3340	32	92
Whole Pizza (8 slices), 640g	1600	6680	64	184

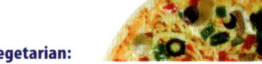

Vegetarian:

Thin N Crispy Crust: 1 slice (⅛ Pizza), 70g	180	750	5	25
½ Pizza (4 slices), 280g	720	3000	20	100
Whole Pizza (8 slices), 560g	1440	6000	40	200
Classic Crust: 1 slice (⅛ Pizza), 75g	190	795	5	25
½ Pizza (4 slices), 300g	760	3180	20	100
Whole Pizza (8 slices), 600g	1520	6360	40	200
Deep Pan: 1 slice (⅛ Pizza), 85g	220	920	6	30
½ Pizza (4 slices), 340g	880	3680	24	120
Whole Pizza (8 slices)	1760	7360	48	240

Also See: Dominos ~ *See Page 189*

Eagle Boys ~ *See Page 190; Pizza Hut ~ Page 204*

Pizza ~ Frozen

	Cal	kJ	Fat	Cb
Casa Barelli *(Aldi):*				
Woodfired Pizzas: *Per ⅛ Pizza, 48 g*				
Four Cheeses	125	525	4.5	46
Mozzarella & Rocket	110	450	3	15
Vegetable	85	365	2	13
Coles:				
Smart Buy:				
Hawaiian, ⅛ pizza, 62g	145	610	3	23
Supreme, ⅛ pizza, 62g	150	620	4	21
Dr Oetker:				
Ristorante Pizza: *Per ½ Pizza*				
Bolognese, 188g	400	1680	18	44
Funghi, 183g	435	1825	23	42
Hawaii, 178g	390	1630	15	46
Mozzarella, 168g	450	1870	23	41
Pepperoni-Salame, 155g	420	1755	22	41
Spinaci, 195g	440	1840	23	42
Vegetale, 193g	390	1635	18	43
International Cuisine *(Aldi),*				
Supreme, ⅛ pizza, 63g	145	605	4.5	18
Lite n' Easy: *Per Pizza*				
BBQ Chicken, 160g	225	945	7.5	31
Pineapple Supreme, 219g	215	890	7	33
McCain:				
Family Pizza: *Per ¼ of 500g Pizza*				
BBQ Meatlovers	300	1240	10	35
Cheese & Bacon, 125g	285	1190	9	34
Ham & Pineapple	290	1205	8	38
Margherita, 125g	330	1375	13	36
Meat Lovers, 125g	280	1170	9.5	32
Supreme, 125g	285	1195	8.5	38
Perfection: *Per ⅛ of Family Pizza*				
House Special, 84g	195	805	8	20
Meatlovers, 84g	200	825	8	22
Perfection: *Per Single Pizza*				
Hawaiian, 270g	640	2670	21	76
House Special, 270g	630	2640	27	62
Meat Lovers, 270g	735	3065	33	89
Ultra Thin: *Per ¼ Pizza*				
Mushroom & Garlic, 86g	170	710	7	16
Spinach & Mozzarella, 87g	195	815	8	20
Tandoori Chicken, 80g	165	695	7	16
Pizza Subs: *Per Sub, 135g*				
BBQ Chicken	280	1170	4.5	48
Ham & Pineapple	295	1220	7.5	42
House Special	290	1205	8	40
Meatlovers	315	1325	10	41
McCain (Cont)				
Pizza Pockets: *Per Pocket, 100g*				
Cheese & Bacon	245	1030	8	32
Ham & Pineapple	235	990	7	34
Supreme	245	1030	10	30
Pizza Singles: *Per Pizza, 100g*				
Cheese & Bacon	235	975	7.5	27
Ham & Pineapple	225	935	6.5	28
Meatlovers	230	950	7.5	27
Supreme	210	885	6	27
Pizza Slices: *Per Slice, 100g*				
Cheese & Bacon	230	960	7	28
Ham & Pineapple	215	890	5	31
Margherita	260	1090	11	28
Meatlovers	235	980	7.5	29
Supreme	195	815	6	23
Pizza Base (12"):				
1 Base, 233g	660	2750	7	126
¼ Base, 58g	165	685	2	32
Made for You,				
Supreme, 265g	365	1520	6	5
Papa Guiseppi's: *Per ¼ Pizza*				
BBQ Chicken, 111g	250	1040	8.5	30
Creamy Mushroom, 125g	290	1205	12	36
Hawaiian, 111g	250	1045	8	32
Hot Special, 112g	255	1060	10	28
Margherita, 103g	240	1010	9	27
Panini, Tomato & Cheese, 125g	290	1200	11	37
Pepperoni, 103g	265	1105	11	28
Supreme, 111g	260	1085	11	27
Remano *(Aldi):*				
Pizza Slices: *Per Slice, 69g*				
Ham & Pineapple	135	575	4	18
Supreme,	130	550	4	17
Weight Watchers:				
Calzones: *Per 160g Calzone*				
Capsicum, Zucchini, Mushroom & Cheese	240	1000	3	41
Chicken, Tomato & Cheese	270	1140	3	43
Thin Crust Pizza: *Per Pizza*				
Chkn w/ BBQ Sauce, 175g	285	1190	3.5	46
Supreme, 175g	260	1085	3.5	42
Woolworths: *Per ⅛ 500g Pizza*				
Homebrand, average all flavours	135	560	3.5	19
Select: Woodfired, Mushr. & Mozzarella	110	450	3	15
Roasted Mediterranean	100	415	2	16

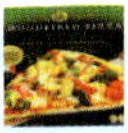

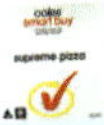

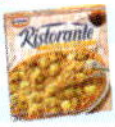

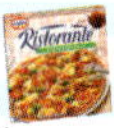

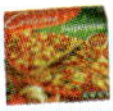

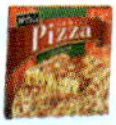

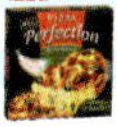

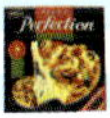

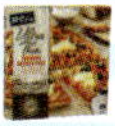

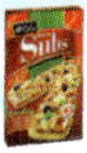

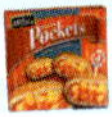

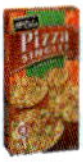

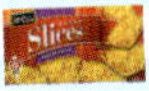

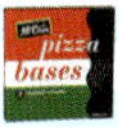

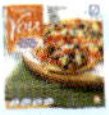

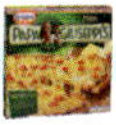

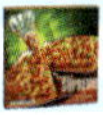

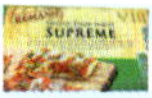

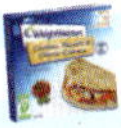

Updated Nutrition Data ~ www.CalorieKing.com.au
Persons with Diabetes ~ See Disclaimer (Page 22)

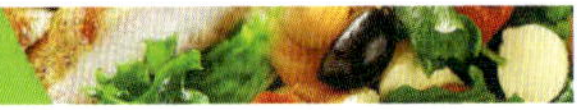

Salads ~ Canned & Packaged

Salads ~ Brands | Cal | kJ | Fat | Cb

Fast Food Outlets:

	Cal	kJ	Fat	Cb
Bean Salad, small, 120g	170	710	6	17
Coleslaw, small, 120g	135	560	6	19
Potato Salad, small, 110g	135	555	6	7.5

Coles: *Per Serving*

	Cal	kJ	Fat	Cb
Baby Potatoes, Tuscan, ½ packet, 200g	170	705	4	26
Caesar Salad Mix, ½ packet, 145g	205	850	14	10
Coleslaw Mix, ⅙ packet, 80g	20	90	0	3
Diced Vegetable Mix, ¼ packet, 100g	25	110	0	4
Mixed Leaves: 4 Leaf, ⅓ packet, 60g	20	80	0	2
Asian, ½ packet, 50g	15	50	0	1
Baby Mesclun, ¼ packet, 30g	10	35	0	1.5
Baby Spinach, ⅕ packet, 30g	10	30	0	1.5
Classic Salad, ¼ packet, 40g	10	30	0	0.5
Italian Salad, ¼ packet, 50g	10	40	0	1
Summer Crisp, ¼ packet, 50g	10	35	0	1
Stir Fry Mix, ½ packet, 200g	60	240	0	7

Mrs Crocket's: *Per 100g Unless Stated*

	Cal	kJ	Fat	Cb
Caesar Salad, 125g	150	620	8.5	10
Coleslaw	135	560	9	13
Creamy Pasta	190	795	10	22
Creamy Potato	150	625	10	15
Crunchy Asian Salad, 250g	240	995	16	20
Greek	45	190	3	2
Light: Alfresco, 275g	280	1175	3.5	55
Bean, 100g	130	540	1.5	23

Simply Less *(Coles): Per Salad*

	Cal	kJ	Fat	Cb
Chicken w/ Indian Rice Pilaf & Chutney, 225g	340	1410	5	50
Falafel & Tabouli w/ Yoghurt Dress., 225g	310	1290	13	37
Beef with Rstd Veg & Chipotle Dress., 225g	290	1215	10	35
Bowls: Mediterranean, 190g	160	655	10	6
Mexican, 190g	90	370	1	12

Woolworths:

	Cal	kJ	Fat	Cb
Coleslaw: Without Dressing, 100g	30	120	0	5.5
Sweetslaw with Dressing, 100g	85	360	5	10
Mashed Potato: Plain, 475g pkt	460	1930	20	58
With Roasted Garlic, 475g packet	415	1730	16	54
Rainbow Salad, ½ packet, 125g	35	145	0.5	6
Vegetables: *Per Serving, without Dressing*				
Baby Spinach, 50g	15	65	0	1
Italian Salad, 100g	20	80	0	2
Deli Salads: Coleslaw, ½ tub, 125g	135	560	6	19
Coleslaw, Low Fat, ⅓ tub, 134g	90	365	2	15
Creamy Pasta Salad, ½ tub, 125g	260	1090	15	26
Creamy Potato Salad, ½ tub, 125g	140	575	6	19
Light & Tasty Pasta Salad, ½ tub, 200g	240	1005	3.5	43
Pasta Salad: W. Mushrooms & Aioli, 150g	290	1210	20	20
W. Sundried Tom. Pesto & Bocconcini, 150g	250	1035	12	23

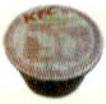

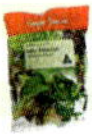

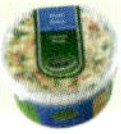

Gourmet Deli Foods | Cal | kJ | Fat | Cb

Antipasto in Oil: *Per ¼ Cup, 50g*

	Cal	kJ	Fat	Cb
With Green Olives, Sweet Potato, Mushrooms and Red Peppers, 50g	60	255	4.5	3.5
With Black Olives & Sundried Tomatoes	90	365	7.5	3
With Fetta, Olives & Sundried Tomatoes	120	495	9.5	4.5

Artichokes:

	Cal	kJ	Fat	Cb
In Brine, 50g	15	65	0.5	0.5
Marinated in Oil, 50g	50	195	4.5	7

Capsicum,

	Cal	kJ	Fat	Cb
Red, roasted, ¼ cup, 50g	20	75	0	3

Dolmades:

	Cal	kJ	Fat	Cb
Vine Leaf stuffed: With Rice, in oil, (1), 30g	45	195	2.5	6
With Sundried Tomatoes & Fetta (1), 30g	45	180	2.5	4.5

Eggplant:

	Cal	kJ	Fat	Cb
Marinated in Oil, grilled, (4 pieces) 55g	45	180	2	4
Strips, in oil, 1/4 cup, 45g	45	195	2.5	0.5

Marinated Dipping Sticks:

	Cal	kJ	Fat	Cb
Carrot (2), 30g	20	85	0	4.5
Cucumber (1), 30g	20	80	0	4
Mixed Chillies in Brine, 20g	5	20	0	0.2

Mushrooms:

	Cal	kJ	Fat	Cb
In Brine, ¼ cup, 30g	20	75	0	2.5
Marinated in Oil, 30g	15	60	1	1.5

Olives: *Per 5 Olives, 5g*

	Cal	kJ	Fat	Cb
Plain, in Lemon/Vinegar/Chilli & Garlic	50	210	3.5	3
Stuffed Green: With Anchovies	60	260	5	1
With Blue Vein Cheese	70	280	4.5	5
With Parmesan	65	275	4.5	4.5
With Salmon	65	270	5	1.5
Kalamata (Black), pitted, in Brine, Chilli/Lemon/Garlic, (5), 10g	20	80	1.5	1.5

Sun-Dried Tomatoes: *Per Serving*

	Cal	kJ	Fat	Cb
Natural, 5-6 pieces, 10g	20	90	0	5
Always Fresh: In oil, 22g	50	205	2.5	5
Spread, 1 Tbsp, 25g	65	270	5.5	3
Sun Dried, in Oil (5 pieces) 22g	50	205	2.5	5
Semi Sun Dried: In Oil (5 pieces), 22g	45	180	2.5	4
99% Fat Free, 22g	25	105	0	4

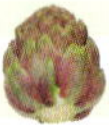

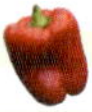

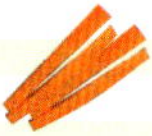

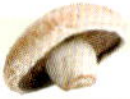

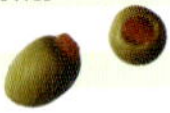

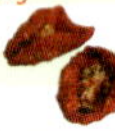

Sushi: Japanese ~ *See Page 182*

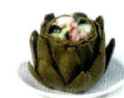

146

Salads ~ Deli ◆ Dressings

Deli-Style & Home Salads — Cal | kJ | Fat | Cb

Medium Serve:
Per ½ cup, 140g. For Large Serving, Double the Figures

Item	Cal	kJ	Fat	Cb
Apple & Celery	70	290	3	8
Bean	170	710	6	17
Bulghur	70	290	2	12
Button Mushroom	120	500	8	10
Carrot & Raisin	70	290	1	5
Caesar	190	795	13	15
Chicken	170	710	8	7
Coleslaw: Regular dressing	150	625	7	18
Light dressing	80	335	1.5	11
Crabmeat	280	1170	14	12
Cucumber: Non-Oil Dressing	60	250	0	14
With Oil Dressing	140	585	9	8
Egg, with mayonnaise	200	835	16	8
Fettuccini, with vegetables	120	500	5	15
Fresh Fruit	60	250	0	14
Greek	150	625	13	6
Pasta/Macaroni	210	880	11	16
Potato: With Mayonnaise	180	750	11	16
With Yoghurt Dressing	140	585	4	16
Rice	160	670	10	13
Shrimp	240	1005	22	8
Spinach	40	165	0	3.5
Tuna	300	1255	25	5
Tabouli	180	755	13	14
Waldorf	150	625	12	10

Note: To minimize cal/kJ/fat in salads, use low-fat or fat-free salad dressings in place of regular dressings.

Salad Dressings ~ Brands — Cal | kJ | Fat | Cb

Per Tablespoon, 20g

Item	Cal	kJ	Fat	Cb
Beerenberg: Blue Cheese	50	200	4.5	2
Caesar Creamy Parmesan	50	205	4.5	2.5
Honey Mustard	40	175	3	5
Ranch Gourmet	65	280	6.5	3
Taka Tala	60	260	5	3
Cardini's, Caesar, 1 Tbsp	110	455	12	0.5
Coles: *Per Tablespoon*				
99% Fat Free, Balsamic	10	35	0	2
98% Fat Free, Greek	10	45	0	2
Asian	65	270	4	6.5
Balsamic Vinaigrette	50	200	5	1.5
Caesar	80	320	8	1
Coleslaw	70	300	5.5	6
Italian	65	270	5	6
Mango Chilli	50	190	3	5.5
Smart Buy: French	15	65	0	3.5
Italian	20	75	0	5.5
Edmonds *(Aldi):*				
Classic: French, 100% fat free	15	65	0	4
Italian, 100% fat free	10	40	0	2
Eta, Potato Salad, 20g	50	210	4	3
Heinz:				
Salad Cream, 25g	115	475	11	4
Lite Salad Cream, 25g	60	260	5	4
Kraft: *Per Tablespoon, 20g*				
Regular: Caesar	65	265	6	1.5
Coleslaw	75	315	6	5
French	40	165	3	2
Italian	40	160	3.5	2
Pasta: Basil & Herbs	70	285	6	3.5
Tangy Tomato	90	375	8	5
Potato	75	300	6.5	3
Thousand Island	70	285	6	3.5
99% Fat-Free: Balsamic	15	60	0	3
Caesar	20	70	0	3
Chilli & Lime	15	55	0	3
Coleslaw	30	115	0	6
French	10	40	0	2
Italian	15	50	0	2.5
Miracle Whip, 1 Tbsp, 20g	75	320	7.5	2.5
Potato Salad, Original Style	70	285	6	3

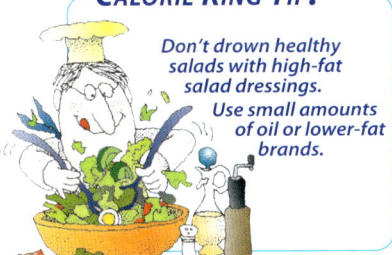

CALORIE KING TIP!

Don't drown healthy salads with high-fat salad dressings. Use small amounts of oil or lower-fat brands.

Updated Nutrition Data ~ www.CalorieKing.com.au
Persons with Diabetes ~ See Disclaimer (Page 22)

Salad Dressings

Salad Dressings (Cont)

	Cal	kJ	Fat	Cb
Ozganics: *Per 20ml*				
Avocado	35	150	3.5	2
Creamy Caesar	30	135	3.5	0.5
Italian	20	80	0	5
Lemon Myrtle	35	145	3.5	1
Paul Newman's Own: *Per 20g*				
Balsamic	35	150	3.5	2
Classic	30	120	3	1
Classic Asian	40	170	3	3
Creamy Caesar	110	455	12	1
Ranch	120	495	13	1
South West	100	425	11	2
Light: Honey Mustard	45	195	3	5
Balsamic	30	130	3	1
Perfect Additions *(Aldi): Per Tbsp, 20ml*				
Balsamic	45	180	3.5	3.5
Caesar	65	270	5	4
Praise: *Per Tbsp, 20ml*				
Thousand Island	55	235	4	5
Coleslaw	85	360	7.5	5
French	45	185	3.5	3
Italian	40	165	3.5	2
99% Fat-Free: Balsamic	10	40	0	2.5
Caesar; Coleslaw	25	100	0	5.5
French; Ranch	15	65	0	4
Italian	10	35	0	1
Deli Style:				
Balsamic & Roasted Garlic	40	175	3.5	2
Honey & Dijon Mustard	45	195	3.5	3.5
Spritz: *Per 2-3 Second Spray, 5ml*				
All varieties	2	5	0	0.5
S&W: *Per Tbsp, 20ml*				
Blue Cheese	40	165	4	1
Honey Mustard	45	190	4	2.5
Simply Less *(Coles): Per Tablespoon, 20ml*				
Aioli: Whole Egg	80	330	8	2
97% Fat-Free: Asian	20	90	1	3
Caesar	30	135	0.5	6
Balsamic Honey Mustard	25	110	0.5	4.5
Mango Chilli	20	75	0.5	3
Taylor's: *Per Tablespoon, 20ml*				
Avocado & Garlic	75	300	6	5
Balsamic Vinaigrette	20	80	0	4.5
Caesar	45	195	3.5	3.5
Creamy Italian	75	315	6	5
French	20	80	0	4.5
Mango Vinaigrette	25	100	0	6
Woolworths: *Per Tbsp, 20ml*				
Home Brand: French	15	65	0	3.5
Italian	20	75	0	5.5
Thousand Island	55	225	3.5	5

Salad Dressings (Cont)

	Cal	kJ	Fat	Cb
Woolworths (Cont): *Per Tbsp, 20ml*				
Select: Balsamic	40	175	3	4
Caesar	80	325	7	4
Coleslaw	70	295	5.5	5
Honey Mustard	80	345	6	7
Italian	50	215	4.5	3
Ranch	120	510	12	2
Zesty Portuguese	90	375	7.5	5.5
99% Fat-Free: Balsamic Italian	20	85	0	5
French	20	75	0	4.5
Greek	15	60	0	3.5
Italian	15	65	0	4

Mayonnaise ~ Brands

Per Tbsp, 20ml, Unless Indicated

	Cal	kJ	Fat	Cb
Best Foods, Real Mayonnaise	140	590	16	0.5
Coles: Whole Egg Mayonnaise	145	605	16	0.5
97% Fat Free Mayonnaise	25	105	0.5	5
Colway *(Aldi):*				
Squeezy: Creamy Mayonnaise	60	255	5	4.5
Light Mayonnaise	30	125	0.5	6
Mayonnaise	40	160	2	5
Real Mayonnaise	150	615	16	0.5
Heinz: Whole Egg, 25g	170	720	19	0.5
Mayonnaise Aioli with Dill	170	720	19	0.5
Hellmann's: Real Mayonnaise	140	595	16	0.5
Light	55	235	5	1.5
Kraft: 97% Fat-Free	25	100	0.5	4.5
Classic	50	195	4	2.5
Creamy	100	410	10	3
Egg with Omega 3	140	585	16	0.5
Melrose: Organic	75	320	7.5	3
Organic Dijonnaise	75	320	7.5	3
Nando's:				
Perinaise: Original	45	195	3.5	4
Hot	40	155	3	3
Norganic: Organic	45	190	4.5	1.5
Golden Soya	130	550	15	0.5
Paul Newman's Own:				
Aioli: Whole Egg	140	585	15	0.5
Whole Egg, Lime & Chilli	130	550	15	1
Whole Egg	150	615	17	0.5
Praise: *Per Tablespoon, 20g*				
Dijonnaise, 97% Fat Free	25	100	0.5	5
Traditional Mayonnaise	135	560	15	2
Whole Egg Mayonnaise	150	620	17	0.5
Light Whole Egg Mayonnaise	65	270	5.5	3
Weight Watchers, 20g	25	100	0.5	5
Woolworths/Select: Whole Egg	145	610	16	1
97% Fat-Free Mayonnaise, 20g	30	130	0.5	6.5

Sauces ◆ Cooking/Seasoning S

Sauces/Condiments
	Cal	kJ	Fat	Cb
Per 1 Tbsp, 20ml				
Apple Sauce, average	30	125	0	5
Bechamel Sauce	35	145	2	2
Bernaise Sauce	70	295	7	0.5
BBQ Sauce: *(Fountain; Rosella)*, average	35	145	0	9
Honey BBQ	40	170	0	10
Smokey BBQ	40	170	0	10
40% Lower Sugar	25	110	0	6
Beetroot in Red Currant	35	145	0	8
Black Bean Sauce	20	85	0.5	4
Cheese Sauce, average	45	185	3.5	1.5
Chilli Sauce:				
Hot Chilli *(Fountain)*	40	165	0.5	8
Mild Chilli *(Fountain)*	15	65	1	3
Sweet Thai Chilli *(Chang's)*	35	150	0	9
Sweet Chilli *(Fountain)*	40	165	0	10
Sweet Chilli *(Trident)*	45	195	0	11
Cranberry Jelly, 40g	60	250	0	16
Cranberry Sauce, 15g	35	145	0	9
HP Sauce: Original	30	115	0	6.5
BBQ	30	130	0	7.5
Hoisin Sauce	15	60	0	2
Hollandaise Sauce	70	295	7	4
Honey & Soy: *Kan Tong*, 30g	45	180	0.5	9
Ayam, 30g	45	180	0	10
Horseradish Cream *(Masterfoods)*	35	155	2	4
Marinades:				
Taylor's: Thai Satay	50	210	3	5.5
Other varieties	55	230	0	5
Masterfoods ~ See Page 155				
Mint Jelly *(MasterFoods)*, 25g	65	280	0	17
Mint Sauce: Average	20	85	0	4
Fountain	15	65	0	4
Mustard, average all types, 1 tsp	5	25	0	1
1 Tbsp, 20g	25	100	1	2
Oyster Sauce	30	115	0	5.5
Pepper Steak	30	130	0	7.5
Pesto: Classic, average, 1 Tbsp, 20g	85	360	9	1
½ cup, 125g	540	2255	55	5.5
Picalilli *(Crosse & Blackwell)*, 20g	60	255	1.5	10
Plum Sauce, average	50	210	0	12
Red Currant Jelly, average, 20g	55	235	0	14
Satay Sauce, average	70	285	5	5
Seafood Cocktail: *McCormick*,	55	230	4	4
MasterFoods, average, 30g	65	265	3.5	7
Soy Sauce: Regular, average	10	45	0	0.5
Light	10	40	0	1.5

Sauces/Condiments (Cont)
	Cal	kJ	Fat	Cb
Per 1 Tbsp, 20ml				
Spicy Red/Plum Sauce, average	50	210	0	12
Steak Sauce, average	40	165	0	10
Sweet & Sour: *MasterFoods*	30	125	0	7.5
Empower, 20ml	10	40	0	2
Tabasco Sauce	2	10	0	0.5
Taco Sauce	5	25	0	1
Taco Seasoning Mix, 3g	10	35	0	1.5
Tamari *(Pureharvest)*,	20	75	0	1.5
Tartare Sauce: *Taylors*, 20g	80	340	7.5	4
MasterFoods: Tartare, 20g	125	515	13	1.5
Portion Control, 14g	85	360	9	1
Teriyaki: Marinade	20	75	0	3
Sauce, 20ml	40	175	0	12
White Sauce, average, 1 Tbsp	35	145	2	3
Worcestershire Sauce, 1 Tbsp	20	85	0	4.5

Tomato Sauce & Products
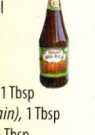
	Cal	kJ	Fat	Cb
Tomato Sauce: 1 Tbsp, 15ml	15	65	0	3.5
¼ cup, 63ml	65	275	0	16
Big Red, 1 Tbsp	20	95	0	5
Rosella, Low Joule, 1 Tbsp	10	50	0	2
No Added Salt *(Fountain)*, 1 Tbsp	25	110	0	6
40% Lower Sugar *(Fountain)*, 1 Tbsp	20	75	0	4
Tomato Ketchup *(Heinz)*, 1 Tbsp	25	100	0	5
Tomato Paste:				
Average, 100g	70	300	1	9
Ardmona, 150g Tub	90	385	0	14
Fountain, 100g	70	290	1	12
Leggo's:				
Tomato Paste, 140g Tub	95	385	0.5	16
Garlic & Herb, 140g Tub	95	400	0.5	16
No Added Salt, 140g Tub	95	385	0.5	15
Tomato Puree: average, 100g	30	120	0.5	4.5
410g Can	120	490	0	17
Pizza Sauce:				
Ardmona, 140g Tub	45	190	0	6
Leggo's, 140g Tub	75	310	0.5	11
Canned Tomato ~ See Page 172				

Vinegar, Balsamic Vinegar
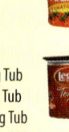
	Cal	kJ	Fat	Cb
Vinegar, average all types, 1 Tbsp, 20ml	5	10	0	1
Honey & Apple Cider Vinegar *(Wescobee)*, 1 Tbsp, 20ml	0	2	0	0

Updated Nutrition Data ~ www.CalorieKing.com.au
Persons with Diabetes ~ See Disclaimer (Page 22)

S Sauces ◆ Gravy ◆ Salsa ◆ Seasoning

Gravy

	Cal	kJ	Fat	Cb
Homemade: *Prepared*				
Thin: 1 Tbsp, 20ml	10	40	0	2
¼ cup, 60ml	30	125	0.5	6
Thick: 1 Tbsp, 20ml	20	85	0	5
¼ cup, 60ml	60	250	0.5	15
Gravox ~ *See Page 152*				
Maggi, all flavours, ¼ packet, average	25	105	0.5	6
Massel, ¼ cup, made up	20	80	0	4.5
White Wings, ¼ cup, made up	20	95	0.1	5

Salsa ~ Brands

	Cal	kJ	Fat	Cb
Average all Types:				
No oil added, 1 Tbsp, 20g	10	45	0	1.5
With Oil, 1 Tbsp, 20g	25	105	1.5	1.5
Doritos, Salsa Dip, avg., 20g	10	35	0	1.5
El Tora *(Aldi)*,				
Salsa Dip, Medium/Mild, 30g	20	80	0	4
Lite N' Easy, 28g	20	85	0	4
MasterFoods ~ *See Page 155*				
Old El Paso, avg all flavours, 1 Tbsp, 25g	10	40	0	1.5

Sauces ~ Brands

	Cal	kJ	Fat	Cb
Abundant Earth:				
Organic Soy Tamari: 2 tsp, 10ml	5	20	0	0.5
Reduced-Salt, 2 tsp, 10ml	10	35	0	1
Asia at Home:				
Stir Fry Paste:				
Green Curry, 14g	25	110	2	1.5
Pad Thai, 21g	55	235	1	12
Red Curry, 14g	20	95	2	1.5
Stir Fry Sauce:				
Black Bean, 75g	70	285	0.5	13
Szechuan, 75g	90	380	3	14
Teriyaki & Honey, 75g	90	385	0.5	21
Thai Satay, 75g	155	640	7.5	20
Ayam: *Per 3 tsp, 18g*				
Black Bean	15	70	0	3.5
Fish	1	5	0	0.1
Hoi Sin /Plum	35	140	0.5	7
Honey Soy Marinade	30	110	0.5	6
Oyster	25	95	0.5	5.5
Soya	10	45	0.5	2
Sweet Chilli, 24g	60	260	0	16
Teriyaki	5	25	0	1

Beerenberg:

	Cal	kJ	Fat	Cb
Apple, 50g	55	225	0	15
BBQ, 20g	30	125	0	7
Chilli, 20g	30	120	0	7
Coopers Ale BBQ, 20g	25	115	0	7
Cranberry, 20g	40	165	0	10
Garlic, 20g	60	250	6	2
Hot Tomato, 20g	20	90	0	5
Peppercorn, 20g	60	245	0	1
Pepper Steak, 20g	20	75	0	4.5
Spicy Plum, 20g	35	135	0	8
Sweet Mustard, 20g	20	90	0	4.5
Smokey Bourbon, 20g	40	175	0	9
Sticky Rib, 20g	40	155	0	9
Taka Tala, 20g	50	205	1.5	8.5
Tomato, 20g	20	80	0	4.5
Worcestershire, 20g	30	130	0	7
Campbell's: *Per ¼ of 415g Can, 140g*				
Spaghetti Sauce: Bolognese	90	380	3	11
With Beef	155	650	6.5	14
Casa Barelli *(Aldi): Per ¼ of 500g Jar*				
Basilico, 125g	75	310	4	7.5
Bolognese, 125g	75	315	4	6
Napoletana, 125g	70	300	2.5	9
Chang's: *Per Tablespoon, 20ml*				
Beijing	25	95	1	3
Black Bean	15	65	0	3
Fish	15	70	0	1.5
Hoisin	15	60	0	2
Hot Chilli	15	60	0	2
Light Soy	10	35	0	1.5
Mongolian	25	95	0.5	3.5
Oyster	15	65	0	3.5
Ponzu	30	135	0	7.5
Soy	10	30	0	1.5
Spicy Sichuan	25	115	1	4
Sweet Manchurian	20	90	0.5	3.5
Tasty Sichuan	20	70	0	3
Thai Sweet Chilli	35	150	0	9

Sauces ◆ Cooking/Seasoning S

Chicken Tonight: Per ¼ 475g Jar:	Cal	kJ	Fat	Cb
Apricot Chicken, 125g	75	310	0.5	17
Butter Chicken, 123g	145	605	10	11
Chicken Honey Soy, 125g	95	400	0.5	21
Country French Chicken, 118g	135	570	13	5.5
Creamy Chicken with Mushrooms	120	505	11	4.5
Creamy Lemon Chicken, 120g	125	525	10	8.5
Malay Satay, 126g	90	370	3.5	12
Lite: Butter Chicken, 121g	90	380	3.5	14
Creamy Chicken with Mushroom, 120g	55	230	3.5	5.5
Golden Honey Mustard, 122g	95	390	3.5	14

Coles:
Organic: Per ¼ of 500g Jar, 125g

	Cal	kJ	Fat	Cb
Garlic Lovers	65	275	0.5	14
Italian	45	195	1	8
Nice N Spicy	55	240	0.5	12
Traditional	65	265	0.5	12

Pasta Sauce: Per ¼ of 500g Jar, 125g

	Cal	kJ	Fat	Cb
Arrabbiata	65	265	3	7.5
Basillico	75	310	3.5	7.5
Bolognese	65	265	3.5	6
Napoletana	100	415	6	8.5
Romana	120	500	8	8

Continental:
Recipe Bases: Per ¼ Sachet, Prepared as Directed

	Cal	kJ	Fat	Cb
Apricot Chicken Curry	495	2070	23	20
Bangers & Mash	820	3430	58	44
Beef & Red Wine Casserole	255	1070	10	12
Beef Goulash	310	1290	10	22
Beef Stroganoff	280	1170	14	10
Butter Chicken	400	1670	21	10
Chilli Con Carne	320	1330	12	19
Chow Mein Mince	375	1570	12	33
Chunky Beef Pie	520	2170	25	28
Creamy Chicken & Vegetable	460	1930	18	33
Creamy Chicken Curry	465	1940	12	54
Creamy Mushroom Chicken	320	1330	17	11
Creamy Potato Bake	375	1570	22	33
Creamy Tuna Mornay	425	1780	6	31
Curried Sausages	635	2650	50	19
Devilled Sausages	660	2750	50	25
Homestyle Meatloaf	290	1220	15	7
Rissoles	280	1170	15	7.5
Smokey Beef Casserole	390	1640	16	17

Continental (Cont):

Lite Recipe Bases: Per ¼ Sachet, Prepared as Directed

	Cal	kJ	Fat	Cb
Beef Stroganoff	250	1040	10	11
Beef & Vegetable Casserole	300	1250	7.5	25
Country Chicken Casserole	290	1210	7.5	23
Mediterranean Chicken	250	1050	7.5	14
Malayasian Creamy Satay	335	1400	18	11
Mild Mince Curry	275	1140	13	10
Rich Beef Casserole	270	1130	7.5	18
Rich Beefy Mince	280	1160	12	15
Shepherd's Pie	445	1860	16	40
Spaghetti Bolognaise	490	2040	12	58

Instant Sauce Mixes: Per ¼ Sachet, Prepared as Directed

	Cal	kJ	Fat	Cb
Cheese	50	215	2	8
Cheese, Bacon & Chives	40	165	1	6.5
Four Cheeses	35	150	1	6.5
Hollandaise	60	260	3	8.5
Mushroom	35	155	1.5	6
Pepper	35	145	0.5	7.5
Steak Diane	35	150	0.5	8
White Sauce	45	190	1.5	8

Cornwell's:
Mint Sauces: Per 30ml

	Cal	kJ	Fat	Cb
Regular	20	90	0	5.5
Thick Mint	25	95	0	5.5

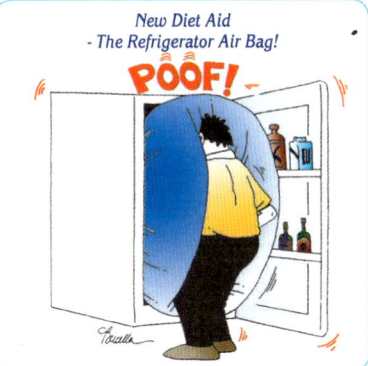

New Diet Aid - The Refrigerator Air Bag!

POOF!

Updated Nutrition Data ~ www.CalorieKing.com.au
Persons with Diabetes ~ See Disclaimer (Page 22)

Sauces ♦ Cooking/Seasoning

Dolmio:

Pasta Sauce: *Per 580g Jar*

	Cal	kJ	Fat	Cb
Carbonara, ¼ Jar	150	620	10	13
Creamy Mushroom, ¼ Jar	150	610	10	12
Lasagne: Extra Cheese, ⅙ Jar	105	450	7.5	8.5
Thick Tomato, ⅙ Jar	75	310	2	11

Extra: Bolognesse

	Cal	kJ	Fat	Cb
Bolognesse	90	370	2.5	14
Creamy Mushroom	145	605	10	12
Creamy Sundried Tom. & Garlic	115	485	6.5	13
Four Cheese	85	360	3	12
Garden Vegetable	75	305	0.5	14
Garlic	90	375	2.5	14
Italian Herb	80	325	1	15
Mushroom	70	295	1	13
Spicy Peppers	80	340	2	14
Red Wine & Italian Herbs	85	360	1	15
Rustic Farmhouse Vege	80	335	0.5	15
Tomato, Onion & Garlic: Reg.	80	340	1	15
Salt Reduced	80	345	0.5	15

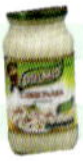

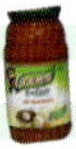

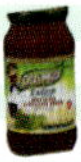

Italian Meal Base: *Per ¼ of 170g Pouch*

	Cal	kJ	Fat	Cb
Carbonara	30	120	1.5	3.5
Cheesy Bolognese	40	170	2.5	5
Chicken Alfredo	25	105	0.5	4.5
Homestyle Macaroni Cheese	20	80	0.5	4

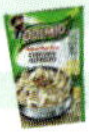

Pasta Bake: *Per ¼ of 530g-540g Jar*

	Cal	kJ	Fat	Cb
Creamy Tomato & Mozzarella	135	565	8	13
Three Cheese	160	665	11	13
Tomato with Cheese	120	505	6	14
Tuna Bake	165	685	11	13

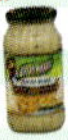

Traditional All Natural: *Per ¼ of 550g Jar*

	Cal	kJ	Fat	Cb
Basil	90	375	2	15
Classic Tomato	90	380	2	17
Salt Reduced	90	385	2	15

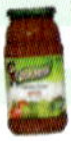

Pesto: *Per ¼ of 165g Jar*

	Cal	kJ	Fat	Cb
Basil	55	225	4.5	2.5
Sundried Tomato	85	360	6.5	6

Eastern Classics (Aldi): *Per ¼ Jar*

Stir Fry: Satay, 125g

	Cal	kJ	Fat	Cb
Satay, 125g	255	1060	20	14
Sweet Chilli, 137g	160	670	0.5	37
Sweet Soy & Garlic, 137g	145	600	0.5	33

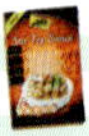

Five Brothers:

Pasta Sauce: *Per ¼ of 500g Jar*

	Cal	kJ	Fat	Cb
Bolognesse	65	275	1.5	9
Five Cheeses	75	300	1.5	10
Grilled Summer Vegetable	65	275	0.5	12
Oven Roasted Garlic with Wine	65	265	0.5	10
Oven Roasted Garlic & Onion	60	250	0.5	10
Portobello Mushroom & Garlic	65	270	1	11
Summer Tomato Basil	55	230	0.5	10

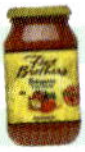

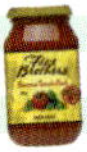

Gourmet Garden:

Herb Paste: *Per 1 teaspoon, 5g*

	Cal	kJ	Fat	Cb
Basil	10	45	0.5	1.5
Chilli, Hot/Mild	10	35	0	1.5
Chives/Dill	15	55	0.5	2
Coriander	10	30	0.5	1
Garlic	10	45	0.5	1
Ginger	10	45	0	2.5
Italian Herb Blend	10	45	0.5	1.5
Lemongrass	15	60	1	2
Mint	10	40	0	2.5
Oregano	10	50	0.5	1.5
Parsley	10	45	0.5	1.5
Rosemary	15	60	1	2

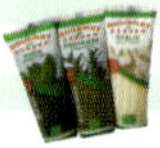

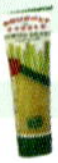

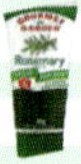

Gravox:

Gravy, Liquid: *Per ⅓ of 165g Pouch*

	Cal	kJ	Fat	Cb
Brown Onion	20	80	0.5	4
Chicken & Herb	25	95	0.5	3
Lamb & Rosemary	15	60	0.5	3
Roast Meat w. Red Wine & Garlic	20	80	0.5	3
Roast Pork	15	70	0.5	3

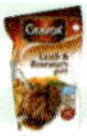

Box Powder: *Per ¼ Cup, 62.5ml, Prepared as Directed*

	Cal	kJ	Fat	Cb
Fuller Flavour	20	75	0.5	4
Lite Supreme	20	75	0.5	4
Supreme Chicken	20	70	0.5	4
Supreme	15	65	0.5	4
Traditional	15	65	0.5	4

Mix Sachet, all flavors,

	Cal	kJ	Fat	Cb
¼ cup, 62.5 ml, prepared	25	105	0.5	4

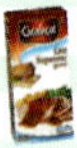

Sauces: *Sachets, per ¼ Cup, 62.5ml, Prepared as Directed*

	Cal	kJ	Fat	Cb
Cheese	30	130	1	5
Mushroom & Garlic	25	100	0.5	5
Pepper	25	115	0.5	5
White	35	135	1.5	4.5

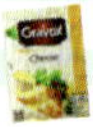

Gourmet: *Per ⅓ of 165g Pouch*

	Cal	kJ	Fat	Cb
Peppercorn & Cream	45	185	3	4
Roast Beef with Shiraz	30	120	1	3

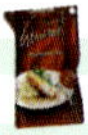

Heinz:

Sauces: *Per Tablespoon, 20 ml*

	Cal	kJ	Fat	Cb
Big BBQ	25	110	0	6
Dijon Mustard with Orange	40	170	2.5	4.5
Peppered	40	165	0	9
Tomato: With Capsicum & Chilli	30	115	0	6
Big Red	20	90	0	5
Lite	20	90	0	4
Ketchup	25	100	0	5

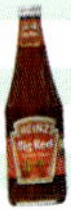

Sauces ♦ Cooking/Seasoning S

	Cal	kJ	Fat	Cb
Indian Tonight:				
Sauces: *Per ¼ of 495g Jar*				
Butter Chicken	145	605	10	11
Creamy Tandoori	110	455	7.5	9
Lite Butter Chicken	90	380	3.5	14
Just Organic *(Aldi): Per ¼ of 500g Jar*				
Basil & Garlic, 125g	90	380	2	16
Traditional, 125g	90	375	2	15
Kan Tong:				
Inspirations: *Per ½ of 160g Pouch*				
Chicken & Cashew Nut	145	615	2.5	30
Chow Mein	65	275	1.5	10
Fragrant Thai Green Curry	65	280	1	13
Honey, Soy & Garlic	65	275	1.5	10
Lemon Chicken	90	385	0	22
Malaysian Satay	120	495	5.5	15
Massaman Curry	75	305	2	13
Sizzling Black Bean	65	270	2.5	8
Sizzling Mongolian	95	385	2	17
Sweet Thai Chilli Noodles	110	460	3.5	18
Teriyaki Sesame	105	435	3.5	17
Simply Stir Fry: *Per ¼ of 350g Bottle*				
Chilli, Garlic & Soy	50	205	0.5	10
Honey & Garlic	95	400	0.5	21
Honey Teriyaki	140	575	2.5	28
Sweet & Sour	120	495	0	29
Sweet Plum	95	400	0.5	23
Stir Fry: *Per ¼ of 575g Jar*				
Black Bean	130	530	4.5	18
Butter Chicken	195	800	15	13
Chinese Barbecue	145	610	1.5	31
Honey, Sesame & Garlic	195	800	4	43
Lemon Chicken	160	655	0.5	38
Peanut Satay	175	735	8.5	20
Sizzling Mongolian	150	635	3.5	28
Sweet & Sour	140	590	0	34
Lite	115	475	0.5	28
Pineapple	150	625	0.5	36
Plum	140	585	0	34
Sweet Soy & Garlic	115	480	0	27
Latina Fresh:				
Pasta Sauces: *Per ¼ of 425g Tub*				
Beef Bolognese	65	270	2.5	5.5
Creamy Carbonara	160	665	11	7
Creamy Sundried Tomato	75	310	5.5	3.5
Italian Tomato & Garlic	60	240	3	5.5

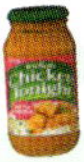

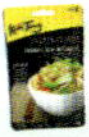

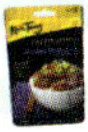

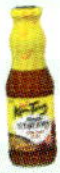

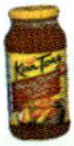

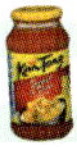

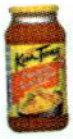

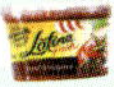

	Cal	kJ	Fat	Cb
Leggo's:				
Pasta Sauces:				
Chunky: *Per ¼ of 575g Jar*				
Bolognese: With Bacon	95	385	3	12
With Mushrooms	85	360	2.5	12
With Red Wine	105	445	4	13
Creamy: Alfredo	175	725	15	8
Carbonara	135	555	10	8
Grilled Vegetables	70	290	1.5	11
Napoletana	100	400	4	12
Hidden Veg: Bolognese	70	295	0.5	11
Cheesy Tomato	70	290	0.5	13
Classic Tomato	70	290	0.5	13
Pasta Bake: *Per ¼ of 575g Jar*				
Creamy Sundried Tomato	105	435	6	10
Creamy Tomato & Mozzarella	100	420	3.5	12
Tomato, Ricotta & Spinach	125	510	7.5	9
Tuna, Spinach & Garlic	140	585	11	7.5
Spaghetti Sauce: *Per ⅓ of 425g Can*				
Sauce with Beef, 141g	105	425	4.5	8.5
Stir Through: *Per ¼ of 350g Jar*				
Chargrilled Vegetables	105	430	7.5	7.5
Roasted Tomato & Bacon	75	305	4.5	5.5
Spinach & Ricotta	135	570	12	4
Sundried Tomato & Roasted Garlic	110	450	8	7
Simmer Sauce: *Per ¼ of 450g Jar*				
Italian Chicken Parmigiana	70	290	2	10
Italian Chicken Scallopini	115	470	8	6
Pesto: *Per ¼ of 190g Jar*				
Traditional Basil	115	485	11	3
Sundried Tomato	100	415	8	4.5
Sugo di Pomodoro: *Per ¼ of 700g Bottle. 175g*				
Premium: Classic Tomato	70	300	0.5	11
Italian Herbs with Basil	75	310	0.5	12
Macro:				
Pasta Sauces: *Per ¼ of 375g Jar*				
Arrabiata	50	195	0	9
BBQ	20	85	0	5
Mediterranean	50	215	0	10
Sweet Chilli	40	175	0	10
Sauce, Tomato, 1 Tbsp, 20ml	20	80	0	4

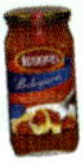

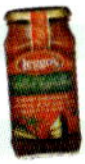

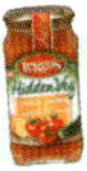

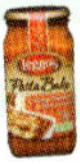

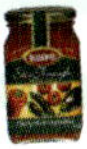

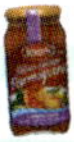

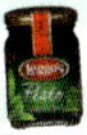

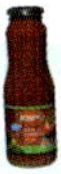

Updated Nutrition Data ~ www.CalorieKing.com.au
Persons with Diabetes ~ See Disclaimer (Page 22)

153

Sauces • Cooking/Seasoning

McCormick:

	Cal	kJ	Fat	Cb
Dinner Winner, Beef, ¼ pkt, prepared	325	1345	12	26
Herbs & Spices,				
Cheesy Pasta Sprinkle; Garlic Granules, 1g	5	15	0	0.5
One Pot: *Per ¼ Packet, Dry*				
Chicken & Leek Casserole	30	135	0.5	6
Herb & Potato Pot Pie	30	120	0	6
Homestyle Meatballs	35	140	1	5.5
Spanish Chicken & Potato Bake	30	130	1	5
Produce Partners: *Per ¼ Pkt, Prep'd as Directed*				
Cauliflower Supreme with Cheese	130	550	5	13
Country Style Roast Potatoes	210	880	4.5	35
Italian Herb Potato	205	845	5	32
Scalloped Potatoes	340	1415	17	38
Sour Cream & Chive Potato	205	855	6	30
Sauce Mix: *Per ¼ Packet, Prep'd as Directed*				
Cheese	85	350	4.5	8
Garlic & Pepper	70	300	4	8
Parsley White	75	305	4	7
Pepper with Peppercorns	35	140	0.5	7
Steak Diane with Garlic	40	175	1.5	7
Slow Cookers: *Per 40g Packet, Dry*				
Beef & Mushroom Ragout	115	475	0.5	26
Beef & Red Wine Casserole	115	480	0.5	27
Chicken, Bacon & Potato	125	515	2.5	21
Chunky Beef Stroganoff	120	495	1	23
Country Chicken Casserole	110	455	1	23
Garlic & Herb Lamb Shanks	110	465	0.5	23
Lamb & Vegetable Casserole	110	455	3.5	18
Mild Chicken Curry	95	400	1.5	17
Mild Indian Beef Curry	120	490	2.5	24
Moroccan Lamb Casserole	60	260	1.5	10
Osso Bucco	115	475	1	21
Portuguese Chicken	115	475	2	23
Roast Beef with Onion Gravy	125	525	1	28
Tomato, Onion & Sausages	140	595	1	31

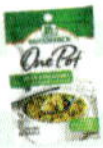

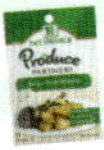

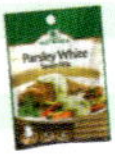

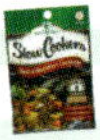

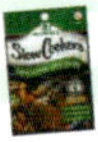

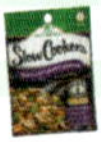

Maggi:

	Cal	kJ	Fat	Cb
Asian Sauces: *Per Tbsp, 20ml*				
Chilli	35	150	0	9
Fish	10	50	0	1
Liquid Seasoning	10	35	0	1
Oyster	25	105	0	5.5
Sweet Chilli	40	170	0	11

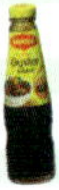

Maggi (Cont):

	Cal	kJ	Fat	Cb
Asian Sauce Mix: *Per ¼ Packet, Dry*				
Mince Chow Mein	35	140	1	6.5
Satay Chicken	40	160	1	7.5
Bakes: *Per ¼ Packet, Prepared*				
Bolognese	540	2260	17	57
Mince Cottage Pie	480	2000	20	42
Tuna	390	1630	7	55
Tuna & Potato Pie	450	1890	12	41
Favourites: *Per ¼ Packet, Dry*				
Apricot Chicken	35	150	0	8
Beef Goulash	35	150	0.5	6.5
Beef Stroganoff	45	190	1.5	7
Butter Chicken	25	100	0.5	4.5
Chicken Chasseur	35	135	0.5	5.5
Chilli Con Carne	40	170	1	8
Devilled Sausages	35	140	0	7
Lamb Casserole	35	155	0.5	7
Lamb Ragout	35	140	0.5	6.5
Instant Sauce Mix: *Per ¼ Packet, Prepare as Directed*				
Cheese & Garlic	45	195	2.5	5.5
Creamy White	35	150	1	4.5
Hollandaise	80	330	4	11
Tasty Cheese	45	195	2	6.5
Just One Pan: *Per 1/4 Pouch, Dry*				
Beef Stroganoff	70	300	5	6.5
Chinese Beef Stir Fry	75	315	3.5	11
Garlic & Parsley Chicken Rice	80	325	4	9
Honey Mustard Chicken	80	325	4	9
Honey Soy Chicken Stir Fry	80	320	3	11
Satay Chicken Rice	70	300	3.5	9
Spaghetti Bolognese	60	255	3.5	7
So Crispy: *Per ¼ Packet, Dry*				
Classic	80	345	1.5	15
Lemon & Herb	80	340	1.5	14
Parsley & Lemon	85	350	1.5	15
So Tender: *Per ¼ Packet, Dry*				
Chicken-in-Bag: Garlic	30	130	0.5	6
Oriental Soy	30	130	0	7
Ribs-in-Bag, BBQ	45	185	1	8.5
Roast-in-Bag, Mixed Herbs	30	130	0.5	5
Ten Minute Marinades: *Per ¼ Packet*				
BBQ	80	340	2.5	15
Honey Soy	85	350	3	14
Portuguese	60	255	2.5	9
Satay	65	270	2.5	11
Teriyaki	105	440	2.5	19

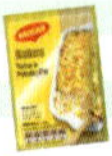

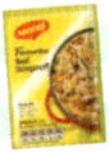

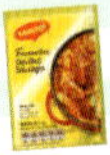

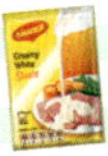

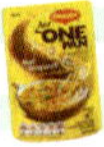

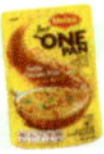

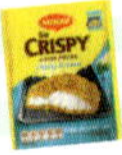

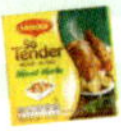

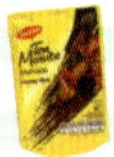

Sauces ◆ Cooking/Seasoning S

Maggi (Cont): | Cal | kJ | Fat | Cb
Vegetable Sides: *Per ¼ Packet, Prepare as Directed*

	Cal	kJ	Fat	Cb
Cheese & Bacon Potato Bake	20	75	0.5	4
Cheesy Cauliflower	30	120	1	3
Creamy Cheese & Garlic	25	95	1	3
Sour Cream & Chives	25	105	1.5	3
Tasty Cheese Vegetable Bake	30	125	1	4.5
Three Cheeses Potato Bake	25	95	1	3

Maggi Beer: *Per 1 Tbsp, 20g*

Sauce: Barossa Tomato Sauce	70	295	0.5	4
Cabernet Sauce	150	630	0.5	8.5
Ginger Chilli Sauce	150	630	0.5	8.5
Pastes, fruit, avg., 10g	25	110	0	6
Verjuice, 30 ml	15	65	0	4

MasterFoods:
Salsa, Chunky, Mild/Med., 30g	10	50	0	2.5
Bacon Chips, flavoured, 20g	75	305	3.5	5.5

Finishing Sauce: *Per ⅓ of 165g Pouch*

Bearnaise	70	300	6	4.5
Caramelised Onion w. Red Wine	35	140	0	7
Creamy White	80	320	6	5
Hollandaise	70	300	6	4.5
Mushroom & White Wine	70	295	5	5.5
Wholegrain Mustard w. Honey	85	360	4	12

Marinade: *Per 1/10 of 375g Bottle*

Honey BBQ	55	230	0	13
Moroccan	30	120	0.5	6
Mustard, Honey & Herb	55	225	0.5	11
Portuguese	25	100	0.5	5
Red Wine & Garlic	45	190	0	12
Satay	65	265	2	11
Smokey BBQ	50	215	0	13
Soy, Honey & Garlic	55	235	0	15
Sweet Plum	55	235	0	15
Teriyaki	65	260	0	15

Recipe Bases: *Per ¼ of 175g Pouch*

Classics: Apricot Chicken	25	100	0	5.5
Beef Stroganoff	45	180	2	6
Country Beef Casserole	20	90	0.5	4.5
Devilled Sausages	50	205	0	12
Italian Chicken Casserole	35	135	1	4.5
Spaghetti Bolognaise	35	135	0.5	5.5
Thai Green Curry	40	170	0.5	8

MasterFoods (Cont): | Cal | kJ | Fat | Cb
Recipe Bases (Cont): *Per ¼ of 175g Pouch*

	Cal	kJ	Fat	Cb
Master Mix: Chilli Con Carne	30	130	1	5
Lemon, Garlic & Herb Fish	25	105	0	4
Mild Chicken Tikka Masala	30	130	1	5
Moroccan Chicken	30	120	1	5

Slow Cooker:

Beef & Red Wine Casserole	30	120	0	6
Farmhouse Chicken Casserole	30	125	0	6.5
Garlic & Herb Lamb Shanks	35	145	0.5	7.5
Lamb Casserole	20	80	0	4
Mild Chicken Curry	40	165	0.5	9

Nando's:
Marinades: *Per Tablespoon, 20g*

Hot Peri-Peri	20	70	1	2.5
Lemon & Herb	15	65	0.5	2.5
Honey, Soy & Ginger	20	95	0.5	4.5
Portuguese BBQ	20	80	0.5	4
Roasted Red Pepper	25	110	1.5	2.5

Sauces: *Per Tablespoon, 20g*

Peri-Peri: Hot	20	70	1	2.5
Garlic	10	50	1	1.5
Lemon & Herb	20	85	1.5	2
Sweet Chilli with Lime	30	125	1	5.5

Simmer Sauces: *Per ¼ Jar*

Curry Coconut	60	230	3	7.5
Mediterranean Tomato	45	190	2	6
Mild Peri-Peri	55	220	2	9

Patak's:
Pastes: *Per 35 g Serving*

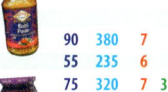

Balti	90	380	7	5
Butter Chicken	55	235	6	4
Korma, Coconut & Coriander	75	320	7	3.5
Rogan Josh	85	350	8.5	2.5
Tikka Masala	95	385	5.5	7
Vindaloo	95	395	2.5	8.5

Simmer Sauces: *Per ⅓ of 350g Jar*

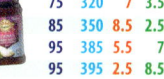

Butter Chicken	140	580	10	13
Korma	185	760	15	11
Mango Chicken	120	495	6.5	14
Rogan Josh	80	335	4	9
Tikka Masala	140	590	12	7.5
Vindaloo	140	570	10	10

Updated Nutrition Data ~ www.CalorieKing.com.au
Persons with Diabetes ~ See Disclaimer (Page 22)

155

Sauces ♦ Cooking/Seasoning

Paul Newman's Own:	Cal	kJ	Fat	Cb
Pasta Sauces: *Per ⅕ of 680g Jar*				
Homestyle Bolognese	75	310	2	12
Red Wine Bolognese	70	300	2.5	10
Roasted Garlic & Basil	75	310	2	12
Tomato, Basil & Garlic	110	450	4	15
Passage Foods:				
Passage To China, Stir Fry Sauce,				
Honey, Soy & Garlic, ¼ 200g pouch	50	215	0	12
Passage To India:				
Simmer Sauce: *Per ¼ of 375g Pouch*				
Balti Cury	135	565	11	7.5
Butter Chicken	160	670	12	13
Rogan Josh	130	540	11	6.5
Vindaloo	125	510	11	5.5
Passage To Italy:				
Simmer Sauce: *Per ¼ of 375g Pouch*				
Cherry Tomato Bolognese	90	360	6.5	6
Cherry Tomato Marinara	90	360	6	6
Cherry Tomato Napoletana	100	420	8	6
Stir-Fry Sauce: *Per ¼ of 200g Pouch*				
Pad Thai	80	335	0.5	18
Thai Basil & Sweet Chilli	60	240	0.5	12
Passage To Malaysia, Simmer Sauce,				
Beef Rendang, ¼ 200g pouch	85	350	1.5	16

Passage Foods (Cont):	Cal	kJ	Fat	Cb
Passage To Morocco:				
Simmer Sauce: *Per ¼ of 200g Pouch*				
Apricot Chicken	80	340	3	14
Honey Lamb	65	275	2.5	10
Lemon Chicken	55	230	3	7
Raguletto:				
Classic Tomato Sauces: *Per ½ Cup, 125g*				
Bolognese	50	215	0.5	8.5
Napolitana	65	270	0.5	12
Romano	60	245	0.5	10
Sicilian	65	275	0.5	12
Venetian	65	275	0.5	12
Red Wine Sauce,				
avg. all types, ½ cup, 125g	65	275	0.5	12
Remano *(Aldi):* *Per ½ of 700g Bottle*				
Chunky Garden Vegetable, 125g	70	300	1	13
Passata, 100g	30	130	0	5
Passata, Tomato, 100g	40	165	1	6
Pasta Bake, Red Wine & Mushroom, 125g	95	400	4	12
Traditional Tomato, 125g	85	355	1	17
Rosella:				
Sauces: *Per Tbsp, 30ml*				
Tomato Sauce: 1 Tbsp	30	130	0	7
Low Joule	10	50	0	2
No Added Salt	30	135	0	7

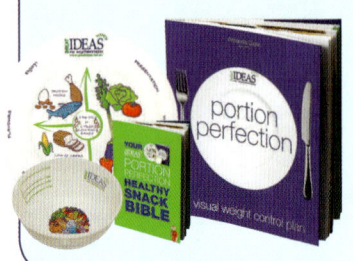

SEE HOW MUCH IS RIGHT TO EAT
.....with 'Portion Perfection'

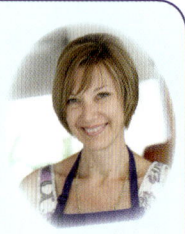

By Amanda Clark
(Dietitian, Adv. APD)

Portion Perfection Pack includes pictorial book, plate, bowl and pocket snack guide.

Bariatric Version Now Available Plus Hypnotherapy Audio (MP3)

Orders: Tel. (07) 5536 6400
www.greatideas.net.au

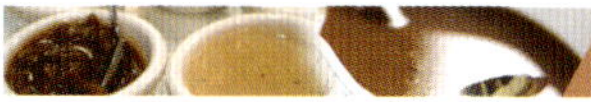

Sauces ◆ Cooking/Seasoning S

San Remo:
Fresh Pasta Sauces: *Per ¼ of 420g Jar*

	Cal	kJ	Fat	Cb
Creamy Bacon & Mushroom, 100g	225	945	21	5
Spicy Tomato & Bacon, 105g	75	315	5	7
Tomato, Onion & Garlic, 105g	80	325	4.5	8
Traditional Carbonara, 100g	240	1000	22	5
Traditional Napoletana, 105g	80	325	4.5	8

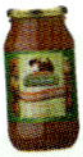

Sharwood's
Curry Pastes: *Per Tbsp, 15g*

	Cal	kJ	Fat	Cb
Korma	55	230	5	1.5
Madras	70	285	6.5	2
Rogan Josh	60	260	6	1.5
Tandoori	35	140	2	3
Tikka Masala	30	110	2	1.5
Vindaloo	55	230	4.5	2

Easy 2 Step Sauces: *Per ⅓ of 420g Jar, 144g*

Biryani: Coconut & Curry Leaf	80	330	4	9
Mint & Coriander	65	275	2.5	10
Tomato & Cumin	65	270	2.5	10

Simmer Sauce: *Per ⅓ of 420g Jar, 140g*

Butter Chicken	160	670	10	14
Korma	230	970	15	23
Madras	140	570	12	7
Rogan Josh	120	500	6.5	12
Tikka Masala	180	745	12	15

Mango Chutney, average, 1 tsp, 5g	10	50	0	3

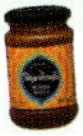

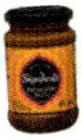

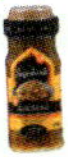

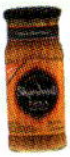

Puppodums ~ *See Page 56*

Silks (Aldi): *Per ¼ of 500g Jar*

Butter Chicken, 125g	218	910	16	16
Korma, 125g	160	675	11	13

Simmer Sensations (Aldi): *Per ¼ Jar*

Classic Stroganoff, 119g	130	530	12	5
Honey Mustard, 121g	140	565	8	15

SPC:
Fruit Sauce: *Per ⅓ of 375ml Jar*

Cranberry	255	1070	0.5	62
Plum	315	1315	0	76
Smooth Apple	95	395	0	22

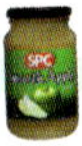

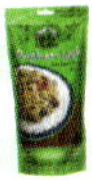

Updated Nutrition Data ~ www.CalorieKing.com.au
Persons with Diabetes ~ See Disclaimer (Page 22)

St. Dalfour:
Sauces: *Per 1 Tablespoon, 17.5g*

	Cal	kJ	Fat	Cb
Blueberry; Strawberry	50	220	0	13
Caramel	60	235	0	13
Chocolate; Raspberry Chocolate	60	235	0	13
Coffee Chocolage	55	230	0	13

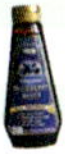

Tandaco:
Coating Mix: *Per ¼ of 75g Packet*

Chicken, 19g	60	255	0.5	12
Fish, 19g	60	260	0.5	13
Southern Fried Chicken, 19g	60	255	0.5	12

Stuffing Mix: *Per Serving, Dry*

Sage & Onion Seasoned, 20g	65	275	0.5	12
Suet Mix, ¼ cup, 32.5g	195	805	15	13

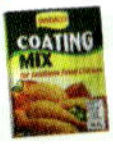

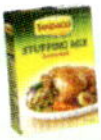

Taylor's:
Marinades: *Per ⅕ of 375g Jar*

Barbeque, 75g	90	375	1	21
Honey Soy, 75g	85	355	0	19
Satay, 75g	135	560	12	14
Sweet Chilli & Garlic, 75g	95	385	0	23
Sweet Soy, Chilli & Sesame, 75g	125	510	1.5	25
Tandoori, 75g	85	340	4	19

Sauces: *Per 1 Tablespoon, 20g*

Mustard & Dill	85	360	8	4
Seafood Cocktail	20	90	6	5
Tartare	20	80	7.5	4.5

Simmer Sauces: *Per ⅕ of 485g - 525g Jars*

Kashmiri Butter Chicken, 97g	115	470	7.5	10
Massaman Curry, 100g	105	435	5.5	12
Peanut Satay, 105g	205	865	13	17
Thai Green Curry, 100g	80	335	5	8

Stir Fry Sauces: *Per ⅒ of 350ml Jar*

Black Bean, 35ml	55	230	0	13
Honey & Chilli, 35ml	75	300	0	18
Sweet & Sour, 35ml	60	250	0	15

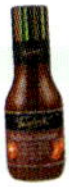

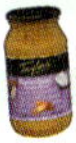

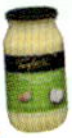

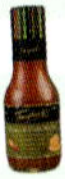

The Curry Makers:
Sauces: *Per ⅙ of 375g Packet*

Butter Chicken	85	360	7	4.5
Chicken Mango	70	290	1	14
Korma	105	435	9	4.5
Roghan Josh	70	285	5	5.5
Thai Green Curry	75	320	4.5	8
Tikka Masala	105	425	7.5	7.5

Sauces • Cooking/Seasoning • Pickles

Trident:	Cal	kJ	Fat	Cb
Curry Paste: Green, 1 Tbsp., 12g	15	50	0	2
Other varieties, 1 Tbsp., 12g	20	70	0.5	3
Sauce: *Per 1 Tablespoon, 20ml*				
Fish	10	40	0	0.5
Hoisin	40	170	1	8
Light Soy	5	25	0	0.5
Oyster	15	50	0	3
Sweet Soy	40	170	0	10
Thai Hot Chilli	5	10	0	0.5
Sweet Chilli Sauce: *Per 1 Tablespoon, 20ml*				
Plain	60	255	0	15
Hot	65	260	0	15
With Ginger	60	255	0	15
With Lime	60	250	0	14
With Mango	60	240	0	14
Woolworths:				
Homebrand: *Per 1 Tablespoon*				
Oyster, 20ml	40	165	0	10
Tomato, 20ml	20	70	0	4
Woolworths:				
Select, Pasta Sauce: *Per ¼ of 540g Jar, 135g*				
Arrabbiata, 135g	75	315	2	12
Bolognese/Tomato & Basil, 135g	80	335	3	12
Tomato & Mushroom, 135g	55	235	2	7.5
Sauces: *Per 1 Tablespoon Unless Indicated*				
Apple Sauce, 2 Tbsp, 50g	40	160	0	9
Cranberry Sauce, 20g	30	130	0	7
Balsamic Glaze, 15ml	20	85	0	4
Barbecue, 15ml	35	140	0	8
Fish, 20ml	10	40	0	1.5
Mint, Thick, 20ml	35	135	0	8
Oyster, 20ml	34	145	0	8
Seafood, 20ml	80	325	6.5	5.5
Soy, 1 teasp., 5ml	10	45	0	2
Steak, 15ml	35	135	0	8
Tartare, Light, 20ml	35	135	0.5	6.5
Tomato, 15ml	25	105	0	6
Worcestershire, 20ml	20	80	0	4

Pickles, Relish	Cal	kJ	Fat	Cb
Per Tablespoon, 25g Unless Indicated				
Beetroot, pickled, 30g	30	120	0	6.5
Capers, 1 serve, 20g	5	25	0	1
Chillies, Hot/Mild), 1 serve, 20g	10	50	1	2
Chutney, Fruit: Avg., 1 Tbsp	45	185	0	11
Hot Tomato *(Beerenberg)*, 30g	30	115	0	6.5
Mango *(Cafe Series)*, 20g	30	120	0	6.5
Low Joule *(Rosella)*, 30g	15	60	0	3
Cranberry Sauce, average:				
Whole Berry, 20g	30	130	0	7
Jellied, 20g	30	130	0	7
Dill Pickle: 1 large, 100g	10	40	0	2.5
Gherkin, 1 medium, 30g	30	135	0	7.5
Sliced Cucumber, 30g	30	135	0	7.5
Mustard: *Per Teaspoon, 5g*				
Average all brands	10	40	0.5	0.5
Wasabi *(Michael's)*	25	110	3	0.1
Masterfoods: French	5	20	0	0.5
Hot English	10	35	0.5	0.5
Mild English	5	25	0.5	0.5
Wholegrain	5	25	0.5	1
Onion, pickled, 1 medium, 20g	10	40	0	2.5
Pickles: *Per 30g*				
Branston *(Crosse & Blackwell)*	45	185	0	11
Hot Mango *(Patak's)*	80	320	6.5	2.5
Mustard *(Beerenberg)*	35	145	0.5	7
Mustard Pickles *(Aristocrat)*	25	110	0	5.5
Sweet Mustard *(Rosella)*	20	90	0	5.5
Relishes: *Per Tablespoon, 20g*				
Beerenberg, Balsimic Beetroot	30	130	0	7
Masterfoods: Corn	20	85	0	5
Gherkin	30	125	0	7
Gourmet Barbecue	20	95	0	5.5
Gourmet Tomato	20	85	0	5
Green Tomato	30	120	0	7
Sauerkraut, ¼ cup, 40g	10	40	0	1

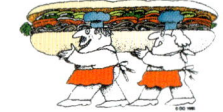

158

Snacks

Snack ~ Quick Guide

	Cal	kJ	Fat	Cb
Average All Brands: Plain/Flavoured				
25g packet	130	550	8.5	12
30g packet	160	660	11	14
50g packet	265	1105	18	23
100g packet	530	2210	35	46
200g packet	1055	4415	69	92
Multipak (250g), 21g pkt	110	465	7.5	10
Potato Straws/French Fries, 50g	260	1090	16	26
French Fries: *Snack Brands*				
Original, 45g packet	235	990	15	23
Salt & Vinegar, 45g	225	950	14	22

Potato Crisps ~ Brands

	Cal	kJ	Fat	Cb
Coles:				
Crinkle Cut: Salt & Vinegar; Chicken, 50g	260	1075	15	28
Original, 50g	270	1120	16	27
Freedom Foods, Low Salt, 50g	275	1140	18	27
Kettle Chips: 50g packet	245	1030	13	29
100g packet	490	2060	26	58
Pringles: Original, 25g (13 crisps)	135	560	9	13
Cylinder, 190g	1020	4275	69	93
Salt & Vinegar, 25g	130	550	8.5	13
Real McCoy, average, 50g	270	1125	17	24
Red Rock Deli: 28g packet	135	575	6.5	18
Average other Flavours, 50g packet	245	1025	11	32
Samboy, Original/Flavours, 45g	235	980	14	26
Slim Secrets, average, 40g	140	590	1	27
Smith's: Extra Crunchy, av., all	240	1005	14	25
Original, 50g	255	1065	16	23
Thinly Cut, 50g	255	1070	15	26
Sprinters *(Aldi): Per ¼ of 160g Canister*				
Flix: Roast Chicken/Turkey, 40g	210	870	11	24
Roma Tomato w. Vinegar, 40g	200	835	10	25
Thai Sweet Chilli, 40g	210	880	11	24
Crinkle Cut, Original, 50g	260	1090	15	28
Thins, 45g packet	230	970	15	22
Vege Chips *(Ajitas):* Deli Crisps, 80g pkt	415	1730	21	45
Vege Chips, 50g	235	980	10	34
Vege Crisps, 80g	415	1735	21	47
Vege Twists, Cheese Max, 21g	100	410	6	13

Rice & Chick Pea Chips ~ Brands

	Cal	kJ	Fat	Cb
Aussie Bodies, Protein Crisps, avg., 30g	130	545	6	6
Freedom Foods, Chick Pea Chips, 50g	240	1000	13	26
Red Rock Deli, Sour Cream & Chives, 125g	660	2765	38	73
Sprinters *(Aldi):*				
BBQ/Cheese, 25g	120	510	5	15
Sour Cream & Chives	125	525	6	14

Updated Nutrition Data ~ www.CalorieKing.com.au
Persons with Diabetes ~ See Disclaimer (Page 22)

Corn Chips ~ Brands

	Cal	kJ	Fat	Cb
Corn Chips, large/thick, 50g	250	1040	15	26
C.C.'s: Nacho Cheese, 50g	255	1070	14	29
Original; Tasty Cheese, 50g	260	1075	13	30
Coles: Original, 50g	250	1050	13	32
Cheese Supreme, 50g	255	1065	14	30
Doritos: Average, 50g packet	260	1090	14	30
230g packet	1195	5005	62	135
Red Rock, average all flavours, 27g	140	580	7.5	15

Cheezels, Twisties ~ Brands

	Cal	kJ	Fat	Cb
Burger Rings: 50g packet	265	1115	15	30
Multipak (250g), 20g packet	105	445	6	12
100g packet	525	2200	29	60
Cheetos: Cheese & Bacon Balls, 50g	280	1155	17	28
Multipak (250g), 20g packet	110	460	7	11
Cheezels: 45g packet	240	995	14	25
125g box	660	2765	38	70
21g Packet (Multipack)	110	460	6.5	12
Minis: 50g serving	265	1105	15	28
125g packet	660	2765	38	70
Cheesters, 20g	115	490	7	11
Coles, Cheese Rings, 50g	265	1095	16	28
Toobs *(Smith's),* 35g packet	160	665	7.5	21
Twisties: 30g packet	150	625	7	20
50g packet	250	1040	12	33
100g packet	500	2080	23	65

Beef & Pork Snacks

	Cal	kJ	Fat	Cb
Beef Jerky *(Jack Link's),* 25g	70	300	1	5
Biltong *(D Jays),* 25g	85	360	2	0.5
Droeworse, 25g	90	365	4.5	1
Twiggy Stick (1), 20g	85	360	6	2
Pork Crackle *(Nobby's),* 25g	130	540	7	1
Porky Bits: Gold Medal, 25g	130	545	7	0
Nobby's, 25g packet	130	545	7	1
Steak Bar *(Jack Link's),* 25g	70	300	0.5	5

Pretzels ~ Brands

	Cal	kJ	Fat	Cb
Average All Brands: 10 sticks, 8cm, 6g	25	95	0.5	4
Parker's Oven Baked Pretzels:				
Regular (97% Fat-Free): Twists (10), 19g	75	310	0.5	15
Sticks	45	180	0.3	9
Flavoured Pretzels (5), 20g	80	325	0.5	16
Pretzel World: *Without Topping*				
Californian Cinnamon; Orig. Low-Fat, avg	335	1400	3	67
Swiss Cheese	415	1725	8.5	68

159

Snacks

Popcorn

	Cal	kJ	Fat	Cb
Air-popped: Without oil, 1 cup, 7g	30	115	0	4.5
Real McCoy, Butter, 25g	105	440	3	15
Commercial, oil-popped: 30g	145	590	7.5	15
1 cup, 8g	40	160	2	4
Butter Flavour, 25g	115	480	6	12
Caramel-coated, ¾ cup, 40g	175	720	5	32
Home-popped (in oil), 1 cup, 7g	35	140	2	3.5
Sugar-coated, 1 cup, 35g	135	565	1.5	22
Microwave Popcorn:				
Uncle Toby's:				
Butter: 1 cup, (popped), 7g	30	135	2	3.5
100g pkt	460	1920	25	46
Poppin *(Greens):*				
Butter Flavour, ¼ pkt, 25g	115	480	6	11
Butter Lite, ¼ pkt, 22g	85	355	3	11
Theatre/Movies:				
Small (4 cups), 36g	170	710	9	19
Medium (5 cups), 45g	215	900	11	24
Large (13 cups), 115g	545	2280	29	61
Maxi (22 cups), 200g	945	3950	50	105

Fruit & Nut Snacks

	Cal	kJ	Fat	Cb
Apricot Delight/Slices *(Plain):*				
Average, 1 piece, 10g	35	150	0.5	8
5 pieces, 50g	175	730	2.5	40
Bite'z *(Back To Nature),* avg., 25g bite	100	420	2.5	17
Ducks Nuts, Endurance Mix, 40g	205	855	14	13
Frugo's *(Go Natural):*				
Berry/Apricot, avg., 30g pkt	150	615	7	19
Clusters (1), 22g	100	410	5.5	11
Fruit & Nut Mixes, avg., 50g	230	960	14	22
Fruit Fix, (1), 22g	75	315	0	18
Fruit Nibbles, average, 22g	120	505	0	28
Fruit Salad Bites *(Golden Days),* 35g pkt	125	530	1.5	27
Fruit Straps: Avg., Small, 15g	50	210	0	11
Large, 30g	100	420	0	22
Fruit Wraps *(Hillcrest/Aldi),* (1), avg, 14g	45	180	0	9
Ginger, Choc/Carob-coated, 10g	45	195	2	6.5
Ginger Nibbles *(Buderim),* 25g	85	360	0	21
SPC, Chewbie, Fruit Bars, 20g	70	300	1.5	14
Roll-Ups, 1 roll, 16g	50	220	0.5	11
Sunbeam: Fruit Flakes, 20g	70	300	0	17
Fruit Bites, 50g	185	775	0.5	42
Fruit 'N'ut: Original, 40g bag	185	765	15	17
Almond Plus, 40g bag	160	675	7	21
Tropical Fruit & Nut, 50g	200	835	10	34
Zipp 'Ems *(Coles),* 1 fruit roll	35	150	1	9

Crackers, Cookies

	Cal	kJ	Fat	Cb
Crackers (Plain/Savoury): *See Pages 51-55*				
Bagel Chips, baked, 30g, 7 pieces	95	400	2.5	15
Bagel Crisps *(Abe's),* 6 crisps, 24g	95	400	2.5	15
Bhuja/Oriental Mix:				
Maharajah's Choice, 50g	165	690	7	17
Majans, 100g	455	1900	15	63
Broad Beans, roasted in oil, 25g	125	530	6	12
Chic Nuts, 1 cup, 100g	385	1580	9	46
Corn Kiks *(Mamee),* 20g	100	420	5	13
70g pkt	360	1500	18	46
Cracker Mix *(Majans),* 100g	455	1900	15	63
Ajitas: Delie Chips, 25g	30	125	6.5	17
Grain Chips, 25g	115	490	4.5	17
Vege Chips, 25g	115	475	4.5	17
Fortune Cookie, (1), 8g	35	140	0.5	7
French Fries, Potato Straws, 50g	265	1100	17	25
Noodle Crisps/Snacks, 50g, average	275	1150	19	22
Oreo, Mini Cup, 115g	540	2260	23	75
Pita Crisps, baked, 6 pcs, 30g	105	440	2	11
Pork Crackle *(Gold Medal),* 25g	135	565	6.5	0
Prawn Crackers *(Chang):* Fried, 20g	125	510	7.5	12
Microwaved, 20g	75	320	0	18
Quaker, Oat Cookies, avg., 30g pkt	130	560	4.5	20
Rice Crackers ~ *See Page 55*				
Soya Crisps/Chips/Multigrain, 25 Crisps/Chips, 50g	270	1130	15	33
Sweet Potato Crisps, 30g	155	645	9.5	16
Vegetable Crisps, 50g	260	1080	16	26

CALORIE KING TIP!

Be aware that salty foods can create a thirst for hours after you stop eating.

This can exacerbate calorie intake if calorie-laden drinks such as soft drinks, fruit juices and beer are consumed liberally.

Limit salty snacks and substitute fresh fruit or unsalted nuts.

Soups

Homemade & Restaurant Soup

Average of Recipes
Per 250ml Cup Serving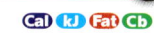

	Cal	kJ	Fat	Cb
Chicken & Vegetable	75	315	0.5	14
Chicken Noodle (w. chicken)	295	1230	11	21
Cream of Mushroom	215	905	12	16
Kumera	120	500	4	16
Lentil & Vegetable	105	440	3	15
Minestrone (w. Beans)	260	1090	8.5	29
Minestrone (w/out Beans)	215	880	8	23
Mushroom (w/out cream)	140	575	8	10
Pea & Ham	415	1740	13	43
Potato & Leek	200	830	4	32
Pumpkin	205	885	5	29
Split Green Pea	325	1365	5	43
Spring Vegetable	80	330	3.5	11
Tomato:				
Mediterranean	110	460	6	10
Roasted with Pine Nuts				
& Parmesan Cheese	315	1320	14	32

Note: Recipes available at CalorieKing.com.au

Stock Cubes & Spices

	Cal	kJ	Fat	Cb
Bonox (Beef/Chicken) 1 round tsp, 8g	10	35	0	1
Bouillon/Stock Powder 1 tsp, 5g	10	45	0.5	1.5
Bovril, 1 round tsp, 8g	15	60	0	1.5
Herbs, Spices, Flavourings:				
(Negligible cal/kJ/fat per serve)				
Average, 1 tsp	10	40	0	1
Parsley, dried, 1 tsp	5	10	0	0.5
Mustard; Nutmeg, ground, 1 tsp	15	70	1	1
Curry Powder, 1 tsp, 3g	5	30	0.5	1.5
Salt, all types	0	0	0	0
Soup Cubes (*Oxo, Maggi, Continental, Massel*):				
Stock Cubes, average	15	70	0	1.5
1 small cube	10	40	0.5	1
Liquid Stocks ~ *See Brand Listings*				
Average all types, 250ml	15	60	0	2

Soup ~ Brands

Ainsley Harriott:
Cup of Soup: *Per Sachet, Prepared as Directed*

	Cal	kJ	Fat	Cb
Country Style Shropshire Pea, 226ml	100	425	2	17
Minestrone, 222ml	85	350	0.5	18
New England Style Vege. Chowder, 225ml	95	405	2.5	16
Southern Cajun Gumbo, 224ml	80	335	0.5	16

Brands (Cont)

Basco:
Instant Soup, Gluten Free: *Per Packet, Prepared as Directed*

	Cal	kJ	Fat	Cb
Creamy Chicken & Veg.	120	505	3.5	20
Pumpkin	115	475	1.5	22

Campbell's:
Chunky: *Per ½ of 505g can, 250g*

	Cal	kJ	Fat	Cb
Beef	130	545	2.5	16
Beef & Potato Curry	180	740	6.5	22
Ham & Pea	175	735	2.5	25
Hearty Chicken & Corn	145	605	4	19
Hearty Irish Stew	145	605	6	15
Potato & Bacon	205	855	10	23
Roast Chicken & Vegetable	125	530	2.5	17
Stockpot	125	520	2.5	15

Chunky Fully Loaded: *Per ½ of 505g can, 250g*

	Cal	kJ	Fat	Cb
Angus Beef & Red Wine Casserole	145	595	3.5	18
Beef Stroganoff	170	715	6.5	18
Chicken & Mushroom Carbonara	195	810	6.5	21
Chilli Beef	195	805	4	22
Hearty Chicken Casserole	155	655	3.5	18
Lamb Hot Pot	165	675	4	21
Morocan Lamb	185	765	5.5	21
Outback Steak & Bacon	160	670	4	19
Peppered Steak & Gravy	145	610	4.5	17
Rigatoni Meatballs	205	850	6	25
Stockman's Lamb Casserole	190	780	5.5	20

Condensed: *Per ⅓ of 420g can, Prep'd, 250g*

	Cal	kJ	Fat	Cb
Chicken Noodle	60	255	1.5	10
Cream of Asparagus	125	515	6	13
Cream of Chicken	135	550	7	13
Cream of Chicken & Corn	145	595	6	17
Cream of Mushroom	110	465	5.5	11
Cream of Pumpkin	140	580	5	19
Rich Tomato	80	335	0.5	18
Tomato	80	335	0.5	19
Vegetable & Beef	70	280	1	11

Country Ladle: *Per ½ of 505g can, 250g*

	Cal	kJ	Fat	Cb
Butternut Pumpkin	90	380	2.5	13
Chicken & Pasta	105	435	1.5	16
Chicken & Sweet Corn	120	500	1.5	19
Chicken Noodle	115	470	2	15
Creamy Chicken	125	530	6	13
Farmhouse Vegetable	85	360	0.5	14

Continued next page...

Updated Nutrition Data ~ www.CalorieKing.com.au
Persons with Diabetes ~ See Disclaimer (Page 22)

161

Soups

Brands (Cont)

	Cal	kJ	Fat	Cb

Campbell's (Cont):

Country Ladle (Cont): *Per ½ of 505g Can, 250g*

	Cal	kJ	Fat	Cb
Hearty Beef & Vegetable	135	570	3.5	18
Minestrone	95	400	0.5	16
Pea & Ham	140	585	2	15
Potato & Leek	160	670	6.5	20
Potato & Sweetcorn Chowder	165	690	6	22
Rich & Creamy Pumpkin	120	500	4	17
Roast Chkn & Winter Vegetables	135	565	3.5	20
Spring Lamb & Vegetable	120	490	3.5	15
Wholegrain:				
Chicken & Mushroom w. Rice	135	555	6.5	13
Garden Vegetable with Barley	85	345	0.5	15
Hearty Vege with Pasta	80	335	0.5	13
Minestrone with Wholegrain Pasta	100	420	0.5	16

Tetra Pak: *Per ½ of 500g Tetra Pak, 250g*

	Cal	kJ	Fat	Cb
Creamy Mushroom with Cracked Pepper	155	640	11	11
Pumpkin with Sour Cream & Sweet Chilli	140	585	6	15
Rustic Vegetable with Herbs	130	530	3	20
Smashed Butternut Pumpkin with Parsley	110	450	3	15
Spiced Autumn Vegetables	105	430	2	16
Vine-Ripened Tomato with Spinach & Feta	140	570	3.5	21

Chunky Microwaveable: *Per 430g Tub*

	Cal	kJ	Fat	Cb
Beef	230	955	5	28
Ham & Pea	265	1100	4	37
Hearty Irish Stew	250	1040	10	25
Roast Chicken & Vegetable	215	900	4.5	30
Stockpot	230	950	5	28

Country Ladle Cafe Style: *Per ½ of 505g Can*

	Cal	kJ	Fat	Cb
Chicken, Mushroom & Wild Rice	140	570	3.5	18
Moroccan Vegetables with Chickpeas	150	630	2.5	22
Pumpkin, Red Lentil & Spoinach	120	505	3	16
Tuscan Tomato, Vegetable & Beans	140	575	0.5	21
Vine Tomato with Spinach & Ricotta Ravioli	130	530	1.5	22

Country Ladle Microwaveable: *Per 430g Tub*

	Cal	kJ	Fat	Cb
Butternut Pumpkin	160	660	3.5	24
Chicken & Sweet Corn	200	820	2.5	31
Chilli Beef	345	1430	7	39
Minestrone	170	700	1	27
Outback Steak & Bacon	285	1195	7	33
Rigatoni Meatballs	360	1500	11	44
Stockman's Lamb Casserole	330	1375	9	35
Lunch Specials:				
Creamy Pumpkin	200	840	7.5	26
Spring Vegetable & Chicken	140	585	2	17
Tomato & Parmesan & Herbs	230	950	5	38
Winter Vegetable Medley	230	970	4.5	39

Campbell's (Cont):

Real Consomme: *Per Cup, 250ml*

	Cal	kJ	Fat	Cb
Beef	90	375	0.5	2.5
Chicken	50	200	0.5	4.5

Real Stock: *Per Cup, 250ml*

	Cal	kJ	Fat	Cb
Beef	30	130	0.5	4
Beef, Salt-Reduced	30	125	0.5	4
Chicken	20	85	0.5	3
Chicken, Salt-Reduced	20	85	0.5	3
Fish	10	45	0.5	1
Vegetable	20	85	0.5	5
Vegetable, Salt-Reduced	20	85	0.5	5

Coles:

Condensed: *Per ¼ of 420g Can*

	Cal	kJ	Fat	Cb
Cream of Chicken, 105g	105	435	4.5	12
Cream of Pumpkin, 105g	110	450	3	16
Tomato, 105g	70	285	0.5	15

Cup a Soup: *Per 250ml Sachet*

	Cal	kJ	Fat	Cb
Chicken Noodle	35	140	0.5	6.5
Cream of Chicken with Croutons	90	375	3	14
Cream of Mushrooms with Croutons	105	435	2.5	18

Dried Soup Mix: *Per ¼ Packet*

	Cal	kJ	Fat	Cb
Chicken Noodle	40	155	0.5	7
French Onion	30	120	0.5	6

Microwave: *Per 430g Bowl*

	Cal	kJ	Fat	Cb
Beef & Vegetables	250	1035	4.5	38
Chicken & Sweetcorn	250	1050	5	38
Creamy Butternut Pumpkin	230	960	8.5	29
Creamy Mushroom	245	10.5	10	31
Creamy Tomato	360	1500	13	51
Minestrone	163	670	1	31

Chefs' Cupboard ~ Aldi:

Ready to Serve: *Per Half Can*

	Cal	kJ	Fat	Cb
Classics, Vegetable, ½ can, 268g	140	580	1	23
Premium:				
Chicken & Sweetcorn, 250g	115	475	2	17
Chunky Chicken, 250g	120	505	3.5	16
Minestrone, 268g	70	295	0.5	10
Pumpkin, 250g	105	440	6.5	13

Condensed, Tomato, ¼ can, 105g | 100 | 420 | 0 | 22 |

Sachet: *Per 250ml, Prepared as Directed*

	Cal	kJ	Fat	Cb
Chicken Noodle	40	165	0.5	6.5
Cream of Chicken	80	340	1.5	15
Cream of Mushroom	105	430	3.5	17

Soups

Brands (Cont)

	Cal	kJ	Fat	Cb
Continental:				
Cup-a-Soup: *Per Sachet, Prepared as Directed*				
Asian: Chinese Chicken & Corn	130	535	2	26
Laksa	145	600	4	24
Thai Red Curry	135	550	3	23
Classic: Chicken & Vegetables	60	235	0.5	13
Chicken Noodle	45	190	1	9
Cream of Chicken	90	360	3	15
Cream of Mushroom	85	345	3	14
Hearty Beef	55	215	0.5	11
Pea & Ham	80	330	2	13
Pumpkin	80	325	1.5	15
Spring Vegetable	60	235	0.5	14
Croutons: Creamy Chicken & Corn	140	575	4	25
Creamy Chicken	145	610	6	22
Creamy Mushroom	125	515	3.5	22
Creamy Potato & Bacon	115	480	4	19
Creamy Pumpkin	125	510	3.5	22
Creamy Seafood Bisque	150	625	6	22
Creamy Vegetable	130	540	5	19
Mushroom Bacon & Sour Cream	130	530	4.5	21
Hearty: Chilli Con Carne	110	450	1	22
Dutch Curry & Rice	125	515	3.5	22
Garden Vegetable	155	650	4	27
Italian Minestrone	145	610	1	32
Pea & Ham	115	475	3	19
Roast Chicken	170	695	4	30
Spanish Tomato	140	575	1	30
Tomato, Bacon & Chilli	145	610	1	29
Vegetable & Beef	135	550	1	28
Winter Vegetable	130	545	1.5	26
Lots-a-Noodles:				
BBQ Chicken	125	515	1.5	29
Beef	115	485	0.5	25
Chicken	115	480	0.5	24
Chinese Chicken & Corn	145	600	3	27
Cream of Chicken	130	550	3	23
Creamy Chicken & Mushroom	130	530	3	23
Mild Chicken Curry	125	525	2.5	22
Vegiful:				
Eight Vegetable	105	425	2.5	18
Potato & Leek	95	395	2.5	16
Winter Vegetable	130	545	1.5	26
Xtrafull:				
Beef Stroganoff	135	555	2.5	24
Flame Grilled BBQ Chicken	125	510	1	24
Pepper Steak	130	530	3.5	21
Smoky Beef'n Bacon	125	510	2	23
Country Cup:				
Per Sachet, Prepared as Directed				
Croutons: Chicken & Mushroom	90	375	3	14
Cream of Chicken & Corn	100	415	3	16
Cream of Chicken	100	420	3.5	16
Cream of Mushroom & Chives	90	365	3	14
Cream of Pumpkin	105	440	4	16
Cream of Tomato	105	435	3.5	18
Pea & Ham	100	420	3	16
Pepper Steak & Mushroom	105	435	3.5	17
Potato & Bacon	105	435	3.5	17
Pumpkin & Ham	110	460	4	18
Roasted Pumpkin & Garlic	105	440	3.5	17
Asian: Chicken & Corn	125	530	2.5	22
Tom Yum	75	320	0.5	16
Noodles: Beef	100	430	0.5	21
Chicken	115	465	2	20
Chicken & Corn	110	450	2	19
Wholegrain Noodles:				
Beef	100	410	1	19
Chicken	115	465	2.5	19
Minestrone	100	415	1	18
Gravox:				
Tetra Pak: *Per 250ml*				
Beef Stock	10	45	0.5	1
Chicken/Salt Reduced	5	30	0.5	0.5
Vegetable	10	50	0.5	1.5
Heinz:				
Big 'N Chunky, Ready To Serve: *Per ½ of 535g Can*				
Bacon Steak & Potato	145	610	3.5	18
Beef Bolognese	205	860	5.5	28
Beef & Vegetable	145	595	3	15
Beef Stockpot	140	585	3	17
Butter Chicken	240	995	14	19
Chicken & Corn	160	655	4	22
Chicken Pasta and Vegetable	135	570	2.5	20
Chilli Meatballs	125	515	2.5	15
Flamin' Chicken	135	570	2.5	19
Peppered Steak	165	690	3.5	18
Ravioli with Beef Tomato	215	890	5.5	31
Tex Mex Beef	225	930	5	29

Updated Nutrition Data ~ www.CalorieKing.com.au
Persons with Diabetes ~ See Disclaimer (Page 22)

Soups

Brands (Cont)

	Cal	kJ	Fat	Cb

Heinz (Cont):
Classic:

Microwave: *Per 430g Tub*
	Cal	kJ	Fat	Cb
Creamy Pumpkin	215	885	10	24
Tomato & Basil	165	690	3.5	28

Ready To Serve: *Per ½ 530g Can*
	Cal	kJ	Fat	Cb
Chicken & Sweetcorn	160	650	6	19
Country Chicken	140	585	6	13
Creamy Chicken	150	623	7	16
Creamy Chicken & Mushr.	135	560	6	14
Creamy Pumpkin	145	600	5	20
Creamy Tomato	135	570	6	18
Italian Minestrone	110	450	0.5	18
Pea & Ham	145	600	2	18
Potato & Leek	110	450	3.5	15
Winter Vegetable	95	400	2	16

Condensed: *Per ¼ of 420g Can, Prepared*
	Cal	kJ	Fat	Cb
Big Red: Spicy Tomato	60	250	0	13
Tomato	65	265	0	13
Tomato, Salt Reduced	60	250	0	13
Cream of Chicken	120	505	4	14
Cream of Mushroom	65	265	1	10
Cream of Pumpkin	100	410	0.5	17
Minestrone	70	295	0	14
Pea & Ham	90	390	0.5	13
Vegetable	50	210	0	10
Vegetable & Beef	70	295	2	11

Soup For One: *Per 300g Can*
	Cal	kJ	Fat	Cb
Big Red Tomato	110	450	0.5	23
Big Red Creamy Tomato	195	810	7	28

Squeeze & Stir: *Per 70g Sachet, Prepared as Directed*
	Cal	kJ	Fat	Cb
Big Red Tomato	75	315	2	12
Mediterranean Vegetable	90	365	3	13
Rich Tomato with Basil	75	315	2.5	12
Ripe Tomato & Vegetable	80	340	2	13

Very Special, Ready To Serve: *Per ½ of 535g Can*
	Cal	kJ	Fat	Cb
Beef & Barley	130	545	2	17
Beef, Vegetable & Pasta	95	400	0.5	13
Chicken Hot Pot	135	570	2.5	19
Creamy Pumpkin with Bacon	160	650	5.5	22
Hearty Vegetable	100	410	0.5	17
Homestyle Veg. & Barley	135	560	0.5	23
Potato & Spinach	120	490	4	15
Pumpkin Minestrone	165	690	4	26
Rich Beef & Vegetable	95	400	1.5	13
Ripe Tomato & Basil	115	480	1	22
Spicy Lentil	175	730	1	29
Sweet Potato & Pumpkin	135	570	2.5	25

Home Brand ~ *See Woolworths*

	Cal	kJ	Fat	Cb

LaZuppa: *Per 420g Bowl*
	Cal	kJ	Fat	Cb
Chicken & Corn Chowder	180	760	3	30
Creamy Chicken & Vege	150	615	3.5	21
Creamy Chicken with Asparagus & Herbs	135	565	2	21
Hearty Chicken & Vege	165	690	3	27
Minestrone	170	700	1	33
Moroccan Pumpkin w. Chickpeas	205	865	2	40
Pumpkin	130	545	0.5	28
Ribbolita Tuscan Vegetable	120	490	0	23
Spinach & Chickpea	190	790	2	35
Spring Vegetable & Wholegrain Rice	150	635	2	27

Maggi:
2-Minute Noodles: *Per 85g Packet*
	Cal	kJ	Fat	Cb
Beef	330	1390	13	47
Chicken	330	1370	13	46
Oriental	280	1170	5	51
99% Fat-Free: Beef; Chicken	280	1180	2	57

Fusian 2-Minute Noodles: *Per Block, Prepared*
	Cal	kJ	Fat	Cb
Hot & Spicy; Satay	360	1500	17	45
Soy & Mild Spice	350	1570	17	44

Cup: *Per Cup, Prepared*
	Cal	kJ	Fat	Cb
Mi Goreng Singapore	315	1310	16	39
Satay	320	1340	16	40
Soy & Mild Spice	315	1305	15	38

Noodle Cup:
Instant Noodles: *Per Cup, Prepared*
	Cal	kJ	Fat	Cb
Asian Beef; Chicken	270	1120	10	38
Beef	265	1110	10	38
Indian Curry	270	1115	11	37
Laksa; Oriental	270	1135	11	38
98% Fat-Free: Beef; Chicken	265	1105	1	55

Massel:
Gourmet Plus: *Per 250ml Cup*
	Cal	kJ	Fat	Cb
Beef	20	80	0	3
Chicken Style	20	80	0	3.5
Vegetable	25	95	0.5	4.5

UltraCube Stock Cubes:
	Cal	kJ	Fat	Cb
Average, 1 cube	30	130	2	3
1 serve, 150ml	10	40	0.5	1

Macro:
Refrigerated: *Per ½ 300g Pouch*
	Cal	kJ	Fat	Cb
Organic: Golden Pumpkin	85	355	2	14
Spicy Tomato & Caposicum	100	430	4	13
Tuscan Vegetable	100	430	1	19

Soups ◆ Soy ◆ Tofu — S

Brands (Cont)

	Cal	kJ	Fat	Cb
OptiSlim VLCD:				
Soup: *Per 55g Sachet*				
Chicken	225	945	7	20
Pumpkin	210	875	3.5	25
Tomato	205	860	2	26
Orgran,				
Tomato, 200g pkt, prepared	60	255	0	13
Rosella, Tomato Soup,				
Condensed, ½ 500g Can, 250g	85	340	1.5	18
The Soup Company *(Aldi): Per Sachet, Prepared as Directed*				
Chicken & Sweetcorn with Croutons	150	620	7.5	17
Pea & Ham with Croutons	90	370	2	13
Pumpkin with Croutons	105	440	3	16
Tony Ferguson:				
Meal Replacement,				
average all flavours, 1 sachet	205	860	2	31
Trident:				
Thai Soup: *Per Serving, 400ml, Prepared as Directed*				
Chicken	205	850	1.5	43
Hot & Spicy	180	760	1	39
Laksa	165	680	3	29
Tom Yum Goong	200	840	2	41
Woolworths:				
Select:				
Fresh Soups: *Per ¼ of 1kg Pouch*				
Chicken & Corn	140	585	5.5	17
Chicken Noodle	145	610	7	15
Classic Pea & Ham	140	590	1	25
Pumpkin	100	415	4.5	13
300g Tub:				
Garden Pea & Ham	150	630	4.5	17
Minestrone	155	650	4.5	25
Red Thai Chicken	185	770	11	16
Sweet Pumpkin & Potato	130	555	2	25
Tomato, Lentil & Bacon	185	780	7	17
Microwaveable Soups: *Per 420g Tub*				
Beef & Vegetables	195	810	7	16
Chicken & Sweetcorn	230	945	3.5	37
Minestrone	150	640	2.5	19
Pepper Steak	180	750	8.5	6.5
Pumpkin	105	440	1.5	16
Winter Vegetable	105	435	3	12

Miso, Tempeh, Tofu

	Cal	kJ	Fat	Cb
Miso: Liquid, 100ml	15	65	0.5	2
Dry, 100g	35	145	1.5	3
Tempeh, (Cultured/Fermented Soybeans):				
Average all brands, 1 cup, 166g	320	1340	18	16
Flavoured, 100g	170	715	8	9
Fried in oil, 100g	450	1870	34	12
Nutrisoy, Tempeh, 100g	140	590	4.5	10
TLY Joyce, 75g	45	190	1.5	4.5
Tofu: *Average All Brands*				
Firm/Hard, 100g	105	450	5	0
Stir fried, 100g	270	1135	20	11
Soft/Silken, 100g	45	190	2	2

Tofu Brands

	Cal	kJ	Fat	Cb
King Land: Organic Tofu:				
Firm, 100g	130	545	7.5	2.5
Silken, 100g	130	540	7.5	2.5
Pureland: Firm, 100g	130	545	7.5	2.5
Organic, 100g	145	605	9	4
Burger: Raw, 100g	215	910	13	16
Cooked, 100g	255	1070	15	19
Nuggets, 100g	210	880	12	15
Soya King: Hard/Firm, 100g	105	445	5	4
Silken (Soft), 100g	45	185	2	2
Nigari, 100g	100	415	5	4
Super Soy, 125g	125	520	6.5	6
Soyco: Chinese Honey Soy, 100g	170	715	8.5	8
Thai, 100g	175	730	10	5
Sweet Chilli:				
Tofu Nuggets (350g pkt),				
100g portion	200	825	11	11
TLY Joyce: Firm Tofu, 100g	60	255	2	5.5
Silken Firm, 100g	45	190	2	2

Updated Nutrition Data ~ www.CalorieKing.com.au
Persons with Diabetes ~ See Disclaimer (Page 22)

Spreads ~ Honey ◆ Jam ◆ Peanut Butter

Honey

	Cal	kJ	Fat	Cb
Average All Varieties				
Honey (Liquid or Creamed):				
1 level tsp, 6g	20	75	0	6
1 rounded/dipped tsp, 12g	40	160	0	10
1 Tbsp, 25g	80	330	0	21
100g quantity	310	1320	0	82
½ cup, 160g	495	2110	0	131
Coles, Spreadable Honey Jelly,				
1 Tbsp, 25g	75	320	0	19

Jams, Fruit Spreads

	Cal	kJ	Fat	Cb
Average all Brands:				
1 level tsp, 6g	15	65	0	4
1 rounded tsp, 10g	25	100	0	6.5
1 heaped tsp, 15g	40	170	0	10
1 level Tbsp, 25g	60	250	0	16
½ cup, 160g	400	1670	0	105
Sugar Reduced/Diet: *Per Heaped Teaspoon, 15g*				
Diet Cottee's	5	20	0	1
IXL, 50% Less Sugar	20	85	0	5
Weight Watchers	20	85	0	5

Chocolate/Nut Spreads ~ Nutella

	Cal	kJ	Fat	Cb
Average All Brands:				
(Cottee's, Duo, Coles, IGA, Nutella, Nutino)				
1 tsp, 5g	25	105	1.5	3
1 heaped teasp, 10g	50	210	3	5.5
1 Tbsp, 20g	105	435	6	11
2 Tbsp, 40g	210	870	12	22

Chocolate Spreads~ Nut Free

	Cal	kJ	Fat	Cb
Pantalica, 1 Tbsp, 20g	70	290	5.5	4
Sweet William, 1 Tbsp, 20g	100	420	7.5	6.5

"Success is 1% Inspiration and 99% Perspiration"

Peanut Butter

	Cal	kJ	Fat	Cb
Average All Brands				
(Dick Smith's, Green's, Kraft, Sanitarium)				
Smooth or Crunchy:				
1 level tsp, 5g	30	130	2.5	0.5
1 heaped tsp, 10g	60	255	5	1.5
1 Tbsp, 20g	120	505	10	2.5
100g quantity	605	2530	51	13
Single Serve Package, 11g	70	290	5.5	1.5
Super Crunchy: 1 level tsp, 5 g	30	125	2.5	0.5
1 Tbsp, 20g	120	505	11	2
Woolworths, Light Peanut Spread, 1 T., 20g	115	480	7.5	8

Other Nut & Seed Spreads

	Cal	kJ	Fat	Cb
Eskal, FreeNut Butter,				
(Made from Sunflower Seeds)				
Smooth/Crunchy, 1 T., 20g	125	525	10	4.5
Nut Spreads *(Melrose):*				
Almond, 1 Tbsp, 20g	115	480	11	1
Almonds, Brazils & Cashews, 1 T., 20g	130	545	12	1.5
Brazil Nut & Linseed, 1 Tbsp	140	580	14	5
Hazelnut, 1 Tbsp, 20g	130	545	13	1
Hoummus, average,				
1 Tbsp, 20g	45	190	4	1.5
Tahini (Sesame Seed Paste):				
1 rounded tsp, 10g	65	270	6	0.5
1 Tbsp, 25g	160	655	15	0.5
¼ cup, 80g	510	2130	48	1.5

Vegemite, Promite ~ Yeast Spreads

Per ½ Teaspoon

	Cal	kJ	Fat	Cb
Vegemite, 3g	5	25	0	0.5
Marmite, 3g	5	20	0	0.5
MightyMite (333), 3g	5	20	0	1
OmegaMite, 3 g	5	20	0	1
Ozemite (Dick Smith's), 3g	5	25	0	1
Promite, 3g	5	25	0	1
Vege Spread (Freedom), 3g	5	20	0	1

Other Sandwich Spreads

	Cal	kJ	Fat	Cb
Vegemite Cheesybite:				
(Mix of Vegemite & Cream Cheese)				
1 heaped teaspoon, 10g	25	105	1.5	12
1 Tbsp, 22g	55	230	3.5	2.5

Spreads ◆ Syrups ◆ Sugar S

Other Sandwich Spreads (Cont)

	Cal	kJ	Fat	Cb
Avocado, mashed, 1 Tbsp, 20g	40	170	4	0
Cheese Spread:				
Bramwells (Aldi): 1 Tbsp, 20g				
Cheddar Cheese	60	240	5	1
Cream Cheese	65	270	6	0.5
Kraft Easy Cheese: 1 Tbsp, 20g				
Cheddar Cheese	60	240	5	1
Light	50	200	3.5	1.5
Cream Cheese	60	260	6	0.5
Light	55	230	4.5	1
Fish Spreads:				
John West, Spreadable Tuna, 40g	65	275	4	2.5
Pecks: Anchovette, 25g	30	125	1	1
Salmon & Lobster, 25g	35	135	1	1.5
Jam/Marmalade, 1 heaped tsp, 15g	40	170	0	10
Lemon Butter/Spread, 2 tsp, 12g	35	140	1	7
Mayonnaise:				
Kraft: 1 Tbsp	45	190	4	2.5
97% Fat-Free, 1 Tbsp	25	95	0.5	4.5
Meat Spread: *Per 2 tsp (10g)*				
Peck's: Chicken & Ham, 25g	60	240	4.5	1
Devilled Ham, 25g	45	190	3	1.5
Paté, average, 1 Tbsp, 20g	60	250	5	0.2
Soy Spread *(Woolworths)*	110	450	12	0
Soya Lecithin, 1 Tbsp, 20g	155	650	17	1.5
Sundried Tom. Pate *(Always Fresh),* 20g	60	245	4.5	2.5

Sandwich Fillers ~ Always Fresh

Per ¼ of 185g Tub, 46g

	Cal	kJ	Fat	Cb
Curried Egg	110	455	9	3
Grilled Vegetables & Feta	90	370	7.5	4
Ham & Wholegrain Mustard	135	560	13	2
Tuna & Sweet Corn	100	415	7	5

Syrup & Molasses

	Cal	kJ	Fat	Cb
Golden Syrup *(CSR):*				
1 level teaspoon, 7g	20	85	0	5
1 level Tbsp, 28g	85	355	0	21
Malt Extract, syrup, 1 Tbsp, 24g	75	315	0	17
Maple Flavoured Syrup:				
Green's, 1 Tbsp, 15g	45	180	0	11
IGA, 1 Tbsp, 20ml	75	315	0	19
Log Cabin/Karo, 1 Tbsp, 20ml	80	335	0	2
Queen, Sugar Free, 1 Tbsp, 20ml	10	45	0	4
Molasses, Blackstrap, 1 Tbsp, 15g	45	180	0	11
Pancake Syrup *(Green's),* 1 Tbsp, 15g	45	180	0	11
Treacle, 1 Tbsp, 20ml	85	360	0	20

Sugar ~ Quick Guide

	Cal	kJ	Fat	Cb
White, granular:				
1 level teaspoon, 4g	15	65	0	4
1 rounded teaspoon, 5g	20	85	0	5
1 heaped teaspoon, 6g	25	100	0	6
1 level Tablespoon, 16g	65	220	0	16
1 cube (small), 4.5g	18	80	0	4.5
100g quantity	400	1670	0	100
½ cup, 115g	460	1925	0	115
1 cup, 230g	920	3845	0	230
Sachets, rectangular, 1 tsp, 4g	15	65	0	4
Stick Sachets: *CSR,* stick, 3g	12	50	0	3
Coffee Shop, average, 1 tsp, 4g	15	65	0	4
Other Sugar:				
Brown Sugar: 1 Tbsp, 12 g	45	190	0	12
Loosely packed, 1 cup, 150g	570	2365	0	147
Packed hard, 1 cup, 240g	925	3865	0	235
Caster Sugar, ½ cup, 110g	450	1870	0	110
Coffee Crystal Sugar, 1 Tsp, 4g	15	70	0	4
Demerara, same as sugar				
Fructose/Fruit Sugar *(Fruisana),* 1 tsp, 5g	20	85	0	5
Icing Sugar, ½ cup, 70g	285	1190	0	70
LoGiCane, Low GI, 1 tsp, 4g	15	65	0	4
Palm Sugar, 1 Tbsp, 19g	60	250	0	16
Raw Sugar: 1 Tbsp, 16g	65	270	0	16
½ cup, 110g	450	1870	0	110
Stick Sachet *(CSR),* 3g	12	50	0	3
Sugar Cane Juice, ½ cup, 125g	100	420	0	25
Dextrose/Glucose/Fructose/Low GI: Same as sugar on weight basis				
Smart Sugar *(CSR),* 50% less sugar:				
½ tsp, 2g (= 1 tsp sugar)	8	35	0	2
½ cup, 57g	230	965	0	57
Stick Sachet, 2g	8	35	0	2

Sugar Substitutes

	Cal	kJ	Fat	Cb
Tablets: Equal/Sugarine	0	0	0	0
Powders: *(Equal Stevia Spoon for Spoon, NutraSweet Spoonful, Splenda)*				
1 level tsp	2	8	0	0.5
1 Tbsp, 2g	8	30	0	2
½ cup, 12g	50	200	0	11
Equal, Sachet, equivalent 2 tsp sugar	5	15	0	1
Stevia: Powder, 1 tsp	1	5	0	0.5
Equal, Stevia, Tablets	0	0	0	0
Xylitol, *(Perfect Sweet),* 1 tsp, 4g	10	40	0	1
Liquid, Sugarine/Sugarless	0	0	0	0

Updated Nutrition Data ~ www.CalorieKing.com.au
Persons with Diabetes ~ See Disclaimer (Page 22)

Vegetables & Legumes

Vegetables

Edible Portion, Raw Weight Unless Indicated

Item	Cal	kJ	Fat	Cb
Alfalfa/Bean Sprouts, 100g	30	115	0	1
Aniseed (Fennel), 50g	10	40	0	2
Artichoke: Globe (French), 200g	110	470	0	3
Jerusalem (Sunchoke), 100g	30	125	0	11
Asparagus, 3 medium spears, 60g	15	65	0	1
Bamboo Shoots, raw: 1 cup, 130g	35	150	0.5	7
Canned, 1 cup, 130g	20	75	0	2
Basil, fresh, 5 leaves	1	5	0	0
Bean Sprouts, 1 cup, 100g	20	85	0	2
Beans: *Fresh, Raw or Cooked, Per ½ Cup*				
Green/French/Runner, 60g	20	85	0	2
Borlotti, 80g	90	375	0	16
Broad Beans, raw, 55g	40	165	0	1
Butter/Lima, 70g	90	385	0	11
Kidney Beans, 80g	105	440	0	12
Purple Bean, 70g	20	85	0	2
Snake Bean (Yard-Long) 70g	35	140	0	6
Dried: Black Eye, Borlotti, Cannellini, Haricot, Kidney, Lima, average:				
Raw, 100g	335	1390	1	35
Cooked, ½ cup, 85g	105	440	0.5	20
Soya Beans: Raw, 100g	375	150	0	13
Cooked, 100g	145	600	8	1.5
Beetroot: 1 medium, 120g	35	155	0	6.5
1 baby, 40g	15	50	0	2
Cooked, 2 slices, 30g	15	60	0	2.5
Bok Choy (White Cabbage), 75g	10	35	0	0.5
Broccoli: 2 florets, 45g	15	55	0	0.5
1 head (13cm diam), 300g	55	225	0.5	1
Broccoflower, 1 cup, 65g	20	85	0	4
BroccoSprouts, ½ cup, 30g	10	40	0	0.5
Brussels Sprouts, raw, 4-5 medium, 120g	30	125	0.5	2
Burdock (Gobo) Japanese Roo, Vegetable, cooked, ½ cup, 100g	90	370	0	1
Cabbage, Green/Red/Savoy, shredded:				
½ cup, 40g	10	40	0	1.5
Chinese shredded, ½ cup, 40g	5	20	0	0.5
Capsicum, raw: Green/Red/Yellow, average all colours:				
1 medium, 140g	30	130	0	3.5
Chopped, 1 cup, 120g	25	110	0	3
Salad Rings (5mm thick), 3	5	30	0	1

Edible Portion, Raw Weight Unless Indicated

Item	Cal	kJ	Fat	Cb
Carrots, raw: 1 baby, 30g	10	40	0	1.5
1 small, 100g	30	130	0	5
1 medium, 140g	45	185	0	7
1 large, 180g	60	240	0	9
Diced/Slices, ½ cup, 70g	20	90	0	3.5
Grated, ¼ cup, 114g	35	150	0	6
4 Sticks, 28g	10	40	0	1.5
Cassava: White, flesh, 100g	140	58	0	31
Yellow, flesh only, 100g	140	585	0	31
Cauliflower:				
Raw, ¼ medium, 145g	35	145	0.5	3
Cooked, ½ cup, 100g	25	105	0	2
Celeriac Root, 100g	40	175	0	3
Celery, 1 piece, 15cm long, 30g	5	15	0	0.5
Celtuce, 100g	10	40	0	0
Chard (Swiss Chard) ½ cup, 100g	25	105	0	1
Chick Peas: Dry, 100g	320	1340	5	55
1 Cup, 220g	705	2950	11	120
Cooked: 100g	160	660	2.5	28
1 Cup, 200g	315	1315	5	55
Chilli Peppers: Red pod, 20g	10	30	0	1
Green pod, 20g	10	35	0	0.5
Chives, chopped, 2 Tbsp, 20g	5	15	0	0.5
Choko (Chayote), ½ medium, 60g	10	40	0	3
Choy Sum (Flower Cabbage), 80g	10	40	0	0.5
Collards, ½ cup, 100g	30	125	0.5	6
Coriander, fresh, 9 sprigs	5	15	0	1
Corn: 1 medium cob, 170g	160	670	3	21
Cobbette, 100g	95	395	2	13
Cucumber: Apple, ½ medium, 150g	10	50	0	2
Green: 1 medium, 500g	60	240	0.5	6
4-5 slices, 30g	5	15	0	0.5
Lebanese (short), 1 medium, 100g	10	50	0	2
Telegraph/Burpless, ¼ medium, 100g	10	50	0	1.5
Dandelion Greens, ½ cup, 100g	45	190	0	9.2
Dill Pickles, 1 large	10	40	0	3.5
Edamame, shelled, ⅔ cup, 85g	120	500	5	9.5
Eggplant (Aubergine):				
2 slices (1cm thick), 60g	10	40	0	1.5
Fried in oil, 100g	140	585	14	1.5
Endive, 30g	5	10	0	0.1
Fennel, (Florentine, sweet), 50g	10	40	0	1.5
Fern (Fiddlehead), 50g	15	7	0	3
Gai Choy/Mustard Cabbage, 75g	10	45	0	0.5
Garbanzo Beans ~ *See Chick Peas*				
Garlic: Fresh, 1 clove 3g	5	10	0	1
Dried, 1 tsp	15	65	0	3.5
John West, Jar, 1 tsp	5	25	0	1

Vegetables & Legumes

Vegetables (Cont)
Edible Portion, Raw Weight Unless Indicated

Food	Cal	kJ	Fat	Cb
Gherkin: 1 medium, sour/sweet, 30g	5	15	0	1
1 medium, sweet/spiced, 30g	25	115	0	6.5
Ginger: Fresh, grated, 1 Tbsp	5	15	0	0.5
Crystallised, 30g	100	420	0	24
Ground, 30g	75	315	0	20
Salad Slices (Bugerim), 1 tsp	5	20	0	0.5
Gow Chai (Garlic Chives), 5g	1	5	0	0
Horseradish, 30g	15	60	0	2.5
Jicama, shredded, 1 cup	50	210	0	11
Kale, ½ cup, 70g	35	145	0	7
Kang Kong (Water Spinach), 75g	15	65	0	2
Kohlrabi, diced, ¾ cup, 100g	35	140	0	4
Kumara ~ *See Sweet Potato*				
Leen Ngow (Lotus Root), 50g	25	105	0	9
Lettuce: Common, 3 leaves, 30g	5	10	0	0
Shredded, 1 cup, 35g	5	10	0	0
Cos, 2 leaves, 30g	5	20	0	0.5
Mignonette, 2 leaves, 30g	5	15	0	0.5
Leeks: bulb & leaf, 30g	10	40	0	1
Lentils: Dried, 100g	290	1200	2	35
Cooked, 100g	80	325	0.5	9.5
Lima/Butter Beans: Dry, 100g	290	1200	2	35
Cooked, 100g	80	340	0.5	10
Lotus Root, 6 slices, 50g	35	155	0	8.5
Lupins/Lupini Beans:				
(13), 30g	110	465	3	13
½ cup, 90g	335	1395	9	37
Mai Tai (Water Chestnuts), 50g	50	200	0	12
Marrow, ½ cup diced, 100g	20	75	0	2
Mung Beans:				
Sprouts, ½ cup, 45g	10	40	0	3
Seeds, mature, dry, 30g	105	445	0	18
Mushrooms (Funghi):				
Button, ½ cup, 60g	15	60	0	0
Field, 140g each	30	125	0	8
Umbrella, ½ cup, 60g	15	55	0	2.5
Wild: Black Fungi, 100g	50	200	0	8
Oyster, (Abalone) 100g	35	140	0	6.5
White Coral/Enoki, 100g	40	170	0	8
Mustard Greens, ½ cup, 70g	15	60	0	3.5
Nopales (Cactus Leaf):				
1 medium leaf, 130g	20	85	0	4
1 cup, thin slices, 85g	15	65	0	3
Okra: Raw, 4 pods, 60g	15	60	0	3
Cooked, ½ cup, 85g	20	85	0	4
Onions ~ *Next Page*				
Peas ~ *Next Page*				

Food	Cal	kJ	Fat	Cb
Potatoes, average all types (raw weight):				
Baby, gourmet, 50g	35	145	0	7
Small, 100g	70	290	0	14
Medium, 150g	105	440	0	21
Large, 200g	140	585	0	28
Extra Large, 250g	175	730	0	37
Mashed: *Per scoop, 50g*				
with butter & milk	55	225	3	5.5
with milk, no fat	30	125	0.5	3.5
Dehydrated Flakes:				
30g dry, reconstituted	105	445	0	51
Roasted in Fat: *Per 100g*				
Small pieces/wedges	150	630	8	18
Whole, 100g	125	525	5.5	15
Baked in Jacket:				
1 medium, 150g:				
with 2 tsp fat	175	730	8	37
with 2 Tbsp Sour Cream	180	750	7	39
with 2 Tbsp Cottage Cheese	170	710	4	38
with ¼ cup Grated Cheese	220	920	10	37
Sautéed, Slices, ½ cup, 100g	150	630	8	18
Hashed Browns/Strips, 75g	130	550	6.5	16
Potato Chips:				
Deep or Pan-Fried:				
Straight-Cut: 100g	200	835	7	27
Large Serve, 200g	400	1670	14	54
Crinkle-cut: 100g	240	1005	10	28
Large Serve, 200g	480	2010	20	56
French Fries: 100g	290	1210	15	28
Large Serve, 200g	580	2420	30	56
Oven Fries: Baked, average, 100g	160	670	4	27
Fried, average, 100g	210	880	10	28
Tefal ActiFry Cooker:				
(Low Fat Method ~ Using				
14ml oil to 1kg fresh chips)				
100g quantity, cooked	150	630	2.5	18
Wedges/Skins/Chunky Chips:				
Oven-fried, average:				
100g serve	180	750	9	42
Large serve, 200g	360	1500	18	84
1 medium wedge, 15g	25	115	1.5	7
Deep-fried: 100g	320	1350	22	30
Large Serve, 200g	640	2700	44	60
Sautéed, 100g	100	420	5	18
Sprayed (e.g. Pure & Simple),				
Oven Baked, 100g	75	315	0	18

Updated Nutrition Data ~ www.CalorieKing.com.au
Persons with Diabetes ~ See Disclaimer (Page 22)

169

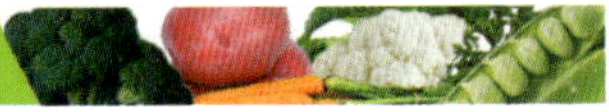

Vegetables & Legumes

Vegetables (Cont)	Cal	kJ	Fat	Cb
Onions, average all types: Small 60g	20	75	0	3
Medium, 120g	30	120	0	4.5
Large, 180g	45	185	0	6.5
Diced, raw, ½ cup, 60g	20	75	0	3
Fried: Lightly oiled pan/BBQ. 100g	120	500	6	7.5
Heavily oiled pan/BBQ, 100g	170	710	12	7.5
Pickled, 1 medium, 20g	10	40	0	2.5
Spring, raw, 1 only, 15g	5	15	0	0.5
Peas:				
Green: Raw, without pod, 100g	60	255	0.5	9
Cooked: ¼ cup, 40g	35	140	0	3
½ cup, 80g	50	200	0.3	5
Snow Peas, 10 pods, 33g	10	45	0	1.7
Sugar Snap, 10 pods, 30g	10	45	0	1.5
Pimentos, canned, 3 medium, 100g	25	105	0	5
Pumpkin: Common/Qld Blue				
Raw, without skin, 100g	45	190	0	8.5
Baked with fat, 100g	120	500	7	8
Mashed, 1 scoop, 50g	25	105	0.5	4.5
Butternut, raw, without skin, 100g	40	175	0	7.2
Golden Nugget:				
Raw, without skin, 100g	30	120	0	4
1 whole, (400g with skin)	110	450	2	16
Purslane, 100g	20	85	0	3.5
Radish, average all types,				
1 small, 20g	2	10	0	0.2
Rocket (Arugula), leaf salad, 1 cup	10	40	0	1
Salsify (Scorzonera, oyster plant),				
1 cup, 100g	80	345	0	19
Sauerkraut, canned, dr., ⅔ cup, 100g	20	85	0	4.5
Seaweed: Fresh, average, 100g	30	125	0	10
Dried, average all types, 100g	240	1100	0	22
Shallots, 3 only, 20g	5	15	0	0.5
Silverbeet, ½ cup, 100g	15	55	0	1.5
Sorrel, 1 cup	30	120	0	4.5
Soy Beans: Green, raw, 100g	150	615	7	11
Cooked, ½ cup, 100g	130	545	8	1.5
Spaghetti Vegetable, raw, 100g	30	130	0.5	7
Spinach:				
English, raw: 1 bunch, 350g	55	240	1	3
Chopped, 1 cup, 35g	10	35	0	0.5
Cooked, ½ cup, 100g	25	105	0.5	1
Baby Spinach Leaves,				
1 cup, 25g	5	25	0	0
Split Peas:				
Dry, ½ cup, 100g	350	1465	1	46
Cooked, ½ cup, 100g	65	275	0.5	7

Vegetables (Cont)	Cal	kJ	Fat	Cb
Spring Onion, 1 only, 15g	5	15	0	0.5
Sprouts:				
Alfalfa, 1 punnet, 125g	30	115	0	0.5
Mung Bean, 1 cup, 90g	20	75	0	5.5
Squash, button, 100g	25	105	0	3
Sugar Snap Peas, 100g	35	145	0	4.5
Swede (Rutabagas), 100g	35	150	0	8
Sweetcorn: 1 large cob, 200g	190	790	4	25
1 medium cob, 100g	95	395	2	13
Kernels only, ½ cup, 60g	55	235	1	7.5
Baby Corn, 1 piece, 10g	5	10	0	0.5
Sweet Potato (Kumara), flesh only:				
Orange flesh, ¼ small, 100g	65	280	0	15
Purple skin, ¼ small, 100g	85	360	0	20
White flesh, ¼ small, 100g	60	250	0	14
Tampala Leaves, 100g	35	145	0	4
Taro, diced, ¾ cup, 100g	110	460	0	24
Tomatoes, 1 medium, 150g	30	115	0	4
Other Listings ~ See Fruit, Page 104				
Canned ~ See Page 172				
Paste/Puree/Sauce ~ See Page 149				
Turnip, white, 1 med., 100g	20	95	0	3.5
Turnip Greens, 100g	30	130	0	7
Watercress: 10 sprigs, 10g	2	10	0	0
1 punnet, 80g	20	90	0	0.5
Water Chestnut, Chinese (4), 25g	25	100	0	6
White Radish, 60g	15	60	0	2
Witloof, (Belgium Endive, Chicory),				
1 medium, 80g	15	55	0	0.5
Yam, ½ cup, 100g	100	420	0	28
Yucca Root, diced, ½ cup, 100g	160	670	0.5	31
Zucchini:				
Raw: 1 small (3cm diam), 125g	15	55	0	2
1 med. (5cm diam), 250g	30	125	0	5
Cooked, ½ cup slices, 100g	10	40	0	2

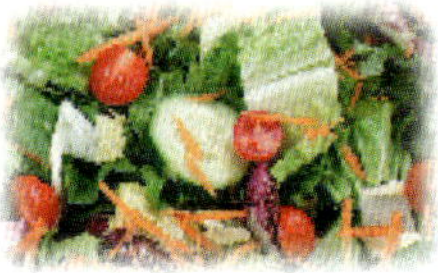

Vegetables ~ Frozen

Potato Chips/Products

	Cal	kJ	Fat	Cb
Frozen/Uncooked:				
Birds Eye:				
Pommes, ¼ Packet, 87g	155	645	6.5	20
Potato Bites, 54g	100	425	4.5	13
Potato Curly Fries	200	845	10	24
Potato Gems, 100g	155	645	7.5	18
Potato Swirls, 100g	160	675	5	24
Golden Crunch Potato: Chips, 100g	125	525	4.5	18
Chips in Beer Batter, 100g	110	450	5.5	12
Crinkles, 100g	155	645	6	20
Monster Chips in Beer Batter, 100g	105	435	4.5	14
Steakhouse Chips, 100g	115	475	5.5	13
Wedges, 100g	135	565	5	18
Hash Browns: Original, 62.5g	110	460	6	11
Golden Crunch, 62g	110	455	6	11
Oven Bake Chips: French Fries, 100g	125	525	4.5	17
Crinkle Cut, 100g	125	520	4.5	17
Seasoned Straight Cut, 100g	155	640	6.5	19
Steakhouse Cut, 100g	120	490	4	17
Straight Cut, 100g	120	490	4	17
Wedges, 100g	180	745	7.5	24
Oven Roast Potatoes:				
Country Style, 100g	135	565	4	21
Traditional; Rosemary & Garlic, 100g	145	595	4.5	22
Coles:				
Potato Royals, 100g	150	615	6.5	19
Chunky Wedges, 100g	175	730	7.5	24
Oven Fries: Crinkle Cut, 100g	125	520	4.5	17
French Fries, 100g	125	525	4.5	17
Straight Cut, 100g	120	490	4	17
McCain: *Per 125g Unless Indicated*				
Chips: Beer Batter varieties	190	785	7	27
Original Fries	190	785	5.5	30
Hash Browns: Original, 75g	130	550	6.5	16
Healthy Choice: Chunky Cut	155	645	4	25
Straight Cut Fries, 100g	125	520	3	21
Mini Roasts, all flavours	180	740	5.5	26
Nuggets, ⅙ packet, 125g	220	920	10	25
Potato Snack, Mash Bites, 100g	180	735	7	25
Purely Potato: 125g				
Potato Chunks/Cubes/Slices	110	450	0.5	22
Sweet Potato Cubes	80	340	1.5	15

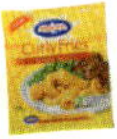

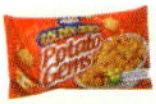

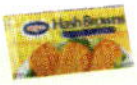

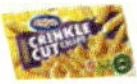

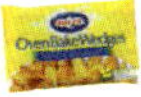

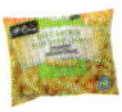

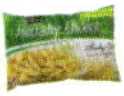

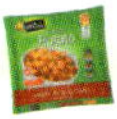

Potato Chips/Products (Cont)

	Cal	kJ	Fat	Cb
McCain (Cont): *Per 125g Unless Indicated*				
Smiles, ⅙ packet	220	925	10	27
Superfries: Chunky Cut	155	645	4	25
Crinkle Cut	195	805	6	30
Extra Long French	180	740	5.5	27
Straight Cut	195	810	5.5	30
Sweet Potatoes: Crinkle Cut, 90g	155	655	6.5	22
Thin Cut, 90g	170	700	6.5	25
Wedges: Beer Batter	195	815	6	29
Hot Bandito	190	785	5.5	30

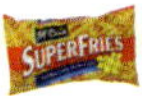

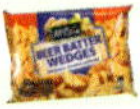

Other Frozen Vegetables

	Cal	kJ	Fat	Cb
Birds Eye:				
Create-a-Meal: *Per ⅓ of 200g Packet*				
Black Bean	85	355	1.5	13
Honey Soy	115	490	0.5	21
Korma Curry	120	510	3.5	16
Teriyaki	105	445	2.5	14
Stir Fry Vegetable Mix: *Per ¼ of 125g Packet*				
Cantonese	45	185	0.5	5
Chow Mein	40	165	0.5	4
Malaysian	65	275	0.5	9
Thai Style	45	175	0.5	5
Steam Fresh: *Per Serving*				
Carrots, Peas & Corn, 75g	50	200	0.5	7.5
Carrot, Broccoli & Corn, 75g	35	155	1	4
Broccoli/Cauliflower, 100g	30	115	0.5	2.5
Oven Roast Mix: *Per ¼ Packet*				
Italian Herb, 143g	110	460	2.5	17
Rosemary & Garlic, 143g	135	550	2.5	22
Pommes, ¼ packet, 87g	155	650	7	20
Vegetables in Cheese, ¼ packet, 125g	155	645	5.5	19
Heinz:				
Beans: Broad, 100g	55	225	0.5	2
Whole Baby, 100g	25	110	0	2.5
Mixed Veggies: *Per Serving, 100g*				
Baby Peas & Supersweet Corn	80	320	1	11
Cauliflower & Broccoli	25	110	0	1.5
Romano	35	135	0	4.5
Peas: Plain/Minted, 100g	85	360	1	9
Baby, 100g	70	290	0.5	9
SteamFresh: *Per 150g Pouch*				
Baby Beans, Carrots & Broccoli	45	190	0.5	4
Broccoli, Carrot & Cauliflower	45	180	0.5	4
Carrots, Corn & Broccoli	75	325	1	10

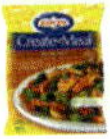

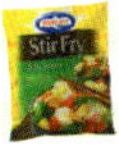

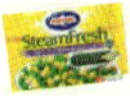

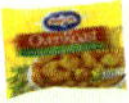

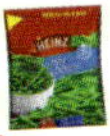

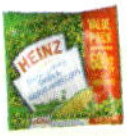

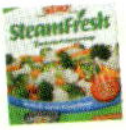

Updated Nutrition Data ~ www.CalorieKing.com.au
Persons with Diabetes ~ See Disclaimer (Page 22)

171

Vegetables ~ Frozen/Canned/Jars/Dried

Other Frozen Vegetables (Cont) | Cal | kJ | Fat | Cb

McCain: *Per 100g Unless Indicated*

Item	Cal	kJ	Fat	Cb
Beans, Green, average	40	160	0.5	5
Broccoli, 1/5 packet	30	130	0.5	2
Brussel Sprouts, 1/5 packet	50	215	0.5	6.5
Carrots, all varieties, 1/5 packet	35	145	0.5	6
Cauliflower, 1/5 packet, 100g	25	105	0.5	2.5
Corn Cobettes, 125g	140	575	2	22
Corn Kernels, Super Juicy	95	390	2	14
Mini Roasts Potatoes, 1/8 packet, 125g	180	740	5.5	26
Peas; Mint Peas; Baby Peas	80	330	1	12
Mixes: Defence	55	225	1	7.5
Baby Beans, Baby Carrots & Peas, 100g	45	185	0.5	6
Cauliflower & Broccoli, 1/5 packet, 100g	30	110	0.5	2.5
Garden Greens	60	260	1	6
Mixed Vegetables: Peas, Corn & Carrots	80	335	1	13
Peas & Corn	90	380	1.5	14
Stirfry Supreme Vegetables	35	135	0.5	4.5
Vision	75	305	1.5	11
Winter Vegetables	30	130	0.5	4

Cans & Jars

Average All Brands

Item	Cal	kJ	Fat	Cb
Artichoke Hearts, 55g each	15	60	0	1
Asparagus: 3 spears, 60g	15	60	0	1
Marinated, 85g, 1/4 jar	45	185	0	8
Bamboo Shoots (Chang's), drained, 142g	45	180	4	0
Beans, e.g. Kidney/Butter, drained average, 1/2 cup, 100g	90	375	0.5	14
Green Beans, 100g	30	125	0	6.5
Broad Beans, 100g	65	270	0.5	2.5
Baked Beans ~ *See Page 122-127*				
Always Fresh: Baked Beans, 90g	15	70	0.5	0.5
Soy, drained, 100g	100	425	5.5	2
Four Bean Mix, 100g drained	120	500	0.5	16
Mixed Bean Mix, 100g drained	100	410	0.5	14
Beetroot: 2 slices, 30g	15	55	0	3
Baby Beets; Wedges, 30g	20	80	0	3.5
Capsicum (*Edgell*), 45g drained	15	60	0.5	2.5
Carrots, 1/2 cup, 90g	25	105	0	3.5
Chick Peas: 100g drained	130	535	1.5	18
Edgell, 75g drained	95	400	1	13
Chillies, 2-3 pieces, 30g	10	35	0	0.5
Corn: Kernel, drained, 1/2 cup, 75g	55	230	1	8.5
Creamed, 1/2 cup, 125g	85	350	1	16
Young Corn, spears/cuts, 125g	25	95	0.5	1

Cans & Jars (Cont) | Cal | kJ | Fat | Cb

Average All Brands

Item	Cal	kJ	Fat	Cb
Dolmade, (2), 40g	60	255	3	7
Garlic/Onion/Chilli/Ginger, Minced, 1 tsp	5	15	0	1
Giardiniera, Pickled Veges, 1/2 cup, 125g	30	125	0	7.5
Hearts of Palm, 1 piece, 50g	10	45	0	2.5
Lentils, Brown (*Edgell; Sanitarium*), 100g	90	385	0.5	13
Mushrooms/Champignons:				
SPC, In Butter Sauce, 1/2 cup, 100g	30	130	1	4.5
Always Fresh, Marinated, 1/2 cup, 60g	35	150	1	5
Olives ~ *See Page 146*				
Onions: Pickled, 1 med., 20g	10	50	0	2.5
Cocktail, 1 only, 7g	5	15	0	1.5
Peas, green, 1/2 cup, 90g	60	255	0.5	7.5
Potatoes: Drained, 100g	55	220	0	12
Edgell, Tiny Taters, all types, 100g	70	285	0	14
Sauerkraut, 2/3 cup, 100g	15	65	0	3
Soya Beans, 100g drained	100	420	5.5	2
Stir Fry Veges:				
Baby corn Mix, 125g	35	145	0	7
Champignon Mix, 125g	30	120	0.5	4
Water Chestnut/Bamboo Shoot, 125g	45	180	0	8
Tomatoes: *Whole, Peeled/Pieces/Diced. Per 1/2 Cup, 125g*				
Ardmona: 1/2 cup, 125g	30	130	0	6
Chopped with Herbs	35	140	0.5	4.5
No Salt, No Sugar	30	115	0	5.5
Coles:				
Diced, 1/2 of 400g can, 200g	40	160	1.5	7
Whole, Italian Style, peeled, 1/2 of 400g can, 200g	40	170	0.5	7
SPC: Crushed	30	135	0	6
Whole/Diced, average	30	115	0	6
Water Chestnuts, 142g	50	205	0	9.5

Dried Vegetables

Item	Cal	kJ	Fat	Cb
Fried Onion, chopped, 30g	140	595	7.5	15
Peas/Carrots, average, 10g dry	15	50	0	2
Corn/Mixed Veges, average, 10g dry	10	45	0	2
Shitake Mushrooms, 10g	30	135	0	7.5
Instant Potato, Plain/onion, reconstituted with milk, 190g	150	635	3	26

Vegetables in Oil

(e.g. Sandhurst; Always Fresh),
Includes Capsicums, Eggplant,
Artichoke, Tomato, avg. drained, 30g | 75 | 315 | 5 | 7

Yoghurt

Yoghurt ~ Quick Guide

	Cal	kJ	Fat	Cb
Yoghurt				
Average All Brands				
Plain: Natural, 200g	170	705	8.5	10
Non-Fat/Skim, 200g	115	480	0	12
Fruit Flavoured: 200g	185	770	6	22
Diet/Non-Fat (no sugar) 200g	80	330	0	11
Light/Reduced Fat, 200g	155	650	2	27
Greek Style: Natural, 200g	240	995	17	13
Fruit Flavoured, 200g	260	1075	13	27

Yoghurt ~ Brands

	Cal	kJ	Fat	Cb
Activia (Danone):				
4-Pack: *125ml Cup*				
Natural	95	385	2	11
Fruit Flavours, avg.	105	430	2	16
6-Pack, Favourites, avg, 125ml	110	450	2	17
Singles, avg., 70g	150	630	2.5	23
Pouring, avg, ½ cup, 125ml	105	440	2	16
Dessert Yoghurts, avg, 125g	140	580	4.5	18
B.-d. Farm Paris Creek: *Per 200g*				
Indulgence: Dessert Style	200	840	5.5	30
Greek Style	125	520	7.5	9
Lemon Myrtle; Tiramisu	235	980	5.5	38
Organic: Apricot	185	760	6	26
Blueberry	175	720	5.5	27
Bush Honey & Vanilla	150	620	6.6	17
Low Fat	65	260	0.5	9
Mango	175	720	5	26
Raspberry	185	760	6.5	26
Strawberry	195	820	6	28
Barambah Organics: *Per 200g*				
All Natural	135	575	7	10
Banana	155	635	6	16
Blueberry/Cherry	145	590	6.5	13
Bush Honey	170	705	6.5	18
Greek	215	900	10	18
Low Fat Natural	100	420	0.5	12
Mango	145	605	6	15
Passionfruit	135	570	6.5	10
Strawberry	140	575	6	13
Vanilla Bean	180	745	7	20
Black Swan:				
Greek Style, (500g Tub):				
Breakfast, ¾ cup, 200g	195	815	5.5	21
Low Fat, ¾ cup, 200g	200	825	4	24
No Fat, ¾ cup, 200g	135	565	0	18
375g Tub, Vanilla Bean, ⅓ tub, 125g	125	520	4	12

Brands (Cont)

	Cal	kJ	Fat	Cb
Brooklea (Aldi):				
Natural, Fat Free Tub Set, 150g	80	330	0	11
Yogurt Squishy, 70g pouch, avg.	60	240	1	10
Brownes (WA): *Per 175g Tub*				
Deluxe: Creamy Vanilla	180	750	5.5	26
Peaches & Cream	190	800	5	30
Diet, avgerage all flavours, 175g	85	345	0	12
Light: Mixed Berry, Strawberry	145	590	2	23
Peach Banana Passion	155	635	2	27
Natural	130	550	5.5	13
Traditional, Muesli	185	770	5	27
Bulla,				
Crunch, average all flavours, 225g	320	1340	5	56
Casa (WA):				
Pot Set: Natural, 200g	160	655	7	10
Gourmet: With Mango, 200g	235	970	5.5	33
With Strawberries. 200g	235	970	5.5	33
Greek Style *(350g Tub):*				
Dessert, Honey, 200g	210	880	6	31
Natural, ½ tub, 175g	175	730	8	8.5
Fruit flavours, average, ½ tub, 175g	185	770	5	29
Chobani: *Per 170g Tub*				
Greek:				
Fat-Free (0%): Plain	110	455	0	8
Fruit flavours, average	140	590	0	21
Honey	135	580	0	18
Low-Fat (2%), avg. all flavours	165	690	3	20
Chris', Greek Style, Natural, 200g	295	1230	20	17
Coles:				
Lite: Peach & Mango, 200g	180	740	3.5	28
Strawberry, 200g	170	720	2	28
Swirl (720g Tub):				
Average all flavours, ¾ cup, 200g	290	1200	11	37
98% Fat-Free (1kg Tub):				
Peach & Mango, 200g	195	820	3.5	32
Summer Berry	190	800	3.5	30
Vanilla, 200g	190	800	3.5	30
1kg Tub: *Per ¾ cup*				
Vanilla, 200g	235	975	7.5	30
Greek Style, average	290	1200	20	16
Dairy Farmers:				
Greek, ¾ cup, 200g	270	1125	20	15
Thick & Creamy: *Per 170g Tub*				
Regular, avg. all flavours	190	800	5.5	27
98% Fat Free, avg. all flavours	175	730	3	28

Updated Nutrition Data ~ www.CalorieKing.com.au
Persons with Diabetes ~ See Disclaimer (Page 22)

173

Yoghurt

Brands (Cont)

Product	Cal	kJ	Fat	Cb
Danone: *Per 125g Tub*				
Oikos (0%): Black Cherry; Blueberry	105	430	0	15
Activia ~ See Activia				
Evia: *Per 200g Carton*				
Classic, average all flavours	270	1120	8	30
Skinny, average all flavours	225	950	1.5	33
Farmers Union:				
Greek Style: Natural, 200g	270	1120	19	15
Light (50% less Fat), 200g	200	840	10	18
Strained: Honey	140	590	0	22
Strawberry	130	540	0	19
European Style, Natural, 200g	150	620	6.5	13
Five:am:				
Organic: *Per 170g Tub*				
Coffee Bean; Dark Caramel	185	770	9	22
Honey Cinn; Vanilla Bean, avg.	190	800	9	20
98% Fat-Free: *Per 170g Tub*				
Orange, Lemon + Ginger	155	645	3	24
Mango; Strawb. & Guava., avg.	145	600	3	21
Smoothies, avg., 240 ml	195	810	6.5	30
Gippsland Dairy:				
Organic: *Per 200g Carton*				
Blueberry; Raspberry; Wildberry	220	930	9	21
Natural	160	670	7	11
Peach Mango & Passionfruit	230	970	12	21
Fat-Free Natural	105	440	0	15
Vanilla	220	910	9	24
Other Fruit flavours	230	945	12	20
Twist, average all flavours,				
¾ cup, 200g	220	925	10	25
300ml cup, avg	330	1385	15	51
Mini Organics, avg, 70g pouch	70	285	2	10
Island Pure (Kangaroo Island),				
Sheep Milk, ¾ cup, 200g	210	880	15	9.5
Jalna: *Per 200g Carton*				
Genuine Leben European Style	170	700	8	14
Whole Milk Natural	155	650	10	7
Premium Creamy: Fruits Of The Forest	235	965	9	28
Honey Vanilla	260	1085	10	32
Natural	205	845	10	17
Strawberry	255	1055	7	30
Vanilla	245	1025	10	29
Fat Free: BioDynamic	100	405	0	14
Natural	105	440	0	15

Brands (Cont)

Product	Cal	kJ	Fat	Cb
Jalna: (Cont): *Per 200g*				
Low-Fat: Berry Fruit	180	745	4	25
Greek	200	845	6	17
Strawberry	190	790	4	24
Vanilla	210	880	4	34
BioDynamic: Blueberry	225	940	9	25
Bush Honey	210	890	9	26
Whole Milk	170	700	9	13
King Island Dairy:				
Plain, 300g Tub	390	1635	19	38
Honey Cinnamon, 200g	275	1150	12	30
Kingland:				
Soy Yogurt, average, 250g	255	1070	8	37
Liddells, Lactose Free, Plain, 140g	120	500	4	14
Lite n' Easy: *Per 100g*				
Fruit of the Forest	115	480	3	16
Mango	110	460	3	14
Passionfruit	115	485	3	16
Vanilla	125	525	3.5	20
Margaret River Dairy Co (WA): *Per 200g*				
Creamy Pot Set: Greek	205	860	11	17
Mixed Berry	195	810	3.5	31
Natural	120	495	0	18
Passionfruit	180	750	3	29
Peach & Mango	175	730	2.5	30
Mundella (WA):				
Premium: *Per 250g*				
Natural	250	1050	10	16
Sunkissed Fruits	300	1245	9	41
Woodland Fruits	250	1030	8	38
Fat Free, Natural, 250g	165	685	0.5	28
Reduced Fat:				
Natural, 250g	190	780	4.5	20
Vanilla, 250g	260	1075	5	34
Greek Yoghurt:				
500g/1kg Tubs: Natural, 250g	300	1245	21	16
Honey; Vanilla, avg., 250g	330	1375	20	28
300g Tubs: Banana Mango Bliss	365	1515	19	36
Blueberry Blitz	355	1480	19	33
Honey Heaven	355	1480	18	34
Little Greek Ones: *Per 140g tub*				
Blueberry	180	755	10	19
Honey	185	775	11	19
Passionfruit	185	770	10	19
Vanilla	185	770	11	16

Yoghurt

Brands (Cont)	Cal	kJ	Fat	Cb
Nestlé:				
Soleil Diet: *Per 150g Tub*				
Black Cherry; Peach Mango	60	250	0	7
Blueberry Apple Crumble	60	245	0	7
Passionfruit; Strawb.; Van.	60	250	0	7.5
Squeezie Pouch,				
Strawberry/Vanilla, 170g pouch	60	260	1.5	10
Pauls:				
All Natural,				
Original, 200g carton	150	625	6	13
Lite: *Per 175g Carton*				
Fruit Salad	145	605	0	28
Strawberry/Passionfruit	140	575	0	26
Vanilla	160	655	0	32
Full Fat: *Per 75g Tub*				
Fruit Salad; Passionfruit	75	315	2	11
Strawberry	70	300	2	12
Vanilla	80	330	2	12
Dora The Explora: Avg, 90g	80	340	2.5	11
Kids Pouch, 70g	65	275	2	9
Roaming Cow:				
Natural, 180g tub	140	575	4	15
Vanilla, 180g tub	165	685	3.5	23
Shaw River Buffalo Yoghurt,				
Plain, ¾ cup, 200g	195	815	14	9
Simply Less (Coles): *Per 170g Tub*				
Greek Style: Blueberry & Muesli	220	900	5	33
Blueberry Swirl	160	670	4	22
Honey & Muesli	240	1000	5	39
Light	150	620	4	17
Passionfruit & Muesli	225	940	5	35
Passionfruit Swirl	170	700	4	24
Peach & Mango Swirl	165	685	4	23
Ski:				
Activ: *Multi Pack, Per Single 125g Tub*				
Mango	115	480	1	20
Mixed Berry	115	480	1	19
Passionfruit	110	460	1	18
Strawberry	110	465	1	19
Vanilla Sensation	155	750	1	26
D'Lite: *Per 200g Tub Unless Otherwise Stated*				
Blueberry Burst	180	745	2	30
Honey Buzz	195	815	2	34
Peach & Mango	175	735	2	30
Vanilla Creme	180	760	2	30
99% Fat-Free: Mango Splash	185	760	2	31
Passionfruit	170	715	2	28
Peach Melba	175	735	2	30
Vanilla Boysenberry	175	715	2	29
Wild Strawberry	175	730	2	29

Ski (Cont):	Cal	kJ	Fat	Cb
Divine: Berry Heaven; Mango	210	875	6.5	28
Passionfruit	195	825	7	25
Tropical Fruit Salad	205	850	6.5	27
Vanilla Creme	205	855	6.5	28
Strawberry	200	835	6.5	26
Double Up: *Per 165g Tub*				
Apple Crumble	220	910	3.5	37
Crunchy Muesli	235	985	3.5	41
Smashed Berry, 185g	220	920	1.5	45
Soy Life: *Per 175g tub*				
Apricot & Mango/Boysenb.	140	585	1	25
Blueberry	145	605	1	27
Vanilla Crème	140	570	1	25
Springbrook: *Per 170g tub*				
Gourmet: Mango/Passionfruit	190	795	8	27
Mixed Berry	185	780	8.5	26
Greek	185	770	9	18
Low Fat, avg, all flavours	125	530	3	23
Tamar Valley:				
Classic: *Per 200g Tub*				
Apricot	170	700	4	22
Mango; Natural	165	680	4	21
Greek Style: *Per 230g Tub*				
Honey	275	1145	6.5	40
Passionfruit	270	1130	6	40
Strawberry	275	1150	6	42
No Added Sugar: Mango	170	690	4	20
Passionfruit	165	685	4	19
Raspberry	160	670	4	18
Strawberry	155	640	4	17
Lite: Apricot, 200g	155	640	2	22
Mixed Berry, 200g	150	630	2	22
Natural, 200g	145	600	2	21
No-Fat, Natural, 200g	145	600	0	20
Tasmanian Creamy: *Per 170g Tub*				
Creamy Passionfruit & Mango	160	670	3	24
Creamy Vanilla	160	670	3	24
The Collective (N.Z.): *Per Serving*				
Gourmet: (500g Tubs), avg, 200g	280	1160	11	36
Skinny Twin Pot, avg, 170g	135	560	1.5	18
4 Pack, 1 tub, avg, 100g	110	455	5	15
Straight Up, (900g Tubs),				
unsweetened, 200g	205	860	11	16
Vaalia:				
Light: Passionfruit, 150g tub	100	405	1.5	12
French Vanilla, 150g tub	100	400	1.5	12
Lactose-Free: *Per 175g Tub*				
French Vanilla	155	650	2.5	24
Passionfruit	160	675	2.5	25
Strawberry	165	690	2.5	27

Updated Nutrition Data ~ www.CalorieKing.com.au
Persons with Diabetes ~ See Disclaimer (Page 22)

Yoghurt ◆ Drinking Yoghurt

Brands (Cont)

	Cal	kJ	Fat	Cb
Vaalia (Cont):				
Low-Fat: *Per 160g Tub*				
Apricot Mango Peach	145	595	2	23
French Vanilla	160	670	2.5	27
Lemon Crème, 160g	170	720	2	30
Luscious Berries	155	650	2.5	25
Natural, 200g	160	670	4	18
Passionfruit	165	685	2	27
Strawberry	160	660	2	26
Strawberry & Raspberry, 160g	150	630	2	24
Vanilla Blueberry	155	645	2	26
Kids, Squeeze, avg., 140g	125	525	3.5	17
My First Yoghurt, all flavours, 90g	80	320	2.5	8.5
Woolworths: *Per 200g*				
Select: Greek Style	295	1230	22	15
Thick & Delicious, average	205	855	4	32
Yalla:				
Banana, 150g tub	250	1050	14	26
Banana Prune, 155g	285	1195	11	40
Guava, 135g	220	915	15	16
Mango, 155g tub	270	1135	19	21
Prune & Vanilla, 155g tub	320	1350	17	37
Strawb. & Pomegranate, 135g tub	250	1050	16	23
Vanilla, 175g	350	1450	24	26
Breakfast With Granola:				
Banana, 130g tub	330	1390	14	42
Mango, 130g tub	260	1085	16	24
Yoplait:				
98% Fat-Free:				
Average all flavours,				
175g Tub	170	705	3.5	26
1kg Tubs, 200g serve	190	800	4	29
Cal-tivate: *Per 175g Tub*				
Honey	150	630	2	24
Passionfruit	150	625	2	24
Strawberry	150	615	2	24
Duets: *Per 150g Tub*				
Plain Yoghurt: w. Apple & Cinn Puree	165	690	2	29
with Choc Bites & Banana	245	1020	10	31
with Choc Cherry Bites	230	960	7	34
with Choc Honecomb Bites	220	920	5	36
with Mixed Berry Puree	160	670	2	28
with Passionfruit Puree	170	695	2	29
Forme Satisfy: *Per 170g Tub*				
Berry Cheesecake	90	380	0	13
Caramel Tart	90	380	0	13
Passionfruit	95	395	0	14
Peach & Apricot Crumble	90	390	0	13
Strawberry	85	360	0	12
Vanilla	90	375	0	13

	Cal	kJ	Fat	Cb
Yoplait (Cont):				
Forme, No Fat: *Per 175g Tub*				
Apple Pie	75	300	0	11
Banana & Creamy Honey	75	305	0	11
Black Cherry	70	290	0	10
Boysenberry	70	285	0	9
Field Berries	70	300	0	10
French Vanilla	70	285	0	10
Passionfruit	70	305	0	10
Peach Mango	70	290	0	10
Strawberry	65	280	0	9
Strawb. Banana; Tropical	70	290	0	10
Go-Gurt:				
Tubes, 70g	75	310	1.5	14
Freeze 'N Go, Smooth,				
average all flavours, 150g pouch	130	535	2.5	21
Petit Miam, average all flavours, 60g tub	70	290	3	8
Smackers, Strawberry, 70 g tube	75	315	1.5	13
Squeezie, all flavours, 70g pouch	60	250	1.5	10
Yoplus, Natural, 100g	75	305	2	8.5

Drinking Yoghurt/Probiotics

	Cal	kJ	Fat	Cb
Bulla, Fruit 'n Yogurt,				
avg, all varieties, 200g bottle	140	590	1	26
Coles, Pro-B Fermented, 62ml	45	195	0	11
Mundella (WA),				
Probiotic, 250ml	195	800	2.5	31
The Collective (N.Z): *Per 250ml*				
Berrystart	195	815	4.5	32
Mango	220	925	4	43
Smooth Banana	175	730	3.5	31
Strawberry	190	780	4	32
Vanilla + Honey	225	940	5	38
Vaalia: Innergy, 90ml	70	300	1	12
Banana & Honey, 200g	180	765	3	28
Yakult: Original, 65ml bottle	50	220	0	12
Light, 65ml	35	155	0	9
Woolworths, Probiotic, 62ml	45	190	0	11

Yoghurt Mix Powder ~ EasiYo

Per 200g Prepared as Directed

	Cal	kJ	Fat	Cb
Natural, unsweetened	135	565	7	11
Bio Life, reduced Fat	120	510	3.5	15
Greek, unsweetened	165	690	9	14
Low Lactose	120	495	3	12
Reduced Fat, unsweetened	115	480	3.5	14
Strawberry; Mango, average	215	890	7	31
Vanilla	205	860	7.5	28

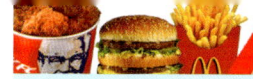

Eating Out & Fast-Foods

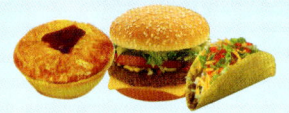

For More Restaurants & Full Nutritional Data ~ See CalorieKing.com.au

©2014 Allan Borushek

Cafe-Style & Take-Away Foods

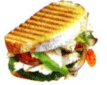 ❏ 178-179

International Foods

- ❏ Asian 180
- ❏ French 181
- ❏ German 181
- ❏ Greek 180
- ❏ Indian/Pakistani 180
- ❏ Italian 181
- ❏ Japanese 182
- ❏ Jewish 193
- ❏ Lebanese/Mid. Eastern . 183
- ❏ Mexican 184
- ❏ Polish 184
- ❏ Thai 184
- ❏ Vietnamese 184

Fast-Food Chains

- ❏ Bakers Delight 185
- ❏ Baskin Robbins 186
- ❏ Brumby's 186
- ❏ Carl's Jr. (N.Z.) 186
- ❏ Chicken Treat 186
- ❏ Donut King 188
- ❏ Domino's 189
- ❏ Eagle Boys 190
- ❏ Grill'd 191
- ❏ Healthy Habits 191
- ❏ Hungry Jacks 191
- ❏ Jesters 192
- ❏ KFC 193
- ❏ McDonald's 196
- ❏ McCafe 197
- ❏ Muffin Break 200
- ❏ Nando's 201
- ❏ New Zealand Natural .. 201
- ❏ Noodle Box 202
- ❏ Oporto 202
- ❏ Pie face 203
- ❏ Pita Pit (N.Z.) 203
- ❏ Pizza Hut 204
- ❏ Red Rooster 204
- ❏ Subway 206
- ❏ Sumo Salad 207
- ❏ Wendy's 207

Cafe-Style & Take-Away

Average All Outlets ~ Estimates only

Food	Cal	kJ	Fat	Cb
Antipasto, 2 slices Salami, 3 Olives, ½ cup Vegetables	180	750	13	4.5
Bruschetta, 2 slices, Tomato/Onion/Pesto	635	2655	41	53
BLT, Bacon, Lettuce, Tomato and Mayo	475	1970	24	31
Beef Burger:				
With Salad & Mayo	495	2060	27	35
With French Fries	750	3130	41	64
Bagel: Plain, large, 115g	320	1340	2	65
With Salmon, Cream Cheese	435	1815	6.5	62
With Turkey, Cranberry & Alfalfa	410	1710	3	78
Cheese Triangle (Filo/Fetta), 170g	500	2090	38	41
Chicken: Crumbed, fried, 1 piece, 130g	430	1800	28	13
Rotisseried/BBQ'd:				
¼ Chicken with stuffing	350	1465	21	7
¼ Chicken, without stuffing	300	1255	16	0
Without skin or stuffing	220	920	7	0
Chicken Nuggets, average (6)	300	1255	18	14
Chiko Roll, deep-fried, 160g	370	1550	17	42
Chips, 1 cup (bucket), 150g	370	1545	20	38
Cornish Pastie, 200g	450	1880	23	47
Croquette, Vegie., large, 190g	390	1630	30	
Dim Sim: Fried, 70g	160	670	7	19
Steamed, small, 50g	75	315	3	13
Doner Burger/Kebab, 300g	625	2610	34	50
Eggs Benedict:				
With Bacon, 330g	1310	5480	107	48
With Spinach & Mushroom, 322g	980	4095	77	47
Fish & Chips: Deep-fried, 1 serving, 350g	930	3885	55	80
Fish, battered, 1 piece, 150g	345	1435	19	21
No batter, fish only	150	630	1	0
Chips, 20 medium, 100g	245	1025	14	25
Falafel Balls: 2 small/1 large, 40g	105	430	6	7
2 Patties, 86g	225	925	13	15
Flans: Cheese & Vege/Savoury, average all types, 210g	565	2370	37	24
Focaccia Sandwiches:				
Bacon, Avocado & Tomato, 300g	660	2745	32	70
Chicken & Salad, 390g	370	1545	7.5	52
Ham, Cheese & Spinach, 200g	560	2340	19	68

Food	Cal	kJ	Fat	Cb
Focaccia Sandwiches (Cont):				
Small: *Per Average 250g*				
Beef, Avocado & Relish	505	2115	14	74
Chicken, Lettuce & Mayo	490	2040	18	56
Turkey with Salad	245	1020	4.5	35
Medium: *Per Average 350g*				
Beef, Avocado & Relish	710	2960	20	103
Chicken, with Salad & Mayonnise	685	2855	25	78
Turkey, with Salad	345	1430	6	48
French Fries:				
Small serve, 72g	255	1070	14	29
Medium serve, 104g	370	1540	20	41
Georgie Pie (McDonald's, N.Z.)	540	2260	35	41
Hamburger: Deli-type	430	1795	13	59
With Cheese & Egg	550	2300	30	59
Hot Dog, with medium roll	365	1520	16	40
Lasagne, 1 serve, 300g	400	1670	17	40
Muffins, Savoury:				
With Ham & Cheese, 170g	575	2410	34	47
With Cheese, Zucchini & Tomato, 170g	540	2255	32	48
Mushroom, Parmesan & Pesto, 165g	465	1930	25	48
Sundried Tomato, Parmesan & Olives, 165g	300	1250	11	36
Nachos, Corn Chips with Tomato Salsa, Beans, Cheese, Sour Cream	890	3715	60	75
Pasta/Fettucine (large): *2 cups Pasta +Sauce*				
Bolognaise (Meat & Tomato Sauce)	620	2585	19	73
Carbonara (Cream/Bacon/Eggs/Parmesan)	950	3980	45	85
Marinara (Mixed Seafood/Tomato Sce)	650	2715	22	70
Pesto (Basil, Pinenuts, Olive Oil & Parmesan)	830	3470	40	65
Pastie: Regular, 175g	390	1615	18	48
Cornish, 250g	605	2525	31	67
Traditional, 200g	525	2200	29	50
Pastizzi (Filo/Ricotta), 90g	310	1285	22	18
Pie Floater (S.A.), Pie in Pea Soup	550	2300	28	43
Pies: Meat, average, 175g	450	1880	24	43
Chicken, creamed, 180g	450	1880	25	43
Pork Pie, 175g	450	1880	25	43
Steak Mushroom/Onion, 175g	475	1985	25	43
Vegetarian, average:				
With Pastry Top, 200g	400	1670	19	45
With Potato Topping, 200g	525	2180	25	58
Pita Burger, 1 large	550	2300	20	37
Pizza: Average, ½ medium	600	2510	26	70
1 small lunch pizza	400	1670	18	50

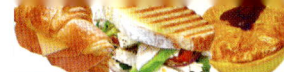

Cafe-Style & Take-Away

Average All Outlets ~ Estimates only

	Cal	kJ	Fat	Cb
Potato Wedges:				
1 small, 4g	5	25	0.5	0.5
1 medium wedge, 15g	20	85	0.5	3
1 large wedge, 25g	35	140	1	5
1 large bowl, 600g	810	3385	30	110
Wedge Dips/Sauces: *Per Small 100g Bow*				
Aioli (Mayonnaise with Garlic)	560	2350	60	2
Mayonnaise	375	1550	33	20
Sour Cream, Light	190	800	18	5
Sweet Chilli	215	900	0	45
Tomato/Ketchup	120	500	0	25
Quiches, average all types, 150g	465	1950	33	27
Rissoles, Lentil, Fried, 190g	335	1405	15	23
Samosa, with vegetables:				
Small, 40g	110	445	5	12
Large/Indian, 190g	515	2150	25	57
Sausage, large, deep-fried, 80g	250	1045	18	6
Sausage Roll: Small, 40g	120	500	9	8
Large, 130g	485	2030	27	48
Extra Large, 176g	505	2120	32	42
Saveloy, battered, 100g	310	1280	21	19
Scotch Egg, 125g	300	1240	21	13
Spinach & Feta Slice, 250g	360	1500	20	25
Spinach & Ricotta Roll, 175g	520	2175	25	57
Spring Roll: Small, 170g	400	1670	17	48
Large, 230g	540	2260	23	65
Souvlakia, 1 skewer, 60g	120	500	7	1
Sushi ~ *See Japanese Foods Page 193*				
Taco Salad, with meat/cheese	250	1045	11	12
Triangles (Filo): Cheese, 170g	495	2065	28	42
Vegetable Slice, 100g	140	575	8	12
Vegie Patty, with Rice, large, 300g	480	1995	21	36
Salads: *Large with Dressing*				
Caesar	380	1590	26	30
Chicken	350	1465	20	14
Chicken & Avocado	325	1360	18	14
Greek	300	1250	26	12
Spinach	275	1150	22	10
Small/Side Garden, without dressing	20	80	0	3
Sandwiches: *Per Sandwich ~ 2 Slices of Wholmeal Bread, 70g Calculations based on 3 tsp fat used and dressings if indicated*				
Bacon, Lettuce, Tomato with Mayonnaise	470	1970	24	32
Chicken, Egg, Bacon Club	620	2590	38	51
Egg & Salad	380	1595	20	37
Ham & Salad	320	1340	14	37
Steak Sandwich, with Onion, Lettuce & Tomato & Sauce	560	2340	22	60
Tuna & Salad	375	1560	14	37

	Cal	kJ	Fat	Cb
Sandwiches (Cont.)				
Toasted:				
Cheese & Tomato	375	1575	20	30
Egg & Bacon	505	2110	32	28
Ham, Cheese & Tomato	430	1800	21	37
Ciabatta :				
Medium: *Per 280g*				
Bacon, Avocado, Tom. & Lettuce	585	2450	31	56
Chicken, Bacon, Avocado & Lettuce	840	3500	55	52
Large: *Per 430g*				
Bacon, Avocado, Tomato & Lettuce	900	3765	48	86
Chicken, Bacon, Avocado & Lettuce	1285	5375	84	80
Croissants:				
Cheese & Tomato, 170g	495	2080	29	41
Chicken & Salad	540	2255	31	52
Ham, Cheese & Tom., 210g	530	2230	30	44
Flatbread: *Includes Lettuce & Tomatoes. Cheese & Dressing Only Where Indicated*				
Cajun Chicken, with Cajun Sauce, & Sour Cream, 317g	445	1850	14	57
Chicken Schnitzel:				
With Mayo, 280g	520	2180	17	73
With Bacon & Mayo, 320g	645	2700	28	73
With Parm. Cheese, Caesar Dressing, and Mayo, 300g	600	2520	24	72
Grilled Eggplant/Capsicum/Sundr. Tomatoes, with Swiss Cheese & Mayo, 320g	430	1790	13	60
Ham, Ched. Cheese & Tom. w. Mayo, 225g	430	1790	13	57
Roast Beef, with Swiss Cheese, Mustard Sce & Mayo, 290g	445	1870	13	58
Pita: With Salad	255	1070	12	33
With Ham, Cheese & Salad	425	1780	22	34
Wraps: *Includes Lettuce & Tomatoes. Cheese & Dressings Only Where Indicated*				
Satay Chicken, with Cheddar Cheeese and Satay Sauce, 290g	585	2450	26	59
Sweet Chili Thai Chkn, with Ched. Cheese, Sweet Chilli Sauce & Mayo, 325g	580	2440	22	66
Tuna, with Cheddar Chse, Onion & Mayo, 250g	500	2080	18	52
Turkey, with Swiss Cheese, Cranb. Sauce, and Mayo, 230g	475	1980	17	52

Subway Sandwiches ~ *See Page 206*

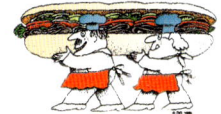

Updated Nutrition Data ~ www.CalorieKing.com.au
Persons with Diabetes ~ See Disclaimer (Page 22)

179

International Foods

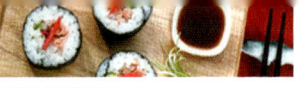

Asian Food Markets

	Cal	kJ	Fat	Cb
Combination Chinese Meals				
High Fat: (e.g. Fried Rice/Noodles				
Spring Roll/Lemon Chicken/				
Sweet Sour Pork), 1 plate	970	4050	50	94
Medium Fat:				
Mix of low & high fat items, 1 plate	720	3160	36	15
Medium-Low Fat: (e.g. Steamed Rice/				
Veges/Chicken & Alm/Beef Black Bean Sce),				
1 plate	550	2300	13	40

Asian Meals

	Cal	kJ	Fat	Cb
Appetisers:				
Curry Puff (Beef), Deep-fried, small, 35g	90	370	5	6.5
Dim Sims: Fried (1), 50g	115	485	4.5	14
Steamed, 50g	105	440	4	13
Fortune Cookies (1)	30	130	0.5	6.5
Prawn Crackers (3), large	45	190	2	6
Prawn Cutlet (1), 30g	80	335	4	4
Spring Rolls (1), 65g	155	640	6.5	19
Wantons (fried): Mini, 15g	55	230	4	4
Medium size, 30g	110	460	8	7
Satay Sticks: Beef/Chicken/Pork, average				
Without Sauce, 1 stick, 72g	145	595	6	0
With Satay Sauce, 2 tsp	175	725	8.5	4
Soup: *Per Medium Bowl*				
Chicken Laksa	285	1190	16	17
Crab/Chicken & Corn	265	1105	15	19
Miso	35	150	1	5
Wanton Soup	240	1005	13	26
Beef: *Per Cup*				
Beef in Black Bean Sauce	365	1630	11	29
Satay Beef	520	2180	30	19
Beef Curry	350	1470	19	15
Beef in Oyster Sauce	320	1345	7	34
Chicken: *Per Cup*				
Chicken & Almonds	360	1510	25	9
Chicken Chow Mein	365	1525	24	16
Chicken Chop Suey	260	1080	16	3.5
Chicken Satay	480	2005	20	38
Lemon Chicken	430	1800	24	18
Duck Dishes:				
Braised/Roast Duck, 1 plEce, 100g	260	1080	18	3.5
Peking Duck, 1 serve	750	3135	50	15
Steamed w. Mushrooms, 1 cup	410	1710	30	11
Sweet & Sour Duck, 1 cup	565	2370	35	43

Asian Meals (Cont)

	Cal	kJ	Fat	Cb
Pork Dishes: *Per Cup*				
BBQ Pork, 230g	650	2710	35	22
Pork in Black Bean Sauce	375	1570	27	10
Pork Chop Suey	275	1145	19	4.5
Pork in Plum Sauce	295	1230	9.5	21
Sweet & Sour Pork	485	2025	25	47
Fish & Seafood:				
Crumbed Prawns (3), 50g	140	580	8	11
Fish Ball (3), 36g	30	115	0.5	1.5
Garlic/Satay Prawns, 1 cup	345	1435	20	7.5
Honey King Prawns, 3 only	300	1250	18	38
Sweet & Sour Fish, 1 cup	510	2140	25	46
Sweet & Sour Prawns, 1 cup	280	1160	10	35
Omelettes:				
Prawn/Chicken, ½ whole, 200g	435	1820	36	5
Combination, ½ whole, 200g	360	1500	28	18
Egg Sambal, ½ whole, 70g	70	295	4	1
Rice: Steamed, 1 serve, 100g	115	480	0	26
1 cup, 160g	185	775	0	42
1 medium dish, 350g	405	1695	0	91
Fried: 1 cup, 165g	360	1500	14	49
1 medium dish, 350g	770	3195	30	104
1 large, 500g	1100	4600	42	148
Nasi Goreng, 2 cups, 330g	595	2490	15	90
Rice Noodles, fried, 100g	180	745	8.5	19
Rice Paper Roll, not fried, 71g	80	335	2	10
Noodles: *Per Cup*				
Noodles: Plain, boiled	135	570	1	29
Fried, plain	285	1195	18	40
Egg, boiled	260	1090	1	29
Chow Mein, Chicken	380	1590	26	18
Beef/Prawn/Combination, average	330	1380	22	18
Indonesian Fried Noodles	370	1550	18	37
Vegetables:				
Gado Gado with Peanut Sauce				
½ serve, 225g, 1 cup	285	1185	18	17
Combination Veges, with oil, 250g	540	2255	8	97
Vegetables, steamed, 250g	200	845	1.5	43
Vegetables & Fried Bean Curd,				
with Satay Sauce, 250g	415	1725	28	18
Desserts:				
Almond Jelly, ½ cup, 120g	75	315	1	15
Banana Fritter, 1 small, 70g	140	585	9	14
Fried Ice Cream Balls, each	170	710	10	21
Lychees (1), 20g	15	64	0	3.5
Snacks/Dumplings:				
Moon Cake, 95g	405	1680	20	43
Pork Dumpling, steamed, 85g	185	760	6	18
Pork Dumpling, fried, 185g	465	1935	26	40
Prawn Dumpling, steamed, 97g	135	560	3	19
Steamed Meat Dumpling, 70g	125	520	4.5	15

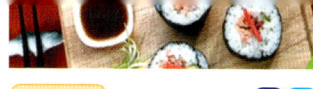

International Foods

French

	Cal	kJ	Fat	Cb
Blanquette d'Agneau, (Lamb Stew)	800	3340	30	17
Brioche, 1 cake	280	1170	14	34
Bouillabaisse	400	1670	15	10
Coq au Vin	800	3340	30	16
Coquilles St. Jacques	320	1340	13	36
Crème Brulée, 1 serving	460	1925	40	21
Baguette, 3 slices, 62g	150	625	1	35
Creme Caramel, (Caramel Custard)	260	1085	10	38
Crepe Suzette, 1x15cm crepe with sauce	220	920	10	13
Duck a l'Orange	780	3260	35	47
Escargot, in garlic butter (6)	200	835	10	4
Frog Legs, fried, 4 med. pairs	400	1670	20	10
Lamb Noisettes, fried, 2 chops	500	2090	40	1
Potage Creme Crecy, (Carrot Soup)	360	1505	18	14
Salade Nicoise, (Tuna/Olives/Vegs)	450	1880	13	14
Veal Cordon Bleu, (Veal/Ham)	650	2715	25	18
Vichyssoise, (Potato/Leek Soup), 1 cup	200	835	9	15

German

	Cal	kJ	Fat	Cb
Bavarian Bread Dumpling, 3 small	330	1380	10	28
Beef Goulash, with Veggies	520	2175	20	46
Black Forest Cake, 1 slice	380	1590	16	30
Bratwurst, grilled, 1 med.	450	1880	37	2
Chicken: Fried, Viennese-style	530	2215	20	28
Livers w/ Apple/Onion, 170g	460	1925	28	10
Herring, Pickled: Rollmops, 113g	260	1085	16	4
With Sour Cream, 113g	310	1295	20	3
Hot Sausage Curry	300	1255	7	6
Kugelhupf Cake, 1 large slice, 113g	400	1670	20	44
Sauerbraten Pork, (Pot Roast)	650	2715	35	15
Torte: Linzer (Almond/Raspb. Jam)	430	1800	18	58
Sacher, Chocolate/Apricot Jam	260	1085	12	23
Weiner Schnitzel, 1 medium	750	3135	35	38

Greek

	Cal	kJ	Fat	Cb
Baklava Pastry: Small	240	1005	13	32
Large, 106g	400	1670	21	45
Calamari, deep fried, 1 cup	300	1255	13	17
Chicken Kebob Plate	345	1440	13	8
Dolmades, (Stuffed Grape Leaves)				
2 rolls, 170g	200	835	5	13
Galaktoboureko, 1 only				
(Filo, Custard, Pastry in Syrup)	360	1505	15	48
Greek Chicken Salad	400	1670	18	9
Gyros: 15cm Pita, 227g	475	1985	32	35
19cm Pita, 240g	680	2840	40	55

Greek (Cont)

	Cal	kJ	Fat	Cb
Hummus & Pita, 113g	260	1085	12	30
Kataifi, (Filo, Nut, Pastry in Syrup)	350	1465	11	56
Moussaka: Small serving, 227g	350	1465	22	22
Large serving, 454g	700	2925	44	44
Soup, Avgolemono				
(Egg Lem. Soup w. Chicken & Rice), 1 cup	85	355	6	5
Souvlaki (Lamb), each, 57g	120	500	6	1
Stuffed Tomatoes, 2	250	1045	12	17
Taramosalata, 1 T., 14g	40	165	3	2
Tyropita, (Filo/Egg/Cheese Pastry)	350	1465	26	31

Indian & Pakistani

Per Serve: (Meat dishes - 120g meat/serve)

	Cal	kJ	Fat	Cb
Aloo, (Potato) Samosa, each	150	630	12	12
Aloo Gosht, Kari (Meat/Potato Curry)	600	2510	40	23
Butter Chicken	450	1880	30	4.5
Chicken Korma	500	2100	35	6
Chicken Pilaf, (Murgh Biriyani)	700	2930	53	50
Chicken Tikka	260	1090	16	2
Chicken Vindaloo	400	1675	20	8
Chapati/Roti, 17 cm diam. piece	60	250	0.5	11
Cucumber Raita, ¼ cup	45	190	2	5
Dhal, (Lentil Puree): 1 cup, without oil	230	960	1	37
1 Tbsp Tadka (oil topping)	120	500	13	0
Dhakla, 3 cm square, 3g	105	440	5.5	14
Dhansak, ½ cup	105	440	3.5	11
Goan Fish Curry	460	1925	25	35
Gosht Kari, (Meat Curry/Tomato/Potato)	460	1925	25	17
Lamb Korma, (in Cream Sauce)	430	1800	28	3
Lamb Pilaf	520	2175	35	40
Lassi, (Sweet or Mango), 250ml	160	670	4	24
Masala Gosht, (Beef/Tomato/Gravy)	400	1675	25	18
Mulligatawney Soup, average	300	1255	15	4
Murgh Tikka, 1 cup	300	1255	4	7
Naan Bread, ¼ (20cm x 5cm), 30g	75	315	2	12
Palek Paneer, 185g	355	1480	31	0
Pappadum, 1 large/2 small	50	210	5	5
Pork Vindaloo Curry	620	2590	47	3
Rogan Josh, (Lamb/Yoghurt Sauce)	500	2100	30	3
Tandoori Chicken: Breast	260	1090	13	5
Leg/Thigh portion	300	1255	17	6

Updated Nutrition Data ~ www.CalorieKing.com.au
Persons with Diabetes ~ See Disclaimer (Page 22)

181

International Foods

Italian

	Cal	kJ	Fat	Cb
Antipasto, 2 sl. Salami/3 Olives/½ c. Veg.	180	750	13	4.5
Bruschetta, Tomato/Onion/Pesto, 1 slice	315	1315	20	26
Chicken Parmigiana, 200g	360	1505	24	3.5
Ciabatta, Plain, 2 slices, 80g	180	745	2	34
Cannelloni, 2 tubes, 250g	385	1615	14	38
Chicken Cacciatore, 300g	385	1620	23	4
Gnocchi, Potato, 197g	295	1220	2	58
Lasagne with Meat: Small/Entrée, 220g	315	1325	14	31
Large/Main, 400g	575	2395	25	56
Manicotti, Cheese/Tomato, 1 serve	230	960	14	29
Minestrone Soup, 1 cup	135	565	3.5	14
Osso Buco, (Shanks/Stock/Oil/Tom/Veg.)	550	2300	28	4
Pasta: Plain, 1 cup, 150g	210	875	0.5	43
2 cups, plain, 300g	420	1755	1	85
+ Bolognese (Meat Sauce)	620	2585	19	73
+ Carbonara (Cream/Bacon/Chse/Egg)	950	3980	45	85
+ Marinara Sauce (Seafood, Tom. Sce)	650	2715	22	70
+ Pesto (Basil/Pine Nuts/Oil/Cheese)	830	3470	40	65
Pizza, average, ½ medium	600	2510	26	70
Polenta, 5 pieces, fried, 200g	240	1005	15	20
Ravioli: With Meat, 250g	340	1430	14	39
Spinach & Ricotta, 250g	275	1150	7	40
Risotto, (Chicken), 1 serve	565	2350	16	78
Saltimbocca, (Veal/Ham/Cheese/Wine), 1 serve, 200g	440	1830	28	4.5
Tortellini, 200g	395	1645	9	58
Veal Marsala	290	1205	10	14
Veal Parmigiana, 300g	590	2465	38	18
Desserts: Cassata, 1 scoop, 80g	150	625	7.5	19
Zabaglione Dessert	190	790	4	14

Japanese

	Cal	kJ	Fat	Cb
Sushi Rice: Cooked, 1 Tbsp	25	105	0	7
1 cup, 160g	210	870	0.5	46
Sushi (Maki) Rolls: *Per Piece, Average all Types*				
(California Rolls; Eel; Salmon; Tuna; Prawn; Vegetable)				
Small (3cm diam. x 3cm high), 25g	20	70	0.5	3
Large (5.5cm diam. x 2cm high), 60g	40	165	0.5	7.5
Sushi Packs: *Average all Types*				
1 piece, 36g	45	190	0.5	8
3 Pieces, 110g	140	585	1.5	25
6 Pieces, 220g	280	1170	3	49
Flower Cone: Seafood Stick, 70g	90	375	2	16
Tuna, 70g	110	460	3.5	16
Hand Roll: Chicken, 125g	170	710	3.5	24
Seafood Stick, 125g	150	625	2	24

Japanese (Cont)

	Cal	kJ	Fat	Cb
Sushi Plate: Assorted 6 pieces	370	1545	4.5	54
Combination (Sushi & Sushi Rolls) 2 Sushi + 6 small & 3 med. rolls	400	1680	5	69
Sashimi, average all types, 113g	130	545	3.5	0
Dipping Sauces: Average, 2 Tbsp	30	125	0	7
Ginger Vinegar Dressing, 2 Tbsp	20	85	0	5
Bento Box, (Beef/Chicken w. Rice & Salad)				
Chicken	650	2720	13	40
Beef	765	3200	33	40
Bubble Tea, avg. 375ml cup	210	865	3.5	45
Edamame, (young green soybeans):				
Steamed/Salad (in pods), 120g	60	250	3	5
Boiled beans (without pods), 120g	160	670	7	12
Gyoza, (Dumplings): Chicken (1), 15g	35	150	1.5	4.5
Pork & Chives (1), 15g	40	165	1.5	5.5
Katsu-don Pork, w. Rice, avg	1100	4600	39	141
Miso Soup, with Tofu pieces, 1 cup	85	355	3	11
Miso Soup, 1 cup	35	130	1	5
Noodles:				
Soba, plain cooked, 1 cup, 150g	180	750	0.5	24
Hokkien Stir Fry, w. Chicken + Veg., 400g	640	2675	25	52
Ramen, plain , cooked, 1 cup, 150g	180	850	0.5	26
Udon, plain, cooked, 1½ cup, 220g	335	1400	2	50
Sake Wine, (16% alcohol), 100 ml	115	800	0	5
Seaweed Salad, 45g	20	85	2	4
Soy Sauce: 1 mini bottle, 5 ml	2	10	0	0.5
1 sachet, 10 ml	5	20	0	1
Sukiyaki, (Beef/Tofu/Veg.), 250g	400	1680	24	32
Tempura, (batter-fried Prawns & Veg.), 3 large Prawns & Vegetables	320	1340	18	25
Teppan Yaki, 300g serving	470	1970	30	15
Teriyaki: Beef only, 120g	350	1470	25	4
Chicken only, 120g	260	1090	9	7
Fish only, medium, 120g	270	1130	8	3
Teriyaki Meal: *With Rice & Vegetables*				
Beef Meal (120g Beef)	650	2720	25	72
Chicken Meal (120g Chicken)	590	2340	10	75
Fish Meal (120g Fish)	570	2385	8	71
Tofu Meal	260	1080	16	2
Udon Noodle Soup: *Per Bowl*				
Beef & Noodles	560	2340	20	70
Chicken & Noodles	500	2100	10	70
Tofu & Noodles	470	1965	5	72
Wasabi, (Japanese Horseradish), 1 tsp. 5g	15	65	1.5	1
Yakatori, Chicken, 1 skewer, 75g	140	590	5	0

International Foods

Jewish

Food	Cal	kJ	Fat	Cb
Bagel/Bialy, ½ small, 30g	80	225	1	18
Beiglach, (Cheese Knish)	350	1460	17	35
Blintzes, (with Cottage Cheese), 1 only	120	500	1	25
plus Sour Cream & Jam	370	1550	10	30
Borscht: W/o Cream, 1 cup	90	375	3	14
With 1 Tbsp Light Sour Cream	130	540	7	15
Cabbage Roll, (Meat/Rice), 150g	170	710	6	21
Chicken Broth: Unskimmed, 1 cup	80	335	8	0
With Vegetables, 1 cup	100	420	8	5
With Noodles, 1 cup	150	630	9	16
Skimmed/Fat-Free, 1 c.	25	105	1	0
Cholent, 1 med.serve, 1 cup	350	1465	16	48
Chopped Liver, with Egg/Onion, ¼ cup, 60g	100	420	7	3
Farfel, dry, ½ cup	90	375	0.5	21
Gefilte Fish:				
1 medium ball, 50g	50	200	2	3.5
With Jellied Broth	80	335	2	6
Hallah, (Yeast Bread), 1 slice, 30g	85	355	2	14
Herring, pickled, 30g	60	250	4	0
Kasha, cooked, ½ cup	100	420	0.5	20
Kipfel, (Vanilla Almond Biscuit), 1 piece	60	250	2	7
Knaidlach, 1 medium ball	40	170	2	5
Kimchee, (Cabbage Relish), ½ cup	30	125	0	6
Knish: Kasha Potato, 1 only	130	540	4	22
Cheese, 1 only	350	1460	17	35
Kreplach, beef, 1 piece	40	170	1	6
Kugel, 1 serve	300	1255	20	25
Latkes, (Potato Pancake): 60g	200	835	11	22
3 Latkes & Sour Cranberry/Apple Sauce	750	3130	25	95
Lockshen: Plain, 1 cup	130	540	2	26
Pudding, 1 cup	380	1590	13	48
Lox, (Smoked Salmon), 30g	35	145	1	0
Mandelbrot, (Almond Bread), 1 sl., 6mm thick	45	190	2	5
Matzo, 1 sheet (17.5cm sq.), 34g	135	570	0.5	28
Matzo ~ Extra Listings See Page 55				
Matzo Ball Soup: With 2 medium balls	150	625	6	24
With Chicken & Noodles	325	1360	13	34
New York Cheesecake, 120g	375	1555	26	28
Pierogi, Potato/Cheese, 1 iece	90	375	4	11
Piroshki/Pierogi (Potato/Cheese), 1 piece	90	375	4	11
Reuben Sandwich, with Corned Beef	920	3845	60	28
Schmaltz (Rend'd Chicken Fat), 1 Tbsp	90	375	10	0
Strudel, Apple/Fruit, 80g	250	1045	17	40

Updated Nutrition Data ~ www.CalorieKing.com.au
Persons with Diabetes ~ See Disclaimer (Page 22)

Lebanese/Middle Eastern

Food	Cal	kJ	Fat	Cb
Baba Ghannouj, 2 Tbsp, 28g (Eggplant/Sesame Dip)	70	295	6	2
Baklava, 1, 50g	245	102	5	18
Cabbage Rolls, 1 roll, 85g (Cabbage Leaf, Meat, Rice)	100	420	3	12
Cous Cous (Semolina, Milk, Fruit, Nuts,) 1 serving	400	1670	21	43
Falafel, (Chick Pea Fritter), fried, 1 medium, 28g	60	250	4	4
Hummus, ¼ cup, 62g	105	440	3	5
Fried Kibbi, 1 piece, 85g (Wheat, Meat, Pinenuts)	180	750	8	15
Kafta, 1 skewer, 43g (Ground Lamb Sausage on Skewer)	85	355	5	2
Kibbeh Nayeh, 1 cup, 155g (Raw Lamb, Bulgur & Spices)	450	1880	18	28
Lebanese Omelet, 1 serve, 113g (Egg, Spinach, Pinenuts, Onion)	200	835	12	13
Pilaf (Rice, Onion, Raisins, Apricot, Spice), 1 cup	400	1670	11	60
Shawourma (Spit-Roast Beef), 1 serving, 113g	280	1170	15	2
Shish Kabob, 1 stick, 70g	130	545	7	2
Spinach Pie, 1 piece, 100g	290	1210	21	20
Sweet Almond Sanbusak, 1 piece (Pastry, Almonds, Spices)	200	835	15	11
Tabouli, 1 serving, 113g	125	525	7	13
Tahini Sauce, average, 1 Tbsp	90	375	8	2

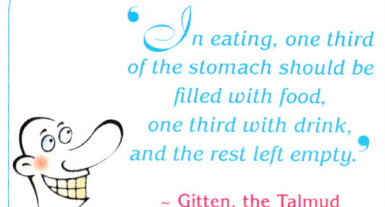

"In eating, one third of the stomach should be filled with food, one third with drink, and the rest left empty."

~ Gitten, the Talmud

183

International Foods

Mexican

	Cal	kJ	Fat	Cb
Per Average Serve				
Arroz Abanda, (Fish with Rice)	340	1420	8	31
Black Bean Soup, 1 bowl	200	835	3	34
Burrito: Bean	370	1545	10	55
Beef/Supreme	440	1840	18	50
Chilli con Carne: With Beans, 1 cup	310	1295	17	15
Without Beans, 1 cup	370	1545	28	10
Chorizo Sausage, 60g	265	1110	23	0
Churros, 45g	150	630	8	18
Corn Chips, average, ½ cup, 30g	160	670	10	17
Empanadas, average, 1 small, 60g	230	960	10	28
Enchilada, Beef, average	330	1390	10	49
Fajitas, Chicken/Beef, each	200	835	7	20
Gazpacho Soup, 1 bowl	60	250	0	15
Guacamole, 2 Tbsp, 40g	70	290	8	3
Margarita, w. 45ml Tequila	160	670	0	6
Nachos: With Beans, Cheese, Avocado, CC's & Cream, 330g	675	2820	39	57
With 500g Beef, Beans, Cheese, Avocado, & Cream	1120	4690	63	75
Paella Valenciana, Chicken/Shellfish	900	3765	42	70
Papas Fritas, 175g	325	1360	18	40
Refried Beans, ¾ cup, 175g	160	670	3	26
Taco, w. Meat/Cheese/Salad	250	1045	11	14
Taco Shells: Regular, 11g	54	225	3	7
Large/Super, 18g	85	355	4.5	11
Tamales, Beef/Chicken, 130g	250	1045	11	27
Tomato Salsa, 2 Tbsp, 40g	20	85	0	5
Tortillas/Tostados, each	70	295	1	14
Tostada: 1 serve	200	835	10	29
With Beef	250	1045	12	29

Polish

	Cal	kJ	Fat	Cb
Cabbage Rolls, with Sour Cream, 2 sm.	220	920	10	30
Chicken Casserole, w. Mushrooms, 1 cup	520	2175	27	5
Kielbasa, Fried, 2 large	350	1465	28	2
Meatballs in Sour Cream, 3 meatballs (40mm)	300	1255	16	11
Piero`gi, Fruit/Vegetables, 75mm ball	80	335	2	15
Pork Goulash, Pork/Vegetable Stew	550	2300	21	38
Pot Roast, with Vegetables	630	2635	21	28

Thai

	Cal	kJ	Fat	Cb
Entrees: *Per Serving*				
Satay Beef, 1 stick, 30g	65	270	4	2
Satay Pork, 1 stick, 30g	105	445	4.5	2
Spring Roll, 35g	110	460	6	13
Soups: *Per Cup*				
Tom Yum: With Seafood	100	420	3	4
Vegetarian	50	210	0	11
Mud Crab, with Coconut	400	1670	30	16
Salads: *Per Serve*				
Green Papaya	160	670	0	40
Spicy Prawn	170	710	3	15
Thai Beef	260	1085	9	15
Thai Chicken	330	1380	9	17
Thai Noodle	410	1715	13	45
Stir Fry: *Per Cup*				
Combination: With Fried Rice Noodles	470	1965	33	30
with Steamed Rice Noodles	360	1500	10	42
Combination Stir Fry & Vegetable, without Rice	410	1720	15	6.5
Stir Fry Vegetables	100	420	2	18
Curries: *Per Cup*				
Chicken, with Ginger	390	1630	34	4
Thick Red Curry, with Beef	600	2500	50	7
Thai Chicken Curry	340	1420	23	4
Thai Beef Curry	500	2090	32	5

Vietnamese

Cal/kJ/fat of dishes are only approximate. Large variations occur with serving size, ingredients and cooking method.

Per Whole Dish, Serves 2-3

	Cal	kJ	Fat	Cb
Beef Satay, 2 only + Sauce	265	1110	9	4
Chicken Satay, 2 only	240	1000	11	4
Crispy Skin Chicken, in Plum Sauce	900	3760	40	105
Curried Lamb, Vegetables in Coconut	900	3760	35	80
Ginger Beef, with Onion & Fish Sauce	750	3135	30	10
Marinated Chicken, with Vegetables	800	3345	26	100
Pork Stuffed Cabbage Roll	200	835	7	11
Stir-fried Vegetables, in Soy Sauce	400	1670	9	65
Whole Schnapper, with Ginger	600	2510	16	6
Soup: *Per Bowl, 1½ cups*				
Chicken & Rice Noodle	400	1675	3	55
Pho Bo (Beef Noodle)	410	1715	7	59
Vegetable Soup, with Bean Curd	80	335	3	13

Fast-Foods & Chains

Bakers Delight® (Sept '13)

Savoury Items:

Item	Cal	kJ	Fat	Sat'F	Carb	Pro	Sod
Savoury Bite, 80g	230	970	11	5.5	22	12	585
Focaccia: Cheese, Herb & Garlic, 120g	625	2605	38	4.5	58	11	640
Bacon Supreme, 180g	455	1905	14	6.5	60	20	1440
Herb & Garlic, 125g	320	1325	5	1	55	10	645
Mushroom & Capsicum, 170g	405	1690	11	6	57	16	970
Traditional, 150g	435	1815	13	7	57	18	890
Mini Twist: Cheese & Bacon, 120g	325	1360	10	5	43	15	880
Chives & Garlic, 120g	330	1370	10	5.5	42	14	690
Pesto, Sundried Tomato & Capsicum, 105g	250	1050	4.5	0.5	43	8	6550
Spinach & Feta, 120g	290	1200	8	4	41	8	610
Sweet Chilli, 120g	340	1405	10	5.5	47	13	755
Tomato, 120g	330	1380	11	6	43	14	705
Pide: Olive & Feta, 105g	285	1190	8.5	3	41	9	920
Two Cheese & Herb, 95g	265	1100	8.5	3.5	35	10	700
Pizza: BBQ Bonanza, 165g	450	1880	18	8	50	22	1525
Hawaiian, 175g	440	1840	16	9	52	21	1310
Supreme, 165g	360	1505	12	6	48	16	1150
Veggie, 165g	370	1550	14	8	45	16	1080
Pullapart: Cheese & Bacon, 65g	180	740	4	2	26	7.5	445
Cheese & Chive, 65g	195	805	6	3	26	8	385
Cheese, Herb & Garlic, 65g	190	795	5.5	3	26	8	385
Cheese, Spinach & Feta, 65g	185	775	5.5	3	26	7.5	385
Cheese & Sundried Tomato, 78g	225	945	7	2.5	32	8	430
Roll: Cheese, 85g	260	1070	8	5	33	11	510
Cheese & Bacon, 85g	290	1210	10	5.5	35	14	810
Cheese & Mushroom, 85g	265	1100	8.5	5	34	11	615
Cheese & Olive, 85g	270	1125	10	5	34	11	645
Cheese & Pineapple, 85g	280	1165	8.5	5	39	11	515
Mini, Cheese & Tomato, 55g	170	690	5	3	22	8	375
Scroll: BBQ, Mini, 55g	190	790	6	3	24	8.5	545
Cheesymite: Regular, 110g	340	1410	10	6	39	15	790
Mini, 55g	160	665	4.5	2.5	22	7.5	410
Chilli & Red Onion, 110g	325	1355	10	6	42	13	670
Country Grain Cheese & Herb, 110g	340	1420	12	7	40	16	605
Sweet Chilli & Cheese, 115g	375	1565	12	7	49	14	825
Wholemeal: Cheesymite, 110g	280	1180	8.5	4.5	34	15	660
Country Grain Cheese & Herb, 110g	325	1355	12	6.5	34	18	615
Spinach & Feta, 120g	315	1310	11	6	35	16	545
Twirl: Ham & Mayo, 125g	360	1515	13	7	42	18	1015
Ham & Mustard Pickle, 125g	360	1515	12	6.5	42	18	1000
Twisted Delight: Cheese & Bacon, 46g	130	540	4	2	17	6	350
Chives & Garlic, 44g	130	550	4	2.5	17	5.5	280
Pesto, Sundried Tomato & Capsicum, 40g	100	420	2	0.5	17	3	260
Salami, Capsicum & Feta, 44g	110	460	3	1	17	4	290
Spinach & Feta, 42g	120	490	3.5	2	16	5	250
Sweet Chilli, 46g	140	575	4	2	19	5.5	300

Bread ~ See Page 58
Cakes/Buns/Pastries ~ See Page 66

Updated Nutrition Data ~ www.CalorieKing.com.au
Persons with Diabetes ~ See Disclaimer (Page 22)

Fast-Foods & Chains

Baskin Robbins® (Sept '13)

Drinks: Per Regular

	Cal	kJ	Fat	Cb
Blast: Cappuccino	350	1465	13	51
Caramel	395	1645	14	57
Cookies 'N Cream	390	1630	17	51
Mocha, regular	435	1820	14	72
Yoghurt Smoothie:				
Banana Buzz	645	2685	6.5	138
Mango-Licious	595	2480	9	120
Very Strawberry	570	2380	7.5	118
Wildberry Delite	585	2440	8	119

Ice Cream ~ *See Page 109*

Brumby's® (Sept '13)

	Cal	kJ	Fat	Cb
Croissant, Ham & Cheese, 93g	235	980	19	7
Deli Roll, Asparagus & Cheese, 125g	280	1170	8.5	39
Pasties: Beef, 170g	455	1905	24	48
Cornish, 170g	460	1920	29	37
Pie, Beef & Mushroom, 215g	550	2295	33	48
Roll, Cheese & Spinach, 160g	545	2275	36	44
Sausage Roll, 164g	470	1955	26	46
Scrolls: Cheddarmite, 122g	300	1260	6	48
Cheese & Bacon, 114g	270	1115	6.5	40
Sun-Dried Tom. & Olive, 126g	310	1285	9	44
Tomato & Herb, 114g	265	1115	6.5	42

Breads ~ *See Page 58*
Cakes/Pastries ~ *See Page 67*

Carl's Jr.® (N.Z.) Sept '13

Charbroiled Burgers:

	Cal	kJ	Fat	Cb
Cheeseburgers: Western Bacon, 270g	790	3300	43	67
Double Western Bacon, 320g	950	3960	52	69
Famous Star with Cheese, 285g	665	2770	37	55
Jim Beam Bourbon Burger, single	770	3220	34	85
Portobello Mushroom Burger, 330g	690	2870	39	53
Super Star with Cheese, 360g	840	3500	50	55
The Big Carl, 300g	845	3540	52	54
Thickburgers: Original, 370g	850	3550	50	55
Guacamole Bacon	1015	4240	67	53
Jalapeno, 360g	905	3780	58	51
Portobello Mushroom, 395g	870	3650	53	53
Western Bacon, 390g	1250	5220	75	88
Low Carb, 300g	595	2490	46	8
Kid's: Cheeseburger, 175g	440	1850	20	39
Hamburger, 160g	390	1640	17	37

Carl's Jr.® (N.Z. cont... Sept '13)

Chicken Sandwiches:

	Cal	kJ	Fat	Cb
Charbroiled Chicken Sandwiches:				
BBQ, 195g	270	1120	3	40
Club, 215g	450	1880	23	35
Santa Fe, 210g	495	2070	29	36
Chicken Tender Sandwiches:				
Bacon Swiss Crispy, 285g	730	3040	47	44
Buttermilk Ranch, 255g	590	2460	34	43
Honey Mustard, 250g	565	2360	31	44
Carl's Catch Fish Sandwich, 330g	1080	4510	80	70
Chicken Tenders, Hand Breaded:				
3 pieces, 130g	250	1030	12	7
5 pieces, 210g	400	1670	19	10
Kids, 2 pieces, 85g	160	680	8	4
Dipping Sauces: BBQ, 40g	65	270	0.5	15
Honey Mustard, 40g	210	870	21	7
Ranch, 40g	210	880	23	2
Breakfast:				
Breakfast Burger, 320g	890	3710	51	70
Hash Rounds, 135g	440	1820	29	41
Monster Breakfast Sandwich, 190g	580	2410	16	29
Platters: Deluxe 340g	1090	4540	74	82
Super Deluxe, 640g	1965	8210	112	194
Pancakes: With Bacon, 210g	550	2310	12	96
Without Bacon, 200g	500	2080	9	97
Fries:				
Natural Cut: Small/Kids, 105g	305	1270	15	40
Medium, 150g	435	1820	21	56
Large, 165g	480	2000	23	62
Chilli Cheese, 320g	780	3260	40	93
CrissCut, 140g	450	1890	29	42
Onion Rings, 130g	535	2240	28	62
Fried Zucchni, 140g	330	1380	18	36
Salads: Without Dressings				
Charbroiled Chicken, 330g	140	570	4	8
Crispy Chicken, 350g	220	930	11	8
Side, 80g	125	520	10	1
Salad Dressings: Balsamic; Italian	10	30	0	2
Cheesecakes: Passionfruit, 1 slice, 180g	600	2500	40	51
Strawberry, 1 slice, 180g	600	2520	41	51
Ice Cream Shakes:				
Chocolate; Vanilla, 400g	750	3130	41	82
Oreo Cookie, 400g	825	3450	47	87
Strawberry, 400g	740	3100	41	80

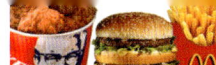

Fast-Foods & Chains

Chicken Treat® (Sept '13)

	Cal	kJ	Fat	Sat'F	Carb	Pro	Sod
Burgers: Chicken Cheeseburger	460	1920	21	6	45	21	1260
Chicken Ham & Cheese	355	1480	14	1.5	35	21	640
Royal Bacon	565	2350	43	7	42	1.5	1220
Royal Boom	495	2065	19	3.5	51	28	1640
Royal Deluxe	450	1870	18	4.5	42	26	1130
Roll, Hot Chicken	615	2565	25	5	57	38	1180
Wraps: Royal	545	2270	26	4	45	31	1595
Royal Boom	550	2285	26	9	49	28	1945
Chicken Packs: Leg with Potatoes	500	2085	19	5.5	45	32	2230
Countrystyle Fried Chicken: 2 pcs Chicken with Chips	970	4040	55	14	72	57	2720
2 pcs Chicken with Garden Salad	625	2610	39	10	29	52	2385
Wing with Potatoes	580	2440	17	5	53	46	2590
½ Chicken & Chips	1175	4905	56	15	93	70	2185
¼ Chicken & Chips, Leg	780	3265	39	23	59	39	1200
¼ Chicken & Chips, Wing	855	3565	37	10	77	52	1540
Hawaiian with Leg	1020	4250	49	8	108	46	350
Hawaiian with Wing	840	3515	35	8	115	57	295
Chicken Pieces:							
Countrystyle Fried: Breast, 160g	345	1435	17	4.5	15	33	1435
Drumstick, 68g	170	715	9	2.5	7	16	695
Rib, 140g	345	1435	21	6	15	30	1435
Thigh, 176g	490	2045	34	9.5	18	29	1750
Wing, 83g	245	1020	14	3.5	10	21	960
Kids Meal: Cheeseburger & Chips	605	2540	28	8	63	20	1375
⅛ Chicken & Chips	445	1865	19	5.5	50	15	645
Dinner	180	755	7.5	2.5	14	13	1090
4 Chicken Nuggets & Chips	725	3030	35	10	75	23	1015
Desserts: Triple Chocolate Mousse	365	1520	27	20	27	3.5	80
Vanilla Cheesecake	340	1420	26	22	22	4	110
Salads: Coleslaw, Small Tub, 110g	105	445	7	0.5	8.5	1.5	275
Garden Salad: With Boom Fillet	230	950	9	0	18	18	800
With Deluxe Fillet	190	790	8	1	13	16	860
Sides: Banana Fritter, 70g	145	595	5.5	3.5	20	2.5	55
Chicken Nugget (1), 16.2g	50	200	2.5	0.5	3.5	3	85
Chicken Twist, regular 128g	450	1870	31	8.5	24	20	1125
Chips, regular 150g	365	1530	16	4	47	6	355
Corn Cobette, (1), 106g	150	620	2	0.5	29	4	15
Garlic Bread, ¼ pack, 45g	150	625	5.5	2	21	3.5	265
Gravy, Small Tub, 130g	70	290	1	0.5	13	1.5	600
Monster Nuggets, (1), 45g	125	515	7.5	1	4.8	8	290
Pineapple Fritter, 56g	120	500	5	1	16	1.5	40
Roast Potatoes, 1 pack, 100g	90	365	2.5	0.5	11	4.5	65

Updated Nutrition Data ~ www.CalorieKing.com.au
Persons with Diabetes ~ See Disclaimer (Page 22)

Fast-Foods & Chains

Donut King® (Sept '13)

	Cal	kJ	Fat	Sat'F	Carb	Pro	Sod
Hot Dogs:							
Basic with Tomato Sauce, 176g	455	1900	20	6	50	20	1525
Classic Aussie, 230g	530	2225	22	10	54	27	1785
El Grande Chilli, 240g	545	2275	22	10	57	27	1790
Original with Tomato Sauce, 205g	500	2090	22	10	51	25	1610
Donut:							
Chocolate Jam Ball, 97g	340	1230	10	5	58	4.5	200
Cinnamon Ring, 46g	150	625	6.5	2.5	21	2	255
Classic Mini Jam, 36g	130	550	5.5	2.5	18	2	95
Iced Ring: Pineapple Icing, 62g	230	960	8.5	4	35	3.5	165
Strawberry Icing w. White Stripes, 59g	200	820	6.5	3	33	2	255
Novelty: Classic Boy or Girl	275	1140	9	4.5	44	4	165
Crocodile, Chocolate, 78g	300	1240	11	5	47	4	255
Dinosaur with Chocolate Icing	265	1100	9	4.5	42	3.5	165
Face, 72g	245	1025	7	3	43	2.5	270
Sweet Talker, Mobile Phone, 79g	305	1265	11	5.5	47	4.5	175
Twinkle Star with Face, 72g	270	1120	9	4.5	43	4.5	165
Sensations: Double Choc Marble, 69g	280	1155	14	8.5	33	4.5	180
Strawberry & Cream, 69g	270	1135	13	6.5	35	4.5	180
White Choc Marble, 69g	280	1160	14	8	34	4.5	180
Eclair: Custard Cream w. Caramel Icing, 79g	245	1020	11	6	38	3.5	180
Iced Cream Bar with Chocolate Icing, 91g	260	1075	13	8	43	4	180
Drinks: *Per Container*							
Frozen Cola, Regular, 490g	255	1075	0	0	64	0	50
Frozen Raspberry, regular, 490g	260	1090	0	0	64	0	40
Fruit Freeze: All flavors, without Cream, 425g	35	150	0.5	0.5	8.5	0.5	2
With Cream, 440g	65	260	1	1	14	1.5	20
Iced Chocolate, 322g	335	1405	16	11	41	8.5	180
Iced Coffee, with Ice Cream, 302g	215	900	14	10	16	7.5	130
Iced Mocha, with Ice Cream, 322g	305	1265	14	9	39	7	150
Quake Shake: *Per Container*							
Cherry Explosion, 473g	410	1700	15	10	61	9	170
Choc Volcano, 465g	390	1615	13	8.5	58	20	185
Honeycomb Lava, 471g	410	1705	13	8	64	9	225
Mint Shock Bubbly, 462g	365	1525	12	8	55	9	155
Sundaes: *Per Cup*							
Caramel Crowne, 207g	235	975	4	2.5	45	3	80
Caramel, with Tiny Teddies, 204g	205	845	3	2	40	3	95
Chocolate Mint Slice, 205g	235	975	1.5	0.5	43	2	90
Cookies & Cream, 160g	100	420	2	1	18	2.5	90
Tee Vee Snack, 205g	225	945	4	1.5	45	3	95
Cakes: *Celebration Pyramid, Per Donut*							
Cars/Fairies, 63g	215	895	6.5	3	37	2	250
Pooh Bear, 66g	225	930	6	2.5	40	2	250
Princess, 62g	210	880	6.5	3	36	2	250
Smiley Face, 62g	225	945	7	3	38	2.5	290
Spiderman, 65g	225	935	7	3	38	2.5	250
Strawberry Delight, 65g	220	910	6	2.5	39	2	250

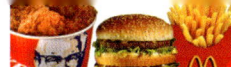

Fast-Foods & Chains

Domino's® (Sept '13)
Pizza: Per Slice, ⅛ Pizza

	Cal	kJ	Fat	Sat'F	Carb	Pro	Sod
Classic Crust, Traditional:							
BBQ Chicken & Bacon, 78g	180	740	6	3	23	8	385
Chicken & Feta, 80g	170	700	5.5	2.5	22	7.5	390
Creamy Chicken & Cherry Tomato, 80g	200	825	9	5	21	7.5	335
Fire Breather, 72g	160	660	4.5	2.5	22	7	385
Garlic Prawn, 76g	170	715	6.5	4	20	7.5	260
Supreme, 76g	165	695	5.5	2.5	22	7.5	360
Cheesy Crust:							
Chicken & Feta, 96g	215	900	9	4.5	21	12	470
Fire Breather, 90g	205	865	8	4.5	22	12	500
Supreme, 93g	215	905	12	9	22	12	480
Vegorama, 90g	190	785	6.5	4	22	10	375
Thin 'n' Crispy Crust: BBQ Chicken & Bacon, 76g	180	750	6	3	24	8	375
Chicken & Feta, 78g	170	710	5.5	2.5	22	7.5	380
Creamy Chicken & Cherry Tomato, 77g	195	820	9	4.5	22	7.5	320
Fire Breather, 70g	160	660	5	2.5	22	7	375
Supreme, 74g	170	715	5.5	3	23	7.5	360
Thin n Crispy: 97% Fat-Free							
BBQ Chicken & Pineapple, 73g	140	580	2	1	23	6	265
Chicken Napolitana, 76g	120	500	2	1	18	7	200
Prawn & Cherry Tomato, 71g	120	500	1.5	1	21	5.5	230
Gluten Free Base: Blue Cheese, 64g	185	770	9	4.5	19	6	365
Chicken & Feta, 73g	160	680	7	2.5	20	6	400
Creamy Chicken & Cherry Tomato, 71g	180	760	9	4	19	6	345
Garlic Prawn, 67g	155	650	6.5	3	18	6	270
Hawaiian, 68g	145	600	4	1.5	20	6	340
Pepperoni, 56g	170	700	8	3.5	19	5.5	375
Vegorama, 66g	135	565	4.5	1.5	20	4	275
Low Carbohydrate Base: Hawaiian, 70g	135	570	5	2.5	7	14	330
Pepperoni, 58g	160	665	8.5	4	5.5	14	350
Supreme, 67g	150	615	7	3	6.5	14	340
Vegorama, 65g	120	495	4.5	2	6	12	235
Chef's Best:							
BBQ Duck & Blue Cheese, 83g	205	855	8.5	4.5	23	8.5	380
BBQ Pork & Hollandaise, 81g	185	770	7.5	3	23	8	375
Shiraz Lamb & Tomato, 91g	185	770	5.5	2.5	23	10	445
Chicken: Chicken Wings, 4 pieces, 288g	665	2785	47	12	21	41	1345
Chicken Kicker: Mild, 1 piece, 24g	45	185	2	0.5	3.5	4	135
Spicy, 1 piece, 24g	45	185	2	0.5	3	4	90
Oven Baked Chicken Wings, 1 wing, 40g	75	305	3	1	5	6.5	150
Sides: Garlic Bread, 24g	85	340	4	1.5	10	1.5	125
Cheesy Garlic Bread, 45g	150	630	8	3.5	17	3.5	285
Chips, Beer Battered, 350g	705	2945	22	14	113	12	1820
Desserts: Chocolate Lava Cake, 92g	390	1620	24	12	38	5.5	120
Chocolate Brownies, 15g	75	305	4.5	4	7	1	10
Dutch Pancakes, 12 pancakes, 107g	440	1840	27	14	44	6	155

Updated Nutrition Data ~ www.CalorieKing.com.au
Persons with Diabetes ~ See Disclaimer (Page 22)

Fast-Foods & Chains

Eagle Boys® (Sept '13)

Gourmet Deep Pan Pizza: Per ⅛ Slice of Whole Pizza

	Cal	kJ	Fat	Sat'F	Carb	Pro	Sod
Bacon, Bocconcini & Brie	150	625	5	2.5	18	7.5	370
BBQ Chicken & Bacon	175	720	5.5	2	23	8	340
Butcher's Block	190	795	7.5	3	22	10	535
Garlic Prawn	125	525	3	1	18	7	280
Peri Peri Chicken	150	630	4.5	2	20	7	370
Prawn & Avocado	140	570	4.5	2	17	7	250
Spanish Tapas	150	615	4	2	20	7	285
The Scorcher	145	605	4	2	21	6.5	335
Vegetarian Bianco	150	620	2.5	0.5	27	23	220

Gourmet Thin Crust Pizza: Per ⅛ Slice of Whole Pizza

	Cal	kJ	Fat	Sat'F	Carb	Pro	Sod
Bacon, Bocconcini & Brie	145	610	6	3	15	8	455
BBQ Chicken & Bacon	175	725	6.5	3	21	8.5	430
Butcher's Block	195	820	8.5	4	19	11	665
Garlic Prawn	110	465	3	1	14	7	250
Peri Peri Chicken	150	620	5	2.5	17	8	435
Prawn & Avocado	135	555	5.5	2	14	7.5	305
Spanish Tapas	145	595	4.5	2.5	17	7.5	350
The Scorcher	140	580	4.5	2	18	7	420
Vegetarian Bianco	140	580	2.5	1	24	29	295

Traditional Thin Crust: Per 1/8 Slice of Whole Pizza

	Cal	kJ	Fat	Sat'F	Carb	Pro	Sod
Aussie Bacon & Egg	175	720	7	3	19	9	360
BBQ Meatlovers	185	775	7	3	23	10	510
Hawaiian	135	560	3.5	1.5	20	6.5	380
Pepperoni	165	695	7.5	3.5	17	7	430
Super Supremo	130	540	4.5	2	17	6.5	295
Vege Delight	120	505	3	1.5	19	5	255

Sides:

	Cal	kJ	Fat	Sat'F	Carb	Pro	Sod
Prawn Skewers: Chilli (1)	70	295	3	0.5	2	8.5	360
Garlic (1)	70	295	3.5	0.5	0.5	9	240
Tandoori (1)	85	355	5	1	1.5	8	490
Ribs, with Smokey BBQ Sauce	175	735	9	3.5	9.5	15	170

Grill'd® (Sept '13)

Burgers:

	Cal	kJ	Fat	Sat'F	Carb	Pro	Sod
Beef Burger: Almighty	805	3365	39	13	57	53	1540
Crispy Bacon & Cheese	705	2935	33	12	54	45	1345
Hot Mama	570	2390	21	9	55	40	1300
Kung Fu Fighter	615	2575	27	7.5	57	35	945
Simply Grill'd	575	2400	25	7	53	33	885
Chicken Burger: Caesar's Palace	700	2925	32	10	46	55	1325
Grill'd Bird & Brie	580	2430	21	6.5	58	38	625
Hot Hombre	615	2580	20	6.5	59	44	895
Simon Says	560	2340	20	5	49	42	945
The Zen Hen	530	2215	18	3.5	53	37	660

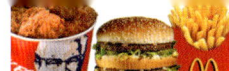

Fast-Foods & Chains

Grill'd® cont... (Sept '13)

Burgers (Cont):

	Cal	kJ	Fat	Sat'F	Carb	Pro	Sod
Lamb Burger:							
Baa Baa	635	2660	29	10	53	40	950
Goats Cheese & Hummus	700	2925	32	11	60	41	1180
Moroccan Lamb	525	2205	16	6.5	56	37	960
Snack Burger: Chicken Licken	420	1760	14	2.5	39	33	460
Mini Moo	390	1630	11	4.5	48	23	695
Veggie Burger: Bombay Bliss	495	2060	6.5	1	85	18	1160
Field of Dreams	495	2070	24	4.5	48	21	735
Garden Goodness	595	2480	21	4.5	77	20	1280

Salad:

	Cal	kJ	Fat	Sat'F	Carb	Pro	Sod
Chicken Caesar	580	2415	31	10	24	51	1145
Chicken, Pomegranate & Goats Cheese	450	1890	24	6.5	22	35	285
Mixed Vegetables & Dukkah	300	1255	12	4	36	9	300

Sides:

	Cal	kJ	Fat	Sat'F	Carb	Pro	Sod
Chips: Regular, 260g	410	1715	22	4.5	44	8	575
Snack, 160g	255	1055	14	3	27	5	355

Healthy Habits® (Sept '13)

Sandwich:

	Cal	kJ	Fat	Sat'F	Carb	Pro	Sod
Classic Crushed Egg	525	2200	20	4.5	58	26	520
Fully Loaded Salad	435	1805	10	2	66	15	500
Hail Caesar	655	2730	29	6	60	36	1200
Hammer Time	545	2285	14	7	72	30	1550
Rajin' Cajun	465	1950	6	1.5	73	27	890
Roastin' Chicken & Avocado	625	2595	29	4.5	60	28	780
Smoked Salmon Sensation	385	1610	15	4.5	60	16	785
Temptin' Tuna	605	2525	26	2.5	59	30	875
The Schnitzel	930	3880	33	12	104	51	1355
Turkey & Cranberry Crush	580	2425	19	11	67	34	1110

Hungry Jacks® (Sept '13)

Burgers/Sandwiches:

	Cal	kJ	Fat	Sat'F	Carb	Pro	Sod
Whopper	690	2885	41	12	49	30	955
With Cheese	780	3250	48	16	50	35	1310
Double Whopper	940	3925	60	20	49	50	1035
With Cheese	1030	4295	67	25	50	55	1395
Double Whopper Ultimate	1170	4880	77	31	51	65	2195
Junior Whopper	360	1500	20	5	30	15	530
With Cheese	405	1685	23	7.5	30	17	710
Angus BBQ Bacon	610	2550	37	14	35	32	1295
Bacon Deluxe	565	2365	35	14	29	33	1040
Big Cheese	780	3260	48	16	50	34	1300
Big Big Cheese	1120	4670	74	30	51	59	1740
BBQ Big Cheese	775	3240	48	16	46	34	1120
Cheeseburger	325	1355	15	6.5	31	18	705
Double Cheeseburger	470	1965	25	12	31	29	910
Grilled Chicken Burger	375	1565	19	4	30	20	850

Updated Nutrition Data ~ www.CalorieKing.com.au
Persons with Diabetes ~ See Disclaimer (Page 22)

Fast-Foods & Chains

Hungry Jacks® Cont... (Sept '13)

Burgers/Sandwiches:

	Cal	kJ	Fat	Sat'F	Carb	Pro	Sod
Hamburger	280	1170	11	4	30	15	530
Tendercrisp Chicken Burger: Classic	590	2455	32	4.5	51	23	825
Spicy	550	2300	28	4	52	23	945
The Aussie	870	3630	53	17	56	41	1715

Breakfasts:

	Cal	kJ	Fat	Sat'F	Carb	Pro	Sod
Hashbrown (1)	160	675	12	2	14	2	205
Muffin: Bacon & Egg	315	1330	14	5.5	28	19	820
Sausage & Egg	400	1660	21	9	28	24	775
Pancakes	755	3160	30	12	110	11	820
Wrap: BBQ Brekky	480	1840	23	11	32	26	1145
Angry Brekky	615	2560	23	11	34	26	1240

Sides:

	Cal	kJ	Fat	Sat'F	Carb	Pro	Sod
Chicken Nuggets: 3 nuggets	120	490	6	1.5	9.5	7	250
6 nuggets	235	975	12	2.5	19	14	500
French Fries: Small	240	1000	13	2	29	3	265
Regular	375	1565	20	3	45	5	410
Angry Onions	410	1700	29	6.5	35	3.5	675
Onion Rings, Regular	300	1260	14	3	39	5	510

Salads:

	Cal	kJ	Fat	Sat'F	Carb	Pro	Sod
Garden	70	290	0.5	0	12	2	395
Chicken Garden Salad with Ranch Dressing	320	1345	22	5	13	16	745

Desserts:

	Cal	kJ	Fat	Sat'F	Carb	Pro	Sod
Soft Serve Cone, ice cream	215	895	9	6	27	6	120
Storm: Cookies & Cream	445	1850	19	12	57	11	325
Flake	460	1920	20	12	54	16	220
Shakes: Chocolate, regular, 305ml	435	1805	11	7.5	70	13	315
Strawberry, regular, 305ml	425	1775	11	7	69	13	250
Vanilla, regular, 305ml	380	1575	12	8	53	14	265

Soft Drinks:

	Cal	kJ	Fat	Sat'F	Carb	Pro	Sod
Coke, regular, 454ml	205	850	0	0	50	0	50
Coke Zero, regular, 480ml	0	0	0	0	0.5	0.5	70
Diet Coke, regular, 454ml	1	10	0	0	2.5	0	70
Fanta, regular, 454ml	265	1100	0	0	65	0	70
Sprite, regular, 454ml	200	835	0	0	50	0	70

Jesters® (Sept '13)

Pies:

	Cal	kJ	Fat	Sat'F	Carb	Pro	Sod
Footy	325	1350	15	8	29	20	510
Morning Glory	450	1875	29	14	27	21	680
Ned	330	1380	14	8.5	35	14	586
Nutty Chook	350	1455	14	11	33	15	320
Pavarotti	325	1360	15	8.5	33	15	425
Popeye	410	1720	20	12	40	17	680
Spud Deluxe	345	1435	18	8.5	34	13	490
Stockmans	315	1310	11	7	34	19	500
Sweet: Blueberry Kiss	295	1235	7.5	4.5	52	4	195
William Tell	290	1200	7.5	4.5	60	4	195

Rolls:

	Cal	kJ	Fat	Sat'F	Carb	Pro	Sod
Bacon & Cheese	540	2255	34	18	41	16	1110
Spinach & 3 Cheese	520	2175	25	8	58	15	845

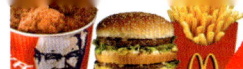

Fast-Foods & Chains

KFC® (Sept '13)

	Cal	kJ	Fat	Sat'F	Carb	Pro	Sod
Original Recipe Chicken:							
Chicken, 2 pieces, 152g	425	1780	27	5.5	15	33	895
Fillet (1), 77g	160	660	6.5	1	5.5	20	505
Fried: Breast (1)	460	1920	29	6	16	36	965
Drumstick (1)	150	620	10	2	5	12	315
Thigh (1)	265	1100	17	3.5	9	21	555
Wing (1)	135	565	8.5	2	4.5	11	285
Extras:							
Crispy Strips, 3 pieces, 114g	265	1100	13	1.5	12	26	550
Grilled, Chicken Strip, 1 piece, 38g	55	225	1	0	1	10	180
Hot & Spicy Pieces, Qld Only, 1 piece, 92g	285	1190	18	3.5	14	17	540
Kentucky Nuggets, 6 nuggets, 119g	305	1270	20	4.5	16	23	800
Popcorn Chicken: Regular, 135g	445	1855	29	5	26	26	755
Maxi, 225g	740	3090	48	8	44	43	1260
Roller, BBQ Bacon	340	1415	16	5	35	14	940
Wicked Wings: 3 pieces, 115g	400	1660	24	5	16	22	620
10 pieces, 383g	1320	5520	79	16	51	71	2065
Meal Box: Per Meal							
2 Piece Feed	1020	4260	42	8.5	121	44	1710
3 Piece Feed	1230	5150	55	12	128	61	2160
Fillets	700	2930	23	2	87	44	1270
Streetwise: Burger Combo	925	3870	22	3.4	132	29	1010
Chicken Combo	810	3390	36	7	91	37	1155
Snack Box: Crispy Strip, 138g	315	1320	14	2	39	13	395
Grilled Taster, 193g	310	1280	11	2	38	15	650
Kentucky Nuggets, 179g	430	1780	22	4.5	45	19	743
Popcorn Chicken, 175g	475	1985	26	4	50	18	635
Wicked Wings, 177g	495	2065	25	4.5	45	18	630
Burgers:							
Original Recipe:							
Burger: 178g	405	1690	11	2	44	29	855
Qld Only	445	1855	16	2	52	22	745
BBQ Bacon & Cheese: 207g	485	2020	16	4.5	49	33	1215
Qld Only	550	2295	24	6	52	30	1085
Bacon & Cheese: 197g	470	1955	16	5	45	33	1130
Qld Only	525	2190	23	5.5	47	31	1125
The Double, 210g	475	1970	22	7	18	51	1970
Tower: 268g	610	2545	25	9	69	35	1640
Qld Only	705	2945	33	6	76	26	1560
Works, 245g	560	2330	24	5.5	57	29	1115
Streetwise Double Crunch, 182g	540	2260	24	2	56	26	750
The Double, Zingin Double, 246g	595	2480	31	9	25	54	2350

Updated Nutrition Data ~ www.CalorieKing.com.au
Persons with Diabetes ~ See Disclaimer (Page 22)

Fast-Foods & Chains

KFC® Cont... (Sept '13)

	Cal	kJ	Fat	Sat'F	Carb	Pro	Sod
Burgers (Cont):							
Zinger:							
Burger: 196g	430	1805	16	3	48	32	1050
Qld Only, 188g	470	1965	19	3	46	29	1090
BBQ Bacon & Cheese: 225g	515	2140	20	6	52	35	1410
Qld Only, 219g	550	2300	24	6	52	32	1370
Bacon & Cheese: 215g	495	2070	20	6	48	35	1320
Qld Only, 208g	550	2290	24	6	50	32	1230
Tower: 285g	660	2740	29	10	72	37	1830
Qld Only, 279g	690	2870	33	6	67	30	1675
Works, 259g	550	2295	23	5.5	52	36	1265
Breakfast: Chicken, Bacon & Egg Twister, 248g	620	2590	26	9	52	41	1965
Donut Sticks with Maple Syrup, 99g	365	1530	14	1.5	54	5	195
Hashbrown, 53g	160	670	9	4.5	17	2	325
Bacon & Egg Roll, 153g	340	1420	11	3	37	22	1480
Twisters:							
Grilled Chicken Twister, BLT	545	2275	24	8.5	41	42	1830
Fiery Grilled, WA/NT only, 218g	410	1720	14	5	44	27	960
Max: Twister	665	2775	29	13	63	36	1655
Qld Only	675	2820	30	13	62	36	1620
Regular, 216g	515	2165	28	5.5	46	24	770
Sweet Chilli, 216g	470	1965	20	5	50	24	830
Sides:							
Dinner Roll, 40g	130	540	2.5	0.5	20	5	160
Chips: Regular serving, 100g	230	955	10	1.5	35	4	215
Large serving, 227g	520	2170	21	3	79	8.5	485
Coleslaw: Small tub, 110g	120	490	6.5	1	12	1.5	140
Large tub, 450g	480	2000	27	3	49	5	565
Gravy, ¼ of large tub, 50g	25	95	1	0.5	3	1	235
Potato & Gravy, regular tub, 110g	80	330	3.5	1.5	10	2	395
Salads:							
So Salad: 205g	50	205	0.5	0	7.5	2	210
With Grilled Chicken Strips	100	430	1.5	0	8	12	390
Desserts:							
Cheesecake, Cookies & Cream, 80g	300	1255	22	13	24	3.5	155
Chocolate Caramel Mousse, 80g	295	1225	19	13	28	3.5	155
Krushers: Per Large Container							
Golden Gaytime	465	1940	17	10	72	4.5	125
Iced Mocha	440	1825	21	13	56	6	290
Kookies 'n Kream	540	2270	27	14	68	6.5	295
Mint Choc	450	1875	17	9	68	5	285
Strawberry	390	1620	7.5	5.5	67	12	285
Triple Choc Crunch	435	1825	13	8.5	66	8.5	330

Fast-Foods & Chains

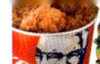

McDonald's® (Sept '13)

	Cal	kJ	Fat	Sat'F	Carb	Pro	Sod
Burgers:							
Big Mac	495	2060	27	11	35	25	860
Cheeseburger: Original	285	1190	13	6	26	15	675
Double Cheeseburger	430	1800	24	12	28	26	980
Filet-O-Fish	305	1270	13	3	31	13	525
Grand Angus	665	2780	34	16	45	43	1200
Hamburger	235	980	8.5	3.5	26	13	480
Mighty Angus	710	2960	36	17	51	45	1400
Quarter Pounder: Original	545	2280	31	16	34	34	1050
Double Quarter Pounder	855	3560	54	28	34	58	1350
Chicken Burgers:							
Chicken 'n' Cheese	395	1640	20	4	33	20	710
Chicken & Mayo	335	1390	16	3	32	13	585
McChamp Chicken	480	2010	23	3	45	22	860
McChicken	410	1710	19	3	38	20	700
McGrilled Chicken	375	1570	14	2	33	27	615
McSpicy Chicken	470	1960	23	3.5	52	22	1080
Wraps:							
Crispy Chicken Sweet Chilli	490	2040	21	5	52	21	850
Grilled Chicken Sweet Chilli	380	1580	3.5	11	41	26	685
Snack Wraps:							
Crispy Chicken	285	1180	13	3.5	29	12	410
Grilled Chicken	225	945	8.5	3	23	14	330
French Fries:							
Small, 72g	255	1070	14	1.5	29	3	245
Medium, 105g	370	1540	20	2.5	42	4	355
Large, 130g	455	1900	25	3	51	5	435
McBites, 10 pieces	160	665	9	1.5	8.5	11	455
McNuggets:							
3 Pieces	140	580	9	1.5	7	8	225
6 Pieces	280	1160	18	3	14	16	445
Sauces: Barbecue	50	200	0.5	0.5	11	0.5	185
Ketchup	10	50	0	0	2.5	0	100
Mayonnaise	90	370	10	2	0.5	0.5	65
Mustard	65	275	3.5	0.5	7.5	0.5	160
Sweet & Sour	50	205	0.5	0.5	11	0	155

Updated Nutrition Data ~ www.CalorieKing.com.au
Persons with Diabetes ~ See Disclaimer (Page 22)

Fast-Foods & Chains

McDonald's® Cont... (Sept '13)

	Cal	kJ	Fat	Sat'F	Carb	Pro	Sod
Happy Meals:							
Apple Slices, 1 bag	40	155	0	0	8	0.5	0
Apple Juice	115	470	0	0	28	0	15
3 McNuggets, Small Fries/Coke	500	2080	23	3	61	11	490
Cheeseburger, Small Fries/Coke	645	2690	27	8	81	18	1030
Crispy Chicken Wrap, Apple Bag & Shake	575	2395	20	7.5	79	19	645
Hamburger, Small Fries/Coke	595	2480	23	5	80	15	760
Chicken Wrap, Apple Bag & Water	265	1100	8.5	3	31	14	330
Shakes, average all flavours, small	295	1240	7	4.5	50	8	195
Breakfast Items:							
English McMuffin: Without Jam	150	620	3	1	25	4.5	270
With Jam	185	775	3	1	34	4.5	270
Hash Brown	155	640	9.5	1	15	1.5	350
Hotcakes: With Butter & Syrup	660	2760	20	8.5	106	12	530
Without Butter or Syrup	400	1660	11	2	63	12	440
McMuffin: Bacon & Egg	300	1240	14	6	26	16	675
Sausage	300	1240	15	7.5	26	16	610
Sausage & Egg	370	1540	20	9	26	22	650
Salads: *Without Dressing*							
Classic Crispy Chicken	300	1250	15	4.5	16	24	630
Classic Grilled Chicken	205	855	6.5	3	6	29	495
Garden Salad	20	70	0	0	1.5	1.5	20
Dressings: Balsamic, 40ml	25	110	1	0	4	0	180
Caesar, 40ml	130	535	13	2.5	2	1	205
Italian, 30ml	15	50	0	0	3	0	70
Desserts:							
Apple Pie	235	970	14	3.5	25	2	145
McDonaldland Cookies, 10 cookies	165	685	5	2.5	27	2	90
McFlurry: Bubblegum Squash	335	1390	8	5	58	7	95
Caramel Crumble	460	1920	11	7	81	8.5	185
Double Chocolate Fudge	470	1960	15	12	74	8	195
Sundae:							
Plain, without Topping, small	210	875	7	4.5	32	5.5	80
Caramel, small	355	1480	8.5	5.5	63	6.5	155
Hot Fudge, small	345	1450	12	9	53	7	135
Strawberry, small	285	1190	7	4,5	50	6	80
Sundae Cone	150	630	4.5	3	22	4	60
Frappe:							
Caramel Crush, small	435	1820	19	3	57	8	120
Choc Whirl, small	395	1650	18	11	52	7.5	100
Coffee Kick, small	380	1570	18	12	46	8	110
Shakes, average all flavours:							
Small	295	1240	7	4.5	50	8	195
Medium	385	1600	9	6	64	11	250
Large	475	1980	12	7	80	13	310
Smoothies, average all flavours:							
Small	185	770	1.5	0.5	40	2	50
Medium	265	1110	2	1	58	3	70
Large	340	1420	3	1	76	4	90

Fast-Foods & Chains

McDonald's® Cont... (Sept '13)

Soft Drinks:

	Cal	kJ	Fat	Sat'F	Carb	Pro	Sod
Coca-Cola, (without ice): Small, 309ml	100	430	0	0	25	0	25
Medium, 410ml	145	610	0	0	36	0	35
Large, 592ml	225	935	0	0	55	0	50
Frozen Coca-Col: Medium	175	725	0	0	43	0	35
Large	225	950	0	0	56	0	45
Fanta, Medium, 410ml	180	750	0	0	44	0	50

Coffee (Espresso Pronto):

	Cal	kJ	Fat	Sat'F	Carb	Pro	Sod
Cappuccino: Small	105	425	5.5	4	8	5	65
Tall	160	665	9	6	13	8	100
Flat White: Small	115	475	6.5	4.5	8	6	70
Tall	205	860	12	8	15	11	130
Latte: Small	110	460	6.5	4	8	5.5	70
Tall	195	820	12	7.5	14	10	125

McCafe® (Sept '13)

Sandwiches:

	Cal	kJ	Fat	Sat'F	Carb	Pro	Sod
Toasted Sandwiches: *On White Bread*							
Cheese & Ham	310	1300	8	4.5	37	21	1170
Cheese & Tomato	265	1110	7	4.5	37	13	515
Cheese, Ham & Tomato	315	1320	8	4.5	38	22	1180
Toasted Sandwiches: *On Wholemeal Bread*							
Cheese & Ham	305	1270	8.5	4	31	23	1100
Cheese & Tomato	260	1090	7.5	4	32	14	440
Cheese, Ham & Tomato	310	1300	9	4	32	23	1100
Turkish Bread: Chicken Troppo	530	2200	14	6	69	28	1170
Ham, Cheese & Relish	530	2220	9	16	68	27	1640
Sweet Chilli Chicken	535	2240	14	5.5	73	28	1250

Cookies: Per Cookie

	Cal	kJ	Fat	Sat'F	Carb	Pro	Sod
Dotty	300	1250	16	10	34	4	135
Triple Choc, Gluten Free	290	1210	15	11	38	3	205
White Choc. & Macadamia, Gluten Free	320	1330	20	12	32	4	235

Cakes/Muffins/Pastries/Slices: Per Slice

	Cal	kJ	Fat	Sat'F	Carb	Pro	Sod
Cakes: Banana Bread	615	2570	26	5	84	10	390
Carrot	680	2830	47	14	57	8	300
Chocolate Truffle	215	895	14	8.5	21	3	55
Double Chocolate	630	2630	37	18	67	7	355
Jaffa Torte	810	3390	56	27	59	17	85
Cheesecakes: Cookies & Cream	670	2790	46	33	57	7	250
Blueberry, mini	230	965	15	11	20	4	165
Mango & Macadamia	720	3010	63	39	36	5.5	175
Raspberry	550	2300	40	28	39	10	350
Custard Tart	360	1510	12	8	58	3.5	300

Updated Nutrition Data ~ www.CalorieKing.com.au
Persons with Diabetes ~ See Disclaimer (Page 22)

Fast-Foods & Chains

McCafe® Cont... (Sept '13)

Cakes/Muffins/Pastries/Slices (Cont): Per Serve

Item	Cal	kJ	Fat	Sat'F	Carb	Pro	Sod
Croissants: Chocolate	385	1600	19	14	47	6	300
Ham & Cheese	360	1500	23	15	26	12	570
Jam & Butter	375	1570	24	16	36	4.5	300
Danish, Apricot & Custard	215	895	8.5	5.5	30	4	200
Donuts: Jam Ball	215	885	7.5	3	32	3.5	210
Iced: Chocolate flavoured	485	2020	23	11	61	8	380
Strawberry	485	2030	23	11	62	7.5	375
Friands: Chocolate; Raspberry, average	370	1540	23	11	32	8.5	45
Lamington	320	1340	11	8	45	6	300
Macarons, average all flavours	110	425	5	2	14	2	20
Muffins: Apple & Cinnamon, mini	90	370	4.5	2.5	11	1	110
Blueberry	580	2420	32	14	66	8	655
Mud	695	2910	34	4	90	8	470
Orange & Poppyseed	320	1320	3	1	57	5	480
Walnut, Carrot & Bran	555	2320	28	6	63	8.5	475
Raisin Toast, with Butter	245	1030	8	5	35	7	180
Scones: Plain	340	1420	10	4.5	53	8.5	760
With Jam & Cream	455	1900	19	10	63	9	765
Slices: Banana & Walnut	480	2010	31	8.5	44	6.5	215
Chocolate Brownie	305	1280	22	13	25	4	30
Mini Caramel	205	850	12	8	22	3	75
Mini Cherry	135	550	7	5.5	16	1.5	45
Mini Mint	120	500	7	5.5	14	1	30
Twist, Vanilla & Sultana	250	1040	11	7	33	5	215

Drinks, Cold: Per Regular Cup

Item	Cal	kJ	Fat	Sat'F	Carb	Pro	Sod
Frappe: Caramel Latte	320	1330	12	8	48	5.5	115
Chai	320	1330	11	7	48	7.5	135
Chocco	330	1370	12	8.5	49	7.5	275
Latte	295	1230	12	8	42	6	125
Mocha	310	1290	11	7.5	45	6.5	180
Iced Chocolate: With Whole Milk	360	1500	19	13	37	11	205
With Skim Milk	275	1140	9	6	37	11	210
With Soy Milk	400	1660	20	7	41	13	265
Iced Latte: With Whole Milk	190	795	8	5.5	23	7	85
With Skim Milk	125	525	0	0	23	7.5	90
With Soy Milk	185	765	7	1	23	7	105
Iced Mocha: With Whole Milk	290	1200	8.5	5.5	44	7.5	170
With Skim Milk	220	925	1	0.5	45	8	175
With Soy Milk	295	1230	7.5	1.5	47	8	200
Smoothie: Mango	315	1320	1	0.5	71	4	80
Strawberry	265	1100	1	0.5	57	4.5	70

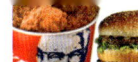

Fast-Foods & Chains

McCafe® Cont... (Sept '13)
Drinks, Hot: Per Regular Cup Unless Indicated

Item	Cal	kJ	Fat	Sat'F	Carb	Pro	Sod
Babycino, with Whole Milk	50	205	2.5	1.5	4.5	2.5	30
Black Tea, all varieties	0	0	0	0	0	0	15
Cappuccino:							
With Whole Milk: Small	120	505	6.5	4.5	10	6	75
Regular	165	690	9	6	13	8	105
Tall	185	780	11	7	15	9	115
With Skim Milk: Small	70	280	0	0	10	6	80
Regular	90	365	0.5	0.5	13	8.5	105
Tall	105	425	0.5	0.5	15	10	120
With Soy Milk: Small	115	470	5.5	1	10	6	90
Regular	160	660	7.5	1	13	8	125
Tall	180	740	9	1	15	9	140
Espresso	0	0	0	0	0	0	0
Flat White:							
With Whole Milk: Small	120	490	7	4.5	8.5	6	75
Regular	170	705	10	6.5	12	8.5	105
Tall	195	815	12	7.5	14	10	125
With Skim Milk: Small	65	265	0	0	9	6.5	80
Regular	90	370	0	0	13	9	110
Tall	105	430	0	0	15	11	130
With Soy Milk: Small	110	465	6	1	8.5	6	90
Regular	160	670	8.5	1	13	8.5	130
Tall	190	780	10	1.5	15	10	150
Hot Chocolate:							
With Whole Milk: Small	200	830	7.5	5	24	7.5	120
Regular	290	1210	11	7	35	11	175
Tall	385	1610	15	10	46	15	230
With Skim Milk: Small	145	595	1	0.5	24	8	120
Regular	210	870	1.5	1	36	12	180
Tall	275	1150	1.5	1.5	47	16	235
With Soy Milk: Small	195	805	6.5	1	25	7.5	135
Regular	285	1180	9.5	2	36	11	195
Tall	375	1560	13	2.5	47	15	260
Latte:							
With Whole Milk: Small	115	475	6.5	4.5	8	6	70
Regular	165	690	9.5	6.5	12	8.5	105
Tall	180	750	11	7	13	9	115
With Skim Milk: Small	60	250	0	0	8.5	6	75
Regular	90	365	0	0	12	9	110
Tall	115	470	0.5	0.5	16	12	140
With Soy Milk: Small	105	445	5.5	1	8.5	5.5	85
Regular	160	655	8.5	1	13	8.5	125
Tall	170	710	9	1	14	9	135
Long Black	1	5	0	0	0	0	0
Macchiato, with Whole Milk	5	15	0	0	0.5	0	5
Mocha: With Whole Milk	245	1030	10	6.5	28	10	150
With Skim Milk	170	705	1	1	28	11	135
With Soy Milk	240	990	9	1.5	28	10	170
Vienna, Regular	85	355	8	5.5	2.5	1	15

Updated Nutrition Data ~ www.CalorieKing.com.au
Persons with Diabetes ~ See Disclaimer (Page 22)

Fast-Foods & Chains

Muffin Break® (Sept '13)

	Cal	kJ	Fat	Sat F	Carb	Pro	Sod
Sandwiches: *Per Sandwich*							
Flatbread: Cajun Chicken, 317g	445	1855	14	5	57	23	1395
Chicken Schnitzel, 281g	525	2185	17	4	73	19	1780
Grilled Vege, 320g	430	1795	13	5	60	16	1170
Roast Beef, 289g	445	1865	14	5.5	58	23	2095
Sandwich: Chicken & Salad, 229g	275	1150	10	5	33	14	650
Curry Egg & Lettuce, 164g	325	1355	17	7	33	15	925
Ham & Salad, 229g	275	1145	10	5	35	11	1000
Salad, 189g	235	985	8.5	5	32	6	385
Toastie: Cheese & Ham, 160g	440	1840	25	16	37	20	1250
Cheese & Tomato, 160g	405	1695	23	16	35	15	605
Cheese, Ham & Tomato, 200g	445	1855	24	16	38	20	1240
Muffin: *Per Muffin*							
Bran: Apple Berry, 167g	490	2055	23	2.5	58	9	305
Banana Nut, 169g	565	2350	29	3	59	10	305
Blueberry Lemon, 165g	485	2030	23	2.5	56	8.5	300
Date & Apple, 169g	530	2215	23	2.5	66	9	305
Mixed Berry, 165g	495	2065	23	2.5	58	9	305
Gluten Free: Apple, 158g	340	1425	6	3	63	7.5	400
Apricot Choc Chip, 158g	385	1615	8.5	4.5	68	8	390
Blackberry, 158g	350	1455	5.5	3	64	7.5	385
Choc Chip, 158g	430	1800	12	6.5	72	8.5	390
Ham, Cheese & Tomato, 165g	385	1605	19	6	39	13	1100
Spinach & Fetta, 165g	365	1515	18	5.5	36	11	1010
Low-Fat: Apple, Bran & Sultana, 145g	380	1595	3	1	69	6	470
Blueberry, 137g	320	1335	2.5	1	57	4	460
Carrot Apple, 135g	315	1310	2.5	1	56	4	465
Strawberry Lemon, 144g	315	1320	2.5	1	57	4.5	460
Premium Delight: Chocolate Bounty, 124g	490	2045	24	10	60	6.5	215
Chocolate Mars, 124g	475	1895	19	5.5	66	7	230
Orange, Date & Pecan, 124g	420	1750	21	2	49	6.5	170
Pear, Honey & Walnut, 124g	390	1625	19	1.5	46	6.5	170
Traditional: Apple Cinnamon, 163g	560	2330	23	2.5	73	10	340
Apple Raisin, 163g	575	2395	22	2.5	83	9	315
Apricot Cream Cheese, 172g	570	2375	25	4.5	73	10	345
Banana Choc Chip, 171g	605	2515	26	5	79	10	330
Blueberry, 160g	510	2130	21	2.5	67	9	310
Butterscotch Pecan, 164g	625	2610	32	3.5	70	11	330
Choc Caramel, 173g	650	2715	29	6.5	83	11	360
Choc Chip, 160g	600	2495	27	6	75	10	315
Date, 165g	570	2375	21	3	82	9	310
Lemon Coconut, 162g	545	2285	24	4	70	9	330
Mixed Berry, 167g	485	2020	20	2	64	8.5	290
Orange Poppyseed, 158g	355	1480	16	1.5	45	6.5	215
Weight Watchers: Chocolate Orange, 119g	235	970	2	0.5	41	4	330
Cranberry & Blueberry, 113g	215	905	1.5	0.5	39	3	320
Peach Cinnamon, 109g	230	965	1.5	0.5	42	3	335
Raspberry Apple, 109g	220	920	1.5	0.5	40	3	325
Raspberry Choc, 109g	235	970	2	0.5	42	3.5	335
Strawberry White Chocolate, 110g	235	980	3	1.5	40	3.5	315

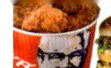

Fast-Foods & Chains

Nando's® (Sept '13)

	Cal	kJ	Fat	Sat'F	Carb	Pro	Sod
Burgers/Sandwiches: *Includes Mayonnaise*							
Classic Chicken Burger	440	1845	13	3	50	33	890
Classic Chicken Pita	330	1365	6.5	1	37	30	895
Classic Chicken Wrap	270	1120	9	3	27	21	705
Supremo Chicken Burger	435	1820	6	1	61	37	715
Supremo Chicken Wrap	290	1210	9	3.5	31	21	810
Supremo Vego Burger	640	2670	18	1.5	102	18	1100
Vege Pita	420	1755	12	1.5	65	13	710
Chicken:							
¼ Chicken, with Skin	290	1210	11	3.5	2	47	940
¼ Chicken, without Skin	255	1055	7.5	2.5	1.5	46	755
BBQ Ribs, 8 ribs	300	1250	19	6	4.5	29	740
BBQ Thighs, 4 thighs	250	1030	11	3.5	3	35	535
Flame Grilled Tenderloins, 4 pieces	235	975	5.5	1.5	2.5	43	785
Portuguese Chicken Skewer, 1 skewer	350	1460	16	5	4	48	860
Salads: *Per Salad, without Dressing*							
Fresh Garden	40	165	0.5	0	6	3	85
Fresh Garden, with Chicken	155	635	3	1	8	24	315
Mediterranean	160	675	12	6.5	6.5	8.5	620
Mediterranean, with Chicken	275	1155	15	8.5	8.5	28	855
Sides:							
Couscous, regular 220g	385	1600	10	2	61	12	1210
Peri-Peri Chips, regular 290g	655	2740	27	7.5	91	12	560
Perinaise/Creamy Chip Dip, 60g	145	600	12	1.5	10	0.5	775
Portuguese Chicken Paella, 400g	495	2070	7	1.5	79	29	1240
Spicy Rice, regular 250g	315	1320	1.5	1	69	6.5	1325

New Zealand Natural® (Sept '13)

	Cal	kJ	Fat	Sat'F	Carb	Pro	Sod
Smoothie: *Per Regular, 660ml*							
Bananarama	405	1690	2.5	1.5	76	17	190
Berry Fling	410	1710	5.5	3.5	70	19	265
Berry'lishus; Paradise Pash	375	1580	4	2.5	80	5.5	95
Calypso Crunch	395	1650	4	2.5	80	6	100
Mango Tango	385	1605	4	2.5	80	5.5	95
Raspberry Rush	390	1630	4.5	3.5	68	17	225
Strawberry Fields	350	1465	4	2.5	73	5.5	95
Tropical Tornado	490	2035	6	3.5	83	22	290

Ice Creams ~ *See Page 111*

Updated Nutrition Data ~ www.CalorieKing.com.au
Persons with Diabetes ~ See Disclaimer (Page 22)

Fast-Foods & Chains

Noodle Box® (Sept '13)

	Cal	kJ	Fat	Sat'F	Carb	Pro	Sod
Box: *Per Regular 710g Box*							
BBQ Sesame Pork, Regular	970	4050	22	4.5	141	51	2415
Blackbean Char Beef, Regular	940	3915	22	3.5	131	45	4545
Combination #8, Regular	930	3890	22	6.5	124	52	2910
Gung-Ho Soy, Regular	925	3850	17	6	149	34	2910
Honey Soy Chicken, Regular	980	4100	28	6.5	122	51	1775
Hot & Spicy Noodle, Regular	830	3460	20	10	103	48	3055
Kway Teow, Regular	1025	4270	31	14	133	42	4615
Mee Goreng, Regula	910	3815	17	5	132	46	2700
Mongolian BeefRegular, 710g	1000	4175	12	2	173	48	2275
Nasi Goreng, Regular, 710g	1215	5085	24	6.5	195	46	2840
Pad Thai, Regular, 710g	1270	5310	36	7	181	54	5540
Satay Chicken, Regular, 710g	1030	4310	32	7	134	50	3340
Singapore Noodles, Regular, 710g	860	3600	21	8.5	110	49	2555
Sweet & Tangy, Regular, 710g	895	3730	19	5	121	49	2840
Teriyaki Beef & Limee: Regular, 710g	895	3730	20	6.5	136	40	2700
Sides:							
Chicken Satay Skewers (1), 130g	310	1295	20	5.5	10	25	740
Dim Sim (1), 100g	180	755	6.5	2	24	7	370
Prawn Crackers, 25g	145	610	10	1	15	0	175
Salt & Pepper Squid, 90g	220	920	13	1.5	15	13	720
Spring Rolls (1), 100g	290	1200	17	3.5	31	5	470

Note: The small 410g Box contains approximately 60% of the calories of the regular 710g box

Oporto® (Sept '13)

	Cal	kJ	Fat	Sat'F	Carb	Pro	Sod
Breakfast:							
Bacon & Egg Rappa, 155g	445	1845	21	4	43	18	1080
Big Breakfast, without Hash Brown, 245g	445	1865	23	6.5	29	31	1240
Brekkie Burger, Bacon & Egg, 120g	275	1140	10	3	27	17	730
Burgers & Sandwiches:							
Bondi, Single Fillet, 155g	415	1735	23	4	29	22	735
Bondi, Double Fillet, 255g	670	2805	33	5	53	38	1020
Chicken BLT, Single Fillet, 195g	425	1775	22	4.5	31	26	985
Chicken BLT, Double Fillet, 285g	650	2710	32	6	45	42	1400
Veggie, 275g	680	2835	38	6.5	61	17	1360
Rappas:							
Bondi with Chilli, 285g	540	2240	20	2.5	46	36	1125
Caesar with Bacon, 300g	760	3180	38	10	52	47	1635
Greek with Feta, 320g	745	3110	37	9	53	47	1505
RappSnacker, Grilled, 155g	400	1710	20	2	38	20	745
Salad, Fresco, 260g	305	1275	20	2	7	22	675
Sauces:							
Chilli, 25g	50	195	4.5	0.5	2	0.5	135
Feisty BBQ, 25g	55	225	1	0.5	10	0.5	280
Prego, 25g	90	370	7	1	6.5	2	190
Sides:							
Bondi Bites (2), 80g	210	860	10	2	13	17	490
Chips, Regular, 165g	490	2045	30	7	47	7	355

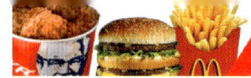

Fast-Foods & Chains

Pita Pit® (N.Z.) (Sept '13)

	Cal	kJ	Fat	Sat'F	Carb	Pro	Sod
Meat Pitas: *Figures include Plain Pita*							
Chicken Breast	285	1200	4	2	35	25	630
Chicken Caesar	380	1600	12	5	35	30	840
Chicken Crave	320	1345	5	1.5	37	30	935
Chicken 'n Fala	330	1390	5.5	2	41	27	730
Ham	280	1180	2.5	0	40	22	1125
Roast Beef	350	1430	3.5	0	38	23	1080
Roast Lamb	310	1305	6.5	2.5	37	22	775
Steak	350	1430	10	1.5	37	25	1200
Tuna	290	1220	0	0	35	32	440
Vegetarian Pitas: *Figures include Plain Pita*							
Cheddar	350	1470	15	8.5	35	16	470
Falafel	280	1180	3.5	0	46	12	415
Feta	270	1135	8	5	35	12	560
Garden	175	735	0	0	35	6	220

Pie Face® (Sept '13)

	Cal	kJ	Fat	Sat'F	Carb	Pro	Sod
Baguette, Ham & Cheese, 215g	470	1960	14	5.5	63	24	1205
Pies:							
Breakfast	605	2520	41	25	40	20	1165
Chicken & Mushroom: Large	425	1760	24	14	29	19	650
Mini (1)	165	680	9	5	14	7	255
Chunky Steak: Large	400	1665	19	11	31	24	830
Mini (1)	155	635	7.5	4.5	15	7	255
Mince Beef: Large	465	1930	27	15	37	17	775
Mini (1)	155	655	8	4.5	16	5	255
Quiche Lorraine, Mini	110	450	7.5	4.5	7.5	3.5	155
Steak & Cheese	445	1855	25	15	39	18	765
Steak & Mushroom	415	1745	19	11	37	24	900
Steak & Pepper	435	1820	23	13	35	23	660
Tandoori Vegetable: Large	450	1885	25	14	48	8.5	815
Mini (1)	155	650	8.5	5	17	3	265
Thai Chicken Curry: Large	425	1770	21	12	38	21	850
Mini (1)	155	650	8	4.5	15	6	270
Sausage Rolls: Large	480	1995	29	16	34	19	850
Mini (1)	215	890	12	7	19	8.5	510
Vegetarian: Large	410	1705	20	12	46	12	600
Mini (1)	215	890	10	6	25	6.5	290
Wrap, Tuna	715	2980	43	6	54	29	955
Brownie, Nutty (1), 119g	625	2605	39	21	60	8.5	220
Lemon Pie, Mini 74g	350	1460	23	14	32	4	90
Muffin, Plain (1), 158g	640	2670	27	20	92	8	350
Pastries, Almond Stick (1), 75g	380	1590	27	17	30	6	340

Updated Nutrition Data ~ www.CalorieKing.com.au
Persons with Diabetes ~ See Disclaimer (Page 22)

Fast-Foods & Chains

Pizza Hut® (Sept '13)
Perfecto Base: Per 1/8 Large Pizza

	Cal	kJ	Fat	Sat'F	Carb	Pro	Sod
Classics: Cheese	195	820	6.5	4	24	11	380
Fresh Tomato Margherita	170	715	5.5	2.5	23	7	255
Ham & Cheese	170	695	5	2.5	22	9	385
Pepperoni	190	780	7	4	22	9	460
Legends: BBQ Meat Lovers	205	845	7.5	3.5	23	11	465
Hawaiian	175	735	4.5	2.5	24	9	440
Hot n Spicy Pepperoni	175	735	6	3	22	9	490
Super Supreme	200	830	7.5	3.5	24	10	460
Veggie	185	770	6.5	3	23	9	275

Light & Delicious: Per 1/8 Pizza

	Cal	kJ	Fat	Sat'F	Carb	Pro	Sod
Chicken	110	470	3	1	17	5	265
Chilli Prawn	110	470	3	1	17	5	235
Veggie	110	450	3	1	16	5	255

Mia: Per 1/8 Pizza

	Cal	kJ	Fat	Sat'F	Carb	Pro	Sod
Beef	175	730	6	3	22	8	370
Cheese	170	700	5.5	3	21	8	320
Ham & Cheese	170	710	6	3	21	9	400
Hot n Spicy	175	720	6	3	22	8	450
Veggie	165	690	5.5	2.5	22	7	345

Signature: BBQ Chicken

	Cal	kJ	Fat	Sat'F	Carb	Pro	Sod
	190	800	6	3	25	10	415
Chicken & Feta	215	900	9	4	23	10	445
Garlic Prawn	180	750	6	2	24	8	330
Surf & Turf	200	825	7.5	3.5	30	12	395
Tandoori Chicken	200	830	6.5	3	25	10	380

Meals: Per Meal

	Cal	kJ	Fat	Sat'F	Carb	Pro	Sod
Pasta: Carbonara	485	2020	15	8.5	55	33	1345
Lasagne	570	2370	20	9	67	28	1110
Mac & Cheese	535	2230	14	9	78	23	1450

Extras:

	Cal	kJ	Fat	Sat'F	Carb	Pro	Sod
Garlic Bread, 2 slices, 40g	135	560	6	2.5	17	3	280
Chicken Wings, Traditional, 2 wings, 80g	240	1000	17	5	3	18	450

Red Rooster® (Sept '13)
Chicken:

	Cal	kJ	Fat	Sat'F	Carb	Pro	Sod
Roast Chicken: Whole Chicken	1950	8135	94	25	55	221	6270
Half Chicken	975	4070	47	13	28	111	3135
Quarter Chicken with Leg	485	2020	33	10	9.5	39	1255
Quarter Chicken with Wing	545	2280	27	8	13	63	1755
Meal: Fish & Chips	740	3120	34	5.5	73	33	935
Spicy Bites (15)	250	1040	13	25	15	18	585
Nuggets: (1) 17g	50	210	3	1	3.5	3	85
Cheesy (1), 18g	60	250	4	1.5	3	3	145
Meal Packs: Classic Half with Chips	1240	5190	67	19	56	99	2930
Classic Quarter with Leg & Chips	785	3270	44	12	52	42	1435
Classic Quarter with Wing & Chips	835	3480	43	12	46	62	2020
Little Red Rooster Meal: Cheeseburger & Chips	590	2465	26	7	64	20	925
Chicken Nuggets & Chips	375	1570	18	4	41	12	745
Tropicana with Leg, Chips & Fritter	1000	4180	51	12	89	40	1260
Tropicana with Wing, Chips & Fritter	1015	4230	46	11	84	56	1680

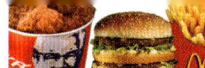

Fast-Foods & Chains

Red Rooster® Cont... (Sept '13)

	Cal	kJ	Fat	Sat'F	Carb	Pro	Sod
Meal Pack:							
Stacked Pack: All-in Pack	1220	5110	55	16	138	41	1900
Legends Pack	1175	4910	51	14	136	39	1780
Power Pack	1235	5160	51	13	114	76	2780
Tropicana	1180	4930	26	11	125	59	1720
Burgers/Sandwiches:							
BBQ Bacon Crispy Burger	430	1850	18	6	41	27	1390
Cheeseburger	360	1510	17	5	34	17	670
Classic Crispy Burger	440	1820	21	8.5	41	20	760
Mayo Cheeseburger	390	1660	21	6	35	17	595
Original Crispy	480	2000	24	3	43	23	950
Peri Peri Burger, with Mayonaisse	315	1300	8.5	1.5	32	25	725
Rooster Roll	550	2290	21	4	54	31	1100
Wraps:							
Flayva: With Mayo	715	2990	46	13	46	27	1655
Peri Peri with Mayo	400	1650	12	2.5	47	25	1155
Baguette, Peri Peri	485	2030	11	2	63	32	1120
Breakfast:							
Rolls: Bacon & Tomato	280	1180	8	3.5	39	14	975
Bacon & Egg	320	1330	13	6	30	19	955
Wrap: Bacon & Egg	365	1530	13	6	40	20	1390
Chicken, Bacon & Egg	420	1750	20	7.5	34	25	985
Hash Brown, (1)	155	640	11	2	14	1.5	230
Rippa Sub:							
Chilli & Garlic Aioli	660	2750	29	6	72	26	1520
Classic	760	3170	39	7.5	72	27	1425
Smokey BBQ	610	2550	21	4.5	79	26	1425
Chips:							
Regular, 150g	315	1315	14	2.5	39	5.5	370
Large, 246g	515	2155	23	4.5	64	8.5	605
Family, 474g	990	4150	44	8	122	17	1160
Salads:							
Coleslaw, regular	145	615	11	1	12	1	165
Garden Salad, regular	15	60	0	0	2	1	55
Potato, regular	155	635	8.5	1.5	18	2	270
Sides: Corn (1), 147g	120	495	2.5	0.5	15	4.5	35
Pineapple Fritter (1), 56g	120	500	5	1	16	1.5	40
Garlic Bread, 2 pieces, 40g	130	550	5.5	2.5	17	3.5	215
Gravy, regular, 120g	55	220	2	1	8.5	0.5	420
Roast Vegies, 3 pieces, 213g	140	585	2.5	0.5	23	3.5	395
Desserts: Chocolate Pudding	245	1010	7.5	6	39	3.5	180
Lemon Cheesecake	345	1440	27	18	21	3.5	115
Sticky Date Pudding	240	1000	6	3.5	44	2.5	270

Updated Nutrition Data ~ www.CalorieKing.com.au
Persons with Diabetes ~ See Disclaimer (Page 22)

Fast-Foods & Chains

Subway® (Sept '13)

	Cal	kJ	Fat	Sat'F	Carb	Pro	Sod
6" Subs: *Figures include cheese & salad, but not dressings*							
Chicken & Bacon Ranch w. Cheese	430	1800	18	6	36	33	1050
Chicken Fillet	345	1430	12	3.5	40	19	845
Italian BMT	375	1560	15	6	37	21	1060
Meatball Marinara	410	1710	16	6.5	47	20	740
Pizza with Cheese	405	1680	18	8	39	20	1030
Seafood Sensation	330	1370	11	2.5	44	12	600
Steak & Cheese	345	1430	9	4.5	36	25	810
Subway Melt w. Cheese	355	1490	12	5.5	38	25	1150
Tuna	330	1380	11	2.5	36	21	560
Veggie Patty	425	1770	9	1.5	68	16	570
6" Subs with 6g Fat or Less: *Figures include salad, but not cheese, dressings or sauces*							
Chicken Teriyaki	305	1280	4.5	1.5	42	23	750
Ham	255	1070	4	1.5	37	16	745
Roast Beef	260	1090	4	1.5	37	17	590
Roasted Chicken	280	1180	4	1.5	36	24	440
Subway Club	270	1120	5	1.5	38	17	725
Turkey	255	1060	5	1.5	36	15	620
Turkey & Ham	265	1100	4.5	1.5	37	17	735
Veggie Delite	205	860	3	1	35	9	285
Breakfast Subs:							
Bacon, Egg & Cheese	370	1550	15	5.5	34	24	940
Cheese & Egg	320	1330	12	4	34	18	665
Ham, Egg & Cheese	345	1440	12	4.5	35	22	895
Wraps: *Figures do not include dressings or sauces*							
Roast Beef	290	1210	7.5	3.5	40	15	855
Chicken	310	1300	7	3	39	22	700
Turkey & Ham	290	1210	8	3.5	40	14	1000
Salads: *Figures do not include dressing*							
Ham	110	455	2.5	1	10	11	540
Roast Beef	110	460	2.5	1	10	11	380
Chicken Strips	125	525	3	1	8	18	345
Subway Club	120	500	3	1	10	12	515
Chicken Teriyaki	155	650	3	1	15	18	540
Turkey & Ham	115	475	3	1	10	11	530
Turkey	105	435	3	1	9	9	405
Veggie Delite	55	230	1	0.5	7	3	75
Dressings: *Per 21ml*							
Ranch	60	240	6	0.5	0.5	0.5	150
Thousand Island	75	310	6	1	5	0.5	85
Sauces:							
Chipotle Southwest, 21ml	95	395	10	1.5	1	1	135
Honey Mustard, 21ml	30	125	0.5	0	6.5	0.5	95
Sweet Onion, 21ml	40	155	0	0	8.5	0	85
Cheese, average all types, 14g	45	185	3.5	3	0	3	200
Cookies, average (1), 45g	210	880	10	5.5	30	2	150
Dessert, Cheesecake, Raspberry	205	860	9	4.5	30	2.5	180
Smoothies: *Average All Flavours*							
Large, 600g	390	1620	3	2.5	73	17	260
Small 420g	275	1140	2	1.5	51	12	180

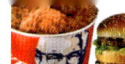

Fast-Foods & Chains

Sumo Salad® (Sept '13)

	Cal	kJ	Fat	Sat'F	Carb	Pro	Sod
Long Rolls: *Per Roll with Dressing*							
Chicken Schnitzel	920	3840	42	14	91	40	1345
Chicken, Bacon & Avocado	820	3435	38	10	73	44	1910
Peri Peri Chicken	620	2595	17	4.5	82	33	1430
Toasties: *Per Toastie with Dressing*							
Bacon & Egg	845	3535	43	14	31	44	1655
Chicken & Avocado	805	3365	43	5	26	36	1350
Ham, Cheese & Tomato	625	2615	22	7.5	30	35	1650
Wraps: *Per Wrap with Dressing*							
Beef & Pumpkin	585	2440	22	6	52	32	1530
Chicken Schnitzel	635	2645	25	6	64	29	1450
Moroccan Lamb	545	2275	14	4	57	35	1180
Toasted Bacon & Egg	480	2005	18	6.5	44	24	1505
Meals: *Per Medium Meal 400g*							
Italian Penne	575	2400	20	2.5	75	18	435
Kasundi Rice & Tandoori Chicken	460	1925	24	3	35	26	1150
Pumpkin & Pinenut Tortellini	730	3065	39	4.5	73	16	620
Spinach & Ricotta Cannelloni	1090	4560	19	11	178	45	800
Deli Salads: *Per Medium 400g Salad with Dressing*							
Asian Greens (Pete Evans)	250	1060	10	1	16	17	300
Basil Chicken Penne	975	1080	71	7.5	62	22	1585
Jamaican Chicken	365	1520	13	2	50	28	1115
Lentil & Tabbouleh	360	1500	13	1.5	37	19	1155
Mexican Bean Salad (Pete Evans)	490	2050	17	2	54	23	1080
Moroccan Roasted Vegetables, 280g (Pete Evans)	300	1255	14	1.5	29	11	490
Pumpkin & Cous Cous	400	1670	30	2	23	5	870
Thai Beef Noodle	745	3115	16	2	129	18	1530
Wild Rice & Chickpea	380	1580	14	1	52	11	1160
Favourite Salads: *Per Large Salad with Dressing*							
Grilled Chicken Caesar, 290g	475	1975	32	7.5	10	36	1270
Grilled Tasmania Salmon, 325g	300	1240	19	4	9	21	520
Man Salad, 457g	675	2800	47	14	15	49	1420

Wendy's® (Sept '13)

	Cal	kJ	Fat	Sat'F	Carb	Pro	Sod
Ice Creams ~ *See Page 113*							
Chillas: *Per Small 460g Container*							
Chocolate	410	1725	6.5	4.5	77	11	185
Coffee; Mocca, average	330	1365	5	4	60	8.5	155
Indulgent Chillas: *Per Small 225g Container*							
Banana Caramel	250	1045	6	4	47	2.5	55
Chocolate Mint	280	1175	10	6.5	45	4	105
Smoothies: *Per Small 450g Container*							
Banana Bliss	360	1500	4	3	71	10	170
Berry Buzz	290	1210	4.5	3	50	10	170
Mango Passionfruit	320	1330	4.5	2	48	11	170
Strawberry Kiss	275	1160	6.5	4	72	10	180
Non-Dairy: Berry Blast	160	660	0	0	38	0	10
Green Apple Bliss	180	745	0	0	43	0	15
Lemon Zest	130	545	0	0	29	0	10

Updated Nutrition Data ~ www.CalorieKing.com.au
Persons with Diabetes ~ See Disclaimer (Page 22)

Fast-Foods & Chains

Wendy's® Cont... (Sept '13)
Supa Shake: Per Small 350g Container

	Cal	kJ	Fat	Sat'F	Carb	Pro	Sod
Choc Mint	485	2030	12	8	84	8.5	190
Crunchie	465	1935	10	6.5	83	8.5	205
Flake	515	2150	17	12	80	11	235

Wok Me® (Sept '13)
Meals: Per Small Box

	Cal	kJ	Fat	Sat'F	Carb	Pro	Sod
Bali Satay, 490g	705	2950	29	11	84	23	1020
Combo, 455g	770	3220	36	6	81	30	1510
Fried Rice, 455g	545	2285	8	2.5	87	28	2180
Hokkien Me, 350	510	2135	12	2.5	80	20	1305
Kuai Tiau, 490g	425	2190	13	2.5	74	27	1395
Mee Goreng, 455g	510	2140	3.5	0.5	87	32	2470
Nasi Goreng, 455g	585	2435	13	3.5	90	28	2070
Oyster Box, 315g	275	1150	2.5	0.5	51	11	1025
Singapore, 455g	460	1925	11	3	62	26	2105
Soy Box, 315g	270	1140	2	0.5	48	13	1855
Spicy Box, 455g	610	2545	15	2.5	89	28	3375
Sweet Chilli, 420g	575	2405	6.5	2	107	21	1275

Large Sizes ~ See www.CalorieKing.com.au

Wokinabox® (Sept '13)
Noodles: Per Regular Serving

	Cal	kJ	Fat	Sat'F	Carb	Pro	Sod
Beef & Black Bean, 363g	755	3150	24	5	107	24	1475
Hokkien Mee, 391g	840	3505	27	4.5	115	30	1945
Hot & Spicy, 401g	615	2565	23	4.5	71	29	2125
Kwai Teow, 429g	875	3650	18	3.5	151	25	1675
Pud Thai, 390g	870	3635	26	5.5	125	31	2230
Satay Chicken, 345g	825	3450	36	10	96	29	2360
Seafood Mee Goreng, 366g	740	3095	21	4	110	26	1935
Singapore	930	3875	17	3	145	33	1325

Rice Dishes: Per Regular Serving

Nasi Goreng, 399g	530	2225	19	3	66	23	1020
Seafood Nasi Goreng, 390g	485	2015	14	3	65	19	1020
Special Fried Rice, 336g	555	2320	19	6	72	20	1515

Soup: Per Regular Serving

Combination, 361	840	3505	8	1.5	141	37	4155
Curry Laksa, 504G	990	4125	39	16	120	35	2905

Stir Fry Meals: Per Regular Serving

Chicken w. Chilli & Basil, 432g	825	3450	44	10	80	19	2055
Honey Soy Chicken w. Cashews, 447g	985	4110	56	12	82	29	995
Mongolian Beef, 448g	845	3515	43	11	86	18	945
Thai Green Chicken Curry, 428g	855	3555	50	14	72	20	890

Entree: Per Regular Serving

Dim Sims (3), 181g	640	2660	47	7	34	13	1560
Fortune Cookie (1), 6g	25	100	0.5	0	5	0.5	5
Gyoza Dumplings (3), 71g	180	740	13	4.5	8.5	6.5	525
Prawn Crackers, 48g	230	970	9	2	35	0.5	625
Prawn Twisters, 109g	535	2235	39	8.5	40	10	470
Salt & Pepper Squid, 185g	830	3460	80	17	8	8	470

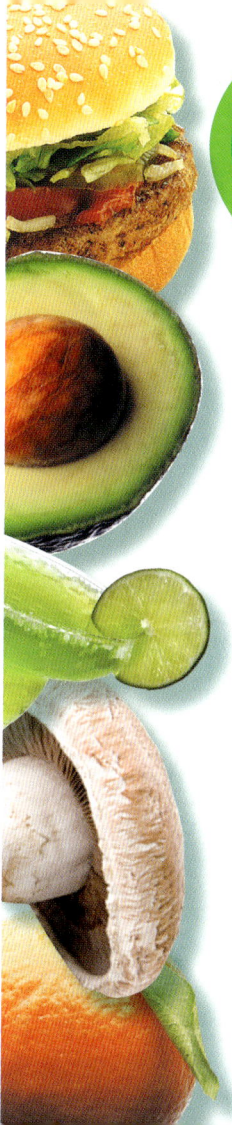

BONUS
DIET GUIDES & COUNTERS

- **Alcohol Guide**....................23-30
  with Alcohol Counter

- **Caffeine Guide**....................210
  with Caffeine Counter

- **Calcium Guide**................211-213
  with Calcium Counter

- **Diabetes Diet Guide**............16-21

- **Fats & Cholesterol Guide**......214-218

- **Fibre Diet Guide**...............219-222
  with Fibre Counter

- **Protein Guide**..................223-226
  with Protein Counter

- **High Blood Pressure Guide**...227-233
  with Sodium Counter

©2013 ALLAN BORUSHEK

Caffeine Guide & Counter

Caffeine Notes:

- **Moderate caffeine intake is probably not** harmful to healthy adults. However, regular large amounts (over 350mg/day) may cause dependency ('caffeinism') and ill-health.

- **Symptoms of excessive caffeine intake include chronic insomnia,** persistent anxiety and depression, restlessness, heart palpitations, stomach upset and increased need to urinate.

- **High caffeine intake,** combined with nicotine and alcohol may increase the risk in men of sperm damage, infertility and birth defects in their children; and may in women, reduce their chances of becoming pregnant.

- **Caffeine-withdrawal headaches,** are more commonly experienced on weekends when any heavy coffee drinking (over 350mg/day) at work is suddenly reduced. Such headaches are relieved by drinking coffee. When ceasing caffeine drinks, withdrawal symptoms may persist up to one week.

- **Sensitivity to caffeine,** may increase during pregnancy and as we age.

To be safe, adults should limit caffeine intake to less than 200mg/day.

Note: Children are highly sensitive to caffeine. They are best to avoid caffeinated coffee, colas and energy drinks.

- **Persons wise to avoid caffeine include:** • those who get irritable and jittery from just one cup of coffee • pregnant and nursing women • children under eight • people with stomach ulcers • people with heart arrhythmia condition (irregular heart beats).

- **Large amounts of cola and energy drinks,** (with caffeine) can also lead to excessive caffeine intake. Caffeine-free colas are available. (Check the ingredients list)

- **Coffee alternatives,** such as Bambu, Caro, Ecco, Dandelion and Teeccino, are caffeine-free and coffee-like in taste. Decaffeinated coffee is also suitable.

- **Alcohol and Caffeine ~ A Dangerous Mix.** Caffeine in coffee and energy drinks does not sober you up if you are inebriated. It simply turns you into a wide-awake drunk, who is more likely to take dangerous risks such as driving.

CAFFEINE COUNTER (Milligrams)

Coffee Instant: Weak, 1 level teaspoon	45
Medium, 1 rounded teaspoon	60
Strong, 1 heaped teaspoon	80
Decaffeinated: 1 round teaspoon	2
Maxwell Lite (25% less caffeine), 1 tsp	45
Brewed: Percolator/Drip, 200ml cup	140
Coffee Shop: Espresso, Regular/Solo	80
Cappuccino: 1 cup, 250ml	80
Take-Out Cups: Tall, 330ml (12 fl.oz)	120
Large, 450ml (16 fl.oz)	160
Cafe Latte, 1 cup	80
Decappuccino, (decaffeinated)	0
Hot Chocolate, 1 cup	10
Mocha, 1 cup	90
Vienna Coffee; Iced Coffee, 1 cup	80
Iced Milk Coffee: Average:	
375ml carton	50
600ml carton	80
Cafecino Double Shot: Espresso: 190ml can	230
Espresso & Milk, 190ml can	120
Coffee Mixes: Average all types	
Jarrah; Nestle; Maxwell House, 1 serve/sachet	50
Coffee Alternatives (Caffeine-Free):	
Bambu; Caro; Ecco; Dandelion; Teeccino, av.	0
Tea (Black/Green): Weak, 1 cup, 250ml	20
Medium Strength, 1 cup, 250ml	40
Strong, 1 cup, 250ml	70
Decaffeinated & Herbal Teas	0
Cola Drinks: *Coca-Cola/Diet Coke,* 375ml can	50
600ml Bottle	80
1.25L Bottle	170
Pepsi/Pepsi Max, 375ml can	40
Energy Drinks: With caffeine:	
Red Bull, V Energy: average	
250ml can	80
330ml bottle	110
500ml can	160
Alcoholic *(Elevate/WKD),* 300ml	100
Chocolate: Milk Chocolate, 50g	10
Dark Chocolate (70%), 50g	30
Baker's/Cooking Chocolate, 50g	40
Cocoa, 1 teaspoon, 5g	5
Chocolate Milk, Hot Chocolate, 1 cup, 250ml	10
Guarana: Powder (BonVit), 5g	170
Tablets, 500mg (1)	40
Medicinals: *No-Doz,* 1 tablet	200
Panadol Extra Caplets, 1 caplet	65

Extensive Caffeine Counter ~ www.CalorieKing.com.au

Calcium & Osteoporosis

Early Prevention of Bone Loss

Gradual loss of bone begins in females in their thirties after maximum bone mass is reached. The stronger the bones at that time, the less trouble that is likely to occur later. The earlier that prevention begins, the greater the benefit.

The key to prevention of osteoporosis is to build strong, dense bones early in life. **By age 16,** some 80% of peak bone mass is already reached.

Young women may lessen the risk by:
- eating high-calcium foods as well as adequate fruits, vegetables, wholegrains and nuts
- drinking less soft drink, and more milk
- not engaging in extreme dieting that results in menstrual period cessation (via less oestrogen)
- being physically active; and not smoking

In menopausal women, hormone therapy as well as calcium supplements and exercise, can help retard osteoporosis. Your doctor can advise you.

Note: While dietary calcium cannot reverse age-related bone loss, it can slow down the process. Other nutrients are also vital for strong bones. Eat a well-balanced diet including adequate fruit and vegetables.

Good Dietary Sources of Calcium

Eat 3-4 servings a day of calcium-rich foods:
- Milk, Yoghurt, Cheese
- Calcium-enriched Milk (e.g. *Anlene, Pura Boost/Tone*)
- Flavoured Milk Drinks & Fruit Smoothies
- Ice Cream (low-fat), Custard (low-fat)
- Soy Drinks (calcium-enriched)
- Tofu (with calcium coagulant)
- Canned Salmon or Sardines (with edible bones)
- Broccoli, Dried Beans, Baked Beans
- Almonds, Brazil Nuts, Hazelnuts, Seeds

RECOMMENDED DAILY CALCIUM REQUIREMENTS

Children:	1-3 yrs	~ 500mg
	4-8 yrs	~ 700mg
	9-11 yrs	~ 1000mg
Teenagers:	12-18 yrs	~ 1300mg
Men:	19-70 yrs	~ 1000mg
	Over 70 yrs	~ 1300mg
Women:	19-50 yrs	~ 1000mg
	Over 50 yrs	~ 1300mg

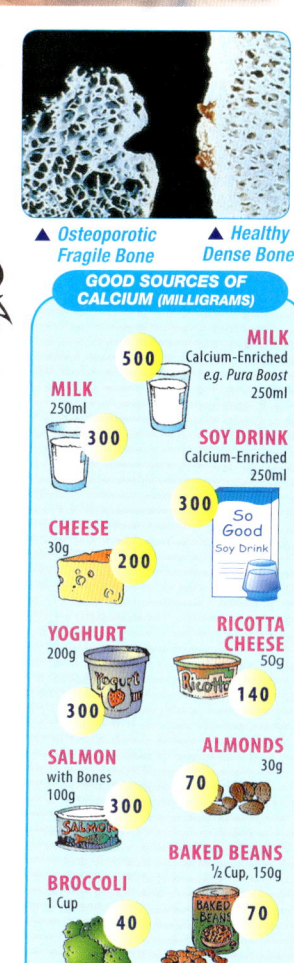

▲ Osteoporotic Fragile Bone   ▲ Healthy Dense Bone

GOOD SOURCES OF CALCIUM (MILLIGRAMS)

MILK Calcium-Enriched e.g. Pura Boost 250ml — 500

MILK 250ml — 300

SOY DRINK Calcium-Enriched 250ml — 300

CHEESE 30g — 200

YOGHURT 200g — 300

RICOTTA CHEESE 50g — 140

SALMON with Bones 100g — 300

ALMONDS 30g — 70

BROCCOLI 1 Cup — 40

BAKED BEANS ½ Cup, 150g — 70

Calcium Counter

Milk: | Calcium
- **Whole/Skim/Nonfat/UHT**, 250ml — 300
- **Reduced-Fat** (e.g. HiLo, Rev), 250ml — 360
- **Calcium Enriched:**
  - *Calcium Plus* (WA), 250ml — 425
  - *Light Start*, 250ml — 315
  - *Pura Tone*, 250ml — 350
  - *Physical*, 250ml — 440
  - *Pura Boost*, 250ml — 500
  - *Smart Plus*, 250ml — 335
- **Buttermilk**, 1 cup, 250ml — 300
- **Flavoured Milks**, average, 300ml ctn — 550
- **Condensed/Evaporated**, 1 Tbsp, 20g — 55
- **Dried Milk:** Whole, 2 Tbsp, 30g — 300
  - Non-Fat/Skim, 2 Tbsp, 30g — 380
- **Goat Milk**, 1 cup, 250ml — 290
- **Other 'Milk' Drinks:**
  - Coconut Milk, 200ml — 35
  - Rice Milk Drinks: Average, 250ml — 30
  - *Pure Harvest*, w/ calcium, 250ml — 275
  - *Yakult*, 65ml bottle — 30

Powdered Milk Drinks, Milo:
- **Akta-Vite:** 3 heaped tsp, 15g — 120
  - With 200ml Whole Milk — 360
- **Cocoa:** 3 heaped tsp, 20g — 25
  - With 250ml milk — 325
- **Malted Milk** (Nestle), 3 heaped tsp, 20g — 130
- **Milo:** 3 heaped Tbsp, 15g — 125
  - With 200ml Skim Milk — 400
- **Nesquik**, average all flavours, dry — 0
- **Ovaltine:** 3 heaped Tsp, 15g — 100
  - W. 200ml Water & 20g Powder — 180

Soy Drinks:
- **Calcium Enriched:** Per 250ml
  - *Liddells*, UHT, Lactose Free — 500
  - *So Good*, Regular — 300
  - *So Good*, Essential — 375
  - *So Natural*, Extra Milky — 300
  - *Pure Harvest*, Nature's Soy — 275
  - *VitaSoy*, Calci-Plus — 400
  - *VitaSoy*, High Fibre — 300
- **Rice/Oat Milk**, Calcium enriched — 300
  - (Vitasoy, Aussie Dream, So Good)

Yoghurt: | Calcium
- **Fruit:** Regular, average, 200g — 310
  - Low-fat/Skim/Diet, avg., 200g — 340
- **Plain/Natural:** Regular, 200g ctn — 340
  - Nonfat/Skim, average, 200g ctn — 360
  - Nestle, Soleil Diet, average, 150g — 185
  - *Yoplait*, Forme, 175g Tub — 315

Cheese:
- **Cheddar:**
  - Avg., 3cm cube, 30g — 240
  - Reduced-Fat (e.g. Coon Light) 30g — 260
- **Blue Vein; Danish Blue, Brie; Camembert** — 160
- **Edam; Gruyere; Mozzarella; Swiss**, 30g — 260
- **Parmesan**, grated, 2 T., 16g — 160
- **Processed Cheese:** 1 sl, 20g — 140
  - *Kraft*, Light n' Tasty Singles, 21g — 165
- **Soft Cheeses:**
  - Feta, 30g — 100
  - Cream Cheese (*Philadelphia*), 30g — 40
  - Cottage Cheese, average, 2 Tbsp, 50g — 40
  - Ricotta, average, 2 Tbsp, 50g — 140
- **Cheese Dishes:** Lasagne, average, 200g — 200
  - Quiche Lorraine, with cheese, 1 serve, 150g — 400
  - Macaroni Cheese, 1 cup 250g — 350

Fats, Oils, Cream:
- **Butter, Margarine, Lard, Oils** — 0
- **Cream:** Fresh, thickened, 1 T., 20g — 15
  - Sour Light, 1 Tbsp, 20g — 30

Ice Cream:
- **Ice Cream:** Regular (10% fat), avg., 1 scoop, 50g — 65
  - Premium/Rich (15%) fat, avg., 1 scoop, 100g — 140
  - Low-Fat (4% fat), avg., 1 scoop, 50g — 75
  - Drumstick; Cornetto, average — 80
- **Fruit Ices**, —
- **Tofu Ice Confection**, avg., 50g — 15
- **Frozen Yoghurt**, ½ cup, 60g — 50
- **Soft Serve**, ½ cup, 125ml — 110

Eggs:
- **Large Egg**, 60g — 50
- **Omelette:** 2 eggs — 70
  - + 30g cheese — 310

Fish & Seafoods: | Calcium
- **Canned:** Anchovies, 30g — 90
  - Pilchards, in Tomato Sauce, 50g — 300
  - Salmon: Pink with bones, 100g — 300
    - Red, with Bones, 100g — 200
    - Australian, with Bones — 350
  - Sardines: With bones, 50g — 250
    - Without bones, 50g — 10
  - Tuna, 100g — 10
- **Fresh Fish:** Cooked, average, 100g — 35
  - In batter (with milk), 100g — 75
- **Crabmeat**, cooked, 100g — 45
- **Crayfish/Lobster**, cooked, 100g — 60
- **Mussels/Oysters**, approx. 10, 100g — 90
- **Prawns**, shelled, 100g — 150
- **Whitebait**, fried, 30g — 260

Meats, Chicken Turkey:
- **Average All Types**, cooked, 100g — 20

Fast Foods:
- **Hamburger:** Average, no cheese — 60
  - With cheese — 150
- **Chicken**, ¼ whole — 20
- **Chips/French Fries**, 1 serve — 10
- **Pizza:** average: Large, 2 pieces — 300
  - w/ extra cheese, 2 pcs — 430
- **Shakes** (McDonald's), med. — 400
- **Taco**, average — 200
- **McDonald's:** Big Mac — 270
  - Bacon & Egg McMuffin — 210
  - Cheeseburger — 200
  - Chicken McNuggets (6) — 13
  - Chocolate Shake, medium — 400
  - Filet-O-Fish — 175
  - French Fries, large — 15
  - Quarter Pounder with Cheese — 300
  - Sausage McMuffin — 190
  - Sundae, average — 230
- **KFC**, Fried Chicken, 3 pieces — 30

Sanitarium Products:
- BBQ Soya Sausages, 40g — 20
- Casserole Mince, 100g — 10
- Country Hotpot, 100g — 20
- Nutolene, 100g — 35
- Soy Beans in Tom. Sce, ½ cup, 150g — 70
- Vegelinks, Rediburger Sausages, 100g — 30
- Soya Mince, dry, 22g — 60

Calcium Counter

Nuts:
Shelled: *Per 30g*

Item	Calcium
Almonds	70
Brazil	55
Coconut, dried	5
Cashews/Hazel/Macadamia	10
Peanuts/Pecans	20
Pistachio	40
Walnuts	30

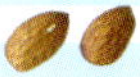

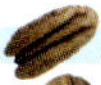

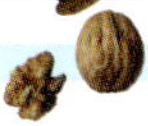

Seeds:
2 Rounded Tablespoon

Item	Calcium
Pumpkin Seeds, dried, 30g	10
Sunflower Seeds, dried, 30g	30
Sesame Seeds, dried, 30g	20
Tahini, 1 Tbsp, 25g	80

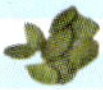

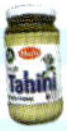

Fruit:
Fresh Fruit: Average all fruits, 1 serve — 20

Item	Calcium
Avocado, 1 medium	20
Orange, 1 medium	50
Rockmelon, ½ melon	30
Strawberries, 1 cup	30

Dried Fruit:

Item	Calcium
Apricots, 5 halves	15
Dates, 5 whole	20
Figs, 1 medium	25
Prunes, 5 large	25

Fruit Juice: Average, 1 cup, 250ml — 25
Berri, Multi-V (with calc.), 250ml pack — 100

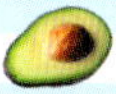

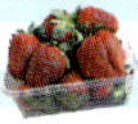

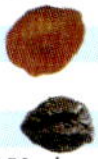

Vegetables:

Item	Calcium
Broccoli, cooked, 1 cup	70
Cabbage, cooked, ½ cup,	25
Collards, leaves, 1 cup	150
Kale, ½ cup	65
Okra, 8 pods	50
Silverbeet, ½ cup	100
Spinach, ½ cup	100
Other Vegetables, average, 1 serve	20

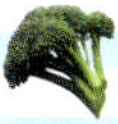

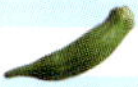

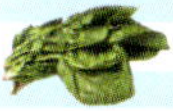

Beans:
Cooked: *Per ½ Cup*

Item	Calcium
Baked Beans in Tom. Sce, 140g	60
Broad Beans	30
Chick Peas (Garbanzo Beans)	75
French/Runner	45
Kidney Beans, Butter Beans	60
Lima Beans	30
Soybeans: Natural, ½ cup, 150g	90
in Tomato Sauce, ½ cup	70

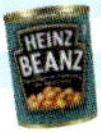

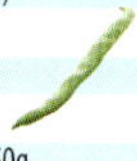

Tofu, Tempeh:

Item	Calcium
Miso, ½ cup	90
Tempeh, 100g serving	90
Tofu: Firm (w. calcium coagulant), 100g	160
Soft (with calcium coagulant), 100g	70
Silken, 100g	15
Tofu Desserts, 100g	10

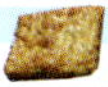

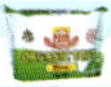

Bread:
Average All Types: 1 thin sl. — 30

Item	Calcium
1 thick slice	40
Bun/Roll: Small	40
Large	90
Pita/Pocketbread, small	50
UP Wraps *(Tip Top)*, Hi Fibre + Calcium, Wrap, 45g	115

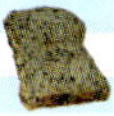

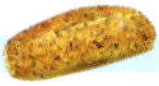

Sandwiches: (mg)
2 Slices Bread: Bread only — 60

Item	Calcium
With 20g Cheese (1 sandwich slice)	160
With 40g Cheese (2 sandwich slices)	320
With Salmon/Sardines (w. bones)	170

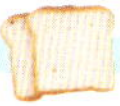

Breakfast Cereals:

Item	Calcium
Average All Types, 30g	10
Granola *(Sanitarium)*, 1 c., 60g	200
Healthwise *(Uncle Toby's)*, 45g	200
Light 'n Tasty *(Sanitarium)*, 40g	200
Lite Start/Sports Plus *(Uncle Toby's)*, 45g	320
Nutri-Grain, 1 cup, 40g	105
Special K, 3/4 cup, 30g	200
Weet-Bix, 4 bisc., 60g	20

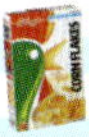

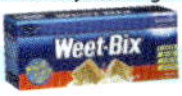

Flours & Grains:
Flour: Wholemeal, 1 cup, 100g — 40

Item	Calcium
Plain/Cornflour, 1 cup, 100g	20
Rice: Cooked: Brown, 1 cup, 150g	5
White, 1 cup, 150g	0
Pasta/Spaghetti, Cooked, 1 cup	12

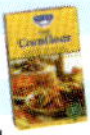

Cakes/Biscuits:

Item	Calcium
Plain cake, 100g	40
Cheesecake, 100g	70
Fruitcake; Fruit Pie, 100g	70
Croissant, each	20
Danish Pastry, average	60
Muffin, large, avg. all varieties, 100g	40
Scone, average, 60g	185
Custard Tart/Pie, 150g	130
Waffles, average	150
Biscuits, average all types, 1 biscuit	20

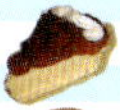

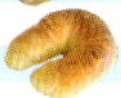

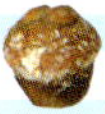

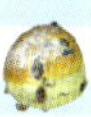

Desserts:

Item	Calcium
Creme Caramel, 150g	200
Creamed Rice, ¾ cup, 200g	200
Dairy, Custards, pouring, 100ml	170
Choc Dessert, 125g Tub	120

Food Bars:

Item	Calcium
Fruit/Nut/Seed Bars, avg.	20-30
Carob, Plain/Fruit/Nut, 30g	110
Yoghurt-coated Confectionary, 30g	40

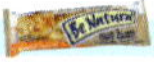

Snacks/Confectionery:

Item	Calcium
Chocolate: Milk/Block, 2 rows, 50g	100
Mars Bar, 53g	80
Lollies, Pastilles, Jubes;	0
Corn/Potato Chips, 25g packet	10
Popcorn/Twisties, 25g packet	0

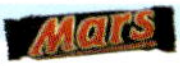

Spreads/Vegemite/Nutella:

Item	Calcium
Jam/Honey/Marmalade	0
Vegemite/Promite/Marmite	0
Nutella, 1 Tbsp, 20g	25
Peanut Butter, 1 Tbsp, 20g	10
Hoummus, 1 Tbsp	15
Tahini, (Sesame Seed Paste), 1 Tbsp, 25g	80

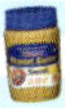

Beverages:

Item	Calcium
Water, (Tap) average, 1 cup	5
Mineral Water, average, 1 glass	20
Beer, Cider, Wine, avg., 200ml	10
Tea/Coffee/Soft Drinks	5

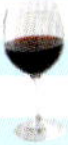

Protein & Diet Shakes:

Item	Calcium
Aussie Bodies, Protein Revival, 375ml	610
Be Good To Yourself, avg, 45g sachet	350
Musashi, SLM High Prot., 250ml t. pak	425
Optifast, VLCD Milk Shake, 1 sachet	300
OptiSlim, VLCD Shakes, 1 sachet	250
Sanitarium, Up & Go:	
Original, 250ml	285
Energize, 350ml	400
Sustagen, 250ml Tetra Pak	400
Tony Ferguson, 375ml Tetra Pak	400

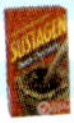

Calcium Supplements:

Item	Calcium
Amway, Nutriway, 1 tablet	200
Bioglan, Calcium Citrate, 2 capsules	160
Calcimax, 1 tablet	300
Caltrate, 1 tablet	600
Healthy Life, Calcium Plus, 1	235
Natures Own, Milk Calcium, 1 tablet	170
Nutra-Life, Calcium Complex, 1 tablet	250
Sandocal 600, 1 tablet	600
Tums, Regular, 1 tablet	200

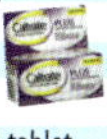

Fats & Blood Cholesterol

Notes on Cholesterol

- **Cholesterol** is a white waxy substance produced mainly by our liver. It is also found in animal food products. Plant foods have no cholesterol.
- **Cholesterol is essential to life.** It is a part of body cell walls and the building block for vitamin D, sex hormones, and bile acids (which help digest dietary fats).
- **The body makes sufficient cholesterol** for its needs and does not rely on cholesterol in the diet. Dietary fats have a major influence on blood cholesterol levels – more so than dietary cholesterol. (See next page)
- **A high blood cholesterol increases the risk of atherosclerosis** – the thickening of arteries that can reduce or block blood flow to the heart muscle, brain, eyes, kidneys, sex organs and other body parts.
  This in turn increases the risk of heart attack, stroke, dementia, blindness, kidney failure, impotence and other blood circulatory problems.
- **Other risk factors** which increase the risk of atherosclerosis include high blood pressure, tobacco smoking, obesity and diabetes (uncontrolled).

BLOOD CHOLESTEROL CHECK YOUR RISK!

Cholesterol Level (mmol/litre)	Risk of Heart Attack
6.5 and above	Very High
5.5 - 6.5	High Risk
4.2 - 5.4	Average
Less than 4.2	Low Risk

♥ Know your cholesterol level, particularly if there is a family history of heart disease or stroke. If your level is high, see your doctor.

♥ All adults should have their cholesterol, LDL, HDL and triglycerides tested at least every 5 years; and every year for adults at high risk.

HEART ATTACK WARNING SIGNS

Many victims die before reaching hospital by ignoring warning signs and delaying medical help.

Symptoms vary and may not always be severe. They commonly include:

♥ **Chest pain,** vice-like squeezing or burning sensation in centre of chest – can be sudden or slowly develop. Pain can be severe or mild.

♥ **Spreading pain** may be felt in the neck and throat, jaw, shoulders, the back and arm(s) – may be an arm or both arms.

♥ **Shortness of breath** or a choking feeling may occur with or before chest discomfort.

♥ **Other signs,** with or without pain, include a cold sweat, nausea or vomiting, light-headedness.

Every Minute Counts!
If you think you may be having a heart attack, call Triple Zero (0-0-0).
The operator will work out if you need an ambulance.

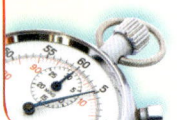

Extra Info: www.heartfoundation.org.au

High Blood Cholesterol increases the risk of atherosclerosis and artery blockage.

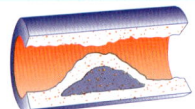

▶ Atherosclerosis can clog arteries and impede blood flow to the heart muscle or other body organs.

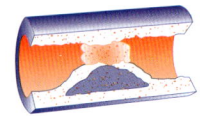

▶ A thrombus (blood clot) can form on unstable, festering atherosclerotic plaque and rapidly block blood flow. A heart attack or stroke can result.

Fats & Blood Cholesterol

The amount and type of dietary fat has the greatest influence on blood cholesterol levels.

Fats in food are a mixture of 3 basic types: saturated, monounsaturated, and polyunsaturated. Animal fats are mainly saturated while plant oils and fish oils are mainly mono- and polyunsaturated.

- **Saturated fats** have subgroups known as long-chain, medium-chain, and short-chain fats. Most of the long-chain fats raise blood cholesterol; and can increase the risk of blood clots and thrombosis leading to artery blockage.

  Long-chain saturated fats are found mainly in full cream milk, cheese, butter, cream, fatty meats and sausages, and processed foods.

- **Monounsaturated fats** tend to more selectively lower 'bad' LDL-cholesterol and maintain the protective 'good' HDL-cholesterol in the blood-stream – but only if they replace saturated fats in the diet.

  Foods rich in monounsaturates include olive, canola and rice bran oils and margarine; peanuts, and avocados.

- **Polyunsaturated fats consist of 2 main classes:**

  (a) Omega-6 polyunsaturates tend to lower blood cholesterol. Rich sources include safflower, sunflower and corn oils.

  (b) Omega-3 polyunsaturated fats can lower blood cholesterol, and also offer extra benefits by lowering blood triglycerides, as well as reducing the risk of thrombosis, heart arrythmias, and artery spasm.

Best practical omega-3 sources include canola oil, canola margarine, soybean oil and fish.

Note: A balanced intake of the two omega classes is important for optimal health. Slightly increasing omega-3 intake by Australians would help to attain a more ideal balance. Adequate vitamin E intake is also important.

Omega-3 fats are also important for brain and retina development in the foetus and infant. They may also benefit inflammatory ailments such as rheumatoid arthritis and psoriasis. Omega-3 fats can also improve blood flow ~ (Also see page 218).

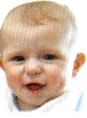
Leah B.

DIETARY FATS COMPARISON

- ■ Saturated Fat
- ■ Monounsaturated Fat
- Polyunsaturated Fats:
- ■ Linoleic (Omega-6)
- ■ Alpha-Linolenic (Omega-3)

OILS — PERCENTAGE CONTENT

Oil	Saturated	Monounsaturated	Linoleic (Omega-6)	Alpha-Linolenic (Omega-3)
CANOLA OIL	8	62	20	10
LINSEED/FLAX OIL	9	19	17	55
SAFFLOWER OIL	9	14	77	
GRAPESEED OIL	10	22	68	
SUNFLOWER OIL	11	23	66	
OLIVE OIL	14	76		10
SOYBEAN OIL	15	23	54	8
PEANUT OIL	19	45	34	2
PALM OIL	51	39	10	

SPREADS & FATS — ▢ Water Content

Spread/Fat	Saturated	Monounsaturated	Linoleic (Omega-6)	Alpha-Linolenic (Omega-3)	Water
BECEL MARGARINE	13	27	29		31
GOLD'N CANOLA LIGHT	14	14	21		51
GOLD'N CANOLA MARGARINE	22	40	13	6	18
DAIRY BLEND/SOFT	42	25	8		25
BUTTER	57	18	2		24
LARD	41	47	12		
BEEF FAT	44	37	4		15

GOOD SOURCES OF OMEGA-3 FATS

PLANT SOURCES — Omega-3 Fats (Grams)

Source	Omega-3 (g)
Canola Oil, 2 tsp (10ml)	1g
Flaxseed Oil, 2 tsp (10ml)	5.5g
Soybean Oil, 2 tsp (10ml)	0.8g
Gold 'n Canola Margarine, 1 Tbsp, 20g	1.2g
Logical/Pro-Active Spreads, 1 Tbsp, 20g	1g
Soybeans, cooked, 1/2 cup, 120g	0.5g
Walnuts, 15g	0.5g

FISH - Per 100g

High Content: Salmon (Pink/Red), Tuna, Sardines, Herring, Mackerel } 2.5g

Medium Content: Mulloway, Trout, Orange Roughy Mullet, Yellowtail, Swordfish } 1.5g

Fair Content: White Fish (eg. Bream/Cod/John Dory Shark Schnapper/Whiting), Shellfish } 0.5g

MILK & SOY DRINKS (with canola or flaxseed)

Dairywise, Farmers Best, 250ml	0.3g
So Good Essential, 250ml	0.5g

How Much Is Needed?
As little as 1-2 grams daily of omega-3 fats may benefit health. Only take high doses of fish oil supplements as directed by your doctor.

Cholesterol ♦ Eggs

Effects of Dietary Cholesterol

Cholesterol in the diet is not the principal factor affecting blood cholesterol levels (BCL). The amount and type of fat is far more important.

Any elevating effect of dietary cholesterol on BCL is more likely to occur when the diet is high in saturated fat. Little elevation, if any, generally occurs when dietary fats are balanced in favour of mono- and polyunsaturated fats.

For example, while fish does contain cholesterol, the omega-3 fats prevent any increase in BCL. Conversely, a meal without any cholesterol but rich in saturated fat, may significantly increase BCL.

Additionally, the body balances its own production of cholesterol with the amount in our food. When dietary cholesterol increases, the body compensates by decreasing its own cholesterol production. This is why changes in dietary cholesterol have little effect on blood cholesterol even when eggs are regularly eaten.

Consequently, the need to be overly concerned about dietary cholesterol is being de-emphasised in favour of a stricter approach to limiting saturated fat, and substituting unsaturated fats.

The Heart Foundation does not limit dietary cholesterol in its recommendations.

Good News for Egg Lovers!

Although eggs are high in cholesterol, they are low in saturated fat; and have little if any effect on blood cholesterol.

There is no link between the eating of eggs and heart disease risk, even in people with high blood cholesterol. Indeed, the Heart Foundation has bestowed its Tick of approval on eggs.

Eggs are a rich source of protein, vitamins and minerals, as well as other vitamin-like substances that can enhance our health. (Extra Notes ~ See Page 93)

Eggs are also ideal for weight control purposes being nutritious, low in kilojoules, and having a high satiety value (hunger is satisfied for a sustained period of time).

> *Avocados (like all plant foods) contain no cholesterol. Their fats are mainly mono-unsaturated and can help to lower blood cholesterol.*
> *They are also rich in antioxidants.*

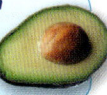

CHOLESTEROL COUNTER

Cholesterol is found only in foods of animal origin. Plant foods contain no cholesterol.

	Cholesterol mg
Meat - Average all types:	
Lean Meat, cooked, 120g	100
Fatty Meat, cooked, 120g	100
Fat, thick strip, 60g	40

Note: While lean meat and fat have similar amounts of cholesterol, choose lean meat to limit fat intake.

Chicken/Turkey, average, 120g	100
Organ Meats: Liver, fried, 4 oz	500
Brains, beef, pan fried, 3 oz	1700
Sausages: Frankfurter, 40g	25
Salami, 2 slices, 55g	40
Bacon: 3 slices, cooked, 30g	20
Fish: Fish fillets, average, ckd, 120g	70
Tuna/Salmon, canned, 100g	50
Scallops, 9 medium, 3 oz	30
Prawns, raw, 100g	110
Oysters, raw, 6 medium, 85g	45
Crayfish, Crab, cooked, 100g	70
Eggs (Chicken), 1 large	210
1 medium	180
Egg White, *Scramblers*	0
Milk/Yoghurt: Whole, 1 cup, 250ml	30
Light/low-fat Milk (1%), 1 cup	10
Skim/Non-fat, 1 cup	10
Soy Milk, Tofu, Tempeh	0
Cheese: Natural/Hard/Cream, 30g	30
Cottage, low-fat, 2 Tbsp, 40g	5
Cream Cheese, 30g	25
Fats: Butter, 1 Tbsp, 20g	45
Margarine, Oils (vegetable)	0
Mayonnaise, 1 Tbsp	10
Cream: Heavy, whipping, 2 Tbsp, 40g	40
Light/Sour, 2 Tbsp	10
Ice Cream: Full-fat (10-11%), 100ml/50g	20
Low-fat (less than 4%), 50g	5
Fruit, Vegetables, Avocados	0
Nuts, Seeds, Grains	0
Coffee, Tea, Beer, Wine	0

Blood Cholesterol Diet Tips

❶ Maintain a healthy weight.
If overweight, lose weight with sensible eating and daily exercise. (See Pages 2-13)

❷ Reduce saturated fat intake.
Note: Food products with added plant sterols can reduce cholesterol absorption from the gut (as can Rice Bran Oil).
Examples: *Flora Pro-Active, Logicol, Kraft Live Active* Cheese.

❸ Increase your 'soluble' fibre intake.
Foods rich in 'soluble' fibre include dried beans, baked beans, lentils, chickpeas, hummus, nuts, seeds, psyllium husks.
Oat bran, rice bran and barley are also useful, as are fruit, veggies and avocados.

❹ Eat more soya bean products
Soy protein (25g/day) in place of animal protein may reduce high blood cholesterol levels. To obtain 25g soy protein, eat 2-3 serves of soy products.
One serving of soy equals:
1 cup Soy Drink
or 2 slices Soy-enriched Bread
or 70g Firm Tofu or 40g Tempeh
or ⅓ cup cooked Soybeans
or *Sanitarium* Soy Sausages (1)
or *Sanitarium* Casserole Mince, 60g
or *Sanitarium* Vegie Roast, 50g

❺ Eat more fruit, vegetables, wholegrains and nuts
in place of high-fat and refined carbohydrate foods. They contain antioxidants that may protect cholesterol in blood from oxidation, and reduce the risk of atherosclerosis and heart disease.

Note: The fat of avocados and most nuts and seeds, is mainly unsaturated and can lower blood cholesterol levels.

TIPS TO REDUCE SATURATED FAT

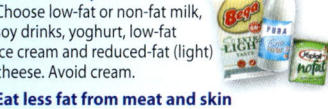

☑ **Eat less dairy fat:**
Choose low-fat or non-fat milk, soy drinks, yoghurt, low-fat ice cream and reduced-fat (light) cheese. Avoid cream.

☑ **Eat less fat from meat and skin of poultry and eat more fish:**
Choose lean meat and skinless chicken. Avoid high-fat luncheon meats, salami and fatty sausages.

☑ **Replace saturated fats** with mono- and polyunsaturated fats/oils. Choose margarine (mainly canola and olive oil types). Cook with oils such as canola, olive, sunflower, soybean and rice bran oil. If overweight, limit all fats and oils.

☑ **Avoid high-fat snacks** such as potato crisps, *Cheezels, Twisties*, savoury snack biscuits (e.g. *Shapes*) and chocolate. Most nuts are fine in moderation.

☑ **Avoid high-fat baked foods** such as cookies, doughnuts, cakes, danish pastries and croissants. Choose low-fat products or home-made with healthier fats/oils.

☑ **Avoid high-fat take-away foods** such as deep-fried foods (e.g. KFC chicken, Chiko Rolls, chips/fries, battered fish, spring rolls, pies, sausage rolls, high-fat pizzas).

For saturated fat content of foods, See www.CalorieKing.com.au.

❻ Spread out your food intake.
Have 4-5 small meals or snacks rather than just 1-2 large meals. Nibbling, versus gorging, favours lower blood cholesterol levels.

How Fats Affect Blood Flow

Fats in the diet not only affect blood cholesterol levels. They can also strongly influence blood clot formation and thrombosis, as well as blood flow and ultimate oxygen delivery to body parts and organs.

While advanced atherosclerosis can impede blood flow to the heart and other organs, it is thrombosis (complete blockage by blood clots) or arterial spasm which commonly result in a heart attack or stroke.

Plant and fish oils rich in omega-3 fats lessen the risk of blood clots, thrombus formation and artery spasm by reducing platelet stickiness and adhesion to artery walls. This reduces the risk of atherosclerotic plaque becoming unstable and reactive.

Omega-3 fats also improve blood flow by reducing blood viscosity; and increasing the flexibility of red blood cells (RBC) that need to flex and twist on themselves in order to squeeze through tiny narrow capillaries often half their diameter.

A diet high in saturated fats has the opposite effect by stiffening RBC membranes and increasing blood viscosity thereby hindering blood flow. The stiffening of the RBC membrane also reduces its ability to release vital oxygen to body cells and take up carbon dioxide.

Stiff, red blood cells may also form aggregates like coin stacks. In narrow blood vessels, this further impedes blood flow and impairs oxygen release (through the much lessened surface area of red blood cell membranes exposed to blood).

Note: Smoking, lack of exercise, and stress can have similar adverse effects on thrombosis, red blood cell flexibility and blood flow.

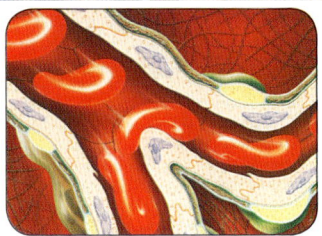

▲ *Picture of Healthy Blood Flow*

Flexible red blood cells twist and slide through tiny capillaries - often half the diameter of red blood cells.

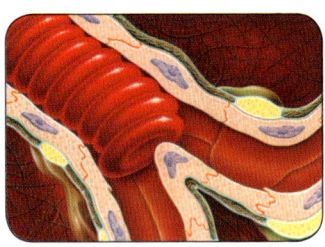

▲ *A Not-So-Healthy Picture!*

Red blood cells have lost their flexibility and ability to twist and slip through capillaries. They are stacked up thereby impeding blood flow.

A diet high in saturated fats can contribute to this picture – as can smoking, lack of exercise and stress.

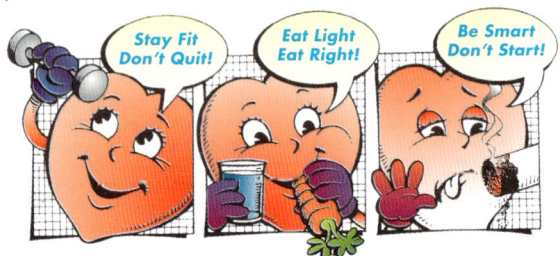

Stay Fit Don't Quit!

Eat Light Eat Right!

Be Smart Don't Start!

Fibre Guide

Fibre & Weight Control

Fibre can assist weight control in several ways. **Fibre-rich** foods such as fresh fruit and vegetables, potatoes and wholegrain bread **contain few calories** for their large volume (due to their low-fat, high water content).

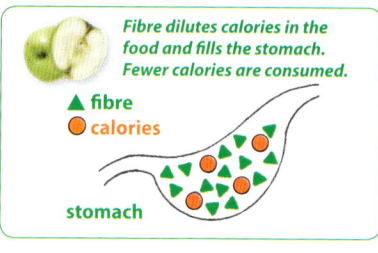

Fibre dilutes calories in the food and fills the stomach. Fewer calories are consumed.

▲ fibre
● calories
stomach

Their bulk **fills the stomach** and satisfies appetite much earlier than fibre-depleted foods. The **extra chewing time** also contributes to satiety, and gives the stomach time to register a feeling of fullness. Excessive calories are less likely to be consumed.

Fibre-depleted foods and drinks are more concentrated in calories; e.g. fats, sugar, lollies, soft drinks, fruit juices, alcohol. They **require little or no chewing.** Thus, large amounts with excessive calories can be consumed before appetite is satisfied.

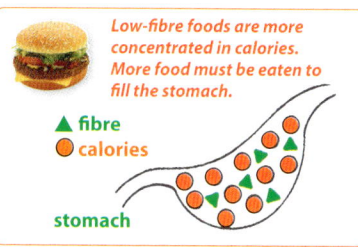

Low-fibre foods are more concentrated in calories. More food must be eaten to fill the stomach.

▲ fibre
● calories
stomach

Example: Whereas one fresh apple might satisfy our appetite, an apple juice drink with the equivalent sugars and calories of 2-3 apples does little to satisfy appetite.

EFFECTS OF REMOVING FIBRE FROM FOOD

2-3 pieces of fresh fruit produces 1 glass of fruit juice.

The removal of fibre concentrates fruit sugars and calories.

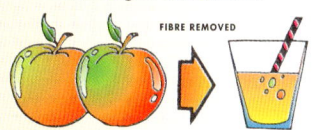

FIBRE REMOVED

Fresh Fruit	Fruit Juice
High Fibre	~ Negligible Fibre
Low Calorie Density	~ High Calorie Density
Long Eating Time	~ No Eating Time (Drink)
Satisfies Hunger	~ Does Not Satisfy Hunger
Sugar Slowly Absorbed	~ Sugar More Quickly Absorbed
Less Insulin Required	~ More Insulin Required

GOOD SOURCES OF FIBRE

- **Bread:** Wholegrain, Rye, Breads with added fibre
- **Breakfast Cereals:** Bran types Rolled Oats, Oat Bran, Muesli, Wheat Germ, Wheat Bran
- **Potatoes, Corn, Rice** (Brown), Pasta (Wholemeal), Barley, Rice Bran, Bulgur/Cracked Wheat
- **Legumes:** Beans (Fresh/Dried), Baked Beans, Soybeans, Lentils, Green Peas, Split Peas, Chickpeas, Nuts, Seeds, Flax Seeds, Psyllium Seed Husks
- **Fresh & Dried Fruit:** Avocados, Apples, Figs, Dates, Prunes
- **Vegetables:** Leafy Greens, Broccoli, Carrots, Brussels Sprouts, Spinach

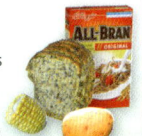
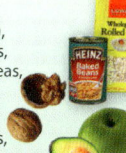
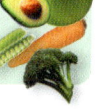

Fibre Guide ~ Constipation

Constipation

Constipation can reasonably be defined as a failure to have a bowel movement at least every second day – and just as importantly, without straining or pain.

Typically, stools are too hard, too narrow, and too small.

The **main cause** is simply a lack of dietary fibre. Other contributing factors include insufficient fluids, too little exercise, emotional stress, gastro-intestinal disease, lack of proper dentition to chew high-fibre foods, and some medications (e.g. some antacids, antidepressants, tranquilisers).

Note: Check with your doctor to rule out any underlying medical problem – especially if you have a change in bowel habits in middle-age or later years.

DESIRABLE FIBRE INTAKE
Adults: 25-35gm per day
Children (under 18): Age + 5gm
Example: 6-year old (6 + 5)= 11gm

SAMPLE FOOD QUANTITIES
For 35 Grams of Fibre/Day — Fibre

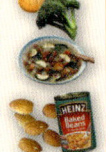

	Breakfast Cereal (higher-fibre)	5g
plus	4 slices wholegrain Bread	6g
plus	3 servings fresh Fruit	9g
plus	1 medium Potato (w. skin)	
or	1 cup Brown Rice	4g
or	½ cup wholegrain Pasta	
plus	3-4 servings Veges/Salad	6g
plus	1 cup Bean Soup	
or	¼ cup Baked/Soy Beans	
or	½ cup Corn/Peas/Lentils	5g
or	35g Almonds (natural)	
or	3 medium Figs	

HINTS TO INCREASE FIBRE AND AVOID CONSTIPATION

1 **Breakfast is an important contributor to daily fibre intake.** Eat high-fibre breakfast cereals (bran-based cereals, oatmeal, etc.) or wholegrain bread/toast and baked beans.

For extra fibre and nutrition, add 1-2 tablespoons of several of these to cereals:
- Unprocessed wheat bran
- Rolled oats
- Wheat germ
- Pumpkin & Sunflower Seeds
- Nuts/Almonds (chopped)
- Linseed meal
- LSA meal (Linseed/Sunflower Seeds/Almonds)
- Dried and fresh fruits
- Psyllium Seed Husks

2 **Drink adequate water and other fluids.** Fibre works by absorbing lots of water.

3 **Eat wholegrain breads,** or fibre-enriched breads. They have over double the fibre of regular white bread.

4 **Eat fruit mainly as fresh fruit** with skins rather than as fruit juice. **Choose wholegrain pasta,** barley, brown rice, nuts and seeds.

5 **Eat more vegetables,** salads and legumes – especially dried beans, baked beans, lentils, potatoes with skins, avocado, broccoli, brussel sprouts, cabbage, carrots, celery, and peas.

6 **Add bran** (barley/rice/wheat) or soy grits to soups, casseroles, yoghurt, desserts, biscuits, cakes. Also use wholemeal flour or soy flour in place of white flour. Use nuts and seeds.

7 **Snack on fresh or dried fruits,** carrot or celery sticks, popcorn, nuts or seeds, wholegrain crackers, high-fibre muesli bars (low-fat). Limit amounts if overweight.

8 **Exercise regularly** to strengthen abdominal muscles and stimulate the gut.

9 **Avoid indiscriminate and regular use of harsh laxatives.** They can overstimulate the intestinal muscles and may make normal bowel activity impossible. It may take several weeks to restore normal bowel function.

Fibre Counter

Desirable Fibre Intake
Adults: 25 - 35 Grams Per Day
Children: 3-18 Years: [Age + 5] grams
Example: A 6 y.o. would need about 11g (6 + 5)

Foods with Nil or Negligible Fibre
Bars, Icecream & Icecream Bars, Cheese, Eggs, Fats & Oils, Sugar & Yoghurt

Breakfast Cereals: | Fib
Be Natural, avg., ½ cup, 50g	5
Coles: Bran Flakes, 30g	4.5
Right Start, ¾ cup, 50g	4
Freedom Food: Ultra Rice, 1 cup, 45g	3.5
Tropico's, 1 cup, 35g	2.5
Kellogg's: All-Bran, ¾ cup, 52g	15
All-Bran Wheat Flakes, 1 cup, 40g	8
Coco Pops, ¾ cup, 30g	0.5
Corn Flakes, 1 cup, 30g	1
Froot Loops, 1 cup, 40g	1
Guardian, 1 cup, 60g	13
Just Right, Orig., ¾ cup, 45g	3.5
Mini-Wheats, 5 Grains, ⅔ cup, 40g	4
Nutri-Grain, 1 cup, 40g	1
Special K, ¾ cup, 30g	1
Sultana Bran, 1 cup, 48g	7
Sustain, ¾ cup, 45g	3
Lowan: Cocoa Bombs, 1 cup, 45g	1.5
Rice Porridge, 50g	4
Nestle: Milo Cereal, 1 cup, 45g	3.5
Nesquick, 1 cup, 45g	2.5
Sanitarium: Corn Flakes, 1 cup, 30g	1
Granola, ¾ cup, 68g	4.5
Light 'n Tasty, 40g	2
Puffed Wheat, 1 cup, 30g	2
Up & Go Drink, 250ml	1
Weet-Bix: Original, 2 biscuits	3
Bites, 14 pieces, 45g	4
Multi-Grain, 2 biscuits	4
Uncle Tobys: Cheerios, 1 cup, 30g	3
Fibre Plus, 1 cup, 45g	7.5
Fruity Bites, 40g	2
Healthwise, For Your Heart, 1 c., 35g	4
Natural Swiss Muesli, 60g	7
Oatbrits, 2 biscuits	5
Oats, Multigrain, 40g	3
Vita Brits, 2 biscuits	4
Vita Weeties 1 cup, 35g	4

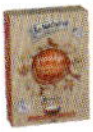

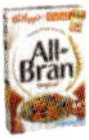

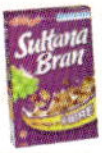

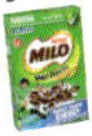

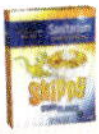

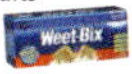

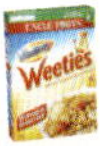

Breakfast Cereals (Cont): | Fib
Vogel's: Fruit & Nut Muesli, ½ cup, 45g	4
Ultra Bran Soy & Linseed, 45g	13
Weight Watchers:	
Bran, ½ cup, 45g	6.5
Fruit & Fibre Tropical, 45g	5
Tropical Breakfast, ½ cup, 45g	3.5

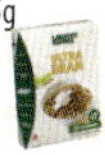

Brans, Oats/Porridge, LSA:
Brans: Barley Bran, 2 Tbsp, 15g	2.5
Oat Bran, 2 Tbsp, 20g	3
Rice Bran, 2 Tbsp, 15g	4
Wheat Bran, 2 Tbsp, 12g	5.5
LSA Meal, 1 Tbsp, 10g	0.5
Psyllium Husks, 2 Tbsp, 12g	9
Rolled Oats, cooked, ¾ cup, 170g	2
Muesli, average, 2 Tbsp, 30g	2.5
Soy Whole-grain Flakes, 40g	4
Wheat Germ, 2 Tbsp, 20g	3

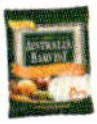

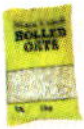

Bread:
White: Thin slice, 30g	0.5
Thick slice, 40g	1
Wholemeal, 1 slice, 30g	2
Multigrain: Thin slice, 30g	2
Thick slice, 40g	2.5
with Soy/Linseed, 47g	2.5
Rye Bread, Light, 30g slice	2
Fruit Loaf: Light, 1 slice, 40g	1.5
Heavily Fruited, 1 slice, 40g	2
Pocket/Flatbread/Pita: White, 42g	1.5
Wholemeal, 1 pocket, 50g	3

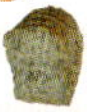

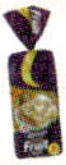

Buns & Rolls:
White, medium, 45g	1.5
Wholegrain, medium, 65g	4

Crackers, Crispbreads:
Arnott's: Salada, Multigrain (2)	2
Sao (2)	0.5
Vita-Weat, Original (4)	3.5
Nabisco, Premium, High Fibre (4)	3.5
Ryvita, Original (2)	3
Matzo, 1 sheet, 34g	5
Ricecakes, 1 Thick/2 Thin, 12g	0.5

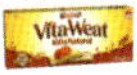

Baked Beans:
In Tomato Sauce, average:
¼ cup, 3 Tbsp, 75g	3.5
½ cup, 150g	7
½ large can (420g), 210g	10
1 large can, 420g	20

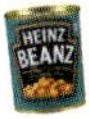

Spaghetti, Canned:
In Tomato Sce: ½ cup 150g	1
Large can (420g), ½ can, 210g	2

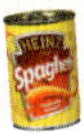

Packaged Meals: | Fib
Lite n' Easy:
Frozen Meals:
Beef & Black Bean, 450g	5
Chicken Schnitzel, 435g	11
Fettuccine Provencale, 480g	6.5
Meatloaf, 430g	9

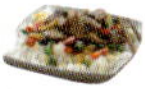

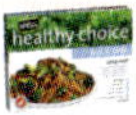

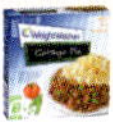

McCain Healthy Choice:
Frozen Meals:
Apricot Chicken	3.5
Beef Lasagne	5
Crmy Chicken Carbonara	3
Honey Mustard Chicken	3
Honey Sesame Chicken	4.5
Spaghetti Bolognese	3

Weight Watchers: *Per Meal*
Frozen:
Beef Burgundy	4
Beef Hot Pot	2
Chicken Risotto	3
Creamy Vegetable Lasagne	3
Thai Chicken Curry	1.5
Wraps, Sweet Chilli Chicken	7

Vegetarian Products:
Sanitarium:
Frozen/Chilled:
Deli Luncheon, Henchen, 62g slice	2
Lentil Patties (1), 75g	3.5
Not Burger (1), 94g	3
Tender Soy Schnitzels, 75g	3.5

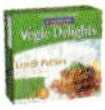

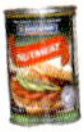

Canned & Packaged:
Casserole Mince, ⅓ can, 138g	1
Nutmeat, 2 slices, 85g	2
Nutolene, 2 slices, 85g	1.5
Sausages, 1 sausage, 40g	1
Savoury Lentils, ⅓ can, 138g	4

Nuts (Shelled):
Almonds, 25-30 nuts, 30g	2.5
Brazil Nuts, 30g	2.5
Cashews, 12-16 nuts, 30g	2
Coconut, Flesh, 30g	2.5
Pecans, 30g	2.5
Macadamia, 30g	2
Peanuts, 30g	2.5
Peanut Butter, 1 Tbsp, 20g	1
Pine Nuts, 30g	1.5
Pistachio Nuts, dried, 30g	3
Walnuts, 15-20 halves, 30g	2

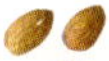

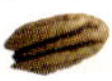

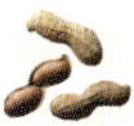

Seeds:
Linseed, 2 Tbsp, 25g	7
Pumpkin, 3 Tbsp, 30g	3.5
Sesame, 2½ Tbsp, 30g	3
Sunflower Kernels, 2½ Tbsp, 30g	3

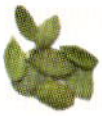

Fibre Counter

Fresh Fruits: | Fib
- Apple, 1 medium, 150g — 3
- Apricot, 1 medium, 40g — 1
- Avocado, ½ medium (240g whole) — 2
- Banana, 1 medium, 170g — 3
- Blueberries, ½ cup, 75g — 1.5
- Cherries, 15 large./25 small, 100g — 1
- Grapefruit, ½ medium, 100g — 1
- Grapes, 1 Medium Bunch, 200g — 7
- Kiwi Fruit, 1 medium, 100g — 3
- Mango, ½ medium, 100g flesh — 1
- Nectarine, 1 medium, 90g — 2
- Olives, pitted, 6 medium, 50g — 1.5
- Orange, 1 medium, 230g — 2
- Passionfruit, 1 med. 45g — 2
- Peach, 1 medium, 115g — 2.5
- Pear, 1 medium, 150g — 4.5
- Pineapple, 1 sl., 2½ cm thick, 85g — 1.5
- Plums, 1 medium (5cm), 100g — 2
- Rambutan, 3 fruit, 120g — 1.5
- Raspberries, ½ cup, 50g — 3
- Rockmelon, ½ small, 400g — 2
- Strawberries, 5 med., 100g — 1.5
- Tomato, 1 medium, 150g — 1
- 1 large, 200g — 2.5
- Watermelon:
  - Thick slice, ¼ circle, 150g — 0.5
  - ½ circle, 300g — 1

Vegetables:
- Asparagus, 3 spears, 60g — 1.6
- Beans, Green/French/Runner, ½ cup, 60g — 2
- Beetroot, 1 medium, 120g — 4
- Broccoli Tips, ½ cup, 60g — 3
- Brussel Sprouts, 4-5 med., 120g — 5.5
- Cabbage, shredded, ½ cup, 40g — 1
- Carrots, 1 medium, 140g — 4.5
- Cauliflower, ½ cup, 100g — 2.5
- Celery, 1 piece, 15cm long, 30g — 1.5
- Corn Cob:
  - 1 medium, 170g — 5
  - Cobette, 100g — 3
- Cucumber, ½ c. slices, peeled, 60g — 0.5
- Garlic, raw, 3 cloves, 9g — 1.5
- Lettuce, average, 3 leaves, 30g — 0.5
- Leeks, bulb & leaf, 30g — 1
- Mixed Veges, frozen, ½ cup, 60g — 4
- Mushrooms: Sliced, ½ cup, 60 g — 1
- Button, 4-5, 60g — 1
- Onion, 1 medium, 120g — 2
- Peas: Shelled, ¾ cup, 100g — 5.5
- Snow peas, 10 pods, 33g — 1

Vegetables (Cont) | Fib
- Potatoes (raw wt):
  - 1 small, 100g — 1
  - 1 medium, 150g — 2
  - 1 large, 200g — 2
- Pumpkin: Without Skin or Seeds:
  - Butternut, 100g — 1.5
  - Golden Nugget, 100g — 2
  - Qld Blue, 100g — 2.5
- Spinach, cooked, ½ cup, 90g — 2
- Squash, button, 100g — 1
- Sweetcorn, Kernels, ½ cup, 60g — 3.5
- Sweet Potato, ¼ small, 100g — 3
- Zucchini, 1 small, 118g — 1.5

Salads (Deli-Style)
- Side Salad, average — 1
- Bean Salad, ½ cup, 120g — 5
- Coleslaw, ½ cup, 120g — 2
- Potato Salad, ½ cup, 120g — 2

Fast-Foods
- Chicken: Rotisseried/BBQ'd,
  - ¼ chicken — 0
  - ¼ chicken, with stuffing — 1
- Chicken Nuggets, 6 pack w. Sauce — 0
- Chicken Roll, 180g — 3
- Chiko Roll, 170g — 3
- Chips, 1 bucket, 150g — 5.5
- Dim Sim, large, 70g — 1
- Fish (200g) & Chips (150g) — 7
- French Fries: Small, 80g — 1.5
- Large, 110g — 2
- Hamburger: Small, 120g — 3.5
- Cheeseburger, 135g — 3
- Hot Dog, 1 — 2.5
- Pastie, 175g — 3
- Pie: Meat, 175g — 2
- Meat, large, 210g — 2.5
- Party Pie, 47g — 1
- Samosa, party size, 50g — 1
- Sausage Roll: Large, 120g — 2
- Party Size, 40g — 0.5
- Spinach Filo, Triangle — 2
- Spring Roll: Small (1), 42g — 1
- Jumbo, 170g — 2
- Sushi Rolls: Small (1), 33g — 0.5
- Large (1), 43g — 0.5
- 1 Pack (6 lge/8 small), 260g — 3
- Taco, average — 1

Fast Food Chains | Fib
- **Domino's:** *Per Slice, ⅛ pizza*
  - Classic/Thin N Crispy, average — 1
  - Deep Pan, average — 1.5
- **Hungry Jack's:** Whopper — 2.5
  - Aussie Burger — 2.5
  - Bacon Deluxe — 2.5
  - Cheeseburger — 2
  - Junior Whopper — 1.5
- **KFC:** Burgers, average — 3
  - Chips, regular, 115g — 3.5
  - Fried Chicken, portions:
    - Drumstick — 0
    - Breast — 0
  - Popcorn Chicken, regular, 135g — 1
  - Nuggets, 6-pack & sauce — 1
- **McDonald's:** Big Mac — 4
  - Cheeseburger — 3
  - Bacon & Egg McMuffin — 3.5
  - Hamburger — 2
  - McChicken; ¼ Pounder w. Cheese — 3.5
  - French Fries, small — 2
  - Wrap, Chilli — 7
- **Pizza Hut:** *Per Slice, ⅛ Pizza*
  - Thin 'n Crispy, average — 1.5
  - Pan/Perfecto, average — 1.5
- **Red Rooster:** Chicken Roll — 2.5
  - Flayva Wrap — 3.5
  - Rippa Sub — 2
  - Quarter Chicken & Chips — 1
- **Subway:**
  - 6g Fat or Less Subs (6"): Roast Beef — 4.5
  - Sweet Onion Chicken Teriyaki — 4.5
  - Veggie Delite — 4.5
  - **12" Subs:** Italian BMT — 9
  - Chicken Fillet — 9
  - Tuna with Cheese — 9
- Wraps, Turkey; Roast Chicken — 3

Fibre Supplements & Laxatives
- Barley Grass dry, 1 tsp, 2g — 0.5
- *Benefiber*, 1 sachet/1 Tbsp, 4g — 3
- *Easy Fibre*, 2 tabs — 8
- *Fibyrax*, 8 tablets, 4.5g — 3
- *Fybogel*, (no added sugar): 1 sachet, 4g — 3.5
- Bulk Pack, 1 heaped tsp — 3.5
- *Metamucil*: Regular, 3 Tbsp, 11g — 3
- Orange, sugar free, 1½ tsp — 3
- Natural Fibre, 12g — 8
- *Nu-Lax*, 10g dose — 3
- *Quick Fibe Plus*, 2 T., 30g — 12
- *Senokot*: Tablets — 0
- Granules (Choc flavoured), 1 tsp — 2

Protein Guide

General Notes

- Protein has many important body functions. It builds and repairs muscle, and is the basis of our body's organs, hormones, enzymes, and antibodies to fight infection.

- Protein is also an emergency fuel in the absence of sufficient carbohydrate and fats. For this reason, weight loss should be gradual so as to preserve protein levels in muscle, the heart and other body organs.

- It is easy to obtain sufficient protein, even if vegetarian. Plant proteins are not inferior to animal proteins. In fact, eating more soy and other plant proteins, and less animal protein, may help to build stronger bones and prevent osteoporosis; and may help to control blood cholesterol levels.

- When changing to a vegetarian diet, include soybeans, and other dried beans, soy milk drinks (calcium-enriched), lentils, tofu, tempeh, nuts, and wholegrain breads and cereals. Milk, yoghurt, cheese and eggs can enhance nutrient intake.

Protein & Muscle

- Although muscles are built of protein, protein is not a special fuel for working muscle cells – carbohydrates and fats are.

- In fact, a diet high in protein (and fat) and low in carbohydrate, can significantly reduce the performance of endurance sports athletes. Carbohydrate is the best fuel for muscles exercised for long periods.

- Any extra protein required by athletes and bodybuilders, can easily be obtained from the extra food eaten to satisfy hunger and energy needs.

- Remember, excessive protein intake will not build bigger muscles. Any excess is converted and stored as fat. Excess protein can also strain the kidneys which excrete the waste products of protein metabolism.

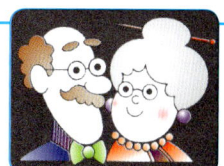

To ensure adequate protein intake, sufficient food must be eaten – particularly by persons on calorie-restricted diets, and by elderly people.

Inadequate protein leads to a drop in immune response with greater susceptibility to illness and infections. Muscle strength and muscle mass also decrease.

Protein needs are easily met with sensible eating. Athletes who eat enough food for their energy needs, can obtain sufficient protein.

RECOMMENDED DAILY PROTEIN INTAKE
~ HEALTHY RANGE ~
(Lower figure is RDI)

Children:	1-3 yrs	14g-26g
	4-8 yrs	20g-38g
Males:	9-13 yrs	40g-70g
	14-18 yrs	65g-100g
	19-70 yrs	64g-100g
	Over 70 yrs	81g-100g
Females:	9-13 yrs	35g-60g
	14-18 yrs	45g-80g
	19-70 yrs	46g-80g
	Over 70 yrs	57g-80g
Pregnancy:		60g-100g
Breastfeeding:		67g-100g

Note: On low kilojoule diets, aim for higher amounts of protein within the Healthy Range.

Protein Counter

Meat: **Pro**

Beef: Average all cuts,
- Lean, raw, 100g — 21
- Cooked, 100g, from 130g raw — 27

Mince, Raw: Regular (80% lean), 100g — 17
- Lean (90% lean), 100g — 20
- Hamburger Patty (added cereal), 85g — 21

Roast Beef, lean, 1 slice, 40g — 11

Steaks (Grilled/BBQ'd): Average All Cuts,
- Small, 120g raw/80g cooked — 25
- Medium, 150g raw/120g cooked — 37
- Large, 220g raw/175g cooked — 54
- Extra Large, 300g raw/240g cooked — 74
- Fillet Steak, grilled, 80g (120g raw) — 25

T-Bone: Medium, 250g raw wt. — 55
- Large, 350g raw wt. — 77

Veal, Similar to Lamb

Liver, grilled, 85g — 23

Lamb: Chump Chop, grilled 85g — 19
- Midloin Chop (95g raw),
- Grilled (65g w. bone + Fat) — 11
- Roast Leg, lean, 1 slice, 40g — 13

Pork: Cooked, lean, 100g — 23
- Bacon, 3 medium slices — 6

Luncheon Meats:
- Ham, average 2 slices, 50g — 8
- Polony, 2 slices, 50g — 5.5
- Salami, average 3 slices, 30g — 6
- Silverside, 2 slices, 50g — 8.5

Spam:
- 1 slice (⅙ can), 56g — 8
- ½ can, 170g — 24

Sausages: Average all types,
- Thin (10/½ kg) (1), 50g — 6.5
- Thick (6/½ kg) (1), 85g — 11

Chicken:
Average white/dark meat,
- Cooked: Lean + Skin, 100g — 25
- Lean only, 100g — 28
- Breast portion, ½ baked, lean only, 80g — 22
- Drumstick, baked/rotisseried, 85g — 13
- ¼ Chicken, rotisseried/take-away, average, 100g edible wt (lean + fat) — 25
- ½ small chicken, 200g edible — 50

Fish: **Pro**

Fresh, Plain: Average all types
- Small serve, 100g raw/80g cooked — 25
- Medium serve, 150g raw/120g cooked — 38
- Large serve, 200g raw/160g cooked — 50

Fish in Batter or Breaded:
- Small fillet, 100g — 12
- Medium fillet, 150g — 18
- Large fillet, 200g — 24

Fish Fingers, (2), 50g — 6

Smoked Salmon, 5 slices, 100g — 23

Seafood: Prawns/Crab/Crayfish, 100g — 17
- Mussels/Octopus, 100g — 17
- Calamari Rings, in batter, 100g — 10

Canned Fish:
Salmon: Pink/Red, avg., drained, 100g — 22
- 100g can (80g drained) — 17
- 210g can (170g drained) — 37

Sardines, in oil/water, 110g can — 28

Tuna: Average, 100g, (drained) — 28
- 100g can, (75g drained) — 20

Eggs:
1 large egg: Whole, 53g — 6
- Egg Yolk only — 3
- Egg White only — 3

Omelette: Plain/Veg & 2 eggs — 13
- With Ham & Cheese, 2 eggs — 17

Milk:
- Whole Milk, 1 cup, 250ml — 8.5
- Low-Fat/Non-Fat: 250ml — 10
- + Fibre, 250ml — 8.5

Flavoured Milk, average:
- 300ml carton — 9.5
- 600ml carton — 19

Rice Milk:
- Average: Regular, 250ml — 1
- Protein Enriched, 250ml — 4

Soy Milk:
Aussie Soy, all varieties, 250ml — 9

Sanitarium, So Good:
- Bliss, average, 250ml — 8
- Essential, 250ml — 8
- Regular or Lite, 250ml — 8

So Natural: Original, 250ml — 5
- Light, 250ml — 7.5
- So Nice, Regular, 250ml — 8

VitaSoy: Original, Light, 250ml — 3.5
- High Fibre, 250ml — 4
- Soy Milky, Regular/Lite, 250ml — 8

Cocoa, Milo, Nesquik: **Pro**
- Cadbury, Drinking Chocolate, 25g — 1
- *Nestle:* Cocoa, 1 Tbsp, 20g — 5
- Milo, 3 Tbsp (¼ Cup), 25g — 3
- Nesquik, 3 heaped tsp, 12g — 0.5
- Ovaltine, 3 heaped tsp, 15g — 1.5

Yoghurt:
- **Natural,** full/low-fat, avg., 200g — 8
- **Fruit Flavoured,** average, 200g — 8
- **Greek Style,** avg., 200g — 12

Cheese:
- **Cheddar:** Average, 30g — 7.5
- Extra Light (50% less fat), 30g — 9.5
- Light Singles Slices (Kraft), 21g — 4
- Reduced-Fat (25% less fat), 30g — 8.5
- **Cottage Cheese,** 2T., 40g — 4
- **Cream Cheese,** 30g — 2
- **Ricotta,** 2 Tbsp, 40g — 2.5

Baked Beans:
In Tomato Sauce, average:
- ¼ cup, 3 Tbsp, 75g — 4
- ½ cup, 140g — 7
- ½ of 420g can, 210g — 10
- 1 large 420g can — 21

Spaghetti/Pasta:
Spaghetti/Macaroni/Fettucine,
- Cooked, 1 cup, 150g — 7.5
- Wholemeal, cooked, 1 cup, 150g — 9
- Canned, in Tomato Sce., ¾ cup, 210g — 4.5

Rice:
- Brown, cooked, 1 cup, 150g — 5
- White, cooked, 1 cup, 150g — 4

Flour:
- Wheat, white, 100g — 13

Grains:
- Barley, cooked, ½ cup, 80g — 2.5
- Bulgar (Cracked wheat), ckd, ½ cup, 90g — 90
- Quinoa: Cooked, ½ cup, 90g — 4
- Raw, ½ cup, 90g — 12

Cup & Block Noodles:
- *Kraft,* Easy Mac, 70g — 8
- *Maggi:* 2-Min. Noodles, avg. — 7
- Cup Noodles, avg., 60g cup — 5.5

224

Protein Counter

Meals, Frozen/Packaged: **Pro**

Lean Cuisine:
- Lasagne — 20
- Satay Beef with Rice — 22
- Thai Red Curry — 15

Blanced Serve: *Per Bowl*
- Beef in Red Wine Sauce with Mash — 14
- Chicken & Vegetable Risotto — 18
- Chicken Florentine with Linguine — 19
- Lamb & Rosemary Hot Pot — 15
- Malaysian Chicken Curry with Rice — 14
- Satay Chicken Noodles — 17

McCain:
HealthyChoice
- Apricot Chicken — 12
- Beef Lasagne — 22
- Fillet of Lamb — 14
- Lemon Chicken — 16
- Stirfry Chicken with Noodles — 14

Quorn:
- Lasagne, 300g — 16
- Schnitzel, 120g — 11
- Tikka Masala — 11

Sanitarium (Vegetarian):
Canned Products:
- Casserole Mince, 1/3 can, 138g — 23
- BBQ Soya Sausages (2), 100g — 15
- Nutmeat, 2 slices (10mm), 85g — 21
- Nutolene, 2 slices (10mm), 85g — 11
- Savoury Lentils, 1/3 can, 138g — 6.5
- Tender Pieces, 1/3 can, 138g — 21
- Vegetarian Sausages (2), 80g — 17

Vegie Delights:
- Burger, 75g — 8
- Hotdogs (2), 100g — 11
- Vegie Roast, 1/4 pkt, 120g — 24

Sara Lee:
- Beef Lasagna, 192g — 14

Weight Watchers:
- Bangers & Mash — 11
- Honey Soy Chicken — 13
- Satay Chicken — 15
- Thai Chicken Curry — 11
- Tuna Bake — 11

Zoglos:
- Vegetarian Burger (1), 75g — 15

Breakfast Cereals: **Pro**

- **Muesli**, average, 1/2 cup, 60g — 5
- **Oatmeal/Porridge:**
  - 1/3 cup uncooked, 30g — 7
  - 1 cup cooked (with water) — 7
  - 1 cup cooked (with milk) — 15

Kellogg's:
- All-Bran, 45g — 7
- Coco Pops, 1 cup, 45g — 3
- Corn Flakes, 1 cup, 30g — 2.5
- Fruit Loops, 30g — 2
- Komplete Oven Baked Muesli, 45g — 4
- Just Right, 45g — 4
- Nutri-Grain, 1 cup, 40g — 4
- Rice Bubbles, 30g — 2
- Special K, 1 cup, 40g — 8
- Sultana Bran, 1 cup, 48g — 4.5
- Sustain, 1 cup, 60g — 5.5

Nestle:
- Milo Cereal, 1 cup, 45g — 5

Sanitarium:
- Honey Weets, 30g — 2.5
- Granola, 30g — 2.5
- Light 'n Tasty, 30g — 2.5
- Puffed Wheat, 30g — 4
- **Weet-Bix:**
  - Original, 2 bisc., 33g — 4
  - Bites, 14 pces, 45g — 4.5
  - Hi Bran, 2 biscuits, 40g — 5

Uncle Tobys:
- Bran Plus, 2/3 cup, 45g — 6
- Cheerios, 1 cup, 30g — 2
- Fibre Plus, 1 cup, 45g — 5
- Healthwise For Your Heart, 35g — 3.5
- Muesli, Swiss Natural, 60g — 6.5
- Oats, Quick, 30g — 3.5
- Protein Plus, 40g — 5.5
- Vita Brits/Weeeties, 30g — 3.5
- Vita Brits Bites, 1 cup, 60g — 4
- Vita Brits, 2 biscuits, 33g — 3.5
- Rolled Oats, raw, 30g — 4

Weight Watchers:
- Berry/Tropical Flakes, avg, 1/2 cup, 45g — 4

Brans:
- Barley Bran, 20g — 2
- Amaranth Breakfast Cereal, 30g — 5
- Natural Wheat Bran, 20g — 3
- Oat Bran, raw, 20g — 3
- Wheat Germ, 2 Tbsp, 15g — 4
- LSA, 1 Tbsp, 20g — 4
- Chia Seeds, 1 Tbsp, 15g — 3

Bread: **Pro**

- **White Bread:** Thin Slice, 30g — 2.5
  - Thin Slice, 40g — 3.5
  - Bun/Roll, 60g — 5
- **Wholemeal/Multigrain:**
  - Thin slice, 30g — 3
  - Thick slice, 45g — 5
- **High Protein**, 2 slices, (18g each) — 5
- **Rye:** Light, 1 slice, 33g — 3
  - Dark, 1 slice, 45g — 4
- **Fruit Loaf** (light), 1 slice, 27g — 2
- **English Muffins**, Plain/Fruit — 7
- **Crispbreads**, average, 2 pieces — 1.5

Sugar, Honey, Jam:
- **Sugar**, all types — 0
- **Molasses**, all types — 0
- **Honey, Jam, Marmalade** — 0

Vegemite, Nutella:
- *Vegemite/Marmite/Promite*, 1/2 tsp, 3g — 0.5
- *Nutella*, 1 Tbsp, 20g — 1.5

Biscuits, Crackers:
Biscuits:
- Sao (2) — 2
- Sesame Wheat (3) — 2
- Sweet, Milk Arrowroot (2) — 1
- Nice; Shortbread (2) — 1
- Cream Biscuits, average (2) — 1
- **Crackers**, Jatz (3) — 1

Cakes:
- Plain, 1 piece, 85g — 4
- Fruit Cake, 1 piece, 45g — 4
- Fruit Pie, 1 piece, 150g — 4

Croissant:
- Plain, 55g — 5
- Doughnuts/Muffin, avg., 55g — 4

Chocolate/Bars & Snacks:
- Chocolate, Milk/Dark/Nuts, avg., 50g — 4
- Cherry Ripe, 52g bar — 3
- Chokito, 55g bar — 3
- Kit Kat, 4 fingers, 45g — 3
- Mars Bar/Milo Bar, 53g — 4
- Picnic bar, 46g — 3
- Fruit & Nut Bar, 55g — 4.5
- Cheezels/Twisties, etc., 50g — 4
- CC's, Corn Chips, 50g — 4
- Potato Crisps, avg., 50g pkt — 3.5

Protein Counter

Health, Muesli Bars: **Pro**

Fruit Bar, 40g	1
Fruit & Nut Bar, 50g	7
Yoghurt Bars, average, 50g	4
Muesli Bars/Slices	
Average: Small (e.g. Uncle Toby's), 30g	2
Large/Meal , 80g	6
Aussie Bodies, Protein FX	20
Be Good To Yourself: Lunch Bars, 45g	11
Snack Bars, 30g	5
Be Natural: Four, 22g	4
Trail, 32g	2.5
Musashi: P, High Protein, 90g	40
P20, Low Carb, 65g	20

Nuts & Seeds:

Almonds, Cashews, average, 30g	6
Mixed Nuts, 30g	5
Peanuts, 30g	7.5
Pistachios, 30g	6
Walnuts, 15-20 halves, 30g	7
Seeds: Sesame, dry, 1 Tbsp	2.5
Sunflower, dried, hulled, 30g	6.5
Tahini/Sesame Butter, 1 Tbsp	3.5
Peanut Butter, avg. all brands, 1 T. 20g	4.5

Fruits:

Fresh Fruit, 1 med./2 small fruit, avg.	1
Avocado, ½ medium	1.5
Dried Fruit: Prunes, 3-4, 30g	1
Apricots, 5-6 pieces, 30g	1
Dates, pitted, 4-5 dates, 30g	0.5
Figs, 3 medium figs, 60g	1
Raisins, 30g	1
Fruit Juice: Average, 250ml	0.5
Prune Juice, 180ml	1

Vegetables:

Beans: Baked Beans	7
Dried, average all types, cooked, 100g	7
Green, cooked, ½ cup, 60g	2
Bean Sprouts, Mung, 1 cup, 90g	3
Broccoli, 2 florets, 45g	2
Cabbage, shredded, ½ cup, 40g	0.5
Cauliflower, raw, 100g	1.5
Corn, ½ cup kernels, 90g	1.5
Lentils, cooked, 30g	2.5
Mushrooms, raw, ½ cup, 60g	2
Peas, green, ¼ cup, 35g	2

Vegetables (Cont): **Pro**

Potatoes:	
1 small, 100g	2
1 medium, 150g	3
1 large, 200g	4
Pumpkin, mashed, 1 scoop, 50g	1.2
Seaweed, kelp, 30g	0.5
Spinach, raw, 100g	2.5
Split Peas, cooked, ½ cup, 100g	8
Squash, 100g	1
Tomatoes, 1 medium, 150g	1.5

Soy, Tofu, Tempeh:

Miso, ½ cup, 150g	17
Soybeans, dry, cooked, ½ cup, 100g	12
Tempeh, 100g	19
Tofu: Raw, firm, 100g	12
Soft/Silken, 100g	4.5

Beer, Wine: Beer, 375ml
Beer, 375ml	1
Wines	0

Soft/Energy Drinks:

Soft Drinks; Red Bull; "V" Energy	0
Gatorade; Powerade	0

Protein, Sports Shakes:

Aussie Bodies, Perfect Protein, 40g	29
Be Good To Yourself (Amcal/Guardian), average all flavours, 45g sachet	20
Betty Baxter, Shakes, 50g sachet	20
Biggest Loser, Shakes, 55g	20
Finding Form, 1 sachet, 54g	18
Horley's, Protein Food, 25g	20
Musashi: Muscle Food, 49g	35
P30 Milk Drink, all flav., 375ml	30
Nature's Way, Sports Edge, 2 Tbsp, 35g	24
Nestle, Sustagen:	
Dutch Chocolate, 250ml,	13
Sports, 100g dry	25
Optifast, Milkshake/Soup, 1 sachet	17
Optislim, VLCD, 40g sachet	16
Slimmm, Shakes, avg., 55g	20
Tony Ferguson, Shakes, 1 sachet	15
Finding Form, 1 sachet, 54g	18
Wonder, Modifast, 1 sachet	23

Coffee: Espresso
Cappuccino/Latte, 250ml	4
Mug, Large, 330ml	7

Hot Chocolate, 250 ml — 7

Milk Shakes, 480 ml (16 oz) — 10

Fast-Foods: **Pro**

Dominos, Hungry Jack's, KFC, McDonalds, KFC, Pizza Hut, Subway ~ See Pages 185-208

General Items:

Cheeseburger, 135g	15
Chicken: Rotisseried/BBQ'd,	
¼ chicken	25
¼ chicken, with stuffing	26
Chicken Nuggets, 6 pack, with Sauce	16
Chicken Roll, 180g	26
Chiko Roll, 170g	10
Chips, 1 bucket/cup, 150g	10
Dim Sim, large, 70g	7
Fish (200g) & Chips (150g)	34
French Fries: Small, 80g	3
Large, 130g	5
Hamburger: Small, 120g	12
Large	34
Hot Dog, 1	9
Pancake: Med., (3), 100g	12
Syrup, 30ml	12
Pastie, 175g	18
Pie: Meat, 175g	19
Meat, large, 210g	22
Party Pie, 47g	3
Vegetarian, avg., 200g	14
Pita, with Filling/Salad	35
Pizza: Average all types	
⅛ pizza, 1 slice	9
½ pizza, 4 slices	36
Whole Pizza, 8 slices	72
Domino's ~ See Page 189	
Pizza Hut ~ See Page 204	
Salads: Bean Salad, 100g	2
Coleslaw/Potato, 100g	2
Samosa, party size, 50g	3
Sausage Roll, large, 120g	10
Spinach Filo Triangle	10
Spring Roll, small (1), 42g	5
Shakes, medium	10
Steakburger, average	40
Sundaes, with topping, average	7
Sushi Rolls: Small (1), 33g	2
Large (1), 43g	2.5
1 Pack (6 large/8 small), 260g	16
Taco, average	10
Wraps: With Chicken, avg.	21
With other meats, average	15

High Blood Pressure Guide

High Blood Pressure

Many Australian adults have hypertension (high blood pressure) and are unaware of it. It is generally symptomless, so **have your blood pressure checked annually** – particularly if it runs in the family.

Untreated hypertension overworks the heart, damages arteries and promotes atherosclerosis. This in turn greatly increases the risk of heart disease, stroke, blindness, kidney disease and impotence. The earlier hypertension is detected, the sooner it can be brought under control.

BLOOD PRESSURE CLASSIFICATION

For Adults Age 18 & Older
(USA Nat'l High Blood Pressure Education Program)

	DIASTOLIC		SYSTOLIC
Normal	▶ Below 80	and	▶ Below 120
Prehypertension:	▶ 80-89	or	▶ 120-139
Stage 1	▶ 90-99	or	▶ 140-159
Stage 2	▶ 100 or more	or	▶ 160 or more

Treating Hypertension

Prehypertension (in the chart above) means you don't have high blood pressure now but are likely to develop it in the future.

You can take steps to prevent it with healthy eating and lifestyle habits such as:

- reducing sodium intake
- eating adequate fruit and vegetables
- losing weight if overweight
- limiting alcohol to 2 standard drinks or less daily
- quitting smoking
- exercising regularly; managing stress

Stage 1 hypertension can often be treated with the above lifestyle changes.

Stage 2 hypertension usually requires drug therapy. However, salt and alcohol restriction, and adopting the above lifestyle changes may improve the success of drug therapy, and enable smaller drug doses to be prescribed.

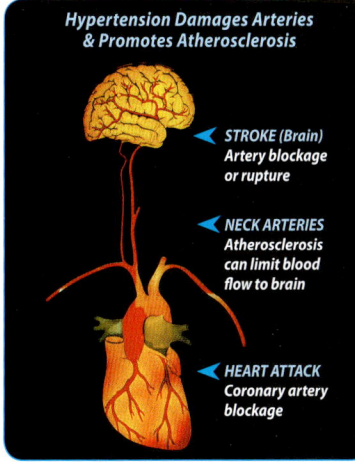

Hypertension Damages Arteries & Promotes Atherosclerosis

◀ **STROKE (Brain)** Artery blockage or rupture

◀ **NECK ARTERIES** Atherosclerosis can limit blood flow to brain

◀ **HEART ATTACK** Coronary artery blockage

S-T-R-O-K-E

KNOW THE WARNING SIGNS

If you notice one or more of these signs, **call your doctor immediately or Triple Zero 0-0-0.** The signs may be signalling a possible stroke or transient ischemic attack (TIA):

- ▶ **Sudden weakness** or numbness in your face, arm or leg on one side of your body.
- ▶ **Sudden dimness,** blurring or loss of vision, particularly in one eye.
- ▶ **Loss of speech,** or trouble talking or understanding speech.
- ▶ **Sudden severe headache** – 'a bolt out of the blue' - with no apparent cause.
- ▶ **Unexplained dizziness,** unsteadiness or a sudden fall, especially if accompanied by any of the other symptoms.

More Info: www.strokefoundation.com.au
www.heartfoundation.org.au

Salt • Sodium & Blood Pressure

- **Sodium is a mineral element** most commonly found in salt (sodium chloride). It also occurs naturally in much smaller amounts in animal and plant foods, and water. This is sufficient for our needs without having to add salt.

- **Sodium is required for nerve** and muscle function and to balance the amount of fluid in our tissues and blood. Sodium acts like a sponge to attract and hold fluids in body tissues.

- **Excess sodium** can cause water retention, and increase the risk of developing hypertension; as well as Meniere's Disease vertigo attacks, PMS (Premenstrual Syndrome), and swollen ankles. Very high salt intake may also increase the risk of stomach cancer.

- **Too little sodium** may cause low blood pressure (hypotension), and decrease blood flow to the heart, brain and kidneys – especially during exercise. (A certain blood volume is required to sustain the blood pressure needed for adequate blood flow in the capillaries.)

Salt-Sensitive Persons

- **Normally, our kidneys excrete excess dietary sodium.** The thirst we feel after a salty meal is the body calling for water to dilute the sodium, and enable the kidneys to flush out excess sodium.

- However, **'salt sensitive' persons** (perhaps more than 50% of adults) tend to retain excess sodium (above approximately 2000mg daily) instead of excreting it. Such persons are more likely to develop hypertension and would most benefit from sodium restriction. Assume you are susceptible if there is a family history of hypertension.

- Although not everyone may benefit, **all Australians are being asked to moderate their salt and sodium intake** as a public health measure – particularly that so many do not know whether or not they have hypertension; and also because we do not know just who is salt-sensitive.

Note: Salt restriction can reduce systolic blood presure by around 4-5mmHg in hypertensive persons.

SAFER SODIUM LEVELS

The Heart Foundation recommends a maximum sodium intake of 1500 mg/day for all Australians, particularly those **with high blood pressure or at risk of cardiovascular disease.**
Persons with hypertension and kidney disease are usually restricted to as little as 1000mg sodium per day. Your doctor will discuss the correct sodium level for you.
(Further Info: www.HeartFoundation.com.au)

FINDING HIDDEN SODIUM

On average, less than 25% of our sodium intake comes from the salt shaker. The rest is hidden in processed foods that have salt added during manufacture.

Sodium compounds added to food or medicinals can also contribute significant amounts of sodium.

Sodium bicarbonate in particular is widely used in antacid tablets and powders; and saline drink powders (e.g. *Eno, Alka-Seltzer, Andrews*).

Sodium bicarbonate contains 27% sodium by weight. Each gram contributes 270mg sodium. Large amounts of sodium can be unwittingly consumed.

**Examples: 1 teaspoon Eno = 800 mg sodium
2 Alka-Seltzer tablets = 1020 mg sodium**

Other sodium compounds include mono-sodium glutamate (MSG), sodium ascorbate, sodium nitrite, and sodium citrate.

POTASSIUM BALANCES SODIUM

Potassium helps to balance sodium by helping the kidneys to excrete excess sodium. Fruit and vegetables are rich sources of potassium – another reason to ensure you have your 5-7 servings every day.

Nuts also provide potassium as well as magnesium and other heart-healthy nutrients and anti-oxidants. Eat them unsalted.

BEWARE ALCOHOL

Excessive alcohol intake contributes to hypertension. Susceptible persons should limit alcohol intake to 1-2 drinks per day.

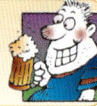

Salt • Sodium & Blood Pressure

Sodium accounts for only 40% of the weight of salt (sodium chloride).

1 gram (1000mg) Salt has 400mg Sodium
1 teaspoon (5g) Salt has 2000mg Sodium

Tips to Reduce Sodium

- **Watch the salt shaker.** Start with an easy 50% cut in sodium by using Lite Salt (e.g. *Diet-Rite*). Then gradually cut back until you can leave the salt shaker off the table.

- **Taste your food before salting.** Use the pepper shaker (small holes) for more controlled sprinkling of salt. Don't salt children's food.

- **Choose 'low sodium', 'no added salt', and 'reduced salt' food products.** To use these terms, labels must conform to:
  - **Low Sodium:** 120mg or less/100g
  - **Salt Free:** Less than 5mg sodium/100g
  - **Reduced Salt:** At least 25% less sodium than the regular food product
  - **No Added Salt:** Made without the salt normally added, but still contains the sodium that is a natural part of the food

  Note: Some European food labels may show sodium as grams in place of milligrams. **Example:** 0.8g sodium = 800mg sodium

- **Avoid retail breads.** Most contain around 1% salt (400-500mg per 100g). This is considered high in view of their significant contribution to our diet (4 thick slices of bread has around 800mg of sodium). Health Food stores often have salt-free breads, or order from your local bakery.

- **Go easy on condiments and sauces** such as tomato sauce, mustard, soy sauce and spaghetti sauces. Salad dressings are also high in sodium. Look for 'no added salt' products.

- **Avoid take-aways** (pizzas, pies, burgers) **and salty snack foods** such as potato crisps, *Cheezels*, salted nuts and pretzels. Choose unsalted popcorn, nuts, seeds, and fruit.

- **Limit or avoid antacids and saline powders** with sodium bicarbonate (e.g. *Eno, Alka-Seltzer*). They are high in sodium.

FOODS HIGH IN SODIUM

- Bread (Retail, 1.2% salt; 200mg/45g slice)
- Cheese, Butter, Margarine
- Pickles, Sauerkraut, Olives
- Condiments, Sauces
- Salad Dressings
- Canned vegetables/salads/beans
- Deli Salads (with dressing)
- Frozen/Packaged Meals/Entrees
- Soups: Canned/Dry/Cubes
- 2-Minute Noodles, Cup Soups
- Meats: Ham, bacon, sausages, luncheon meats, smoked meats
- Canned & Smoked Fish
- Salt & Seasoning Salts
- Snack Foods (potato crisps)
- Tomato Jce (Canned), V8 Vege Juice
- Take-Aways: Pizza, Burgers, Chicken, Pies, Sausage Rolls

MODERATE SODIUM

- Bread (Reduced Salt, 0.5% or less)
- Meat, Fish, Poultry - Unprocessed
- Milk, Yoghurt, Soy Drinks, Eggs
- Peanut Butter
- Breakfast Cereals (<200mg/serve)
- Chocolate Candy, Fruit/Nut Bars

FOODS LOW IN SODIUM

- Products labeled *Low Sodium*, or *No Added Salt* or *Salt Free*
- Bread (No Added Salt)
- Fresh fruits and vegetables
- Canned and Dried Fruits
- Potatoes, Rice, Pasta (No Added Salt)
- Dried Beans & Lentils, Tofu
- Nuts & Seeds (unsalted)
- Corn & Popcorn (unsalted)
- Pepper, Spices, Herbs
- Jam, Honey, Nutella
- Chewing Gum
- Hard & Jelly Confectionery
- Coffee, Tea, Alcohol
- Fresh Fruit Juices, Water

Sodium Counter

Sod ~ Sodium (mg)

Milk, Yoghurt

	Sod
Milk: Whole/Skim, average, 250ml	120
Reduced-Fat/Low-fat, avg., 250ml	140
Powdered: Full cream, 30g	100
Skim, 4 Tbsp, 30g	130
Canned, Cond./Evap., 30g	35
Flavoured Milk, avg., 300ml ctn	150
Soy Drinks:	
So Good, 250ml	115
So Natural, 250ml	225
Vitasoy, Original, 250ml	150
Yoghurt: Avg. all types, 200g carton	140
Soy Life, average, 175g	175

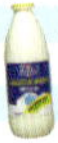

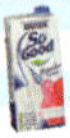

Cheese:

Hard Cheeses:	
Colby, Gouda, Edam, average:	
1 slice, 30g	200
100g quantity	660
Reduced Fat, 30g	210
Reduced Salt, 30g	110
Bocconcini *(South Cape)*, 50g	135
Easy Cheese Spread *(Kraft):*	
Cream Cheese, 1 Tbsp, 20g	250
Light, 1 Tbsp, 20g	280
Feta: Average, 30g	295
Reduced-Fat, 30g	345
Processed Cheddar, 30g	400
Mozzarella; Swiss, 30g	185
Parmesan: 30g	370
Grated, 1 Tbsp, 10g	125
Provolone, Romano, 30g	300
Pizza Cheese, 30g	180
Soft Cheeses: Brie, avg, 30g	180
Camembert, avg. 30g	180
Cottage, 2 Tbsp, 40g	120
Cream Cheese, 30g	120
Cheese Dip, avg., 30g	300
Ricotta: Average, 2 Tbsp, 40g	50
Baked Ricotta, 30g	320

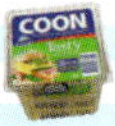

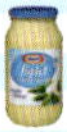

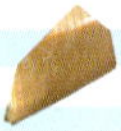

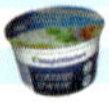

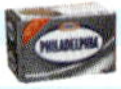

Ice Cream

Average all types, 1 scoop, 50g	25
Novelty Bars, Cornetto, avg.	70
Fruit & Water Ices	10

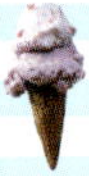

Eggs

Hen, large, 1 egg	65
Egg Omelette:	
2 eggs: Plain	215
with Ham & Cheese	400
Quiche, average, 1 serve	805

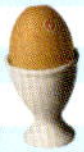

Fats/Oils/Cream

	Sod
Butter: Regular (salted), 1 Tbsp, 20g	125
Reduced Salt *(Western Star)*, 1 T., 20g	60
Unsalted/No Added Salt	5
Butter Blends, average, 1 T., 20g	140
Margarine/Spreads: Reg. 1 Tbsp, 20g	120
Light/Extra Lite, 1 Tbsp, 20g	75
Salt Reduced *(Flora/Logicol)*, 20g	75
Unsalted/No Added Salt, 30g	0
Logicol, Extra Lite, 1 Tbsp	75
Oils (Cooking), Lard/Dripping, 30g	115
Cream, average, all types, 30g	60
Coffee-Mate, 1 tsp	10

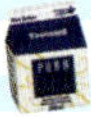

Meats/Sausages

Meat: Average all types, cooked 100g	45
Casserole/Stew, average, salt added	
1 cup, 200g	750
Beefburger/Hamburger Patty, 50g	300
Bacon, fried, 1 rasher, 20g	400
Liver, cooked, 100g	100
Sausages: Avg., 1 thick, 60g	650
Frankfurter boiled (1), 50g	500
Cold Meats: *Per 30g*	
Corned Beef, 1 slice, 30g	415
Ham (Leg), 1 slice, 30g	475
Luncheon Meat e.g. Devon, Fritz,	
Chicken/Ham Roll, average, 30g	250
Mortadella, Cabanossi, Strassburg, 30g	370
Liverwurst, average, 30g	190
Paté, average, 30g	1150
Pepperoni, 5 slices, 30g	440
Salami, average all types, 30g	490
Spam, average all varieties:	
⅙ of 340g can, 56g	580
Lite/50% Less Salt	290

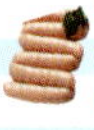

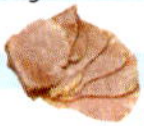

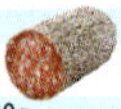

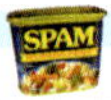

Chicken

Raw, Chicken Meat, 100g	75
Cooked: Unsalted, 100g	75
¼ Chicken: No salt added	100
With salt	400
Stuffing: 1 Tbsp, 20g	120
¼ cup, 70g	425
KFC — *See Page 193*	
Red Rooster — *See Page 205*	

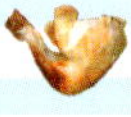

Fish

	Sod
Edible Portion: Per 100g (Unless Indicated)	
Average all types, cooked (no salt):	100
Battered, 100g	450
Crumbed, 100g	160
Fried in Oil, 100g	200
Crab/Lobster, cooked, 100g	400
Mussels/Scallops, 6 medium, 100g	250
Octopus, raw, 100g	280
Oysters, fresh, shelled, 6 medium, 60g	190
Prawns/Shrimps, cooked, ½ cup	140
Roll-Mop/Pickled Herring, 55g	480
Seafood Cocktail: With Lemon Juice	150
With Dressing	350
Seafood Highlighter, 50g	300
Smoked Fish, average, 100g	1200
Fish Fingers: (2), 50g	150
Birds Eye, (2), 50g	120
Fish Cakes, avg, 1 cake, 50g	200
Fish Portions, battered, 100g	400

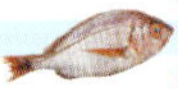

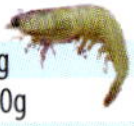

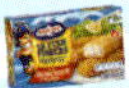

Canned Fish

Salmon: regular, in brine, 100g	600
No Added Salt (John West/Coles), 100g	80
Tuna: Reg. in brine or oil, drained, 100g	350
No Added Salt, 100g	100
Springwater (Weight Watchers), 100g	240
Sardines: In Tomato Sauce, avg., 50g	300
In Spring Water *(Brunswick)*, 50g	130
No Added Salt *(Brunswick)*, 50g	95
Crabmeat, ½ cup, 100g	600
Anchovies, drained, 25 g	1300
Mussels *(John West)*, dr., 60g	215
Smoked Oysters, drained, 30g	400
Fish Spread, avg, 2 tsp, 10g	100

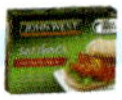

Soups & Stock Cubes

Canned, Condensed Soup:	
Average all brands, undiluted, 100g	450
Reduced Salt, undiluted, 100g	250
No Added Salt, undiluted, 100g	50
Dried Packet Soup: Avg, 200ml	800
Reduced Salt, 200ml, range	400-500
Continental Cup-A-Soup, avg., 250ml	760
Stock Cubes: Average, each	700
Reduced Salt: Salt Skip, each	55
Ultracube, average, 150ml	500
Stock Liquid: 250ml	1120
Reduced Salt, 250ml	625
Stock Tablets, each	740

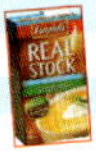

Sodium Counter

Baked Beans

	Sod
Baked Beans: ¾ cup, 200g	540
Salt Reduced, *Heinz*, 200g	480
No Added Salt, *Heinz*, 200g	20

Frozen Meals

Lean Cuisine, Packets, avg.	870
McCain, Healthy Choice, avg.	750
Meat Pie: Family Size, 150g serve	450
Individual Pie, 180g	600

Packet/Cup Meals & 2-Minute Noodles

Easy Mac *(Kraft)*, avg., 70gpkt/bowl	650
Microwave Cup Meals, average	900
Noodles: Single Serve	
Fantastic, average, 70g cup	1300
Maggi: 2-Minute, average, 72g pkt	1100
99% Fat Free, average	980
Fusian Cup, average, 65g	1050
Suimin, average, 70g cup	1870
Woolworths, Homebrand:	
Average, 85g pkt	1450
1 cup, average, 70g	1300

Sanitarium ~ Vegetarian

BBQ Soy Sausages, 50g each	305
Casserole Mince, ⅓ can, 138g	600
Nutmeat; Nutolene, avg., 85g	275
Savoury Lentils, ⅓ can, 138g	490
Tender Pieces, ⅓ can, 138g	525

Fast-Foods/Take-Away

General Items, Average All Outlets

Chicken: Rotisseried, average	
¼ Chicken, no stuffing	400
Chicken & Chips Pack	700
Tropicana Pack	700
Chicken Dinner	1200
Fried Chicken, 100g	430
Chicken Nuggets, 6 Pack + Sauce	630
Chiko Roll, 180g	620
Chips: Potato, unsalted, 150g	10
Salted, 1 cup, 150g	300
French Fries, small serve	150
Chinese: Dim Sim, average (1)	200
Fried Rice, 1 cup, 150g	800
Doner Burger/Kebab, 400g	1200
Fish & Chips, salted, 1 serve	600
Hamburgers, average	1000
Hot Dog, average	900
Meat Pie, average, 175g	900

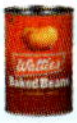

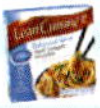

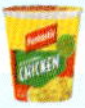

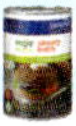

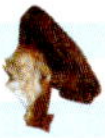

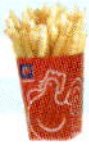

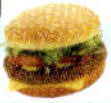

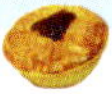

Fast-Foods (Cont)

	Sod
Pastie, average, 170g	700
Pizza: ¼ medium, no meat	1200
With meat/sausage	1500
Pita, meat + salad, average	500
Quiche, average, 1 serve, 170g	500
Sandwiches: Ham & Salad	800
Cheese & Vegemite	700
Peanut Butter	500
Sausage Rolls: Small, 40g	330
Large, 80g	660
Taco, average	400
Tomato Sauce, 10g sachet	110

Bread, Buns, Pita

Bread (Average all types): *Per Slice*	
1 thin slice, 30g	130
1 thick slice, 40g	180
1 extra thick slice, 50g	220
Buns/Rolls: Dinner Roll, small, 40g	200
Large (14cm/6"), 140g	720
Hamburger, 90g	400
Breadcrumbs, average, 30g	200
Chapatis, 30g	200
Crumpet, average, 1 only	290
English Muffin, avg., 67g	300
Garlic Bread, 60g serve	400
Pita Pocket, average	330
Pumpernickel, 26g	180
Raisin Bread, 1 slice, 40g	100
Salt-free Bread, 1 slice	5

Crispbreads, Rice Cakes

Crispbreads, Average, 1 slice	45
Matzo, 1 sheet	5
Rice Cakes, average, 1 cake	5

Peanut Butter, Nutella

Peanut Butter,	
average, 1 Tbsp, 20g	125
No Added Salt *(Coles)*, 20g	5
Nutella,	
1 Tbsp, 20g	10

Vegemite • Jam • Honey

Vegemite, ½ tsp, 3g	165
***My First Vegemite**, ½ tsp, 3g*	55
Cheesybite, 1 heaped tsp. 13g	185
Marmite, Promite, ½ tsp, 3g	100
Ozemite, ½ tsp, 3g	75
Honey, Jam, Marmalade	0
Lemon Spread, 6g	10

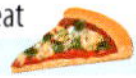

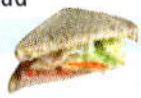

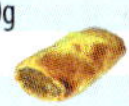

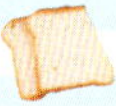

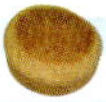

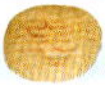

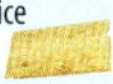

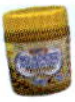

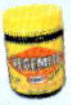

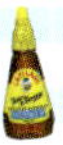

Breakfast Cereals

	Sod
Coles:	
Bran Flakes 30g	120
Corn Flakes, ½ cup, 30g	180
Right Start, ¾ cup, 45g	100
Kellogg's:	
All-Bran, ¾ cup, 52g	200
Coco Pops, 1 cup, 45g	245
Corn Flakes, 1 cup, 30g	195
Froot Loops, ¾ cup, 30g	140
Guardian, 1 cup, 60g	130
Just Right, Original, ¾ cup, 45g	175
Komplete Muesli, ½ cup, 45g	50
Nutri-Grain, 1 cup, 40g	240
Rice Bubbles, 1 cup, 30g	185
Special K, avg., 1 cup, 40g	215
Sultana Bran: 1 cup, 48g	130
Extra ⅔ cup, 45g	135
Sustain, 1 cup, 60g	60
Nestle: Milo Cereal, 1 cup, 45g	65
Nesquik Cereal, 1 cup, 45g	110
Uncle Toby's:	
Oats, 100g	10
Bran Plus, 45g	175
Cheerios, 1 cup, 30g	120
Fibre Plus, ¾ cup, 45g	55
Fruity Bites, 30g	15
Nut Feast, 45g	230
Oat Crisp, 40g	130
Vita Brits, 2 biscuits, 33g	135
Vita Brits Weeties, 1 cup, 35g	140
Sanitarium:	
Corn Flakes, 1 cup, 30g	175
Granola, Clusters, 50g	125
Honey Weets, 1 cup, 30g	10
Light'n'Tasty, 1 cup, 40g	60
Puffed Wheat, 1 cup, 30g	5
Weet-Bix:	
Original, 2 bisc., 33g	95
Bites, avg., 14 pieces, 45g	155
Kid's, 2 biscuits, 30g	35
Hi-Bran, 2 biscuits, 40g	165
Multi-Grain, 2 biscuits, 48g	115
Organic, 2 biscuits, 30g	90
Other Cereals	
Oatmeal/Lecithin/Wheat Grits	0
Muesli, average, 2 Tbsp, 30g	40
Bran, Oat/Rice/Wheat	0
Wheatgerm; LSA, 1 Tbsp	0

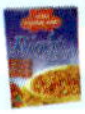

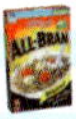

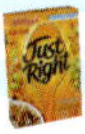

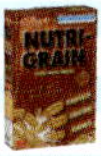

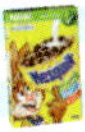

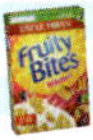

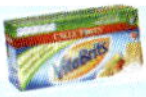

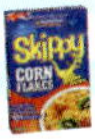

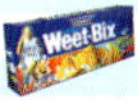

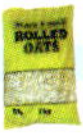

231

Sodium Counter

Sod ~ Sodium (mg)

Flour, Grains, Rice | Sod
Flour: Plain, white — 0
   Self-raising, 100g — 780
   Soybean, Carob — 0
Rice, Wheat, Barley — 0
Rice, cooked with salt, ½ cup, 80g — 250

Spaghetti/Pasta
Dry, No salt added, 30g — 5
Fresh, Vegetable flav. (no salt), 100g — 5
Canned: (In Tomato Sauce),
   Average, ½ cup, 150g — 370
   Salt Red.: SPC, ½ cup, 150g — 360
   Heinz: Regular, ½ cup, 150g — 615
   Big Eat, ½ cup, 150g — 525
   Spaghetti Oops,130g can — 685

Biscuits
Savoury: Shapes, average: 25g — 230
   100g quantity — 920
   Jatz, Chicken, Clix Sticks: 25g — 205
   100g quantity — 820
   In A Biskit, Avg., 10 bisc., 25g — 330
   Soho's Rice Snacks, 13 biscuits, 25g — 200
Crackers: *Per Cracker*
   Arnott's: Cruskits — 50
   Salada, 1 cracker, 4 squares — 140
   Sao — 65
   Sesame Wheat — 70
   Vita-Weat, Original — 25
   Water Cracker — 20
   Matzo, 1 sheet — 5
Sweet Biscuits: *Per Biscuit*
   Granita — 50
   Butternut Cookie/Snap — 65
   Chocolate Biscuits/Tim Tam, average — 30
   Marie, Milk Arrowroot, Morning Coffee — 35
   Monte Carlo — 60
   Scotch Finger — 90
   Tim Tam — 30

Cakes/Pastry/Croissants
Plain, average, 40g — 120
Cupcake, 50g — 150
Cheesecake, average, 100g — 200
Croissants, average — 200
Doughnut, average, 100g — 180
Fruit Cake, 50g — 80
Fruit/Apple/Pie/Tart, 140g — 250
Lamington, medium, 80g — 110
Scone, large, 85g — 590
Sponge Cake, Iced, 50g — 90

Muffins: | Sod
Avg all types: Medium, 60g — 320
   Large, 100g — 530
   Extra Large, 180g — 950

Desserts & Ice Cream
Custard, average, ½ cup — 100
Jelly/Canned Fruit — 0
Pudding, average, 1 serve — 150
Ice Cream, 50g scoop — 40

Sugar • Honey • Jam
Sugar; Sugar Substitutes — 0
Honey, Jam — 0
Molasses, Treacle, 30g — 30

Snack Foods & Crisps
Burger Rings, 50g pkt — 570
Beef Jerky, average, 25g — 500
Cheezels, 50g — 610
Corn Chips: Average, 50g pkt — 220
   C.C.'s, Original, 50g pkt — 285
   Nature's Earth, Natural, 50g — 25
Muesli Bars/Slices, average — 40
Potato Crisps: Avg. all brands, 50g — 400
   Thins, average, 45g pkt — 260
   Ajitas, Vege Chips, avg., 50g — 320
   Red Rock Deli, average, 50g — 300
   Smith's Crisps, 50g — 300
   Sultry Sally, average, 50g — 410
Popcorn: Salted, 1 cup — 300
   Unsalted — 0
Pretzels, 10 twists, 19g — 280
Twisties, Cheese/Chicken, avg., 50g pkt — 560
Vege Deli *(Ajitas),* average, 45g — 265

Nuts • Seeds/Bars
Nuts, Seeds: Unsalted, 50g — 5
   Salted, average, 50g — 210
Fruit/Nut/Seed Bars, average, 1 bar — 20

Chocolate & Confectionery
Chocolate: Milk, 50g — 60
   Dark, plain, 50g — 20
   Mars Bar, 60g — 90
Fruit Gums; Jelly Beans, 30g — 10
Licorice, 50g — 60

Salt, Herbs, Spices | Sod
Salt: Common, 1 tsp, 5g — 2000
   Single serve sachet, 1 g — 400
   Lite Salt *(Diet Rite),* 5g — 975
   Chicken Salt, 1 tsp, 5g — 1600
   Garlic/Onion Salt, 1 tsp, 5g — 1600
   Sea/Rock Salt, 1 tsp, 5g — 1950
   Salt Flakes, 1 tsp, 5g — 1950
Baking Powder, 1 tsp, 5g — 700
   Low Sodium (Salt Skip) — 10
Bicarbonate of Soda,
   1 tsp, 5g — 810
   Potassium BiCarb (Salt Skip) — 0
Meat Tenderizer, 1 tsp, 5g — 1600
Monosodium Glutamate,
   1 tsp, 5g — 500
Pepper, Spices, Herbs — 0
Curry Powder:
   With added salt *(Keen's),* 1 tsp, 4g — 230
   W/out added salt, 1 tsp — 5
Garlic, Onion, Ginger, Mustard Powder — 0
Mustard, Powder — 0
Yeast, nutritional, 1 Tbsp — 10

Sauces & Condiments
Apple Sauce — 0
Balsamic Dressing, avg, 20ml — 250
Balsamic Vinegar — 0
Barbecue Sauce, avg., 1 T., 20g — 200
Black Bean *(Taylor's),* 20ml — 590
Capers, 1 Tbsp, 20g — 375
Chilli Sauce, avg., 1 Tbsp, 20g — 200
Chutney, avg. all types, 1 Tbsp, 20g — 40
Curry Paste, average, 50g — 1400
Curry Sauce, avg., ½ cup, 125g — 520
Father's Favourite, avg, 1 Tbsp, 20g — 200
Fountain, Steak/Spicy /Mstd, 1 Tbsp — 160
Gravox/Gravy Mix:
   Prepared, ¼ cup, 63ml — 370
   Lite (Salt-Reduced), ¼ cup, 63ml — 110
Horseradish, Regular, 1 Tbsp, 20g — 200
Hoisin *(Trident),* 1 Tbsp, 20ml — 385
Hoi Sin *(Fountain),* 1 Tbsp — 420
Minced Garlic, avg all brands, 1 tsp, 5g — 40
Mint Jelly, 1 Tbsp, 20g — 20
Mint Sauce *(Fountain),* 1 Tbsp — 5
Mustard, 1 tsp, 5g — 130
Oyster Sauce: 2 tsp, 10ml — 360
   Kikkoman, 2 tsp, 10ml — 550
Plum Sauce *(Ayam),* 1 Tbsp, 20g — 265
Seafood Cocktail *(MasterFoods),* 1 T., 20g — 275

Sodium Counter

Sauces (Cont) — Sod
Item	Sod
Satay Sauce, 1 Tbsp, 20g	300
Soy Sauce: Avg all brands, 1 T., 20ml	1500
Salt-Reduced, 1 T., 20ml	715
Thick, 1 Tbsp, 20g	1325
Pasta Sauce: average, ½ cup, 125g	570
Leggo's, Stir Through, avg. ¼ jar, 88g	620
Pizza Sauce (Ardmona), ½ cup, 35g	265
Sweet & Sour Sauce (Masterfoods), 20g	110
Sweet Chili (Trident), 1 Tbsp, 20ml	330
Tartare Sauce, 1 Tbsp, 20g	160
Tomato Sauce/Ketchup:	
1 Tbsp, 20ml	250
No Added Salt (Fountain), 1 Tbsp, 20ml	5
Tomato Paste: (Leggo's), ¼ 140g ctn, 35g	295
No Added Salt (Leggo's), 35g	20
Tomato Puree: Canned, average, ½ cup, 125g	400
Ardmona (No Added Salt), 100g	10
Leggo's, 100g	315
Vinegar, Balsamic Vinegar	0
Worcestershire Sauce, avg. 1 T., 20ml	250

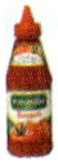

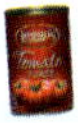

Pickles & Relishes
Item	Sod
Sweet Mustard/Tomato Pickles, 25g	150
Cucumber (Bread & Butter) 6 sl., 50g	220
Dill Cucumber, ½ large, 60g	740
Corn Relish, 20g	70
Gherkin Relish (Masterfoods), 5g	50

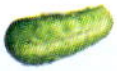

Salad Dressings & Mayo
Item	Sod
Average All Brands: Per Tablespoon, 20g	
Coleslaw	200
French, Italian	300
Salad Cream (Heinz), Regular/Lite, 20g	175
Thousand Island	250
Mayonnaise	250
Miracle Whip	70

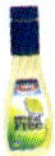

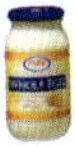

Fruit & Fruit Juice
Item	Sod
Fresh/Dried/Canned Fruit, 250ml	0
Fruit Juices, fresh/commercial, 250ml	0
Tomato Juice, commercial, avg., 250ml	740
V8 Fruit & Veg, Citrus Splash, 250ml	30
V8 Plus Berry, 250ml	45
V8 Vegetable Juice:	
300ml bottle	780
Low Sodium, 250ml	275

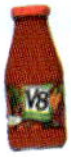

Vegetables — Sod
Item	Sod
Fresh: Average, 100g	10
Celery, 30g	50
Silverbeet, Spinach, ½ cup, 100g	70
Frozen Veges: Average, ½ cup, 100g	10
Chips: Unsalted, ½ medium, 100g	10
Salted, 12 medium, 100g	400
Dried: Similar to fresh vegetables	

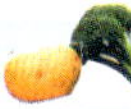

Canned Vegetables
Item	Sod
Asparagus, Canned, 6 spears, 100g	150
Beetroot, 2 slices, 30g	70
Corn Kernels: ½ cup, 100g	150
Cream Style, ½ cup, 125g	250
Cucumber, pickled, ½ medium, 100g	1400
Four Bean Mix (Edgell), 100g	250
Gherkin, 1 medium, 10g	70
Mushrooms:	
In Brine, ½ cup, 60g	530
In Butter Sauce, ½ cup, 100g	290
Olives: pickled, Green, 4 medium, 20g	450
Black, 4 medium, 20g	140
Stuffed, 4 medium, 20g	370
Onion, pickled, 1 medium, 30g	440
Peas, in brine, ½ cup, 100g	230
Red Kidney Beans (Coles), 100g	270
Sauerkraut, ½ cup, 80g	600
Three/4-Bean Mix: average, 100g	300
No Added Salt, 100g	5
Tomatoes:	
Peeled, whole NAS (Ardmona), 100g	5
Crushed (Ardmona), 100g	270
Organic, Chopped, 100g	100
Diced, 100g	100
Italian Roma, 100g	100
Tomato Supreme (Edgell), 100g	300
Tomato Puree, average, 100g	350
Tomato Paste, average, 100g	160

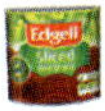

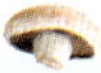

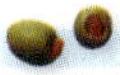

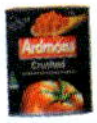

Soft Drinks, Tea, Coffee
Item	Sod
Tea, Coffee & Substitutes	5
Soft Drinks/Cordials, avg., 200ml	20
Soda Water, average, 200ml	20
Fruit & Vegetable Juice, avg., 1 glass	
Mineral Water, average, 1 glass	10
Water (Tap), average, 1 glass	5
Bonox; Bovril, 1 rounded tsp, 8g	460

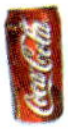

Drinks ~ Energy, Alcohol
Energy & Sports: — Sod
Item	Sod
Gatorade, 600ml	395
Lucozade, 300ml	5
Powerade, 600ml	170
Red Bull, 250ml	100
V Energy Drink, 250ml	280
Alcoholic Drinks: Beer, 375ml	25
Wine, average, 1 glass, 200ml	25
Spirits, Whisky, Brandy	0

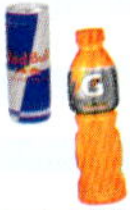

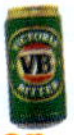

Antacids, Indigestion
Item	Sod
Alka-Seltzer: Reg. 2 tablets, 1 dose	1020
Lemon flavour, 2 tablets, 1 dose	940
Andrews: Antacid Tablets	0
Effervescent, 1 tsp, 7g	420
Dewitt's, 1 rounded tsp	650
Dexs: 1 capful, 15g	1500
Antacid Liquid	
Eno, 1 rounded tsp, 5g	850
Gaviscon Cool: 1 tablet	45
Liquid, 1 dose	260
Lemon Saline, 2 heaped tsp, 10g	470
Mylanta Plus: 1 tablet	70
Liquid, 1 dose, 20ml	150
Mylanta Liquid, regular, 10ml	15
Salvital, 2 heaped tsp, 10g	370
Tums	0

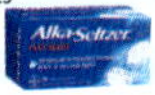

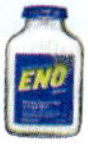

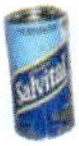

Note: Sodium in above items is mainly from sodium bicarbonate (27% sodium).
1 gram (1000mg) contains 270mg sodium.

Cold & Flu Medicinals
Item	Sod
Lemsip, Cold & Flu Hot Drink 1 sachet	95
Lemsip Max, 1 sachet	120

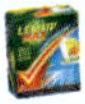

Headache/Pain Relievers
Item	Sod
Aspro, Aspro/Aspirin Soluble, 1 tablet	0
Aspro Clear, 1 tablet	160
Codis, Disprin, Panadeine	0
Panadol, Original	0
Panadol Rapid, 2 caplets	350
Panadol Rapid Soluble, 1 tablet	425

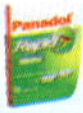

Vitamin Supplements
Item	Sod
Tablets/Capsules, average	0
Effervescent:	
Berocca, 1 tablet	270
Supradyn, Redoxin Vit C, 1 tablet	290
Sandocal, 600/1000	250/400
Caltrate Calcium, 1 tablet	5
Cernovis, Vita-Fizzies. 2 tabs	820
1 tablet	410

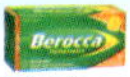

Index A-C

Abalone 95
Acorns 141
Afogatto 36
Agrum 49
Akta-Vite 46
Alcohol 23-30
Alcoholic Sodas 29
All-Bran 61
Almond: Fingers 53
  Jelly 180
  Milk Drinks 47
Almonds 141
Aloo 181
Amaranth 101
Anchovies 97
Angostura 48
Angostura Bitters 28
Anticol 88
Antipasto 146, 178, 181
Anzac Biscuits 52
Apple: 103
  Crumble 65, 90
  Juice 40-43
  Pie 65
  Sauce 149
  Strudel 65
Apricot: 103
  Nectar 40
  Delight 160
Arnott's Biscuits 51
Arrowroot 101
Artichoke: Fresh 168
  in Oil 146
Asian Meals 180
Atkins: Bars 31
  Cereal 60
  Drinks 39
Aussie Bodies Drinks 39
Avocado 103, 216, 222

Babybel Cheese 72
Bacardi 28, 29
Bacardi Breezer 29
Baci 81
Bacon 136
Bagel 57, 178
Bagel Chips 160
Baguette 56, 181
Baileys Irish Cream 28
Bakers Delight:
  Bread 58, 185
  Sweet Buns 66

Bakewell 115
Baking Ingredients 64
Baking Powder 64
Baklava 65
Baklava Pastry 181
Balsamic Vinegar 148
Bamboo Shoots 168
Banana 103
Banana Split 90
Bardies 138
Barley 101
Barley Sugar 85
Barramundi 95
Baskins Robbins 109, 186
Basmati Rice 101
BBQ Pork 180
Bean Sprouts 168
Beans: Fresh 168, 172
Bechamel Sauce 149
Beef 130-132
Beef Goulash 181
Beef Jerky 134
Beef Olives 134
Beef Patties 115
Beer 24-26
Bento Box 182
Berri Juice 40
Berries 103, 105
Betty Baxter:
  Bars 31
  Shakes, Soups 50
Betty Crocker 67
Bi-Carbonate Soda 64
Biggest Loser: Bars 31
  Shakes, Soups 50
Billabong 111
Biltong 159
Birds Eye: Fish 96
  Meals 115
Biscuits 51-54
Bisleri Chinotto 48
Bitter Lemon 48
Black Currant Juice 40
Black Forest Cake 181
Black Pudding 138, 139
Blackberries 103
Blancmange 90
Bloody Mary 27
BLT 178
Blue Cheese 72
Bonox 161
Boost Juice 40

Bouillabaise 181
Bourbon 28
Bovril 161
Brains 136
Bran 63
Brandy 28
Brawn 139
Bread Pudding 143
Bread: Fresh 56-59
  Mixes 57
Breadcrumbs 56
Breaka 45
Breakfast Bars 31-35
Breakfast Cereals: 60-63
Brie 72
Brioche 57, 181
Brisket 131
Brumby's: 58, 186
  Sweet Buns 67
Bruschetta 178, 182
Bubble Gum 85
Bubble Tea 50, 182
Bubble'n Squeak 115
Buffalo 136
Bulgar 101
Bulla Icecream 109
Bundaberg Rum 29
Buns 57
Burgen 58
Burger Rings 159
Burrito 123
Butter 94
Butter Chicken 181
Butter Menthol 85, 88
Buttermilk 46

Cabanossi 139
Cadbury: Chocolates 81
  Drinking Choc 46
  Icecream 110
Caesar Salad 179
Caffe Latte 36
Cajan Chicken 179
Cake Decorations 64
Cakes 65-71
Calamari 181
Calippo Bar 113
Camembert 72
Camp Pie 118, 139
Campari 27
Campbell's Soup 161
Cannelloni 181

Canola 94
Capers 158
Cappuccino 36
Capretto 136
Capsicum 168
Caramel Slice 65
Caramello 81, 110
Caramels 85
Carl's Jr. (N.Z.) 186
Carlton 24
Caro 36
Carob: 79
  Confectionery 88
  Flour 101
  Rice Cakes 55
Carrots 168
Cashews 141
Cassata 108
Casseroles 133
Cassis 28
Cauliflower: 168
  Cheese 93
Cereals 60-63
Chai Tea 38
Challah 56
Champignons 172
Chapati 56, 181
Cheese Triangle 178
Cheese: 72-74
  Snaks 74
  Soufle 93
  Spread 73, 167
Cheesecake Shop 67
Cheestiks 73
Cheetos 159
Cheezels 159
Cherries 103, 105, 107
Cherry Ripe 81
Chewing Gum 85
Chianti 30
Chick Peas 168
Chicken: 75-78
  Cacciatore 182
  Chow Mein 180
  Korma 181
  Treat 186-187
  Dumpling 120
  Fat 94
  Nuggets 178
  Vindaloo 181
Chiko Roll 116, 178

Chilli Peppers 168
Chilli Sauce 149
Chinotto 48
Chipolatas 137
Chips 178
Chitterlings 136
Chocolate: 79-84
  Brownie 65
  Chip Cookie 51
  Cooking 64
  Drinks 38, 45
  Eclair 65, 85
  Mint Slice 51
  Roll 70
Chokito 81
Chop Suey 180
Choux Pastry 143
Christmas Cake 65
Christmas Pudding 143
Chump Chop 133
Chupa Chups 85
Chutney 158
Ciabatta 57, 179
Cider 26
Clam 95
Clarified Butter 94
Claytons 28
Cloves 64
Coca-Cola 48
Cocktails 27
Coco Pops 61
Cocoa 46
Cocoa Butter 94
Coconut: 103, 141
  Desiccated 64
  Milk, Cream 46, 47
  Water 41, 42
Coffee: 36-38
  Liqueur 28
  Scroll 65
Coffee-Mate 46
Cognac 28
Cointreau 28
Cold Lollies 88
Coles: Bars 32
  Biscuits, Crackers 52
  Cakes, Desserts 68
  Canned Fish 97
  Canned Fruit 106
  Cereals 60
  Cheese 72
  Chocs 81
  Desserts 90
  Drinks 48
  Icecream 110
  Juice 41-43

Index C-H

Coles (Cont):		Crispbreads	55	**Eagle Boys**	190	Freddo	82	Granita	49, 51
Meals	116	Crispy Chicken Skin	184	Easter Eggs	80	French Fries	178	Grapefruit	103
Noodles	116	Crocodile	136	Eel	95	French Meals	181	Grapes	103
Pizza	145	Croissants	57, 179	Egg Nog	28, 93	French Onion Dip	92	Grapeseed Oil	94
Potato Products	171	Cronut/Cronot	65	Eggs	93	Friand	65	Gravox	152
Salad Dressings	147	Croquette	178	Eggs Benedict	178	Fried Icecream Balls	180	Gravy	150
Sauces	151	Crostoli	65	Enchilada	123	Frogs Legs	138	Greek Meals	181
Soups	162	Croutons	56	Energy Drinks	39	Fromage Frais	90	Greek Salad	146
Soy Drinks	47	Crumpets	55	Ensure	39	Frosties	61	Green's Cakes, Cookies	68
Coleslaw	146	Crunchie	82	Equal	167	Frozen Meals	115-128	Greenseas: Fish	98
Condensed Milk	46	Crunchie Icecream	110	Escargot	138, 181	Fruche	90	Greewheat Freekeh	101
Confectionery	85-88	Cupcakes	65	Espresso	36	Fruit: Fresh	103-107	Grenada	49
Connoisseur Icecream	110	Currants	105	Europe Bars	32	Juices	40-43	Grenadine	28
Continental: Meals	116	Curry Powder	161	Evaporated Milk	46	Leather	85	Grill'd	190-191
Seasonings	151	Curry Puff	180	**Fairy Floss**	85	Mince	64	Grissini Breadsticks	51
Soup	163	Custard	89	Fajitas	123	Mince Pies	65	Guiness	25
Cookies	51-54	Custard Cream Bisc.	51	Falafel Balls	178	Pectin	64	Gum	85-88
Cooking Choc	79	Custard Tart	65	Falafel Mix	124	Roll	105	**Haggis**	136
Cool Drinks	48-49	Cuttlefish	95	Fanta	48	Sorbet	108, 111	Haloumi	73
Copha	64, 94	**Daiquiri**	27	Fantales	85	Fudge	85	Halva	86
Coq au Vin	181	Dairy Whip	89	Fantastic Noodles	117	**Galactobureko**	181	Ham	139
Cordial	50	Damper	56	Fast-Foods	177-208	Garlic	168	Hamburger Patty	115, 132
Corn	172	Dandelion Drink	36	Fats	94	Garlic Bread	56	Harvey Fresh	41
Corn Chips	159	Danish Pastry	65	Fennel	141	Gatorade	39	Hash Browns	171
Corn Flakes	61	Darrell Lea	80	Ferrero Rocher	82	Gelati	108	Healthy Choice Meals	122
Corn Bread	56	Dates	105	Fetta cheese	73	Gelatine	64, 91	Heart	136
Corn Fritters	65	Deep Spring	48	Fettucine	119	Gelato	110	Hearts of Palm	172
Corned Beef	131, 139	Deli Meats	139	Figs	103	Georgie Pie (N.Z.)	178	Heaven	111
Cornetto	112	Desserts	90-91	Fillet Steak	131	German Meals	181	Heineken	25
Cornflake Crumbs	56	Devilled Eggs	93	Filo Pastry	143	Ghee	94	Heinz:	
Cornflour	64, 101	Dhal	181	Finding Form: Bars	32	Gherkin	169	Baked Beans	118
Cornish Pastie	178	Dhansak	181	Shakes, Soups	50	Gin	28	Big Eat	118
Cornmeal	101	Diet Bars	35-38	Fish & Chips	178	Ginger: Fresh/Dried	105	Spaghetti, Canned	118
Cosmopolitan	27	Dill Pickle	158. 168	Fish:	95-100	Snack	160	Helga's Bread	59
Cottage Cheese	72	Dim Sims	128, 180	Cakes	96	Ginger Beer	26, 48	Herb Butter	94
Cough Lollies	88	Dips	92	Canned	97-100	Ginger Nut	51	Herbs	161
Cous Cous	101, 115	Dolmades	146, 181	Capsules	94	Glace Fruit	64, 105	Herring	95, 181
Crackerbread	55	Dolmio	152	Fingers	96	Gloria Jean's	37	Hoisin Sce	149
Crackers	51-54	Domino's	189	Oil	94	Glucose	167	Hommus	92
Crackling	136	Doner Burger/Kebab	178	Spread, Pastes	97, 167	Gnocchi	142, 182	Honey	166
Craisins	105	Donut King	68	Flambe Desserts	30	Goat	136	Honeycomb	82, 86
Cranberry Juice	42	Donuts	65	Flans	178	Goat Milk	46	Horseradish	169
Cranberry Sce	149, 158	Drambuie	28	Flatbread	179	Goji Juice	41	Horseradish Cream	149
Crayfish	95	Dried Fruit	105	Flora Margarine	94	Gold'N Canola	94	Hot Cross BunS	65, 66
Cream	89	Drinking Chocolate	46	Florentine	65	Gold Bears	85	Hot Dog	178
Cream Bun	65	Dripping	94	Flours	101	Golden Circle Juice	41	Hot Dog Rolls	57
Cream Cheese	73	Drumstick	111	Focaccia	56	Golden syrup	91, 167	Hoummus	166
Cream of Tartar	64	Duck:	78	Focaccia S/wich	178	Goose	78	HP Sauce	149
Creaming Soda	49	Eggs	93	Fortune Cookie	160, 180	Gorgonzola	73	Hudsons Coffee	38
Creative Gourmet	105	Dumpling	56, 180	Four'N Twenty	117	Goulburn Valley	106	Hundreds & Thousands	51
Crème Brulee	181			Frankfurts, Franks	137	Juice	41	Hungry Jacks	191-192
Crepe Suzette	181			Freckles	85	Grains	101		
Crepes	91								

235

Index I-P

I & J Fish 96
Ice Magic 91
Icecream: 108-113
  Soft Serve 108
  Cones 108
Iced Coffee 36
Iced Vo Vo 51
Icing Sugar 64
Icy Pole 111
Indian Meals 181
Irish Coffee 28
Irish Moss 88
Ital Biscuits 53
Italian Meals 182
Italian Shortbread 53

Jack Daniels 29
Jaffas 86
Jaffle 117
Jalapeno 123
Jam 166
Japanese 182
Jarrah:
  Coffee 36
  Chocolate Drinks 46
Jatz Crackers 52
Jelly 91
Jelly Beans 86
Jester's 192
Jim Bean 29
John West Fish 98-99
Jols 88
Juice 40-43
Junket 91
Just Juice 41
Just Right 61

K-Time Twist 33
Kahlua 28
Kan Tong 153
Kavli 55
Kellogg's:
  Bars 33
  Cereals 61
  KFC 193-194
Kidneys 136
Kingston 51
Kipper Fillets 97
Kit Kat 82
Kraft:
  Cheese 73
  Crackers 53
  Meals 119
Krispy Kreme 69
Kugelhopf Cake 181

L.S.A. 63
Lactose-free Milk 44, 46
Lamb: 133
  Noisettes 181
  Pilaf 181
Lamington 65
Lapin 136
Lard 94
Lasagne 182
Lavosh 53, 56
Lean Cuisine 120
Lebanese Flatbread 56
Lecithin 63
Leggo's:
  Meals 120
  Sauces 153
Legumes 168-170
Lemon: 104
  Butter 167
  Juice 40
  Lime & Bitters 48
  Meringue Pie 65
  Peel 64, 105
Lemonade 49
Lenard's: Chicken 76-77
  Meals 120
LeSnak 74
Lettuce 169
Licorice 86
Lifesavers 86
Lime 104
Lindt Choc 82
Linseed 141
Lipton Iced Tea 50
Liqueur Coffees 28
Liqueurs 28
Listerine 88
Lite 'n Easy 121
Liver 136
Liver Pate 136
Liverwurst 138
Lobster 95
Loin Chop 133
Lollies 85-88
Lozenges 88
Lucozade 39
Lychees 104, 180

M&M's 82
Macadamia Nuts 141
Macarons 65 198
Macaroni Cheese 119, 142
Macchiato 36
Maderia 30

Maggi: Meals 122
  Noodles 122
  Sauces 154
Magnum 112
Maison Grape Juice 30
Maize Meal 101
Malt Extract 46
Malted Milk 46
Maltesers 83
Mango 104
Manicotti 182
Manioc 101
Maple Syrup 91
Mararoon, Coconut 65
Maraschino Cherry 105, 107
Margarine 94
Margarita 27
Marinades 149
Marmite 166
Marron 95
Mars Bar 83
Marsala 30
Marshmallows 36, 86
Martini, Dry 27
Marzipan 64
Mascarpone 73
Matzo Meal 55
Mayonnaise 148
McCafe 197-199
McCain: Chips 171
  Meals 121
McCormick's 154
McDonald's 195-197
Mead 30
Meal Replacements 50
Meals 115-128
Meat 130-139
Meat Balls 132
Melba Toast 56
Melons 103-105
Michelina's 122
Midori Melon 28
Milk 44-47
Milk Arrowroot 51
Milkshake 36, 38
Millet 101
Milo: 46
  Icecream Bar 111

Mince, Beef 132
Mineral Water 49
Minestrone 182
Mints 86, 87
Miso 165
Miso Soup 182
Mocha 36
Mocktails 27
Molasses 167
Moon Cake 180
Moove 45
Moreton Bay Bug 95
Mortadella 139
Moussaka 181
Mousse 90
Mousse Mixes 71
Mozzarella 73
Mr Whippy 108
Mrs Mac's Pies 123
Muesli 61-63
Muesli Bars 31-35
Muffin Break 69, 200
Muffins:
  English 55
  Savoury 178
Mulled Wine 30
Multi V Juice 40
Musashi: Bars 33
  Drinks 39
Muscatel 30
Mushroom 169
Mustard: Sauce 149
  Vegetable 158

Naan Bread 56, 181
Nabisco 53
Nachos 178, 184
Nando's 201
Nanna's Desserts 70
Nasi Goreng 101
Nectars 40
Nescafe 36
Nesquik 46
Nestea 50
Nestle: Cereals 62
  Cocoa 46
  Desserts 90
  Icecream 110
Neufchatel 73
NZ Natural 111, 201

Nice 51
Nippy's: 42
  Milk Drinks 45
Noodle Box 202
Noodles 116-123
Norfolk Punch 30
Norgen Vaaz 112
Nougat 86
Nudie 42
Nutella 166
Nutri-Grain Bar 33
Nuts 141
Nuttelex 94

Oat Bran 63
Oat Milk 46, 47
Oats 63
Octopus 95
Offal 136
Oils 94
Old El Paso 123
Olive Oil 94
Olives 146
Omelettes 93
Onions 170
  Fried 138
Oporto 203
Optifast 50
OptiSlim 34, 50, 165
Oranges 104
Orgran: Cookies 53
  Egg Replacer 93
  Spaghetti 124
Osso Buco 182
Ouzo 28
Ovaltine 46
Oysters 95, 97

Paddle Pops 113
Paella 101
Pakistani Meals 181
Pancakes: 91
  Syrup 167
Panini Bread 56
Pannacotta 90
Pannettone 66
Papaya 104
Pappadum 56, 181
Paradise Biscuits 53
Parmesan 74
Passiona 49
Passionfruit 104
Pasta 142
Pasties 115
Pastizzi 178
Pastry 143
Pate 138

Index P-S

Patties Pies 124
Paul Newman's Own 148
Pauls Milk Drinks 45
Pavlova 68, 90
Pawpaw 104
Peach 104
Peanut Butter 166
Peanuts 141
Pearl Barley 101
Peel, Mixed 105
Peking Duck 180
Pepper: Steak 161-165
  Chilli 168
Peppermints 87
Pepperoni 139
Pepsi 49
Perfect Sweet 167
Pernod 28
Perrier 49
Peters Icecream 110
Petit Miam 90
Philadelphia Cheese 74
Pickles 158
Picnic 83
Pide (Turkish) 57
Pie Floater 178
Pies 115
Pigeon 136
Pikelets 91
Pimms 27, 28
Pina Colada 27
Pistachio 141
Pita: Bread 56
  Crisps 160
Pita Pit (N.Z.) 203
Pizza Hut 204
Pizza: 144-145
  Bases 143
Plain Flour 101
Plum Pudding 143
Polenta 101, 182
Pollen Granules 63
Polony 139
Popcorn 160
Poppy Seeds 64, 141
Pork 135
Pork Crackle 160
Porridge 62, 63
Potato: 169
  Crisps, Chips 159
  Flour 101
  Mashed 169
  Salad 146
  Wedges 179
Powerade 39

Powdered Drinks/Milk 46
Powdered Milk 46
Prawn Crackers 160, 180
Prawn Dumplings 180
Prawns 95, 97
Pretzels 56, 159
Profiterole 66
Promite 166
Prosciutto 139
Protein Drinks 39
Prune 105, 107
Psyllium 63, 101
Puddings 70-71, 143
Puff Pastry 143
Pumpernickel Bread 56
Pumpkin 170
Pure & Simple 94
Pure Blonde 25

Quail 136
Egg 93
Quark 74
Quesadilla 123
Quiche 93
Quiche:
  Take Out 119
Quinoa 101

Rabbit 136
Raisin 105
Raisin Bread 58
Raita 182
Ravioli 120
Red Bull 39
Red Rooster 204-205
Redskin 87
Refried Beans 123
Relishes 158
Rhubarb 104
Ribena 43, 50
Rice 101
Rice Bran Oil 94
Rice Wine 30
Rice Bubbles 61
Rice Cookies 51
Rice Cream 91
Rice Milk Drinks 47
Rice Noodles 140
Rice Paper 64
Ricecakes 55
Ricotta Cheese 74
Risotto 101, 182
Rissoles 179
Roast Duck 180
Rockmelon 104
Rocky Road 79, 110

Rogan Josh 181
Rollettes 70
Rolls 57
Roti 56, 181
Rum 28
Rye Bread 58
Ryvita 55

Safcol Fish 99
Sago 101
Sakata 55
Sake 30, 182
Salad Dressings 147-148
Salads 146-147, 179
Salami 139
Salmon 95
Salsa 150
Salsa Dips 123
Salt 161
Saltimbocca 182
Samosa 179
San Remo Meals 124
Sandwiches 179
Sanitarium: Cereals 62
  Meals 124
  Nutmeat 124
  Nutolene 124
  So Good 47
  Up & Go 47
Sao Cracker 52
Sara Lee:
  Cakes & Pastries 70
  Icecream 112
  Lasagna 125
  Quiche 125
Sardines 97
Sarsparilla 48
Sashimi 182
Satay: Beef 180
  Sticks 180
Sauces 149-158
Sauerkraut 158, 170
Sausage Rolls 115
Sausages 137
Saveloy 138
Scallops 95
Schnitzel 134
Scones 66
Scorched Almonds 83
Scotch: 28
  Eggs 93
  Finger 51
Seafood Sticks 96
Sealord Fish 96
Seasonings 149-158
Seaweed Salad 182

Seeds 141
Semolina 101
Sesame: Oil 94
  Seeds 141
Shakes 45
Shandy 26
Shapes, Crackers 52
Shellfish 95
Sherry 30
Shishkebabs 134
Shitake Mushrooms 172
Shooters 27
Shortbread 51-53
Shredded Wheat 63
Shrimp 95
Silverside 131, 139
Skittles 87
Slurpees 49
Slush Puppie 49
Smarties 111
Smirnoff 29
Smoked Mussels 97
Smoothie 38, 40, 45
Snackabouts 74
Snacks 159
Snails 138
Snakes 87
Snickers 83
So Good 47
Soba Noodles 140
Soda 48-49
Soda Water 49
Soft Drinks 48-49
Sorbet 108
Soup 161-165
Souvlaki 181
Souvlakia 179
Soy: Crisps 165
  Grits 63
  Sauce 149
  Cheese 74
  Drinks, Powder 46
  Ice Cream 112
  Sausages 124
Soybean: Flour 101
  Fresh 170
  Oil 94
Spaghetti: Plain 142
  Restaurant Meals 142
Spam 139
Spare Ribs 135
Special K 61
Speculaas 53
Spices 161
Spider 38
Spinach & Ricotta 179

Spirits 28
Splices 113
Split Peas 170
Sponge Roll 66
Sports Bars 31-35
Sports Drinks 39
Spreads 94
Spring Roll 119, 143
Spring Valley Juices 43
Sprite 49
Spritz 49
Sprouts 170
Squid Rings 96
Stagg Chilli 125
Staminade 39
Starbucks 37
Starburst 87
Steak 130
Steggles Chicken 77
Stevia 167
Stewed Fruit 106
Sticky Date Pudding 70, 143
Stock 161-162
Stock Cubes 161
Stone's Green Ginger 29, 30
Stout 25
Strawberries 104
Streets Icecream 112
Strepsils 88
Strongbow Cider 26
Stuffed Tomatoes 181
Stuffing 78
Stuffing Mix 128
Subway 206
Suet 94
Sugar 167
Suimin 125
Sultana 105
Sumo Salad 207
Sun-Dried Tomato 146
Sunflower Seeds 141
Sunraysia 43
Sunrice 101, 126
  Rice Cakes 55
Sushi Rice 182
Sustagen 39
Sweetcorn 170
SweetLife: Bake Mix 70
  Gum 85
Swiss Roll 66
Swordfish 95
Syrups 43, 167

Index T-Z

Tabasco Sce	149	Toppings	91	Vegetarian Sausages	138	Wendy's	
Taco	123	Torquay	49	Vegie Croquette	178	Ice Cream	207

Tabasco Sce 149
Taco 123
Tahini: Paste 166
 Seeds 141
Take Away Foods 178
Tandoori Chick 181
Tang 50
Tapioca 101
Taramosalata 181
Tart Cases 143
Tartare Sce 149
Tarts 66
Tartufo 108
Taylor's Sauces 157
Tea 50
Teddy Bears 51
Tempeh 165
Tempura 182
Tequila 28
Tequila Sunrise 27
The Coffee Club 38
Throaties 88
Tia Maria 28
Tic Tac 87
Tim Tams 51
Tiny Teddy 51
Tip Top Bread 59
Tiramisu 66, 91
Toblerone 79
Toffee 87
Tofu 165
Tofutti: 113
 Slices 74
Tom Piper 127
Tomato: 105
 Canned 172
 Juice 40
 Juice Cocktail 27
 Puree 149
 Sauce 149
 Sun-Dried 146
Tongue 136
Tonic Water 49
Tony Ferguson: Bars 35
 Meals 127
 Shakes, Soups 50
Tooheys 26
Top Taste Cakes 70

Toppings 91
Torquay 49
Torte 66
Tortellini 124, 182
Tortilla 56, 123
Treacle 167
Triangles 179
Trident 127
Trifle 91
Tripe 136
Trout 95
Truffles 108
Tuna: 95
 Tempters 99
Turkey: 78
 Eggs 93
Turkish Bread 56
Turkish Delight 84, 87
Twinings Tea 50
Twisties 159
Tzatziki 92

Udon Noodle 182
UHT Milk 44
Ultra Slim 50
Ultra-C 50
Uncle Toby's: Bars 35
 Cereals 63
 Roll-Ups 105
Up & Go 47

'V' Energy Drinks 39
V8 Juices 43
V8 Vegetable Juice 40
Vanilla Extract 64
Vanilla Slice 66
Veal: 134
 Marsala 182
 Parmigiana 182
Vegemite 166
Vegemite Cheesybite 166
Vegetable: Juices 40-43
 Oils 94
Vegetables: 168-172
 Canned 172
 Dried 172
 In Oil 172

Vegetarian Sausages 138
Vegie Croquette 178
Vegie Patty 179
Venison 136
Vermouth 30
Victoria Bitter 26
Vienna Sausage 138
Viennetta 112
Vinegar 149
Violet Crumble 84, 111
VitaBrits 63
Vitasoy 47
Vive 47
Vodka: Cruiser 29
 Red Bull 27
 Sprits 28
Vol au Vent 119, 143

Wafers 54
Waffles 70, 91
Waffle Cone 108
Wagon Wheels 51
Waldorf Salad 147
Walnuts 141
Wantons 180
Wasabi 182
Water Chestnut 172
Water Crackers 52
Watercress 170
Waterfords 49
Watermelon 105
Weet-Bix 62
Weeties 6
Weight Watchers:
 Biscuits 54
 Cakes, Puddings 70
 Canola 94
 Cereals 63
 Cheese 74
 Crispbread 55
 Drinking Choc 46
 Fish, canned 100
 Icecream 113
 Meals 127, 128
Weiner Schnitzel 181
Weis Icecream 113

Wendy's
 Ice Cream 207
Wheat Bran/Germ 63
Wheat Grass Juice 40
Whey Powder 46
Whisky 28
White Wings: 71
 Custard 89
 Pancakes 91
Whitebait 95
Wild Rice 101
Wine 30
Witchetty Grubs 138
Wok Me 208
Wokinabox 208
Wonka 85
Woolworths: Bars 35
 Biscuits 54
 Cakes, Muffins 71
 Cereals 63
 Chocolate 84
 Deli 138
 Fish, canned 100
 Fruit 107
 Icecream 113
 Meals 128
 Pizza 145
 Salad Dressings 148
 Sauces 158
 Soup 165
 Soy Drink 47
Worcestershire Sce 149
Wraps 179

Xmas Cake 65
Xmas Eggnog 93
Xmas Pudding 143
XXX Mints 87
XXXX 26
Xylitol 167

Yabbies 95
Yakatori 182
Yakult 176
Yeast 64
Yellowglen 30
Yo Yo 51
YoFrost 108
Yoghurt: 173-176
 Frozen 108-113
 Lollies 88
 Soft Serve 108
YoGo 90
Yum Cha 119

Zabaglione 91, 181
Zucchini 170

OTHER COUNTERS
Alcohol 23-30
Caffeine 210
Calcium 211-213
Cholesterol 214-218
Fibre 219-222
Protein 223-226
Sodium 227-233

USA CalorieKing Edition

AMERICA'S BEST!

- Includes 200 U.S. Fast-Food Chains

- #1 Rated by Dietitians & Doctors

Available from:
Barnes & Noble, Amazon.com
Calorieking.com (for USA residents)

Notes

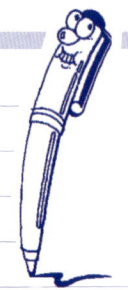

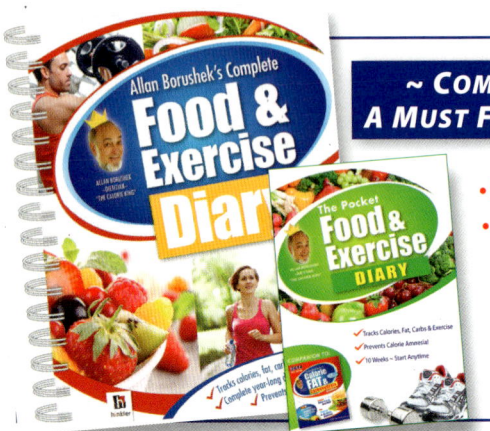

~ COMPANION DIARIES ~
A MUST FOR SERIOUS DIETERS!

- **Pocket Size (10 Weeks)**
- **Larger Size (12 Months)**
  (Extra recording options)

**FROM NEWSAGENTS
& BOOKSTORES**

Extra Info:
hinkler.com.au